Nutrition and Diet Therapy Dictionary

Nutrition and Diet Therapy Dictionary

Third Edition

Virginia S. Claudio, Ph.D., M.N.S., R.D.
Rosalinda T. Lagua, M.P.S., M.N.S., R.D.

VNR VAN NOSTRAND REINHOLD
New York

An AVI Book
(AVI is an imprint of Van Nostrand Reinhold)
Copyright © 1991 by Van Nostrand Reinhold

Library of Congress Catalog Card Number 91-8537

ISBN 0-442-00465-6

Manufactured in the United States of America

Published by Van Nostrand Reinhold
115 Fifth Avenue
New York, NY 10003

Chapman and Hall
2-6 Boundary Row
London, SE 1 8HN, England

Thomas Nelson Australia
102 Dodds Street
South Melbourne 3205
Victoria, Australia

Nelson Canada
1120 Birchmount Road
Scarborough, Ontario M1K 5G4, Canada

16   15   14   13   12   11   10   9   8   7   6   5   4   3   2   1

Library of Congress Cataloging-in-Publication Data
Claudio, Virginia Serraon, 1932-
    Nutrition and diet therapy dictionary / Virginia S. Claudio,
Rosalinda T. Lagua.—3rd ed.
        p.   cm.
    Rev. ed. of: Nutrition and diet therapy / Rosalinda T. Lagua,
Virginia S. Claudio, Victoria F. Thiele. 2nd ed. 1974.
    Includes bibliographical references.
    ISBN 0-442-00465-6
    1. Diet therapy—Dictionaries.   2. Nutrition—Dictionaries.
I. Lagua, Rosalinda T., 1937-   .   II. Lagua, Rosalinda T., 1937-
Nutrition and diet therapy.   III. Title.
    [DNLM: 1. Diet Therapy—dictionaries.   2. Nutrition—dictionaries.
QU 13 C615n]
RM219.L26   1991
613.2'03—dc20
DNLM/DLC   91-8537
                                             CIP

Disclaimer

Extreme care has been taken in preparation of this work. However, author and publisher make no warranty or representation, expressed or implied, with respect to accuracy, completeness, or utility of the information contained in this document; nor do the authors or publisher assume any liability with respect to the use of or reliance upon, or for damages resulting from the use of or reliance upon, any information, procedure, conclusion, or opinion contained in this document.

Mention of products, companies, and services in this book is informational and not an endorsement by authors.

Dedicated
To Our
Husbands

Preface

This reference dictionary presents up-to-date and complete information on terms used in nutrition. Its outstanding feature is the thorough treatment of clinical nutrition and diet in disease. Written primarily for practitioners in the fields of nutrition and dietetics, its contents are at the same time useful to physicians, nurses, professionals in other health care delivery services, educators, and students. To these varied groups we have sought to furnish as much fingertip knowledge as can be offered in a brief and compact volume.

About 3800 terms are presented alphabetically and discussed concisely to give the latest information about each word entry. In choosing the terms to be included, we used as criteria the frequency of use and importance of the terms in nutrition. For greater fullness of coverage, definitions are amplified by materials found in the appendices. There are 48 appendices, and a quick scan of the Table of Contents reveals that some topics, especially those containing international data, are unique. All the appendices are useful and handy for practitioners, educators, and students.

First printed for use in the Philippines in 1969, the second edition (1974) was redesigned for American and international use with a third author, Victoria F. Thiele. This third edition has retained the purposes and main features of the second edition but is revised and enlarged, adding about 30 pages including at least 250 new terms in nutrition and diet therapy.

Virginia S. Claudio
Rosalinda T. Lagua

GUIDE TO THE USE OF THE DICTIONARY

Word entry. The word or term to be defined is set in bold-face and extends slightly to the left of the definition. All entries, including abbreviations and compounds of two or more words, have been entered in strict alphabetical order, regardless of any space or hyphens that may occur between them. If two or more variant spellings of a single word exist, the one most frequently used is entered in boldface and the variants are given in the definition. When usage is about evenly divided, both spellings are entered in boldface.

Subentries. Groups or classes of definitions related by a common root term appear under that term: *anemia, amino acid, dietitian,* etc. The series is slightly indented, and each subentry is set in the same boldface type as the main word entry.

Definitions. Innumerable definitions have been scrutinized, redefined, or expanded to conform to changing concepts of present-day knowledge. The definitions of a term are numbered when there is more than one distinct meaning or use. The most inclusive definition is present first, followed by the more restricted meanings. Definitions restricted to specialized fields are preceded by field labels such as "In nutrition," "In medicine," and so on. Advertently omitted are definitions in certain specialized fields that do not have any application in the field of nutrition. A semicolon after a definition generally means that the material that follows is not part of the definition proper but is additional information enlarging on the factual content.

Abbreviations. Abbreviations with nutritional significance appear in their proper alphabetical sequence in the dictionary. They are defined in full in word entries for which such abbreviations stand.

Cross references. The user is directed to additional or fuller information by such cross reference terms as *see* or *see under.* Cross references to related information are identified by the words *see also.* The word entry to which the user is directed is italicized; when a cross reference appears under a group entry, the user is instructed to look for the subentry under the word entry for the definition of the specific term. Cross references to the appendices are not italicized but presented in the same typeface as the definition; the user, however, is clearly directed to the appendices for additional information.

Italics. Some words are italicized to indicate to users that such words, in case they are not known to them, are defined elsewhere in the text. Cross-referenced words are also italicized.

Nutrient requirements. Unless specified otherwise, nutrient requirements stated are for adults.

Contents

Preface ix

Guide to the Use of the Dictionary xi

Dictionary Terms 1

Appendixes 263

  1   Recommended Dietary Allowances, revised 1989 265

  2   Estimated safe and adequate daily dietary intakes of selected vitamins and minerals 266

  3   U.S. reference daily intakes (USRDI) for nutrition labeling 267

  4   Recommended dietary standards for adults in selected countries and FAO/WHO 268

  5   A daily food guide for the basic food groups 273

  6   Food grouping systems in different countries 274

  7   Dietary guidelines for all healthy Americans over 2 years old 276

  8   Classification of carbohydrates 277

  9   Classification of proteins 279

 10 Classification of lipids 281

 11 Summary of digestive enzymes 283

 12 Utilization of carbohydrates 284

 13 Utilization of proteins 285

 14 Utilization of fats 286

 15 Interrelationship of carbohydrate, protein, and fat 287

 16 Summary of vitamins 288

 17 Summary of minerals 290

 18 Median weights and heights for children from birth to 18 years 292

 19 Average weights for men and women aged 18-74 years 293

20-A Acceptable weights for men and women 294

20-B 1983 Metropolitan height-weight tables 295

 21 Estimation of frame size and stature 296

22   Reference values for triceps skinfold thickness 297

23   Reference values for midarm muscle circumference 298

24   Estimation of energy and protein requirements of adults 299

25   Interpretations and equations for assessing nutritional status 301

26   Physical assessment of nutritional status 304

27   Biochemical assessment of nutritional status 306

28   Plasma lipid concentrations and association with coronary artery disease 308

29   Expected 24-hour urinary creatinine excretion 309

30   Reference values for normal blood constituents 310

31   Normal reference values for urine 316

32   Dietary fiber in selected foods 318

33   Alcohol and caloric content of alcoholic beverages 319

34   Cholesterol and fatty acid content of selected foods (per 100 gm edible
     portion) 320

35   Average caffeine content of selected foods (mg) 322

36   Protein food mixtures in the world 323

37   Composition of milk and selected formulas for infant feeding 324

38   Composition of oral and intravenous electrolyte solutions 325

39   Proprietary formulas for enteral nutrition 326

40   Selected amino acid solutions for parenteral nutrition 330

41   Intravenous fat emulsions 332

42   Suggested intravenous multivitamin formulation 333

43   Caloric values and osmolarities of intravenous dextrose solutions 334

44   Nutritional intervention in inborn errors of metabolism 335

45   Common prefixes, suffixes, and symbols 338

46   Common abbreviations in medical records 339

47   Agencies and organizations with nutrition-related activities 345

48   Sources of nutrition information 350

A

AA. Abbreviation for 1. *adenylic acid* 2. *amino acid* 3. *Alcoholics Anonymous.*

Abetalipoproteinemia. A rare congenital disorder due to a lack of apoprotein B, which is needed to secrete chylomicrons or to export hepatic triglyceride. As a result, fat is not transported from the intestinal cells into the lacteals. The blood lacks the chylomicrons and has very low levels of low-density and very-low-density lipoproteins, cholesterol, triglycerides, and free fatty acids, especially linoleic and arachidonic acids. A low-fat diet is recommended; substitution of medium-chain triglycerides for long-chain fats in the diet may improve fat absorption, since the shorter-chain fats are absorbed by way of the portal vein rather than by the lymph. Supplements of the fat-soluble vitamins A and K are necessary, and pharmacologic doses of vitamin E are now thought to be important for correction of some retinal and neuromuscular abnormalities.

Absorption. Assimilation or taking up of fluids, gases, nutrients, or other substances by the skin, lacteals, mucous membranes, or absorbent vessels.

Absorption, nutrients. After food is digested, the end products (see Appendix 11) are absorbed mainly in the intestines through the *villi.* Each villus is connected to the circulatory and lymphatic systems. Almost all the water-soluble nutrients are absorbed by diffusion or osmosis (passive absorption). Glucose, galactose, and amino acids are absorbed with the help of energy supplied by the enzyme K^+/-ATPase and a cofactor, sodium ion. The process is carried out against a concentration gradient which therefore needs ATP energy (active absorption). Fructose absorption, however, uses a carrier without expending energy. Fructose pulls water with it upon entering the intestines. This type of absorption is called facilitative. The fourth absorption process is pinocytosis or phagocytosis, in which the absorptive cell engulfs the material. This process is used for fat absorption. Below is a summary of absorption in the gastrointestinal tract (GIT):

GIT ORGAN	NUTRIENTS AND OTHER SUBSTANCES
Stomach	Alcohol (20% of the total ingested) Some short-chain fatty acids
Intestines Duodenum	Vitamins A and B_1, iron, calcium, glycerol and fatty acids, monoglycerides, amino acids, monosaccharides and disaccharides
Jejunum	Glucose, galactose, amino acids, glycerol and fatty acids, monoglycerides, diglycerides, dipeptides, copper, zinc, potassium, calcium, magnesium, phosphorus, iodine, iron, fat-soluble vitamins D, E, and K, most of the vitamin B complex, vitamin C, and the rest of the alcohol.
Ileum	Disaccharides, sodium, potassium, chloride, calcium, magnesium, phosphorus, iodine, vitamins D, E, K, B_1, B_2, B_6, B_{12}, and ascorbic acid, and most of the water.
Colon	Sodium, potassium, water, acids and gases, some short-chain fatty acids metabolized from plant fibers and undigested starch, and vitamins synthesized by bacteria (biotin and vitamin K).

Water-soluble nutrients pass directly into the circulatory system, while fat-soluble materials pass through the lymphatic system first before they are transported by the blood. Amino acids and peptides are actively absorbed by the absorptive cells of the villi; peptides are broken down into individual amino acids which then go to the liver via the portal vein for metabolism. Fatty acids that are water-soluble (fewer than 12 carbons) and glycerol pass through the portal vein to the liver. Bile aids in the emulsification of fats to facilitate absorption. Fatty acids of longer-carbon chain (more than 14 carbons) form triglycerides in the absorptive cells and combine with cholesterol, phospholipids, and similar substances with a protein coat (the compound formed is called a chylomicron). The chylomicrons pass through the lymphatic system before entering the bloodstream. Understanding the absorption process gives background knowledge and a rationale for nutritional therapy for disorders associated with *malabsorption syndrome* and *enterostomies*.

Accessory food factors. Earliest name given to vitamins by Hopkins, who demonstrated in 1906 that foods contain, in addition to the nutrients then recognized (i.e., carbohydrates, proteins, fats, minerals, and water), minute traces of unknown substances essential to health and life.

Acesulfame-K. A nonnutritive sweetener which is a potassium salt of the 6-methyl derivative of oxathiazinone dioxides. Its relative sweetness (based on that of sucrose, which is 1.0) is 130, and it is noncaloric. Sold under the brand name Sweet One.

Acetic acid. An organic acid commonly formed in the metabolism of sugars and related substances. As acetylcoenzyme A, it participates in a number of important metabolic processes.

Acetoacetic acid. Monobasic ketone acid formed in the course of normal fatty acid catabolism and oxidized further to acetic acid, which is utilized in various metabolic reactions. It accumulates in the blood when fatty acids are incompletely oxidized. The reduction of acetoacetic acid yields beta-hydroxybutyric acid, and its decarboxylation yields acetone. See also *Ketone bodies.*

Acetohexamide. A sulfonylurea oral hypoglycemic agent used for the management of noninsulin-dependent diabetes mellitus; sold under the brand name Dymelor.

Acetone. Dimethylketone. A colorless liquid with a sweetish, ethereal odor; formed by the decarboxylation of acetoacetic acid. It is normally present in minute quantities in blood and urine but may accumulate when fatty acid degradation is excessive or incomplete. See also *Ketone bodies.*

Acetone bodies. See *Ketone bodies.*

Acetonemia. Presence of large amounts of acetone (ketone bodies) in the blood. See also *Ketosis.*

Acetonuria. Excretion of large amounts of acetone bodies in the urine. While normally present in trace amounts in the urine, their excretion may increase from 0.02 gm/day to as much as 6 gm/day in certain pathologic conditions.

Acetylcholine (ACh). Acetic acid ester of choline. It is released from nerve endings to initiate a series of reactions leading to the transmission of a nerve impulse. Its actions correspond to those of the cholinergic fibers, including a depressant effect on the blood pressure and stimulation of intestinal peristalsis.

Acetylcoenzyme A (acetyl CoA). Acetyl derivative of coenzyme A. An important member of the *Krebs cycle* as a precursor for the biosynthesis of fatty acids and sterols, it gives rise to acetoacetic acid and is the biologic acetylating agent in the synthesis of acetylcholine.

Achalasia. Neuromuscular disorder of the esophagus that causes dyspepsia, esophageal regurgitation, esophageal pain, vomiting, and eventually weight loss. It is also called esophageal dysnergia or cardiospasm. The main problem is failure of the lower esophageal sphincter to relax and open after swallowing to permit food to enter the stomach. The lowest part of the esophagus therefore becomes narrowed and blocked with food. The main treatment is the dilatation of the sphincter or a surgical procedure to cut the circular muscle of the cardiac sphincter. *Dietary management:* depending on the degree of dysphagia, foods and beverages per os have to be carefully selected for each individual; some may require tube feeding. Avoid foods that stimulate secretion of gastrin, the hormone that controls the lower esophageal sphincter. Proteins and carbohydrates promote gastrin production. Fats, chocolate, and coffee lower esophageal pressure. For other dietary guidelines, see *Dysphagia.*

Achlorhydria. Absence or lack of hydrochloric acid in the gastric juice. Primarily due to a reduction of the acid-producing cells in the stomach, as in the elderly. Digestion of protein that needs the enzyme *pepsin* is lessened in achlorhydria.

Acid. Compound capable of yielding hydrogen ion in solution. Also defined as a substance that produces or donates protons.

Acid-ash residue. Inorganic radicals (chiefly chloride, sulfate, and phosphate) that form acid ions in the body. When excreted in the urine, they lower the pH or make the urine more acid.

Acid-base balance. Equalization of total acid and total base in body fluids at levels compatible with life. Normally, the blood is kept within a narrow pH range of 7.35 to 7.45. Adjusting mechanisms come into play to neutralize or remove excess acid or base to maintain the balance. These include the buffer systems of the blood, the excretion of carbon dioxide by the lungs, and the excretion of fixed acid or base by the kidneys.

Acid-forming foods. Foods in which the acidic residue exceeds the alkaline residue. These include meats, fish, poultry, eggs, and cereals. See also *Alkaline-forming foods* and *Diet, ash.*

Acidosis. An abnormal condition characterized by a fall in the pH of the blood or a decrease in the *alkali reserve* of the body. A reduction in blood bicarbonate (alkali reserve) indicates that an excess of fixed acids is being produced or retained in the body at a rate exceeding that of neutralization or elimination. Various acids retained in different conditions are the acidic ketone bodies (as in diabetes mellitus), phosphoric, sulfuric, and hydrochloric acids (as in renal insufficiency), lactic acid (as in anoxia, ether anesthesia, and prolonged strenuous exercise), and carbonic acid (as in respiratory disease).

Acid tide. Temporary increase in the acidity of urine and body fluids after eating while alkali is being secreted into the duodenum.

Acne vulgaris. Skin condition characterized by pimples or eruptions occurring most frequently on the face, back, and chest. An acne pimple is an obstructed and infected oil gland, and the pimples are more numerous where the oil glands are most abundant. For many years, people have associated diets high in fat or carbohydrate (particularly chocolate, nuts, candies, carbonated drinks, and fried foods) with acne. There is no basis for such beliefs. Studies have shown that foods do not produce major flareups of acne. However, some cases respond to high doses of vitamin A (100,000 IU) and retinoic acid applied topically, both of which should be used only under a physician's order.

Acquired immune deficiency syndrome (AIDS). A devastating infectious disease that attacks the immune system of the body. The causative agent is the human immunodeficiency virus (HIV), which destroys the T cells of the defense system of the body. To date there is no known cure for AIDS, and due to its mode of transmission and the increasing mortality rate, it has become a major health problem. *Clinical signs and symptoms:* night sweating, easy fatigability, poor digestion, anorexia, fever, cachexia, and eventually protein-energy malnutrition (PEM). Lymph nodes are swollen, and there is dysphagia, diarrhea, and malabsorption. The two most common problems are *Kaposi's sarcoma,* which is a form of cancer, and pneumonitis carinii pneumonia, which develops in the latter stage of AIDS and usually leads to death. *Mode of transmission:* the Surgeon General's office has listed the ways of becoming infected with AIDS: by having sex with someone infected with the AIDS virus; by sharing needles and syringes with an infected person; by receiving infected blood; or by birth (babies of AIDS-infected mothers can acquire the disease before or during birth) or by breast milk from AIDS-infected women. However, AIDS is *not transmitted* via clothes, drinking or eating utensils, casual contact at work, being in the same room with an AIDS patient, talking to an AIDS patient, from saliva, sweat, tears, urine, or bowel excretion. Nor it is transmitted by flies and insect bites. *Dietary management:* nutritional care should be highly individualized. Determine the most appropriate nutritional support option (enteral or parenteral) for patients experiencing oral lesions, dysphagia, anorexia, and protein-energy malnutrition (PEM). If tolerated, however, encourage feeding by mouth, avoiding foods the patient finds irritating. Serve foods at moderate temperatures and give single-textured meals. Experiment with different flavors if the patient has lost taste acuity. Perk up the appetite with mild spices and favorite foods. In cases of diarrhea, modify the diet accordingly to avoid dehydration and electrolyte imbalance. There are many choices of supplementary feedings to increase nutrient density. Serve foods in small, frequent feedings. Monitor any malabsorption, and restrict raw fruits and vegetables to protect against contamination with microorganisms. Watch out for side effects of drug therapy. The multifunctional role of nutrition in the care of AIDS patients cannot be overemphasized. As with other opportunistic illnesses, longevity may be achieved with a teamwork approach by the medical, nursing, dietary, and other allied health services.

Acromegaly. Chronic condition resulting from the hypersecretion of the growth hormone during adulthood. The characteristic features are overgrowth of the bones of the face and extremities, protrusion of the chin, enlargement of the hands, feet, and fingers, thickening of the scalp, bowing of the spine, glycosuria, and suppression of sexual function. Treatment is by radiation or surgery, usually by partial resection of the pituitary gland. *Dietary management* is directed to surgical care. Maintain an adequate diet and a desirable body weight. If the patient develops diabetes, which has been observed in 20 to 25% of cases, use nutritional therapy to control diabetes mellitus.

ACTH. Abbreviation for *adrenocorticotropic hormone.*

Activator. A substance that renders another substance active, either by being part of the reaction system or by combining with the inactive substance. An enzyme activator is called a *cofactor.*

Active transport. Also called biologic "pump." The process in which a substance is moved across a cell membrane from a lower to a higher electrochemical potential. It involves an expenditure of metabolic energy derived from the breakdown of adenosine triphosphate (ATP). Active transport is mediated by a carrier molecule that combines with the substance to be transported. See *Absorption, nutrients* for examples.

Acute. Having a sudden beginning or onset, short course, or severe symptoms. Examples are *acute renal failure* and acute complications of *diabetes mellitus.*

Acute renal failure (ARF). Sudden deterioration of renal function with retention of nitrogenous wastes which may lead to uremia. The condition is life-threatening and needs immediate, aggressive therapy using a teamwork approach. Possible causative factors are severe trauma like extensive burns and multiple injuries; widespread infections like peritonitis and sepsis; nephrotoxic agents; cardiac transplantation; and shock. Clinical signs are oliguria with proteinuria and/or hematuria; increased blood urea nitrogen (BUN), creatinine, serum potassium, phosphate, and sulfate; decreased sodium, calcium, and bicarbonate ions; anorexia, nausea, and vomiting; hypertension and lethargy. There are two distinct phases of ARF: the *oliguric* phase, which lasts for a few days, and the *diuretic* phase, which is a recovery period. Generally, it takes a year or so before renal function is restored, depending on the rate of renal cell regeneration. In both phases, dialysis is the major remedy. *Dietary management:* during the oliguric phase, monitor closely fluid and electrolyte balance. Fluids are restricted to a basic amount of 400 ml/day, and losses from diarrhea, vomiting, and perspiration should be replaced. Daily records of fluid intake and output, body weight, and food intake are essential in this phase. Serum potassium and creatinine are the most critical; nitrogen, potassium, sulfate, and phosphate restriction is accomplished by providing a protein-free diet for the first few days. Calories are supplied by carbohydrates (about 150 gm/day) and fat sources as oral supplementary feedings. Intravenous glucose is administered as necessary. Later on, supplementation with essential amino acids (30 gm/day) is given using special formulas. Total parenteral nutrition is beneficial to some patients. During the diuretic phase after the initial management and as the patient recovers, food and fluid intake are gradually increased, still maintaining a controlled protein intake of about 0.5 to 0.6 gm/kg/day. Continue to monitor BUN, serum creatinine, and serum electrolytes, especially sodium. If hypernatremia develops, restrict sodium intake to 1 to 2 gm/day. In a controlled protein intake (40 to 50 gm/day), adequate calories (35-40 kcal/kg/day) can be provided by the use of commercial formulas or by careful meal planning using the food exchange lists.

Acute respiratory failure. Sudden failure of the pulmonary gas exchange function. Prolonged pulmonary illness may lead to this disorder, which usually requires mechanical ventilation. Common causes are asthma, myasthenia gravis, muscular dystrophy, pulmonary embolism, and Guillain-Barré syndrome. *Dietary management:* start with tube feedings (low osmolality is recommended) to wean patients from the mechanical ventilator. To avoid overproduction of carbon dioxide, balance 30 to 50% carbohydrate calories with the same amount of lipid calories. Provide protein, allowing 1 to 1.5 gm/kg/day or close to 20% of total calories. For total energy intake, maintain 30 to 40 kcal/kg/day. Reduce sodium if pulmonary edema develops. Choose foods which are easy to eat and are nonirritating to the patient. Vitamins A and C, with phosphorus supplements, may be given.

ADA. Abbreviation for 1. American Dietetic Association 2. American Diabetes Association 3. American Dental Association.

Addison's disease. Metabolic disorder due to adrenal insufficiency. It is characterized by rapid loss of weight, emaciation, weakness, poor appetite, anemia, deep bronzing of the skin, low blood pressure, hypoglycemia, electrolyte imbalance with excessive loss of NaCl in the urine, and retention of potassium. It is a life-threatening disease because of the loss of adrenal cortex functions, which are vital life processes (see *Adrenal glands*). There is failure of the regulation of the autoimmune processes and hemorrhaging of the gland. The main treatment is continued administration of corticoid drugs. *Dietary management:* maintain adequate fluids and a regular diet to meet the nutritional needs of the patient. Monitor blood glucose, sodium, and potassium levels. If the patient has infection or trauma and is underweight, increase the protein and calorie intake to about 1.3 times the recommended daily allowances.

Adenine. One of the major purine bases of nucleic acids. As *adenosine phosphate,* it provides energy for muscular movement.

Adenohypophysis. Anterior lobe of the *hypophysis* or pituitary gland. It secretes vital hormones that regulate other endocrine glands. These are the growth, thyrotropic, adrenocorticotropic, lactogenic, and gonadotropic hormones.

Adenosine phosphates. Adenosine monophosphate (AMP), adenosine diphosphate (ADP), and adenosine triphosphate (ATP) are present in practically all tissues, especially the muscles and liver. Cyclic adenosine monophosphate, also called adenylic acid, is important in the activation of phosphorylase, whereas the di- and triphosphates are important sources of high-energy phosphate for cellular activity.

Adenyl cobamide. One of the coenzyme forms of vitamin B_{12}. See *Cobamide*.

Adenylic acid (AA). See under *Adenosine phosphates.*

ADH. Abbreviation for *antidiuretic hormone.*

Adipose tissue. Fatty tissue that acts as depot fat for storage of energy and serves as insulation against heat loss and padding for protection and support of organs. It is found largely in subcutaneous tissues and around visceral organs. Like other body constituents, it is not inert but is in a *dynamic state.* Fat is constantly being formed and hydrolyzed in adipose tissue. Adiposity is another term for *obesity.*

ADP. Abbreviation for adenosine diphosphate. See *Adenosine phosphates.*

Adrenal glands. Also called suprarenal glands; these two small endocrine glands are located at the upper end of each kidney. Each gland consists of two parts: the *cortex,* which elaborates estrogen, androgen, progesterone, and the adrenocortical hormones, and the *medulla,* which elaborates epinephrine and norepinephrine. The two groups of adrenocortical hormones that maintain nutrient homeostasis in the body are glucocorticoids and mineralocorticoids. Glucocorticoids promote the release of amino acids from muscles and lipolysis as needed and increase glyconeogenesis. Mineralocorticoids maintain electrolyte balance by increasing urinary potassium excretion and retaining sodium by promoting kidney reabsorption of sodium back to the plasma.

Adrenocortical insufficiency. See *Addison's disease.*

Adrenocorticotropic hormone (ACTH). A hormone secreted by the anterior pituitary gland which stimulates the adrenal cortex to produce *corticosteriod.* The ACTH level increases when a person is under stress, during surgery, and in acute hypoglycemia. See also *Hypophysis.*

Adrenoleukodystrophy (ALD). An inherited metabolic defect characterized by an unusual accumulation of very-long-chain fatty acids (VLFA), especially C26:0, a hexacosanate. These are normally present in small amounts in the diet and are also synthesized within the body. Accumulation of the VLFA result in demyelination of the central nervous system (CNS), which leads to loss of voluntary movements and death. While this disorder usually occurs in young children, there is an adult form designated *adrenomyeloneuropathy* (AMN), indicating adrenal insufficiency, one of the clinical signs of ALD. *Dietary management:* restrict intake of very-long-chain fatty acids to less than 3 mg/day and increase intake of monounsaturated fatty acids, especially oleic acid (C18:1). A commercial preparation of oleic acid is available as glyceryl trioleate (GTO). Other nutrient sources are provided by nonfat milk, simple sugars or syrups, and vitamin-mineral supplements. Depending on the individual's progress, give a regular diet adequate for his or her nutrient needs but continue to alter dietary fat, restricting VLFA.

Adsorption. 1. The ability of a substance to attract and concentrate on its surface a thin layer of gas, liquid, or solid by adhesion. 2. Attachment of one substance to the surface of another.

Advance. Registered name of a milk formula used as a transition between infant formula and cow's milk; combines soy protein isolates and cow's milk to help reduce the risk of cow milk-induced enteric blood loss. Available in ready-to-use concentrated liquid. See Appendix 37.

A/E ratio. Number of milligrams of each essential amino acid per gram of total essential amino acids. This ratio is a method of evaluating protein quality.

Aerobic exercise. Physical exercise requiring increased breathing and extra effort by the heart to meet the oxygen needs of the skeletal muscles. Examples of aerobic exercises are vigorous walking, cycling, running, swimming, and jogging. Helpful for weight reduction, glucose control, and physical therapy or rehabilitation in some ailments. See also *Nutrition, exercise,* and *Nutrition, physical health.*

Aging. Theoretically, aging is a continuous process from conception until death. But in the young and growing organism the building-up processes exceed the breaking-down processes, so that the net result is a picture of growth and development. Once the body reaches adulthood, the process is reversed. Aging proceeds at different rates in different individuals. Environmental factors—chemical, physical, and biologic—influence the aging process. Certain physiologic functions show a gradual decrement with age. These include basal metabolic rate, cardiac output, renal blood flow, and lung capacity. However, other physiologic functions remain quite stable over the entire life span unless the individual is subjected to stress factors. For example, fasting blood glucose levels do not change significantly with age, and blood volume and red cell content remain relatively constant. See also *Nutrition, aging process.*

A/G ratio. See *Albumin/globulin ratio.*

AIDS. Abbreviation for *acquired immune deficiency syndrome.*

AIN. Abbreviation for *American Institute of Nutrition.*

Al. Chemical symbol for aluminum.

Alanine (Ala). Alpha-aminopropionic acid, a nonessential amino acid readily formed from carbohydrates by its reversible conversion to pyruvic acid. Beta-alanine is the only naturally occurring beta-amino acid. It is found in pantothenic acid, carnosine, and anserine.

Albinism. Inborn error of metabolism characterized by lack of pigmentation of the hair, skin, and eyes due to inability to form the pigment melanin. The condition is caused by lack of the enzyme tyrosinase, which catalyzes the hydroxylation of tyrosine to dihydroxyphenylalanine (dopa) to form melanin.

Albumen. 1. White of eggs, consisting chiefly of albumin. 2. *Oxford Dictionary* spelling of albumin.

Albumin. A simple protein soluble in water and dilute salt solutions and coagulable by heat. Examples are lactalbumin in milk and ovalbumin in egg. See also *Serum albumin.*

Albumin/globulin ratio (A/G). Ratio of albumin to globulin concentration in the serum.

The normal value ranges from 1.8 to 2.5. See *Serum albumin.*

Albuminoid. Also called scleroprotein; simple protein characteristic of skeletal structures and protective tissues such as skin and hair. It is of three distinct types: *elastin* in tendons and ligaments, *collagen* in tendons and bones, and *keratin* in hair, nails, and hooves.

Albuminuria. Presence of albumin in the urine. It occurs in kidney disease, toxemia of pregnancy, and certain conditions in which circulation to the kidney is inadequate. Normally, the kidneys reabsorb plasma albumin, which filters out from the glomerulus into the Bowman's capsule.

Albuterol. A synthetic sympathomimetic amine; used as a bronchodilator in the symptomatic relief of bronchospasm in obstructive airway diseases. It has an unusual taste and may cause nausea and vomiting; it may also cause hyperglycemia and may aggravate preexisting diabetes mellitus in large doses. The trade names are Proventil and Ventolin.

Alcohol. 1. Aliphatic hydrocarbon derivative containing a hydroxyl (−OH) group. 2. Groups of organic compounds derived from carbohydrate fermentation. 3. Unqualified, it refers to ethyl alcohol (ethanol) in wines and liquors. Except for calories, alcoholic beverages supply few or no nutrients. One gram (or milliliter) of alcohol yields 7 calories. Alcohol is a depressant, affecting the central nervous system and other vital organs. Excessive intake is a prominent contributor to three of the ten leading causes of death in the United States, namely, cirrhosis of the liver, motor vehicle and other accidents, and suicide. Women are generally less able to tolerate alcohol than men because they tend to be smaller and appear to absorb more of the ethanol than men. Individuals who consume alcoholic beverages are advised to drink in moderation. "Moderate" drinking is defined for normal healthy women as no more than one drink per day and for normal healthy men as no more than two drinks per day. Count as a drink 12 oz regular beer, 5 oz wine, or 1½ oz distilled spirit (80% proof). Individuals who are cautioned not to drink alcoholic beverages include women who are pregnant or trying to conceive, individuals using certain medications that should not be taken with alcohol, and those who plan to drive or engage in other activities that require a high level of attention or skill. See also *Alcoholism* and Appendix 33.

Alcoholics Anonymous (AA). An international nonprofit organization that regularly meets for group support of alcoholics. The main purpose is to help its volunteer members cope with abstinence from drinking.

Alcoholism. Chronic excessive use of alcohol, which eventually leads to irreversible disorders affecting the liver, digestive system, pancreas, and nerves. Thiamin, folacin, pyridoxine, and vitamin B_{12} absorption are impaired, causing multiple vitamin deficiencies. Clinical signs and symptoms include Wernicke-Korsakoff syndrome, peripheral neuropathy, pedal edema, ascites, anemia, glossitis, cardiac arrhythmias, and electrolyte imbalance. Liver cells are damaged, resulting in reduced enzyme production and poor nutrient metabolism. Steatorrhea is common due to pancreatic dysfunction. Most alcoholics suffer from malnutrition because of poor eating habits and diets that are usually deficient in calories and essential nutrients. As a consequence, anemias and liver *cirrhosis* are serious problems that need nutritional intervention. Alcohol may induce hypoglycemia in some insulin-dependent diabetics, leading to complications. *Dietary management:* withdrawal from alcohol use is often associated with anorexia, nausea, and gastrointestinal problems, all of which need individualized assessment. If acute alcoholics are overdehydrated, fluid intake is limited. Electrolyte imbalance and severe hypoglycemia are corrected intravenously. When the patient's condition improves, the diet progresses gradually from full liquid to regular meals with vitamin B supplements. Thiamin is given at a dose of about 200 mg/day. Folic acid, niacin, pyridoxine, pantothenic acid, and vitamins B_2 and B_{12} are also prescribed. Protein and calories are increased according to the patient's needs and state of recovery. With alcoholic hepatitis, a minimum of 30 kcal/kg body weight and 1.5 gm protein/kg is ample for liver regeneration and protein anabolism. See *Nutrition, alcoholism* from the public health standpoint. For other dietary guidelines, see also *Cirrhosis* and *Ascites.*

ALD. Abbreviation for *adrenoleukodystrophy.*

Aldosterone. An adrenocortical hormone. It plays an important role in the regulation of electrolyte balance. Aldosterone acts on the distal convoluted tubules of the kidneys to reabsorb sodium and water and excrete potassium.

Alimentary. Pertaining to food, nutrition, or diet.

Alimentary tract. The digestive tract or gastrointestinal tract (GIT) extending from the mouth to the anus. Site of *digestion* and *absorption* of nutrients. See Appendix 11.

Alitame. A nonnutritive sweetener that is sweeter than *aspartame.* Made by chemical synthesis and contains the amino acids L-aspartic acid and D-alanine, along with a novel amide substitute. It is an odorless, nonhygroscopic powder and has no unpleasant aftertaste. Exhibits good stability under a range of baking conditions and has excellent solubility in water. May contribute a theoretical maximum of 1.4 kcal/gm (equivalent to 0.02% of the calories of sucrose on a sweetness basis). Alitame is still under study and could be approved for use in the food industry.

Alkali. Also called base. 1. Any substance that accepts or acquires protons. 2. Any substance that dissociates in aqueous solution to yield $-OH$ ions. 3. Class of compounds that saponify fats, form salts with acids, and form soluble carbonates.

Alkaline-ash residue. Inorganic elements, chiefly sodium, potassium, calcium, and magnesium, that form basic ions in the body. When excreted in the urine, they increase the pH or make the urine more alkaline or basic.

Alkaline-forming foods. Foods in which the alkaline residue exceeds the acid residue. These include milk, vegetables, and fruits, except for cranberries, plums, and prunes. Most fruits, despite their acidity, exert a basic effect on the body since the organic acids in them, such as citric acid and malic acid, can be completely oxidized to carbon dioxide and water, leaving the salts to contribute to the supply of basic elements. Cranberries, plums, and prunes contain benzoic and quinic acids, which are not oxidized in the body but are converted in the liver into hippuric acid and excreted as such in the urine. These fruits are therefore acid-forming. See also *Diet, ash.*

Alkali reserve. Buffer compounds in the blood, e.g., sodium bicarbonate, dipotassium phosphate, and proteins, that are capable of neutralizing acids. Sometimes called blood bicarbonate since bicarbonate is the chief alkali reserve of the body.

Alkaloid. Naturally occurring basic nitrogenous compound, usually of plant origin. It is insoluble in water but soluble in organic solvents and can precipitate proteins. Many alkaloids from plants such as cocaine, strychnine, morphine, and quinine are useful in medicine in regulated amounts.

Alkalosis. An abnormal condition characterized by a rise in the pH or a fall in the hydrogen ion concentration of the blood. It results from excessive loss of acids from the body without comparable loss of base or the formation or supply of base at a rate faster than its neutralization or elimination. Alkalosis is commonly due to persistent vomiting and excessive intake of sodium bicarbonate; it may also be due to hyperventilation.

Alkaptonuria. Inborn error of metabolism characterized by excretion of urine that darkens on contact with air due to the presence of abnormal amounts of homogentisic acid. Phenylalanine and tyrosine are not completely oxidized because of a lack of hepatic homogentisic acid oxidase. The precise dietary treatment is not known, although ascorbic acid supplementation and low intake of phenylalanine and tyrosine may be of some value.

Allergen. An agent or substance capable of producing an allergic reaction. Common allergens are inhalants (pollen, dust, hay), ingestants (food, beverage, condiment, drug), contactants (cosmetics, medicine, environment), and injectants (vaccine, serum, drug). It is also possible to have physical (heat, cold, sunlight) and emotional (feelings, moods) forms of allergy. See also *Food allergen.*

Allergy. Unusual or exaggerated susceptibility to a substance (allergen) that is harmless in similar amounts to most people. See *Food allergen.*

Allopurinol. A structural isomer of hypoxanthine; used in the treatment of gout and other hyperuricemias. Allopurinol has a metallic taste, may decrease iron absorption and cause anemia, prolongs the action of anticoagulants, and may cause anorexia, nausea and vomiting, abdominal pain, and diarrhea. Brand names are Lopurin, Zyloprim, and Zurinol.

All-or-none law. 1. Response of an individual nerve or muscle fiber to an adequate stimulus is always maximal, i.e., a stimulus either causes a full-sized impulse or fails to set up an impulse. 2. Tissue synthesis occurs only when all the necessary amino acids are present in the proper amounts and proportions at the site of tissue formation. Absence of even one amino acid will prevent synthesis, and unless a tissue protein can be synthesized all at once, it is not synthesized at all.

Alloxan. A red crystalline substance produced by oxidation of uric acid. It can cause necrosis of the islets of Langerhans in the pancreas. Alloxan has been used to treat cases of hyperinsulinism due to pancreatic tumors, but it is toxic in high amounts.

Alopecia. Baldness or loss of hair. This is seen in experimentally induced *biotin* deficiency in rats, which begins with dermatitis around the eyes and progresses to general loss of hair. Alopecia in humans is not corrected by administration of biotin. It is due to various causes, including seborrheic dermatitis, dandruff, effect of certain drugs or chemicals, syphilis, and other bacterial, fungal, or viral infections. Baldness is also seen in *myxedema* and other cases of pituitary insufficiency.

Alterna. Brand name of a low-protein milk powder substitute for patients with renal disease; tastes like low-fat milk. Can be used as beverage and in place of milk in cooking. Contains whey protein, dry skim milk, sodium caseinate, corn syrup powder, sucrose, partially hydrogenated soybean oil, and mono- and diglycerides.

Alternative sweeteners. Sweetening agents other than table sugar or sucrose, syrups, honey, and molasses. Grouped as nutritive or nonnutritive sweeteners. The latter are sometimes called "low-calorie sugar substitutes," although most of them have almost no calories and are useful for persons who have to avoid nutritive sugars, such as diabetics and obese persons. The other advantage of nonnutritive sweeteners relate to reduced tooth decay. For nutritive sweeteners, see *Fructose, Glucose, Glycine, Mannitol, Sorbitol,* and *Xylitol.* For nonnutritive sweeteners, see *Acesulfame-K, Alitame, Aspartame, Cyclamate, Dulcin,* and *Saccharin.*

Aluminum (Al). The third most abundant element in the earth's crust; its compounds are widespread in soils. Although present in trace amounts in biologic material, aluminum does not appear to be an essential element. It is very poorly absorbed. Large intake, however, is known to produce gastrointestinal irritation. Aluminum combines with the phosphates present in food to form insoluble aluminum phosphate, which is excreted in the feces. The ability of the kidneys to excrete aluminum is decreased in renal failure. Aluminum poisoning is an important potential hazard to patients with chronic renal failure on hemodialysis; aluminum present in the dialysis fluid may be transferred to the patient. Some aluminum is also absorbed when aluminum hydroxide is used as an antacid or oral phosphate binder to control plasma phosphorus. Accumulation of aluminum may also result from the parenteral administration of nutritional solution contaminated with aluminum. Toxic effects are manifested in neurologic, bone, and hematopoietic functions. Aluminum intoxication intensifies anemia in uremic patients and can cause uremic osteomalacia and encephalopathy. Contrary to earlier beliefs, trace amounts of aluminum from cooking utensils are harmless and do not cause chronic poisoning. There is no evidence that aluminum cookware, foil wrapping, pie plates, or cookie sheets contribute to increased aluminum levels in food.

Alzheimer's disease. Also called senile dementia–Alzheimer type (SDAT). A form of dementia characterized by a group of symptoms which include loss of memory, thinking, and reasoning power; disorientation, confusion, and sometimes speech disturbances. The exact causes of Alzheimer's disease are not yet known, although structural changes in the brain have been observed, consisting of neurofibrillary tangles and neuritic plaques in the cortex. Recent studies have shown an abnormal accumulation of aluminum in the brain cells of persons with Alzheimer's disease. While these patients are generally over 65 years old, a few are in their forties. *Dietary management:* irregularity of mealtimes and snacks, loss of appetite or refusal of food, inability to carry out daily tasks like self-feeding and cooking, and loss of sphincter control and aspiration are nutritional problems. Maintaining good nutrition may delay the progression of the disease. Because of gross behavioral changes, patient needs assistance around the clock, especially during mealtimes. Monitor body weight and guard against dehydration and constipation.

Amantadine. A synthetic compound used in the treatment of parkinsonian syndrome and drug-related extrapyramidal reactions and in the symptomatic treatment of influenza caused by influenza A virus strains.

Constipation and dry mouth may become problems because of its anticholinergic effect. Brand names are Symmetrel and Symadine.

Amblyopia. Dimness of vision. Nutritional amblyopia appears after a period of many months when diets are grossly deficient in nutrients, particularly the B complex vitamins. Common presenting complaints are blurred or dim vision, difficulty in reading, photophobia, and discomfort in the retrobulbar region on moving the eyes. When the symptoms are not severe, they are relieved rapidly by improved nutrition and B vitamin supplementation; little or no improvement results from any form of treatment when vision is already markedly affected.

American Diabetes Association (ADA). A voluntary organization to help improve the well-being of people with diabetes. With a membership of over 225,000 nationwide, the association offers support for research, education, and services to diabetics and their families, including a monthly issue of *Diabetes Forecast.*

American Dietetic Association (ADA). Professional organization whose objectives are to improve the nutrition of human beings, to advance the science of dietetics and nutrition, and to promote education in these and allied areas. It publishes monthly the *Journal of the American Dietetic Association* and the *ADA Courier.* With over 60,000 members, most of whom are registered dietitians, the ADA is an authority on national food and nutrition issues. It is the largest and oldest professional organization concerned with the practice of dietetics.

American Institute of Nutrition (AIN). Professional organization founded in 1928 to develop and extend nutrition knowledge and to promote personal contact between researchers in nutrition and related fields. It publishes the *Journal of Nutrition* and the *American Journal of Clinical Nutrition.*

Agency for International Development (AID). Agency of the U.S. State Department that helps developing countries with their various food, agricultural, and educational programs.

American Society for Clinical Nutrition (ASCN). Division of the *American Institute of Nutrition (AIN)* that aims to promote education about human nutrition in health and disease and to promote the presentation and discussion of research in human nutrition.

American Society for Parenteral and Enteral Nutrition (ASPEN). Group of physicians, dietitians, nurses, pharmacists, nutritionists, and others dedicated to fostering good nutritional support of patients during hospitalization and rehabilitation. By promoting the team approach and by educating health care professionals at all levels, ASPEN encourages the development of improved nutritional support procedures. It publishes the *Journal of Parenteral and Enteral Nutrition (JPEN).*

Amethopterin. A potent metabolic antagonist of *folic acid;* it inhibits the enzyme dihydrofolate reductase and interferes with the conversion of folic acid to its active form, *folinic acid.* Amethopterin is used in the treatment of leukemia. Adverse gastrointestinal side effects include oral lesions, glossitis, stomatitis, abdominal distress, anorexia, nausea, vomiting, and diarrhea. Trade names are Folex and Mexate.

Amiloride. A potassium-sparing diuretic; used concomitantly with other diuretics in the treatment of edema associated with congestive heart failure and hepatic cirrhosis. The potassium-sparing effect of amiloride may cause hyperkalemia, especially in geriatric patients and in those with renal insufficiency and diabetes mellitus; it may also cause hyponatremia, appetite changes, gas pain and abdominal bloating, and heartburn. Brand names are Midamor, Moduret, and Moduretic.

Amin-Aid. Brand name of an instant drink that is high in calories but low in protein, sodium, and potassium for use in renal failure; contains essential amino acids plus histidine, maltodextrins, sucrose, partially hydrogenated soy oil, lecithin, and mono-

and diglycerides. It requires vitamin and mineral supplementation if used as the principal source of nutrition. See Appendix 39.

Amine. Compound that has the characteristic amino (NH_2) group. It is formed by replacing one or more of the hydrogen atoms of ammonia with one or more organic radicals. Amines are classified as *primary, secondary,* or *tertiary,* depending on whether one, two, or three hydrogens are replaced.

Aminess. Brand name of a 5.2% amino acid solution for total parenteral nutrition. Contains essential amino acids plus histidine, based on the minimal requirement for each. It is low in aromatic amino acids (tryptophan, phenylalanine, and tyrosine) and is used for nutritional support of uremic patients, particularly when oral feeding is not possible. See Appendix 40.

Amino acid (AA). Fundamental structural unit of protein with the general formula

$$\begin{array}{c} NH_2 \\ | \\ R-C-COOH \\ | \\ H \end{array}$$ (R is a radical, the basis for classifying amino acids)

Amino acids may be acidic, basic, or neutral, depending on the number of acidic or basic groups in the molecule. According to their structure, amino acids may be aliphatic, aromatic, or heterocyclic. Of the 20 amino acids considered to be physiologically important, 9 are known to be essential for the human adult. The others are dietary nonessential amino acids. For a list of the amino acids and human requirements, see Appendix 9. Amino nitrogen comprises about 16% of the weight of protein. The biological value of protein is based on its amino acids. See *Protein.*

Aliphatic AA. Amino acid with a carbon-to-carbon chain. Examples are threonine, glycine, serine, and alanine.

Antiketogenic AA. See *Glucogenic AA.*

Aromatic AA (AAA). Amino acid in which the carbon atoms are arranged in a ring. Examples are tryptophan, phenylalanine, and tyrosine.

Branched-chain AA (BCAA). Amino acid that is aliphatic but whose side chain is branched. Examples are leucine, isoleucine, and valine.

Dibasic AA. Amino acid that has a second nitrogen atom. Examples are lysine, arginine, and histidine.

Dispensable AA. See *Nonessential AA.*

Essential AA (EAA). Also called indispensable amino acid; an amino acid that cannot be synthesized by the body from materials readily available at a speed commensurate with the demands for normal growth. It must therefore be supplied preformed in the diet. The nine essential amino acids for humans are *histidine, isoleucine, leucine, lysine, methionine, phenylalanine, threonine, tryptophan,* and *valine.*

Glucogenic AA. An amino acid that can be converted to an alpha-keto acid, a carbohydrate former. Examples are glycine, alanine, serine, threonine, aspartic acid, and glutamic acid.

Indispensable AA. See *Essential AA.*

Ketogenic AA. An amino acid that can be converted to acetate or acetoacetate, a ketone body. Examples are leucine, isoleucine, and lysine.

Limiting AA. The essential amino acid that is most deficient in a protein, in comparison with the amino acids of a standard protein. Lysine is the limiting amino acid in rice and other cereals; tryptophan is limiting in corn; and methionine and cystine are limiting in beans.

Nonessential AA. Also called dispensable amino acid; an amino acid that can be synthesized in the body, provided that there is an adequate source of nitrogen. It need not be supplied preformed in the diet. Examples are alanine, arginine, asparagine, aspartic acid, cystine, cysteine, glycine, glutamic acid, glutamine, hydroxyproline, proline, serine, and tyrosine.

Semidispensable AA. See *Semiessential AA.*

Semiessential AA. Also called semidispensable amino acid; an amino acid that, when present in the diet, reduces the need for an essential amino acid. For example, cystine reduces the need for methionine, and tyrosine reduces the need for phenylalanine.

Sulfur-containing AA. Amino acid that contains sulfur in its molecule. Examples are methionine, cystine, and cysteine.

Amino acid, functions. The physiologic roles of amino acids as integral components (building blocks) of protein are summarized under *Protein, functions.* However, some amino acids have specialized functions, and these are discussed under the specific amino acid. For example, tryptophan is a precursor of niacin; methionine is a methylating agent (donates the CH3− radical); cystine is a component of bile acid; and tyrosine is needed for the synthesis of thyroxine.

Amino acid pool. Reservoir or metabolic pool of amino acids that come from the diet (exogenous source), that are synthesized in cells, and that are derived from the breakdown of tissue proteins (endogenous sources). The size of the pool is determined by the quantity of the constituents instantaneously present and available for all of the reactions leading into and from the pool (i.e., anabolic and catabolic reactions).

Amino acid reference pattern. The ideal combination of amino acids in total quantity and proportion to meet all physiologic requirements. The Food and Agriculture Organization reference pattern was derived from the minimal daily requirements for the essential amino acids for infants and adults. Other reference patterns have been based on the amino acids present in egg and human milk.

Amino acid requirement. Established values for the nine essential amino acids are given in Appendix 9, using nitrogen balance as the criterion for adults. See also *Protein requirement.*

Aminoaciduria. Increase in the urinary excretion of amino acids due to elevated concentrations of amino acids in the plasma. The condition is caused by a defect in the renal tubular reabsorption of amino acids. The renal defect may be congenital, or it may be acquired as a result of toxic agents, metabolic disorders such as acidosis and hypercalcemia, and deficiencies of vitamins B, C, and D.

Aminogram. Amino acid pattern showing the quantitative relationship between the essential amino acids in a dietary protein and those found in egg protein. Since egg is an unreasonably high protein standard for the world food supply, the Food and Agriculture Organization uses a theoretical ideal aminogram as the protein standard.

Aminopterin. Folic acid antagonist used clinically in the treatment of leukemia and other neoplastic diseases. See also *Methotrexate.*

Amino sugar. Sugar in which a hydroxyl group has been replaced by an amino group. All amino sugars known to occur in nature are derivatives of aldohexoses, with the amino group on carbon atom 2. Examples are glucosamine and galactosamine.

Aminosyn. Trade name of a standard parenteral amino acid solution in five different concentrations (3.5%, 5%, 7%, 8.5%, and 10%); includes all the essential amino acids and several nonessential amino acids. Also available with high levels of branched-chain amino acids for hepatic diseases, stress, and trauma (Aminosyn-HBC) and with low levels of aromatic amino acids for renal disease (Aminosyn-RF). See Appendix 40.

Amitriptyline. A tricyclic antidepressant. The drug interferes with riboflavin metabolism; it may also cause altered taste acuity, anorexia, stomatitis, dry mouth, constipation, and changes in blood glucose. Brand names include Amitril, Elavil, Endep, Etrafon, and Triavil.

Ammonia. 1. Volatile alkaline gas that is soluble in water. 2. By-product of protein metabolism by deamination of amino acids. In the body, ammonia may be used in the reductive amination of alpha-keto acids to form new amino acids, or it may be used in the synthesis of purines and pyrimidines. Ammonia is toxic in large concentrations and normally is not allowed to accumulate in the cells. It is either excreted directly in the urine or eliminated via glutamine or urea formation.

Amphotericin B. Antifungal antibiotic used to treat severe systemic infections and meningitis caused by susceptible fungi. Weight loss is common with this drug; it may also cause proteinuria, decreased serum potassium and magnesium, increased blood urea nitrogen and creatinine, anorexia, dyspepsia, cramping, and epigastric pain. Brand names are Fungizone and Mysteclin-F.

Amputation. The surgical removal of a part of the body or a limb for medical treatment, as in the removal of malignant tumors, gangrene of the toe, a portion of a limb due to a severe injury, as from an auto accident, and so on. The percentage of body weight loss in amputees is considered in determining desirable body weight. The following data are close estimates:

BODY PART AMPUTATED	(PERCENT OF BODY WEIGHT LOSS)
Whole arm (6.0%)	Total leg and foot (18.8%)
Upper arm (3.6%)	Upper leg (11.6%)
Lower arm (2.2%)	Lower leg and foot (7.2%)
Hand (0.8%)	

Amyotrophic lateral sclerosis (ALS). Also known as Lou Gehrig's disease or motor neuron disease; characterized by progressive spinal muscular atrophy, which may be fatal due to respiratory failure. Early symptoms are loss of reflexes and gait, difficulty in chewing and swallowing, and negative nitrogen balance. *Dietary management:* correct protein losses and other nutritional deficiencies. Provide liberal fluid intake (about 2 liters daily). When the swallowing reflex is severely affected, tube feeding is recommended. A well-balanced, regular diet in six to eight small feedings, consisting of foods that are easy to chew and swallow, should be provided as the patient's condition improves. Supplement with zinc, phosphorus, potassium, magnesium, and vitamins, particularly vitamin E.

Anabolic agent. Compound that promotes synthesis, growth, and weight gain. The endogenous anabolic hormones, produced throughout every human's lifetime, are the steroid hormones—estradiol, progesterone, and testosterone. There are synthetic steroid and nonsteroid hormones which are also anabolic. Those used in the food industry are approved by the Food and Drug Administration. The levels used and the residues left on food (e.g., meats) are closely monitored by the Food Safety and Inspection Service, U.S. Department of Agriculture.

Anabolism. Synthesis; process by which simple substances are converted by living cells into more complex substances. Also referred to as constructive metabolism. Compare with *Catabolism.*

Anaphylaxis. Hypersensitivity or increased susceptibility to a foreign protein or substance. It is characterized by exaggerated reactions and widespread systemic involvement.

Androgen. Generic name for the hormones secreted by the testes that are responsible for the development of male accessory sex organs and secondary sex characteristics. Androgenic hormones also have anabolic influence on nitrogen and calcium metabolism. The two major naturally occurring androgens are androsterone and testosterone.

Anemia. Reduction in the size or number of red blood cells, the quantity of hemoglobin, or both, resulting in decreased capacity of the blood to carry oxygen. The symptoms vary according to the etiologic factors, but the common clinical signs and symptoms include pallor, breathlessness on exertion, easy fatigue, dizziness, insomnia, and lack of appetite. Anemias may be classified according to cell size, which may be *large* (macrocytic), *small* (microcytic), or *normal* (normocytic). Another classification is based on the color index of the blood, which may be *high* (hyperchromic), *low* (hypochromic), or *normal* (normochromic). Anemia may be due to excessive loss of blood; to excessive blood cell destruction as a result of chemical poisons, such as lead or specific infections such as malaria; or to congenital abnormalities of the red cells, as in sickle cell anemia. Anemias may also be due to a defect in blood formation. The defect may be nutritional in origin or may be due to aplasia of the bone marrow, toxic inhibition, or diseases that affect the bone marrow, spleen, liver, or lymph nodes.

Anemia, nutritional. Anemia due to a deficiency of nutrients necessary in the formation of blood. Iron, protein, folic acid, vitamin B_{12}, and vitamin C are the major nutrients essential in blood formation. Copper and cobalt are also essential, but the amounts needed are so small that they are more than amply supplied by the normal adequate diet. The deficiency in these nutrients may be caused by inadequate intake, defective absorption, imperfect utilization, increased requirement, or increased excretion. See also *Hemopoiesis* and *Nutrition, anemias.*

Iron-deficiency a. Form of anemia characterized by small (microcytic), pale (hypochromic) erythrocytes. It is generally due to chronic blood loss, as in excessive or prolonged menstruation, repeated pregnancies, and parasitic infestation; faulty iron intake; impaired iron absorption, as in achlorhydria and chronic diarrhea; and increased blood volume, which occurs during infancy and pregnancy.

Protein-deficiency a. Macrocytic type of anemia seen in association with protein malnutrition. Patients with this type of anemia also show signs of multiple nutritional deficiencies, especially of folic acid, vitamin B_{12}, and iron.

Vitamin B_{12}- and folic acid-deficiency a. Deficiency in either vitamin B_{12} or folic acid interferes with the normal development of erythrocytes, characterized by megaloblastic arrest in the bone marrow and the production of an insufficient number of large erythrocytes that carry a normal complement of hemoglobin (i.e., megaloblastic, macrocytic, normochromic anemia); it may also be hyperchromic (i.e., macrocytic hyperchromic anemia). Vitamin B_{12} deficiency may be due to inadequate intake of animal protein foods, lack of intrinsic factor, reduced absorptive capacity of the ileal mucosa, and competition for the vita-

min from intestinal parasites. Folic acid deficiency may be due to inadequate dietary intake; increased demand for folic acid, as in pregnancy and chronic blood loss; malabsorption syndrome; and administration of drugs that are folic acid antagonists.

Vitamin C-deficiency a. Macrocytic type of anemia seen in severe cases of vitamin C deficiency (scurvy). Vitamin C is necessary for the absorption of iron and the conversion of folic acid to its biologically active form, folinic acid.

Anergy. 1. Lack of energy or activity. 2. Diminished reactivity to specific antigen(s); the total absence of an allergic response under conditions that would otherwise be expected to lead to such a response. Anergy is seen in protein-energy malnutrition, stress, cancer, and sepsis. See *Hypersensitivity skin test.*

Angina pectoris. A sudden, severe pain radiating from the heart region to the left shoulder and down the arm into the fingers. It tends to occur suddenly following emotional stress, physical exertion, and other conditions subjecting the heart to heavy strain. *Dietary management:* maintain desirable body weight. Give small feedings with rest periods when eating. Avoid caffeine and increase dietary fiber. If the angina is associated with coronary heart disease, restrict intake of sodium, cholesterol, and saturated fats.

Angiotensin. A vasoconstrictor substance present in the blood. It is formed from an alpha-2 globulin by the action of the enzyme *renin,* which originates from the kidney. It promotes the release of aldosterone from the adrenal cortex and increases blood pressure.

Angular stomatitis. Inflammation of the oral mucosa at the angles of the mouth, giving the appearance of fissures radiating outward from the mouth. It may extend into the buccal mucosa as whitish patches on the mucous membrane lining the cheeks. The tongue is often red and smooth or has patchy areas of white coating. Angular stomatitis often responds to large doses of riboflavin and sometimes to pyridoxine. It is often seen in patients receiving long-term antibiotic therapy, especially chloramphenicol, and also occurs in association with iron-deficiency anemia. Nonnutritional factors, such as ill-fitting dentures, may also cause angular stomatitis.

Anorexia. Lack or loss of appetite.

Anorexia nervosa. A disorder characterized by an aversion to food and a self-imposed restriction of food intake. There is a preoccupation with food as a fear of getting fat, and the individual denies being excessively thin despite extreme emaciation, denies hunger despite malnutrition, and denies fatigue despite frantic exercise. A spectrum of the disorder occurs, ranging from mild conditions that require little or no intervention to very severe forms that can require hospitalization. Anorexia nervosa is a life-threatening disorder due to the effects of starvation and extreme inanition, which lead to secondary endocrine disorders resulting in amenorrhea, lowered basal metabolic rate, slow pulse, electrolyte imbalance, and other metabolic consequences; immune functions can be compromised. Some individuals with anorexia nervosa go on periodic binge eating, which is followed by self-induced purging by vomiting or the use of enemas or cathartics. Many treatments of anorexia nervosa have evolved, focusing on biologic interventions to bring about weight gain, psychological techniques to deal with personal and family conflicts, or a combination of these methods. The dietary goal is to establish a normal eating pattern. Parenteral or nasogastric feeding should be reserved for life-threatening states and are usually not necessary. See also *Eating disorders.*

Anorexigenic drug. An appetite depressant; used in weight reduction programs; not to be used without a physician's advice. Some of these drugs have undesirable side effects.

Antacid. Inorganic salt that dissolves in acid gastric secretions, releasing anions that partially neutralize gastric hydrochloric acid. Antacids inactivate thiamin, decrease iron and vitamin A absorption, and cause phosphate depletion. Undesirable gastrointestinal effects are bloating, constipation and fecal impaction, and stomach cramps. Brand names include Amphojel, Alu-Cap, Basaljel, Di-Gel, Gelusil, Maalox, and Mylanta.

Antagonist. An agent or substance that counteracts or blocks the effect of another. See also *Antimetabolite* and *Antivitamin.*

Anthranilic acid. Product resulting from the hydrolysis of *kynurenine* by the enzyme kynureninase with pyridoxal phosphate as a cofactor. In pyridoxine deficiency, hydrolysis of kynurenine results instead in the production of *xanthurenic acid,* which is excreted in the urine.

Anthropometry. Scientific measurement of the various parts of the body. This includes the measurement of body weight and height, as well as the chest, arms, head, and other body parts. Anthropometry is a useful aid in assessing the nutritional status of individuals and groups. See also *Nutritional assessment.* See Appendices 18 to 23.

Antibiotic. A substance elaborated by certain microorganisms that has the capacity to destroy or inhibit the growth of other microorganisms. Examples are penicillin, aureomycin, terramycin, and neomycin. See *Nutrition antibiotics.*

Antibody. Specific substance produced in the body in response to invasion by a foreign or antagonistic substance known as an antigen. Antibodies are serum proteins elicited by the lymphoid cell system. These proteins, called immunoglobulins (Ig), protect the body by reacting as agglutinins, lysins, precipitins, or antitoxins.

Anticoagulant. A substance that inhibits or prevents blood coagulation by interfering with the clotting mechanism. Examples are Dicumarol and heparin, which inhibit prothrombin formation, and oxalate and citrate, which combine with calcium. See *Blood clotting.*

Antidiuretic hormone (ADH). A hormone produced by the posterior portion of the pituitary gland (neurohypophysis). It has a marked antidiuretic action by increasing the rate of reabsorption of water from the kidney tubules, thus decreasing water excretion. A deficiency in this hormone results in a condition known as *diabetes insipidus.*

Antiketogenic factor. See *Ketogenic-antiketo-genic ratio.*

Antimetabolite. Structurally related compound that interferes with the metabolism or function of a chemical compound (metabolite) in the body. Also called metabolic antagonist.

Antioxidant. A substance that delays or prevents oxidation. The more common ones are alpha-tocopherol, ascorbic acid, propyl gallate, butylated hydroxyanisole (BHA), butylated hydroxytoluene (BHT), and lecithin.

Antipyrine. A chemical used as an antipyretic and analgesic; also widely used in total body water determinations. See *Water determination, body.*

Antithyroid agents. A large number of substances that inhibit normal thyroid function either by inhibiting the synthesis of thyroid hormones or by preventing their release from the thyroid gland. Examples are thiourea, thiouracil, and *goitrogens* in foods.

Antivitamin. Natural or synthetic substance similar in structure to a vitamin which interferes with its normal functioning by competitive inhibition, inactivation, or chemical destruction. Some of the most common antivitamins are Dicumarol (vitamin K), thiaminase (vitamin B_1), Atabrine (vitamin B_2), aminopterin (folic acid), and avidin (biotin).

Anuria. Suppression of renal secretion; absence of urinary excretion. It may occur in the final stages of glomerulonephritis or after severe trauma, surgery, or transfusion of incompatible blood. Sometimes anuria is nervous in origin.

AOAC. Abbreviation for *Association of Official Agricultural Chemists.*

Aphagia. Loss of ability or power to swallow. See also *Dysphagia.*

Apparent digestibility. Difference between the measured intake of food and the portion recovered in the feces. Expressed as a percentage, apparent digestibility is called *coefficient of digestibility.*

Appetite. Natural desire or craving for food. Loss of appetite (anorexia) accompanies many disorders; certain drugs decrease appetite, e.g., amphetamines, alcohol, and insulin. Some drugs increase appetite, e.g., antihistamines, steroids, and psychotropic drugs.

Applied Nutrition Programs. Practical nutrition programs aimed at strengthening the national nutrition services and group feeding practices of a country; sponsored by the specialized agencies of the United Nations—the World Health Organization, the Food and Agriculture Organization, and the United Nations Children's Fund.

Arabinose. A pentose sugar widely distributed in root vegetables and plants, usually as a component of a complex polysaccharide. It has no known physiologic function in humans, although it is used in studies of bacterial metabolism.

Arachidonic acid. Unsaturated fatty acid containing 20 carbon atoms and four double bonds. It is an important constituent of lecithin and cephalin and occurs in the lipids of the brain, liver, and other organs. This fatty acid is considered one of the essential fatty acids. See *Essential FA* under *Fatty acid.*

Arginine (Arg). Aminoguanidovaleric acid, a dibasic amino acid. Its major metabolic roles include the synthesis of urea and creatine. It is not considered an essential amino acid for humans because the urea cycle provides sufficient arginine for maintenance in adults. However, the need for arginine may be increased in thermal injury, wound healing, sepsis, and trauma. Dietary arginine supplementation may be beneficial under these conditions.

Arginosuccinic acid. Intermediate product in the conversion of citrulline to arginine. It is formed by the condensation of citrulline and aspartic acid in the presence of adenosine triphosphate and magnesium.

Arginosuccinic aciduria. Inborn metabolic defect due to a lack of the enzyme *arginosuccinase.* The condition is characterized by increased excretion of arginosuccinic acid in the urine, hair abnormalities, intermittent ataxia, seizures, coma, mental retardation, and ammonia intoxication. A diet moderately low in protein with arginine supplementation has been recommended.

Ariboflavinosis. Term given to *riboflavin* deficiency. It is characterized by inflammation of the lips with cracking at the angles (cheilosis), sore mouth with purplish red or magenta tongue, and seborrheic dermatitis around the nasolabial folds. Visual symptoms include photophobia, lacrimation, burning and itching of the eyes, dimness of vision, and a normochromic, normocytic anemia.

Arm muscle circumference. See *Mid-arm muscle circumference.*

Arsenic (As). A trace element that is better known as a poison, although minute amounts are essential in maintaining the life span of red blood cells. Arsenic deficiency in animals results in stunted growth, rough hair, anemia, and increased erythrocyte fragility. It remains unclear whether arsenic is also an essential element for humans. Various forms of arsenic are readily absorbed from the diet; seafoods, especially shellfish and shrimp, are rich in arsenic. Intake is quite variable and depends on the amount of seafood consumed, the natural arsenic content of water, and inhalation from environmental exposure. Chronic toxicity is characterized by weakness, prostration, muscle aches, gastrointestinal symptoms, peripheral neuropathy, and changes in the pigmentation of fingernails and skin. Arsenic is fatal in large amounts. Although it is naturally present in foods, the amount usually consumed is too minute to cause toxicity.

Arteriosclerosis. Cardiovascular disease characterized by thickening, loss of elasticity, and hardening (calcification) of the walls of the arteries. It is generally a part of the aging process, although factors other than advancing age are believed to hasten the condition. Among these are high blood pressure, diabetes mellitus, nephrosclerosis, hyperlipidemia, excessive nerve strain, certain infectious diseases, and several other factors not clearly understood. There is no specific treatment except for relief of symptoms. Dietary management depends on the attending disorders and causative factors. See also *Atherosclerosis.*

Arteritis. Also referred to as "cranial or giant-cell arteritis," it consists of chronic thickening of the temporal arteries causing constricted blood flow. Slight but persistent temple throbs with swollen, painful arteries are common symptoms, accompanied by fever and anorexia. *Dietary management:* cut down on sodium and fat intake. Maintain nutritional adequacy, increasing or decreasing the calorie level for weight control. In some cases, high carnitine intake has been effective. Monitor protein (serum albumin) and potassium levels when steroids are used.

Arthritis. Acute or chronic inflammation of a joint. It occurs in varying forms according to the severity, location, deformity, and cause. The most common are rheumatoid arthritis (also called arthritis deformans or atrophic arthritis), osteoarthritis (also called degenerative or hypertrophic arthritis), and gouty arthritis. Arthritis is the principal crippler in the United States, occurring mostly after 45 years of age, with a higher incidence in women. For dietary management, see under the specific form of arthritis.

Artificial feeding. Introduction of food by an unnatural method, such as by *tube feeding* or *parenteral feeding.* In infant feeding, it refers to the nourishment of the baby other than by breast feeding. See *Infant feeding.*

Artificial kidney. Device that removes blood from the artery of an arm, pumps it through a dialyzing membrane that allows accumulated toxic materials to pass into a surrounding bath, and returns clean blood to a vein. It is used in acute and chronic renal failure.

Artificial sweeteners. Synthetic sweetening agents used as sugar substitutes. See *Alternative sweeteners.*

As. Chemical symbol for arsenic.

Ascites. Accumulation of fluid in the peritoneal cavity due to portal hypertension, low blood protein levels, or sodium retention. The condition is often associated with cirrhosis of the liver, cardiac failure, and renal insufficiency. *Dietary management:* institute rigid sodium restriction of 500 mg/day (22 mEq/day) initially until fluid retention subsides. Gradually increase the sodium level to 1000 mg/day and eventually to 2000 mg/day. Fluid intake is restricted to 1500 ml/day if edema is present. See *Diet, sodium-restricted.*

ASCN. Abbreviation for *American Society for Clinical Nutrition.*

Ascorbic acid. Also known as *vitamin C;* a white crystalline compound closely related to the monosaccharide sugars. It exists in two forms: as L-ascorbic acid (reduced form) and as dehydroascorbic acid (oxidized form). Both forms are biologically active, although dehydroascorbic acid is somewhat less stable. They are readily reversibly reduced and oxidized, but further oxidation of dehydroascorbic acid results in complete loss of activity. See *Vitamin C* and Appendix 16.

Ash. Incombustible *mineral* residue remaining after all the organic matter has been burned or oxidized. See also *Diet, ash.*

Asparaginase. An antineoplastic agent; used as a component of various chemotherapeutic regimens for lymphosarcoma and leukemia. Its side effects include impaired pancreatic function and decreased insulin synthesis, hyperglycemia and glucosuria, anorexia, weight loss, and malabsorption syndrome. The brand name is Elspar.

Asparagine. The beta amide of aspartic acid present in most tissues and occurring abundantly in higher plants. It participates in transamination reactions. The enzyme *asparaginase* has anticancer activity in guinea pigs but produces side effects in humans. It depresses protein synthesis and causes nausea, anorexia, and weight loss.

Aspartame. A low-calorie nutritive sweetener composed of the two naturally occurring amino acids aspartic acid and phenylalanine. Its relative sweetness is 200 times greater than that of sucrose. Its sweetness is decreased by heat and acid. Approved for use in about 30 countries, including the United States. Contraindicated in persons with phenylketonuria (PKU). Sold under the brand names Nutrasweet and Equal.

Aspartic acid. Aminosuccinic acid; a nonessential glucogenic amino acid involved in transamination reactions and the formation of urea, purines, and pyrimidines. It is hydrolyzed by the enzyme *aspartase* to fumaric acid and ammonia.

Aspirin. Acetylsalicylic acid; an analgesic, antipyretic, and anti-inflammatory drug. It may cause iron-deficiency anemia due to gastrointestinal blood loss, decreased absorption of glucose and amino acids, and depletion of folate, vitamin C, vitamin K, thiamin, and potassium. Supplementation with these nutrients may be necessary when aspirin is taken in large doses or for long-term use. Brand names include Bayer, Ecotrin, and Empirin; aspirin with buffers includes Ascriptin and Bufferin; and combination drugs with aspirin include Anacin, Excedrin, Midol, Percodan, Talwin, and Vanquish.

Association of Official Agricultural Chemists (AOAC). Voluntary organization of chemists that sponsors the development and testing of methods for analyzing nutrients, foods, food additives, animal feeds, liquors, beverages, drugs, cosmetics, pesticides, and many other commodities.

Atabrine. Antimalarial drug; a riboflavin antagonist.

Ataxia. Inability to coordinate bodily or muscular movements. It is generally due to a disorder in the brain or spinal cord, or it may be due to nutritional deficiencies, especially of the B complex vitamins.

Atenolol. A beta-adrenergic agent used in the management of hypertension or chronic angina pectoris in patients with chronic obstructive pulmonary disease (COPD) and insulin-dependent diabetes mellitus (or type I). Drug uptake is enhanced by ingestion of food; a decrease in dosage is needed if the patient is hypoalbuminemic to avoid central nervous system side effects; the drug may also increase serum triglycerides. Brand names are Tenormin and Tenorectic.

Atherosclerosis. Term denoting a number of different processes resulting in atheroma or patchy deposits of various materials in the intima of the arteries. These deposits are produced by an accumulation of fatty substances (cholesterol, phospholipids, and triglycerides), complex carbohydrates, lipoproteins, calcium and calcified plaques, fibrin, and the formed elements of the blood. Areas of thickening in the intima of affected arteries look like patchy tiny lumps, and lead to narrowing of the lumen and diminution of blood-carrying capacity. Atherosclerosis is the result of an interplay of several factors, including elevated blood lipids, high blood pressure, cigarette smoking, sedentary living, obesity, psychologic tension, and endocrine disorders. Foods influence many of these risk factors. A diet high in saturated fat and cholesterol increases blood cholesterol and lipid levels; habitual overeating coupled with inactivity leads to obesity. Thus the recommended dietary modification for the general public in the prevention of atherosclerotic diseases include adjustment of caloric intake to achieve and maintain healthy weight, reduction of dietary cholesterol intake to about 200 mg/day or less, and control of saturated fat intake to less than 10% of total calories, with calories from fat accounting for no more than 30% of total caloric intake. See *Diet, cholesterol-restricted, fat-controlled;* see also *Hyperlipoproteinemia.*

ATP. Abbreviation for adenosine triphosphate. See under *Adenosine phosphates.*

Atresia. An abnormal condition due to the absence of a body opening or duct, such as the anus, bile duct, external ear canal, etc. In *biliary atresia,* there is total degeneration or incomplete development of one or more bile duct components due to stagnated fetal growth. Clinical signs are jaundice, swollen abdomen, and dark-colored urine. *Dietary management:* use a low-fat diet that is high in medium-chain triglycerides. Maintain normal protein intake with added vitamins A, D, and K. If edema exists, restrict sodium intake.

Attain. Brand name of an isotonic, lactose-free, low-residue liquid formula for oral or tube feeding; made of calcium and sodium caseinates, maltodextrin, and corn oil. Also available in a low-sodium form (Attain L.S.) with only 200 mg or 9 mEq of sodium per liter. See Appendix 39.

Atwater respiration calorimeter. Apparatus for measuring the total energy expenditure of the body by confining the subject inside the chamber. The original Atwater apparatus was later modified by Rosa and Benedict. See *Direct calorimetry* and *Calorimetry.*

Atwater values. Average physiologic fuel values of carbohydrate, protein, and fat based on experiments conducted by Atwater. He found that on a typical American diet, each gram of carbohydrate, fat, and protein yields 4, 9, and 4 calories, respectively. The Atwater values are used extensively in dietary calculations and food analysis. See also *Food, energy value.*

Avidin. A glycoprotein in raw egg white which binds firmly with the vitamin *biotin* and prevents its absorption from the digestive tract. Excessive intake of raw egg whites can result in a biotin deficiency syndrome known as *egg white injury,* which is characterized by loss of hair, scaly dermatitis, and cirrhosis of the liver. Avidin is inactivated by heat and other agents that denature proteins.

Avitaminosis. Literally, it means "without vitamin," but the term is more commonly used in reference to a vitamin lack or deficiency which is more appropriately called hypovitaminosis. The condition may be due to inadequate intake, deficient absorption, increased body requirement or excretion, or ingestion of vitamin antagonists.

Azathioprine. A purine antagonist metabolite used mainly for its immune suppressive activity and as an adjunct for prevention of the rejection of kidney allografts. It is a folacin antagonist and inhibits RNA and DNA synthesis. Large doses may cause macrocytic anemia, anorexia, oral lesions, steatorrhea, diarrhea, nausea, and vomiting. The brand name is Imuran.

Azidothymidine (AZT). An antiviral agent; may cause anorexia, nausea, vomiting, and megaloblastic anemia. The brand name is Retrovir. Used for treating AIDS.

Azotemia. Also called *uremia.* Retention of urea and other nitrogenous substances in the blood. It is a manifestation of kidney disease.

B

B. Chemical symbol for boron.

Baby bottle tooth decay (BBTD). Dental caries of the maxillary incisors and molars rampant among infants and toddlers under two years old. The main causes are prolonged, inappropriate bottle feeding beyond the normal time babies are weaned from the milk bottle and putting the baby to sleep with a bottle. Nutrition education of parents is crucial in preventing this disorder.

Balance study. Quantitative method of measuring the amount of a nutrient ingested and the amount of the same nutrient or its metabolic end product(s) excreted in order to determine whether there has been a gain (positive balance) or loss (negative balance) in the body. At equilibrium, nutrient intake equals output. Balance studies are generally classified into two types: balance of matter (those dealing with nutrients that can be weighed) and balance of energy (those dealing with heat and energy). See *Energy balance, Nitrogen balance,* and *Water balance.*

Bariatrics. The study of *weight control.* See *Nutrition, weight control.*

Baryophobia. An eating disorder resulting in the reduced growth rate of a child caused by underfeeding because the parents are afraid he or she may develop obesity and/or cardiovascular diseases later in life. Nutrition education of the parents is needed immediately.

Basal energy expenditure (BEE). Also called *resting energy expenditure (REE).* Some clinicians or researchers still use BEE as originally used by Harris and Benedict, who devised the formula. For details, see *Harris-Benedict formula* for estimating BEE.

Basal metabolic rate (BMR). The current term used is resting metabolic rate (RMR) and refers to the amount of energy expended per unit of time under basal conditions. The adult basal metabolic rate is approximately 1 kcal/kg body weight per hour. The rate is affected by the size, shape, and weight of the individual, body composition (amount of active protoplasmic tissue), age (highest during infancy, with a gradual decline with advancing age), activity of the endocrine glands, state of nutrition, rate of growth, and pregnancy. Clinically, the BMR is reported as a percentage above or below normal. See also *Resting energy expenditure (REE).*

Basal metabolism. Energy expended in the maintenance of "basal metabolic" processes, or involuntary activities in the body (respiration, circulation, gastrointestinal contractions, and maintenance of muscle tonus and body temperature) and the functional activities of various organs (kidneys, liver, endocrine glands, etc.). It is taken under "basal" conditions, i.e., at complete physical and mental rest, in the postabsorptive state (12 to 16 hours after taking food), and at a temperature within the zone of thermal neutrality (20° to 25°C). Measurement is performed when the person is awake but lying down and relaxed in a quiet atmosphere.

Basal metabolism determination. The amount of heat produced by the body may be measured in two ways: directly, by measuring the amount of heat given off with the use of an apparatus called a *calorimeter,* or indirectly, by measuring the amount of oxygen consumed over a given period of time with the use of a *respirometer.* Basal metabolism may also be determined by using various prediction formulas developed by Boothby, DuBois, Berkson, and Dunn (based on *body surface area*); by Harris and Benedict (based on body weight and standing height); and by Kleiber (based on *metabolic body size*). Another indirect clinical method is to analyze T₃ and T₄ blood levels.

Base. Same as alkali. See *Alkali.*

Basic food groups. Classes of foods listed together under one heading because of their similarities as good sources of certain nutrients. The number of groupings and the foods in the groups may vary in different nations, depending on the food habits, food economics, and dietary needs of a country. The basic food groups are used in planning and evaluating diets for nutritional adequacy. See Appendices 5 and 6.

Basic-forming foods. See *Alkaline-forming foods.*

BEE. Abbreviation for *basal energy expenditure.*

Benedict-Roth spirometer. Closed-circuit apparatus for measuring oxygen consumption over a period of time to determine basal metabolism. The energy equivalent is calculated by multiplying the volume of oxygen consumed by 4.825, the caloric equivalent of 1 liter of oxygen. See also *Indirect calorimetry* under *Calorimetry.*

Benztropine. An antiparkinsonian agent; has an anticholinergic effect and may cause constipation and dry mouth. The brand name is Cogentin.

Beriberi. Nutritional deficiency disease due to lack of thiamin, or vitamin B₁. It is characterized by loss of appetite and general malaise associated with heaviness and weakness of the legs, which may be followed by cramping of the calf muscles and burning and numbness of the feet. There may also be some edema of the legs, heart palpitations, and precordial pains. There are three forms of beriberi: dry beriberi, a form in which polyneuropathy and progressive paralysis are the essential features; wet beriberi, a form characterized by pitting edema, enlarged heart, rapid pulse, and circulatory failure (beriberi heart disease); and infantile beriberi, seen in infants breast-fed by mothers suffering from beriberi. The onset is often acute and is characterized by pallor, facial edema, irritability, and abdominal pain. The infant may suddenly become cyanotic, with dyspnea and tachycardia, and die within a few hours. Recovery with thiamin therapy is dramatic. A daily thiamin dose of 50 to 200 mg/day is the usual range, although some clinicians give multiple-vitamin preparations. See *Thiamin.*

Beta-carotene. A precursor of vitamin A; yields two molecules of vitamin A per molecule. See *carotene.*

Bezoar. Hard ball of vegetable or hair fiber that may develop in the intestines or stomach. Common foods leading to bezoar formation are apples, berries, coconuts, figs, oranges, persimmons, brussels sprouts, green beans, potato peels, and sauerkraut.

Bicarbonate. Salt of carbonic acid, characterized by the radical $-HCO_3$. Blood bicarbonate is the chief *alkali reserve* of the body. It plays a key role in the maintenance of a constant hydrogen ion concentration in body fluids.

Bifidus factor. Collective term for growth factors needed by *Lactobacillus bifidus* var. *pennsylvanicus,* found in human milk and growing in the intestines of breast-fed infants. It is believed to be beneficial to young infants in preventing the growth of less desirable bacteria that cause intestinal putrefaction. See *Breast feeding.*

Bile. Fluid produced and secreted by the liver, stored and concentrated in the gallbladder, and poured into the duodenum at intervals, particularly during fat digestion. It aids in the emulsification and absorption of fat, activates the pancreatic lipase, and prevents putrefaction. Among its constituents are *bile acids, bile salts, bile pigments, cholesterol,* and *lecithin.*

Bile acids. Glycocholic and taurocholic acids formed by the conjugation of glycine or taurine with cholic acid.

Bile pigments. Principally *bilirubin* and *biliverdin,* which are responsible for the color of bile.

Bile salts. Chiefly sodium glycocholate and sodium taurocholate, which are the sodium salts of bile acids.

Biliary. Pertaining to bile or the gallbladder. Some of the biliary disorders are biliary atresia, gallstones or cholelithiasis, cholecystitis, biliary cancer, and obstruction.

Bilirubin. Principal orange pigment of bile formed by the reduction of biliverdin, a product of hemoglobin breakdown. It is normally present in the feces and sometimes in the urine. Its accumulation in the blood results in jaundice. See *Jaundice.*

Bilirubinuria. Presence of bilirubin in the urine. The urine is unusually dark, and the condition accompanies *jaundice.*

Biliverdin. The green pigment of hemoglobin that undergoes reduction to bilirubin in the liver; one of the *bile pigments.*

Bioassay. Also called biologic assay; measurement of the activity of a drug, substance, or nutrient by noting its effect on test animals or microorganisms.

Bioavailability. Descriptive term for the extent of digestion and absorption of a nutrient; therefore the amount actually available for cell utilization.

Biocatalyst. Biochemical catalyst or *enzyme.*

Biocytin. Biotinyl lysine; a naturally occurring complex of biotin and lysine. It is resistant to hydrolysis by proteolytic enzymes in the intestinal tract, as is the complex of biotin and avidin. An enzyme in the plasma and erythrocytes, called biocytinase, catalyzes the hydrolysis of biocytin to yield free biotin.

Bioelectrical impedance. Total body fat measurement using low-energy electric current. Higher impedance to the current indicates more fat tissues stored because fat has resistance to electric flow.

Bioflavonoids. Group of naturally occurring substances belonging to the flavin and flavonoid groups of compounds; originally designated as vitamin P (permeability vitamin) or vitamin C_2 (synergist of vitamin C). Some of the flavonoids exhibit biologic activities, including reduction of capillary fragility and protection of biologically important compounds through antioxidant activity, but none has been shown to be essential for humans or to cause deficiency syndromes. Hence bioflavonoids are now considered to be pharmacologic rather than nutritional agents.

Biologic oxidation. Also called physiologic oxidation; the cellular reactions liberating energy by the transfer of electrons via the *redox systems.*

Biologic value (BV). Relative nutritional value of individual proteins compared to that of a standard protein. It is the amount of protein digested and absorbed from food, i.e., utilized by the body and not excreted in the urine. BV is therefore a measure of how efficiently food proteins are retained to become part of body tissues. BV is calculated as follows:

$$BV = \frac{N \text{ retained}}{N \text{ absorbed}} = \frac{\text{dietary } N - (UN + FN)}{\text{dietary } N - FN}$$

where

N = nitrogen
FN = fecal nitrogen
UN = urinary nitrogen

Biotin. Sulfur-containing, water-soluble vitamin; one of the B complex vitamins. Biotin is an integral part of enzymes that transport carboxyl units and fix carbon dioxide in animal tissues. Biotin enzymes are involved in gluconeogenesis, fatty acid synthesis, and catabolism of branched-chain amino acids. Biotin is widely distributed in low concentration in both animal and plant foods; the best sources are liver, egg yolk, whole-grain cereals, soy flour, and yeast. It is synthesized in the lower gastrointestinal tract by microorganisms; hence, treatment with large doses of antibiotics, notably streptomycin, can decrease biotin levels. Dietary biotin deficiency is rare in humans, with the exception of seborrheic dermatitis seen in infants under 6 months of age and during hemodialysis and long-term total parenteral nutrition without added biotin and following extensive bowel resection. Deficiency has also been reported after long-term anticonvulsant therapy. Ingestion of large amounts of raw egg white can induce biotin deficiency, producing a syndrome characterized by scaly dermatitis, muscle pains, alopecia, glossitis, mental depression, and general malaise. There is one rare disorder with biotin dependency in which an abnormality in the carboxylation of propionic acid leads to a ketotic hyperglycemia. There are no reports of biotin toxicity with excessive intake.

Biotinidase. An enzyme that releases protein-bound biotin and cleaves *biocytin* so that biotin can be recycled. Infants with biotinidase deficiency show features of biotin deficiency, including vomiting, hypotonia, metabolic acidosis, and neurologic changes; the condition responds to treatment with oral D-biotin.

Bisacodyl. A stimulant laxative. Abuse of this drug can cause fluid and electrolyte loss (especially potassium) and malabsorption with weight loss. Undesirable side effects are abdominal cramps, nausea, and belching. Oral bisacodyl should not be taken with milk since milk dissolves the enteric coating, causing gastric irritation. Brand names are Bisco-Lax, Codylax, Dulcolax, Rectolax, and Theralax.

Bitot's spots. Small, triangular, grayish or glistening white plaques, sometimes with a foamy surface, on the conjunctiva. The spots are generally bilateral on the temporal sides of the cornea and are associated with vitamin A deficiency. Bitot's spots may be treated with therapeutic vitamin A (about 20,000 to 50,000 IU/day).

Bleomycin. An antineoplastic antibiotic active against gram-positive and gram-negative bacteria and fungi; used in the treatment of lymphomas and squamous cell carcinomas. Its side effects include nausea, vomiting, oral lesions, anorexia, and weight loss which may persist after therapy is stopped. The brand name is Blenoxane.

Blood. Fluid medium that carries oxygen and nutritive materials to the tissues, removes carbon dioxide and waste products for elimination by the excretory organs, and distributes other substances (such as clotting factors, regulatory agents, and body defense mechanisms) throughout the body for utilization or action. It consists of *formed elements* (erythrocytes, or red blood cells; leukocytes, or white blood cells; and thrombocytes, or blood platelets) and a pale yellow portion, *plasma,* which contains a large number of organic and inor-

ganic substances in solution. A normal adult has a total blood volume of about 8% of body weight. For normal constituents of the blood, see Appendix 30.

Blood clotting. Process of changing liquid blood to a soft gel. Prothrombin is converted to thrombin with the help of vitamin K, calcium, and other tissue factors. Thrombin, in turn, catalyzes the conversion of fibrinogen to a network of insoluble fibrin; the latter immobilizes all the formed elements, resulting in the blood clot.

Blood glucose (BG). See *Blood sugar level.*

Blood lipids. Principally cholesterol, phospholipid, and triglyceride. These lipids circulate in the plasma bound to proteins. As lipoprotein complexes, the otherwise insoluble lipids are solubilized, thus enabling their transport into and out of the plasma. Five major types of lipoproteins in the blood have been identified. Each type contains phospholipid, triglyceride, cholesterol, and protein in varying proportions. For details, see *Lipoprotein.* See also *Hyperlipoproteinemia.*

Blood platelet. Also called thrombocyte; one of the three formed elements of the blood that is necessary in the clotting of blood. Blood platelets liberate small amounts of thromboplastin, which activates the proenzyme prothrombin to its active form, thrombin, the enzyme that catalyzes clot formation. See *Blood clotting.*

Blood pressure (BP). The force that blood exerts against the walls of the blood vessels during each heartbeat. As measured by a sphygmomanometer, it is the pressure of the blood on the walls of the arteries of the upper arm. The human heart pumps intermittently by means of a sudden contraction of the entire ventricular musculature, followed by a period of relaxation. The pressure during the contraction phase is called systolic pressure and the pressure during the resting phase is called diastolic pressure. In recording blood pressure, the systolic pressure is written first, followed by the diastolic pressure. A normal blood pressure reading is 120/80 mm Hg (systolic over diastolic blood pressure). Blood pressure is maintained by homeostatic mechanisms in the body, mainly by the renin-angiotensin-aldosterone system, the kinin-prostaglandin system, and the neuroendocrine adrenergic system. It is affected by blood volume, the lumen of the arteries and arterioles, the force of heart pumping, and any illness or disorder that alters these factors. See also *Hypertension.*

Blood sugar level (BSL). The normal level of sugar (glucose) per 100 ml of blood is about 70 to 100 mg by the Somogyi method or 80 to 120 mg by the Folin-Wu method. A range of normal values for blood sugar is usually given (expressed as milligrams per deciliter) with slight variations, depending on the method of analysis used. Among several factors that *maintain* the blood sugar level are glycogen-glucose interconversion in the liver, conversion of carbohydrate to fat, formation of muscle glycogen and its utilization, and glucose excretion in the urine (renal threshold). Conditions that *increase* the blood sugar level include diabetes mellitus, hyperfunction of the anterior pituitary gland, hyperfunction of the adrenal cortex, insufficient insulin production, hyperfunction of the thyroid gland, head injury, multiple trauma, sepsis, and hypermetabolic states. Conditions that *decrease* the blood sugar level include hyperinsulinism, anterior pituitary deficiency, adrenal insufficiency, hypothyroidism, prolonged undernutrition, tumor of the pancreas, and abnormal kidney function (renal glycosuria). Clinically, the plasma sugar level would be expected to increase moderately (in individuals without a history of diabetes) following general surgery or multiple trauma (BS of 150 ± 25 mg/dl). Sepsis and hypermetabolic states are characterized by markedly elevated plasma glucose (about 250 ± 50 mg/dl). Fasting plasma glucose is normally 80 to 115 mg/dl for adults and is slightly lower during pregnancy (60 to 90 mg/dl). Postprandial levels are 90 to 150 mg/dl 1 hour after meals and 80 to 140 mg/dl 2 hours after meals. See also *Diabetes, Glucose tolerance test, Hyperglycemia,* and *Hypoglycemia.*

Blood urea nitrogen (BUN). The amount of nitrogenous substance present in the blood as urea; measured to indicate kidney function. It is increased in kidney failure, diabetes mellitus, shock, and gastrointestinal bleeding and with some medications. It is decreased during pregnancy, malnutrition, and liver disease. The normal value of BUN is 10 to 20 mg/dl. See Appendix 30.

BMI. Abbreviation for *body mass index.*

BMR. Abbreviation for *basal metabolic rate.*

Body composition. The representative percentage composition of a human adult is about 16% protein, 15 to 20% fat, 0.5% carbohydrate, 4.5% ash, and 60% water. These body components are distributed through four separate compartments: lean body mass, extracellular fluid, mineral of the skeleton, and adipose tissue. Body composition varies with age, sex, and nutriture. Females generally have a higher fat content than males; infants and young children have a relatively higher water content than adults, which decreases as they grow older. The degree of leanness and fatness (e.g., mild, moderate, and morbid obesity) varies widely among individuals. Also, pathologic conditions alter body composition, as in osteopenia, marasmus, edema, and cancer.

Body composition determination. The living body can be partitioned into essentially two compartments: the fat-free portion and the fat portion, or adipose tissue. The fat-free weight of an individual remains relatively constant; variability in total weight is attributed to varying degrees of fatness. Measurements of body composition include *physical methods:* underwater weighing for body density, whole body counter, total body electric conductivity (TOBEC), computed tomography, magnetic resonance imaging, and bioelectrical impedance. *Anthropometric methods* of measuring body composition are more economical and speedier. These include skinfold thickness, midarm muscle circumference, height and weight measurements, ponderal index, and body mass index.

Body mass index (BMI). Or the Quetelet index. Ratio of weight (in kilograms) over height squared (in meters). For adults, normal BMI values are between 19-25 for ages 19-34, and 21-27 for ages 35 and over. BMI values of 30-40 indicate moderate obesity. BMI values above 40 indicate gross or morbid obesity. BMI values below 18 are life-threatening.

Body surface area (BSA). Area covered by the exterior of the body. The surface area of the body was first determined by wrapping the body with a gauze tape, removing the tape, and measuring the area covered. BSA is estimated by plotting a person's height and weight on a standard chart originally developed by DuBois. An improvement was made by Boothby and Sandiford, who devised a monogram for determining BSA.

Bolus. Mass of food ready to be swallowed.

Bomb calorimeter. Apparatus that measures directly the energy value of foods. It consists of an inner chamber that holds the food sample and a double-walled, insulated jacket that holds a can containing water. An electric connection ignites the weighed sample of food. A differential thermometer records the rise in the temperature of the water surrounding the chamber.

Bone. Also called osseous tissue; a mineralized connective tissue consisting of an organic matrix in which inorganic elements (mineral salts) are precipitated in a crystal lattice structure similar to that of the naturally occurring mineral *hydroxyapatite.* The organic matrix consists largely of *collagen* in a gel of cementing substance. The mineral fraction is composed largely of calcium phosphate, carbonate, fluoride, and citrate. Specialized bone cells (osteoblasts, osteoclasts, and osteocytes) control the relationship between the organic matrix and the bone salts. See also *Nutrition, bone* and *Peak bone mass.*

Bone fracture. A break in the continuity of the bone tissue. May be simple, compounded, or comminuted, depending on what bone is involved and the nature of the injury. *Dietary management:* the location of the fracture and the surrounding tissues affected will determine how the diet is modified. Generally, provide an adequate diet supplemented with vitamins and minerals for bone repair. A liberal protein intake will promote healing; give foods as tolerated.

Boron (B). A mineral found in most tissues, especially the brain, liver, and body fat. It is generally accepted as essential for plants. There is also accumulating evidence that boron may be an essential nutrient for animals and humans. Boron complexes with many biologic substances, including sugars and polysaccharides, pyridoxine, riboflavin, dehydroascorbic acid, and adenosine-5-phosphate. Boron may influence parathormone action; metabolism of calcium, phosphorus, and magnesium; and the formation of the active form of cholecalciferol. Boron seems to be beneficial in the prevention of calcium loss and bone demineralization in nutritional disorders characterized by secondary hyperparathyroidism and osteoporosis. The daily intake of boron by humans varies widely. Foods of plant origin, especially fruits, vegetables, and nuts, are rich sources; wine, cider, and beer are also high in boron. Meat and fish are poor sources. Studies on the signs of boron deficiency are not complete; the most consistent manifestation is depressed growth. Boron is toxic in large amounts; signs of toxicity include nausea, vomiting, diarrhea, dermatitis, and lethargy. High boron intake also induces riboflavinuria. Boric acid was formerly used as a food preservative but has been declared unsafe as a food additive by a Food and Agriculture Organization/World Health Organization Expert Committee.

Bowel resection. Complete or partial removal of a section of the intestines. The absorption of nutrients occurs throughout the small bowel, so that there is little disturbance of bowel function when a short length of the bowel is resected. If intestine is resected in lengths that compromise absorption, adaptation of the remaining bowel increases function and restores the ability to absorb normally. However, when over 50% of the bowel has been resected, impairment of absorption tends to be permanent and more pronounced. Ileal resection of less than 100 cm, with the colon intact, usually causes steatorrhea. The degree of malabsorption increases with increasing length of resection. The absorption of fat and carbohydrate can be reduced by 50 to

75% of the intake; nitrogen absorption is reduced to a lesser extent. A vitamin B$_{12}$ study should be done and, if abnormal, monthly intravenous administration of 100 μg of the vitamin should be given to prevent pernicious anemia. *Dietary management:* depends upon the extent of bowel resected. A normal oral diet should be tried if more than 60 to 80 cm of the bowel still remains. Start by giving small feedings of dry solids, with isotonic fluids 1 hour after the meal. The separation of solids from liquids is important because of the increased speed of gastric emptying, resulting in diarrhea. Electrolyte replacement may be required parenterally in order to meet requirements even when oral intake is sufficient. Depending on the patient's tolerance and on the degree of diarrhea, gradually increase the volume of feeding to reach the goal of 1.5 to 2 times the basal energy expenditure for calories and 1.2 to 1.3 gm protein/kg body weight. Total parenteral nutrition may be necessary in resections leaving less than 60 cm of the small bowel and those leaving only the duodenum intact.

Brain injury. Common feeding difficulties encountered in injury of the brain are reduced and ineffective sucking; tongue dysfunction, which affects chewing and swallowing; and a hyperactive or hypoactive gag reflex. A hyperactive gag reflex may lead to vomiting during feeding, and a hypoactive gag reflex may lead to choking. Often a patient may be able to swallow solid foods but will aspirate liquids. *Dietary management:* careful assessment of the patient's chewing and swallowing ability, using a team approach; modification of food consistency; and small, frequent feeding of meals consisting of foods with contrasting colors and flavors to encourage consumption.

BranchAmin. Brand name of a 4% solution of branched-chain amino acids (isoleucine, leucine, and valine) for intravenous administration; does not contain electrolytes and is not intended to be used alone, but rather as an admixture with other amino acid solutions. See Appendix 40.

Breast feeding. Recommended infant feeding for full-term babies due to the benefits of mother-infant bonding and advantages in the composition and bioavailability of nutrients in human milk over other formulas. See *Infant feeding* and *Nutrition, infancy.*

Bronchitis. Acute or chronic inflammation of the membrane lining the bronchial tubes. Acute bronchitis may be due to an extension of infection from the upper respiratory tract. Chronic bronchitis may be caused by irritants in polluted air, particularly smoke or gas fumes. *Dietary management:* provide adequate to liberal calorie and protein intakes to help reduce infection. Avoid milk if it tends to produce mucus. Give small feedings and allow frequent rest periods while eating when there is difficulty in breathing. See also *Chronic obstructive pulmonary disease.*

BSA. Abbreviation for *body surface area.*

BSL. Abbreviation for *blood sugar level.*

Buffer. Agent that resists marked changes in hydrogen ion concentration with the addition of acids or bases. In general, buffer action is exhibited by ions of weak acids or weak bases and their salts, by proteins, and by amino acids. Buffers play a vital role in the regulation of acid-base balance in the body. The principal buffer systems in the blood are the plasma proteins, carbonic acid, sodium bicarbonate, mono- and disodium phosphate, mono- and dipotassium phosphate, oxyhemoglobin, and reduced hemoglobin.

Bulimarexia. An eating disorder in which the individual switches between *anorexia nervosa* and *bulimia.*

Bulimia. An eating disorder also called the "binge-purge syndrome." The person has an insatiable appetite but is afraid to gain weight; binge eating is followed by purging caused by induced vomiting, diuretics, or laxatives. A typical bulimic pattern of eating involves several secretive binges a day for a few days when the individual consumes several thousand kilocalories in an hour or two. The binging ends when abdominal discomfort or sleepiness occurs, and purging is used. Induced vomiting causes complications, such as erosion and decay of teeth, esophagitis, metabolic alkalosis, dehydration, hypokalemia, and other electrolyte imbalances. Protein-energy malnutrition (PEM) in some cases becomes a serious problem that needs immediate nutritional support and hospitalization. *Dietary management:* correct PEM and fluid and electrolyte imbalances. Use foods of high nutrient density given in small, frequent feedings. A team approach is needed to bring about changes in attitudes toward food and coping with stress. See also *Eating disorder.*

Bulk. The indigestible portion of carbohydrates that is not hydrolyzed by enzymes of the human gastrointestinal tract. See also *Crude fiber* and *fiber.*

Bulking agent. A metabolically inert substance, such as nonfibrous cellulose, added to food to increase its volume without any calorie contribution.

Bumetanide. A sulfonamide loop diuretic used for the management of edema associated with congestive heart failure or hepatic or renal disease. It is a potent diuretic and can produce profound diuresis with loss of sodium, potassium, magnesium, and calcium; it may also cause nausea, vomiting, and anorexia. The brand name is Bumex.

BUN. Abbreviation for *blood urea nitrogen.* See *Urea* and Appendix 30.

Burn. Tissue injury or destruction caused by excessive heat, caustics (acids or alkalis), friction, electricity, or radiation. On the basis of the extent of injury, burns are divided into three degrees: *first-degree,* with simple redness of the affected parts; *second-degree,* with the appearance of blisters in addition to redness; and *third-degree,* with actual destruction of the skin and underlying tissues. *Dietary management:* a person with severe burns is in a hypercatabolic state, with an extensive nitrogen deficit, fluid and electrolyte imbalances, and rapid weight loss, unless given nutritional support immediately. The goals of the diet are to prevent protein-calorie malnutrition, restore electrolyte and water balances to avoid shock, promote wound healing, and correct stress hyperglycemia. The basal metabolic rate (BMR) of a burned patient is often twice his or her normal BMR. The protein requirement is usually three times his or her normal recommended dietary allowance (RDA). The caloric supply should be at least 50 kcal/kg body weight per day. Consider selecting commercial preparations of special formulas to meet the patient's increased nutrient needs. Carefully calculate and monitor the daily diet intake. Burns, unlike other disorders, result in a highly accelerated rate of hypercatabolism. Most body stores are used up; therefore, immediately correct massive losses in fluids, protein, nitrogen, vitamins, and minerals in order to hasten the processes of healing and restoration. For details in calculating nutrient needs, see Appendix 24.

Burning feet syndrome. Set of symptoms consisting of listlessness, fatigue, postural hypotension, rapid heart rate on exertion, and numbness and tingling of the hands and feet. As the condition becomes worse, the throbbing sensation intensifies, with sharp burning and stabbing pains. It is due to a deficiency of *pantothenic acid,* a water-soluble vitamin, and has been induced by administering methylpantothenic acid as an antagonist and by feeding a semisynthetic diet virtually free of pantothenic acid. Burning feet syndrome has been reported by prisoners of World War II and by chronic alcoholics whose diets were deficient in protein and the B complex vitamins.

Busulfan. An alkylating agent used in the treatment of leukemia and other forms of cancer. It interferes with DNA replication or RNA transcription and ultimately results in the disruption of nucleic acid formation. Busulfan may cause nausea, vomiting, diarrhea, cheilosis, glossitis, anemia, and weight loss. The brand name is Myleran.

Butyric acid. Short-chain saturated fatty acid containing 4 carbons. It is present as triglyceride in butterfat and milk; other fats contain very small amounts of butyric acid.

BV. Abbreviation for *biologic value.*

C

Ca. Chemical symbol for calcium.

Cachexia. Weakness, extreme weight loss, and severe wasting of tissues due to long-standing chronic diseases, malnutrition, or terminal illnesses. It is often associated with cancer, tuberculosis, and AIDS. See also *Cardiac cachexia.*

Cadmium (Cd). A trace element found in the body in minute amounts, mainly in the kidneys and liver. The essentiality of cadmium in humans remains to be established. Nutritional requirements, if they exist, are very low and easily met by the levels in food and drink. Laboratory animals fed diets low in cadmium have impaired reproductive performance and depressed growth. Cadmium is widely distributed in nature. Oysters, seafoods, and grains are rich sources; appreciable amounts may also be obtained from the air and the water supply. Daily intakes by human adults have been estimated to be 25 to 60 mg/day. About 5% of dietary cadmium is absorbed. In the body, it accumulates mainly in the kidney and liver, and to a lesser extent in bones and teeth. The half-life of cadmium is 15 to 30 years; hence, its level increases with age. Cadmium poisoning is an industrial hazard. Chronic intoxication leads to growth retardation, impaired reproduction, hypertension, and renal dysfunction.

Caffeine. Trimethyl xanthine or methyltheobromine; an alkaloidal purine found in coffee, tea, and cola drinks. It is a cardiac and renal stimulant producing varying pharmacologic effects in humans. To some, caffeine is effective in counteracting drowsiness and mental fatigue; others experience some gastrointestinal distress, increased gastric secretion, insomnia, restlessness, and diuresis. At a rate of 1 gm/day, it may cause cardiac palpitations, tremors, and anorexia.

If it is over 5 gm/day, it can lead to convulsions, coma, respiratory failure, and heart failure. It is contraindicated in certain heart diseases, in peptic ulcer patients who find caffeine irritating, in persons who are undergoing therapy for chemical dependency, and in mothers who are breast-feeding. Caffeine is absorbed by a healthy adult almost completely (99%), and it may take about 5 hours to eliminate half of this amount through the urine. For the caffeine content of selected foods and beverages, see Appendix 35.

Cal. Abbreviation for *Calorie*. If the letter *c* is not capitalized, it refers to a small calorie; if capitalized, it means a large calorie or kilocalorie (kcal).

Calcidiol. 25-Hydroxyvitamin D_3. Also known as 25-hydroxycholecalciferol; previously called calcifediol. A metabolite of vitamin D formed in the liver and further hydroxylated in the kidney to yield 1,25-dihydroxyvitamin D. It is the major circulating form of vitamin D and is the form measured in assessing the vitamin D status of patients.

Calcifediol. Former name for 25-hydroxyvitamin D_3; now called *calcidiol*. Commercially available calcifediol is synthesized for use in the management of hypocalcemia in patients with chronic renal failure undergoing dialysis. The brand name is Calderol.

Calciferol. Former name given to vitamin D_2 or ergocalciferol. Synthetic preparations are used for prophylaxis and treatment of vitamin D deficiency, rickets, and hypocalcemic tetany. Brand names are Calciferol, Deltalin, and Drisdol.

Calcification. Deposition of calcium salts within the tissues of the body. It is a normal process in bone formation or may be abnormal, as in pathologic calcification of soft tissues, particularly arteries, kidneys, lungs, pancreas, and stomach. Deposition of calcium salts also occurs in areas of fatty degeneration and in dead or chronically inflamed tissues. Areas of necrosis, infarcts, scar tissues, and caseous tuberculous areas have calcium deposits. See also *Nutrition, bone.*

Calcinosis. A condition characterized by abnormal deposition of calcium salts in various tissues of the body, including the cartilage and tendon.

Calciol. Formerly called cholecalciferol; vitamin D_3 occurring in animal cells and formed in the skin on exposure of 7-dehydrocholesterol to ultraviolet light from the sun.

Calcitonin (CT). Hormone secreted by the thyroid gland that is concerned with the regulation of calcium ions in the blood. Its action is opposite that of *parathormone.* When the blood calcium level is high, calcitonin is secreted and "shuts off" the release of calcium from bones.

Calcitriol. 1,25-Dihydroxyvitamin D_3 (1,25 $(OH)_2D_3$), also known as "1,25-dihydroxycholecalciferol (1,25-DHCC)." It is the most active metabolite of vitamin D and is formed in the kidney from 25-hydroxycholecalciferol. In addition to ensuring adequate absorption of calcium, calcitriol plays a role in the regulation of plasma calcium by increasing bone resorption synergistically with parathyroid hormone and stimulating the reabsorption of calcium by the kidney.

Calcium (Ca). A major mineral constituent of the body that makes up 1.5 to 2% of body weight. Of this amount, 99% is present in bones and teeth; the remaining 1% is found in soft tissues and body fluids and serves a number of functions not related to bone structure. Calcium is important in blood coagulation, transmission of nerve impulses, contraction of muscle fibers, myocardial function, and activation of enzymes. Calcium deficiency results in *rickets* in children and *osteomalacia* in adults. Good food sources are milk, cheese, and other milk products (except butter) and some leafy green vegetables (such as broccoli, collards, and kale), lime-processed tortillas, and calcium-fortified foods. Intestinal absorption of calcium is influenced by several nutritional and physiologic factors. It is increased during periods of high physiologic requirement, and a higher percentage of calcium is absorbed at low intakes than at high intakes. Vitamin D, ascorbic acid, lactose, and an acid medium favor absorption. Absorption is impaired in the elderly and in the presence of phytate and oxalate, and certain fiber fractions bind calcium and interfere with absorption. Calcium supplementation much higher than the recommended dietary allowance is not advisable. A high calcium intake inhibits the intestinal absorption of iron, zinc, and other essential minerals. Ingestion of very large amounts may result in hypercalciuria, hypercalcemia, and urinary stone formation. See Appendix 1 for the recommended dietary allowances.

Calculus. Pl. calculi. An abnormal stony mass in the body, found principally in ducts, passages, hollow organs, and cysts. It is more commonly called a "stone," such as a kidney stone or a gallbladder stone. Seldom "pure," it is usually a mixture of several substances, such as uric acid, cystine, calcium oxalate, calcium carbonate, and calcium phosphate. Once the stone is formed, no diet is effective in bringing about its dissolution. However, for the predisposed individual, dietary management may help prevent or retard the growth or recurrence of the stones. The type of diet depends on the chief component of the stone. Restrict calcium and phosphorus intake with calcium phosphate stones; maintain an acid urine with magnesium phosphate stones; restrict sulfur-containing amino acids and maintain an alkaline urine with cystine stones; restrict oxalate and calcium intakes with calcium oxalate stones; and maintain an alkaline urine to keep urate stones in solution. A high fluid intake is recommended in all types of stone formation. See *Diet, ash; Diet, calcium-phosphorus-restricted;* and *Diet, oxalate-restricted.*

Caliper. Instrument for measuring linear dimensions. Calipers may be fixed, adjustable, or movable. The three types that are often used in nutrition surveys are skin-fold, sliding, and spreading calipers.

Calorie (Cal). A unit of heat. The amount of heat required to raise the temperature of 1 kg of water 1°C. This is the large Calorie, or kilocalorie (spelled with a capital *C*), which is 1000 times as large as the small calorie (spelled with a small *c*). In nutrition, the kilocalorie (kcal) is used, and this is generally understood whether the word is written with a capital *C* or a small *c*. The small calorie is used in physics. See also *Joule.*

Calorie:nitrogen (C:N) ratio. A method of evaluating the adequacy of a tube feeding formula for protein based on the value of nitrogen × 6.25 = protein; 16% of a protein molecule is nitrogen. Thus,

$$C:N \text{ ratio} = \frac{kcal/day}{gm \ N/day}$$

where kcal/day is the total energy intake. Then

nonprotein kcal/gm N

$$= \frac{total \ kcal - kcal \ from \ protein}{gm \ N}$$

The desirable ratio to promote anabolism in severe stress is 100 to 150 kcal:1 gm N. The ratio is 150 to 200 kcal:1 gm N for moderate stress, and 250 to 300 kcal:1 gm N for normal tissue maintenance.

Calorie-protein malnutrition (CPM). Also called protein-energy malnutrition (PEM) or protein-calorie malnutrition (PCM) or energy-protein deficits (EPD). For further details, see *Protein-energy malnutrition.*

Calorimetry. Measurement of heat absorbed or given off by a system or body. The measurement is carried out in either of two ways: *direct* or *indirect* calorimetry. Direct calorimetry is carried out by measuring the heat produced by a subject or food enclosed in a chamber which has water outside the chamber walls. An example is the bomb calorimeter. Food is weighed and placed on a dish inside a container shaped like a bomb (hence the name), which is filled with oxygen. The container is then immersed in water. The amount of heat produced when food is burned which is absorbed by the surrounding water is then measured. Indirect calorimetry is calculated from the amount of oxygen consumed and the amount of carbon dioxide or nitrogen excreted. An example is the respiratory calorimeter, an apparatus that measures the exchange of gases between a living organism or subject and the atmosphere around it, with the simultaneous measurement of the amount of heat produced by that organism or subject.

Cancer. Common term for a malignant cellular growth that tends to spread due to the inability of the DNA to respond to normal physiologic stimuli. The abnormal (cancerous) cells reproduce without control, crowding out the healthy cells and using up nutrients needed by these cells. There are many kinds of cancer, designated by the organ or part of the body affected. The following account for about 88% of cases: oral and esophageal, lung, skin, prostate, urinary tract, leukemia and other blood cancers, breast and uterine, gastrointestinal tract (intestines, colon, rectum), liver, and pancreatic. The exact cause(s) of human cancer is not definitely established, although contributing or predisposing factors are known in many cases. These include genetics, environmental and occupational hazards, and personal habits like smoking, alcoholism, and dietary factors. *Dietary management:* the most common problems in patients with metastatic cancer which affect food intake are anorexia, nausea and vomiting, constipation, abdominal pain, mucositis, easy fatigability, and weight loss. Individualize caloric level to maintain healthy weight; some patients need a caloric intake at least twice their basal energy expenditure. Appetizing food is emphasized, especially if the patient is undergoing chemotherapy or radiation therapy. Depending on the organ(s) affected, dietary modifications should afford rest to the cells and give nutrients to the normal cells. For example, if the gastrointestinal tract is involved, precluding oral or enteral feeding, parenteral feeding is indicated. With progress to solid foods, a low-fiber diet is given initially, followed by a gradual introduction of fiber to promote motility. A mechanical soft diet consisting of smooth, semisolid foods is indicated in cancer of the esophagus. Tube feeding is often used when there is difficulty in swallowing or when feeding by mouth (per os feeding) is nutritionally inadequate. In breast cancer, restrict fat to 25% of the total caloric intake. Studies on dietary factors in relation to cancer prevention include the following: vitamins A, C, E, and selenium, which are antioxidants, protect the DNA from electron-seeking compounds so that it is not altered; dietary fibers are recommended, since they bind carcinogens in the feces; cruciferous vegetables like cabbage, cauliflower, and Brussels sprout contain indoles and phenols, which are believed to reduce cell division; nitrate-cured and smoked foods are to be eaten in moderation. More studies are needed to confirm the role of diet in cancer prevention. In general, the risk of cancer is lessened by following the dietary guidelines for healthy Americans given in Appendix 7. See also *Nutrition, cancer.*

Cancrum oris. An infective gangrene of the mouth that erodes the lips and cheeks, giving the appearance of harelip. This has been reported chiefly in South Africa and is presumably caused by a combination of malnutrition and infection. See *Synergism.*

CAPD. Abbreviation for *continuous ambulatory peritoneal dialysis.*

Capillary resistance test. Test to determine the tendency of blood capillaries to break down and produce petechial hemorrhages. This is done by applying enough pressure to obstruct venous blood return on an arm and noting the number of *petechiae* produced after 5 minutes. Capillary fragility is a clinical sign of vitamin C deficiency which is measured by this test.

Captopril. An angiotensin-converting enzyme inhibitor used in the treatment of severe hypertension and congestive heart failure. It acts by lowering the concentration in the blood of angiotensin II, which is one of the factors responsible for high blood pressure. Captopril has a persistent metallic or salty taste and may decrease taste acuity. It may also cause hyponatremia, hyperkalemia, hypoalbuminemia, proteinuria, anorexia, and weight loss. The brand name is Capoten.

Carbamazepine. An anticonvulsant drug structurally related to the tricyclic antidepressants; used for control of seizures and relief of pain associated with neuralgia. It may cause anorexia, glossitis, stomatitis, dry mouth, and gastric distress. The brand name is Tegretol.

Carbohydrate. Polyhydroxy aldehyde, ketone, or any substance that yields one of these compounds. The term was originally designated for compounds of hydrates of carbon having the general formula $C_x(H_2O)_y$. Now it includes other compounds having the properties of carbohydrate even though they do not have the required 2:1 ratio of hydrogen to oxygen. Some carbohydrates contain nitrogen and sulfur in addition to carbon, hydrogen, and oxygen. The most important carbohydrates in foods are the digestible sugars and starches and the indigestible cellulose and other dietary fibers. The digestible carbohydrate is the major source of energy, providing about 50% of the calories in the American diet. In the developing countries where protein foods are scarce and expensive, carbohydrate foods may be as much as 80% of the total caloric intake. The chief carbohydrates in the body are glucose ("physiologic sugar") and glycogen ("animal starch"). One gram of digestible carbohydrate yields 4 kcal. A recommended distribution of calories in the daily diet is to allow 50 to 60% of total calories from carbohydrate sources, emphasizing complex carbohydrates and reducing simple sugars. For a classification of carbohydrates and food sources, see Appendix 8.

Carbohydrate by difference. In the *proximate analysis* of food, this is the difference obtained by subtracting from 100 the sum of the percentages of water, protein, fat, and ash content. Included in this value, in addition to the sugars and starches, which the body can utilize almost completely, are the *crude fiber* and some organic acids that the body cannot utilize.

Carbohydrate functions. Carbohydrate is the primary source of heat and energy (1 gm yields 4 kcal). Next to water, carbohydrate is the single largest nutrient in the diet. The sugars are valued for their sweetening power. Carbohydrate has a protein-sparing effect and serves as a carbon skeleton for the synthesis of nonessential amino acids. Glucose is the major energy source of the brain and nervous tissues. As the "physiologic sugar," glucose is the immediate source of energy for all body cells and is stored as glycogen in the muscles and liver. Plants store carbohydrates as starch, which in turn become an inexpensive and readily available energy supply for humans. Lactose increases absorption of calcium from the intestinal tract and provides a medium for the growth of favorable intestinal bacteria. The indigestible carbohydrates (dietary fibers) stimulate peristaltic movement and help prevent constipation, regulate absorption of simple sugars, and control the level of blood cholesterol by preventing or delaying its reabsorption into the bloodstream. Mucopolysaccharides and mucoproteins are compounds related to carbohydrates which are normal constituents of certain body fluids and tissues, such as mucous membrane linings and lubricating fluids. Other compounds in the body that contain carbohydrate are heparin (for blood clotting), galactopins (part of nervous tissues), dermatan sulfate (found in collagen and skin), glycosides (sugar component of steroid and adrenal hormones), and immunopolysaccharides (part of immune bodies). There is no recommended dietary allowance for carbohydrate, but it is a dietary item essential to prevent ketosis. At least 50 gm a day is the minimum amount needed to avoid ketosis, assuming normal homeostasis in the body. Allow 125 to 150 gm carbohydrate/ 1000 kcal per day. Of current interest, especially in public health nutrition is *alcohol,* which is produced by fermentation of glucose in foods (fruit sugars and cereal grains). For additional functions of carbohydrates, see under *Fiber.* See also *Carbohydrate loading.*

Carbohydrate intolerance (malabsorption). A group of conditions in which the absorption of one or more nutritionally important carbohydrates is caused by a deficiency in one or more of the intestinal disaccharidases (lactase, maltase, isomaltase, invertase, and trehalase) or by blockage in the transport mechanism across the gut. Disaccharidase deficiency may be a congenital defect, or it may be acquired in association with certain diseases (celiac disease, enteritis, kwashiorkor, and malnutrition) due to unspecific lesions in the intestinal mucosa. The chief clinical manifestation is diarrhea, which occurs when the sugar that cannot be absorbed is introduced into the diet.

Carbohydrate loading. More appropriately called glycogen loading. It is a 7-day diet and exercise routine prior to an athletic event for the purpose of increasing glycogen stores in the muscles two to three times the norm. A diet in which carbohydrates supply 350 gm/day is given the first 4 days, followed by 550 gm/day during the next 72 hours or 3 days prior to the competition. Heavy physical activity is avoided 2 days before the competition, with a tapered rest regimen to maximize glycogen loading. Due to some adverse effects, however, the practice is limited to two times a year. It is not recommended for young athletes (e.g., children and teenagers), diabetics, persons with muscle enzyme deficiencies and renal disorders, and those prone to heart disease.

Carbohydrate utilization. See digestion, absorption, and metabolism of carbohydrate under *Absorption, nutrients,* and Appendices 11, 12, and 15.

Carbon (C). A nonmetallic element occurring in all organic compounds and widely distributed in nature. Its tetrahedral atom enables it to link with a wide variety of chemical combinations. Radioactive carbon is widely used as a tracer element in metabolic studies.

Carbon dioxide-combining power. Carbon dioxide capacity of the plasma. Normal values range from 53 to 75 vol%. It is increased in alkalosis and decreased in acidosis.

Carbon dioxide fixation. Process of utilizing carbon dioxide to synthesize more complex molecules. It takes place in photosynthesis, whereby plants, in the presence of solar energy, use carbon dioxide from the atmosphere to build carbohydrates and other organic compounds. The ability to fix carbon dioxide is now known to be possessed also by animal tissues even without radiant energy but with chemical energy and the aid of the vitamin *biotin*. This carbon dioxide fixation in the body is referred to as dark-reaction photosynthesis.

Carbonic acid. A weakly ionized acid formed by the dissolution of carbon dioxide in water. It is a good *buffer*, and its salt is the chief alkali reserve of the body.

Carbonic anhydrase. Zinc-containing enzyme that catalyzes the reversible hydration of carbon dioxide. It is found in the tissues and erythrocytes, and facilitates the transfer of carbon dioxide from the tissues to the blood and then to the lungs for elimination.

Carboxyhemoglobin (HbCO). Hemoglobin combined with carbon monoxide, which has a stronger affinity for hemoglobin than oxygen. Carbon monoxide displaces oxygen, causing asphyxia and carbon monoxide poisoning.

Carcinogen. Cancer-producing agent or substance. Carcinogenic compounds such as aflatoxin and cycasin have been identified in some plants. A variety of chemical agents have been used to induce malignancy in animals, but not all of them show the same capability in humans. Some dietary components implicated to be carcinogenic are *N*-nitroso compounds, cyclamates, saccharin, sassafras tea, coffee, some food colors, and smoked products containing significant levels of polycyclic aromatic hydrocarbons (PAHs).

Cardiac. Pertaining to the heart. Cardiac failure is a set of symptoms resulting from the inability of the heart to function as a pumping organ. It may be of sudden or slow onset and may be left-sided, right-sided, or a mixture of the two, depending on which side of the heart is mostly affected. Difficulty in breathing is the most prominent symptom if the left side of the heart is affected. Edema and engorgement of body organs with blood characterize right heart failure, often referred to as *congestive heart failure.*

Cardiac cachexia. A form of coronary heart failure moderately or severely damaging to the heart valves. The main symptoms are weight loss, anorexia, increased fluid retention, and malabsorption (steatorrhea or diarrhea). *Dietary management:* improved heart function can be attained by correcting fluid and electrolyte imbalances. Small, frequent meals are preferred, with high concentrations of folate, thiamin, magnesium, zinc, and iron. A hypermetabolic state can be achieved by allowing sufficient caloric intake calculated as basal energy expenditure (BEE) $\times$ 1.5, keeping the calorie:nitrogen ratio at 150:1 and the protein level at 1.0 to 1.5 gm/kg/day.

Cardiac disease. Also called heart disease. Includes cardiac insufficiency, heart failure, myocardial infarction, pericarditis, and any cardiovascular disease (CVD). *Dietary management:* caloric intake is adjusted to bring about weight loss and consequent lowering of blood pressure, slowing of the heart rate, and reduction in the work of the heart. Rest is the primary consideration in acute heart diseases such as heart failure and coronary occlusion. Fluids are restricted during the first few days. With improvement, soft, easily digested foods are gradually introduced in small amounts as tolerated. Sodium intake is restricted to 500 mg with edema and then maintained at 1000 to 1500 mg/day once the edema disappears. In ischemic heart disease involving hypercholesterolemia and atherosclerosis, the fat in the diet should be predominantly of the polyunsaturated type; cholesterol and saturated fats are restricted. In chronic heart conditions, three small meals with between-meal feedings are recommended to avoid strain on the heart. Constipation should be avoided, and maintenance of normal or slightly below-normal weight is desirable. Sodium may be restricted (2000 mg/day) to prevent edema. See also *Diet, prudent.*

Cardiac transplant. Usually recommended for terminal cardiac heart failure (CHF) patients after thorough assessment and evaluation normally cover chronic coexisting diseases, cardiac status, patient stability, and other medical factors. Transplantees should have normal renal and hepatic functioning, without pulmonary disorders, diabetes, peptic ulcers, or a peripheral heart condition. *Dietary management:* after routine preoperative and postoperative nutritional care, encourage per os feedings. Some transplantees require *tube feeding* initially. Monitor calorie, protein, sodium, potassium, cholesterol, and fat intakes and modify them accordingly, following the guidelines of the prudent diet.

Cardiovascular disease (CVD). Collective term denoting a large group of diseases affecting the heart and blood vessels. The most important of these diseases from the public health point of view are arteriosclerotic heart disease, cerebrovascular disease, and hypertensive disease. See dietary guidelines under *Cardiac disease.*

Caries. Molecular decay of bones and teeth, making them soft and porous. See *Dental caries* and *Nutrition, dental health.*

Carmustine. A cytotoxic agent used in the treatment of brain tumor, multiple myeloma, and malignant lymphoma. It may cause nausea and vomiting within periods ranging from a few minutes to 2 hours and may persist for up to 6 hours after administration. It may also cause anorexia, dysphagia, esophagitis, diarrhea, glycosuria, and hypophosphatemia. The brand name is BiCNU.

Carnitine. Designated as vitamin B_t; a dietary essential nutrient for the mealworm *Tenebrio molitor.* Under normal conditions, humans and higher animals can synthesize carnitine from lysine and methionine; hence, it is not necessary to supply this in food. However, recent studies show that the synthesis of body carnitine may be inadequate for some individuals and that a number of diseases alter levels of carnitine in body fluids and tissues. Since carnitine is formed from amino acids, protein malnutrition will lower carnitine production. Carnitine functions in lipid metabolism as a carrier of long-chain fatty acids into the mitochondria for beta-oxidation. Abnormalities seen in patients with genetic disturbances in carnitine metabolism include muscle weakness, hypoglycemia, and lipid accumulation between muscle fibers. Evidence of carnitine deficiency has been reported in premature infants maintained on intravenous feeding, and low serum carnitine levels have been found in infants fed soy formula and in certain lipid storage diseases of the muscles.

Carnosine. Beta-alanylhistidine, a dipeptide found in vertebrate muscle tissue. Its biochemical function is not known. A protease, *carnosinase,* that attacks the peptide bond of carnosine is present in the liver, pancreas, and kidneys.

Carnosinemia. Inborn error of amino acid metabolism characterized by excretion of large amounts of *carnosine* in the urine, even when all dietary sources of this dipeptide are excluded. The condition is also associated with unusually high concentrations of homocarnosine in the cerebrospinal fluid and with a progressive neurologic disorder characterized by severe mental defects and myoclonic seizures. The defect may be due to a deficiency in the enzyme *carnosinase.*

Carotene. A *carotenoid* present in green leafy and yellow vegetables. It exists in several forms, of which alpha-, beta-, and gamma-carotene are provitamins A. Beta-carotene is the most active of these three forms. In the body, carotene is converted to vitamin A in mucosal cells. See *Retinol equivalent.*

Carotenemia. Presence of large amounts of carotene in the blood, resulting in a yellowish discoloration of the skin. The condition is harmless and should not be mistaken for jaundice. The conjunctivae and urine are not discolored in carotenemia.

Carotenoids. Group of fat-soluble yellow to red pigments occurring widely in plants. Many different carotenoids exist in nature, but only a few are converted to vitamin A in the body. Beta-carotene is the most active provitamin A carotenoid in food. Cryptoxanthin and alpha-carotene yield only half the vitamin A activity of beta-carotene. Other carotenoids, like lycopene, cantaxanthin, and zeaxanthin, do not have provitamin A activity.

Carrier. 1. A person who, without showing symptoms of a communicable disease, harbors and transmits disease-producing germs. 2. A substance that transports another substance or compound; for example, fat is a carrier of fat-soluble vitamins. 3. A naturally occurring element added to a pure substance in minute quantity for ease in handling. 4. In physiologic oxidation, a compound that can accept hydrogen or electrons from a substrate and transfer them to another compound in the transport system.

Casal's necklace. Type of dermatitis seen in *pellagra* as a result of niacin deficiency. The lesions on the face and areas of the neck exposed to the sun are distributed to resemble a necklace.

Casec. Brand name of a powdered protein supplement for infant feeding; may be mixed with cereals, mashed potatoes, and casseroles or blended into milk drinks. It is made of calcium caseinate from skim milk curd; it is low in fat and has only a trace of lactose. Each tablespoon provides 4 gm protein and 75 mg calcium.

Casein. A phosphoprotein; the principal protein of milk. It is converted to calcium caseinate or milk curd by the enzyme *rennin* in the presence of calcium, leaving a residual clear fluid called whey.

Catabolism. Destructive metabolism; the breakdown of complex substances by living cells into simpler compounds with the liberation of energy. It is the opposite of *anabolism*. Together catabolism and anabolism constitute *metabolism*.

Catalyst. A substance that hastens the speed of a chemical reaction without itself undergoing a change. Catalysts in living cells (biocatalysts) are called *enzymes*.

Catecholamines. Substituted diorthophenols synthesized in the brain, sympathetic nerve endings, peripheral tissues, and adrenal medulla. They are discharged into the circulation under conditions of stress, anger, and fear. Catecholamines (chiefly epinephrine and norepinephrine) are pressor substances and can mobilize sources of rapidly utilizable energy from the body's storage depot to prepare the animal for flight or fight. See *Epinephrine* and *Norepinephrine*.

Cd. Chemical symbol for *cadmium*.

CDC. Abbreviation for *Centers for Disease Control*.

CDP. Abbreviation for cytidine diphosphate. See *Cytidine phosphates*.

Celiac. Abdominal; pertaining to the abdomen.

Celiac disease. Also called celiac sprue. Appropriately known as gluten-induced enteropathy because it is an intolerance to gliadin, a constituent of the protein *gluten*. A form of malabsorption syndrome primarily affecting the proximal portion of the small intestine, with destruction of the villi. The principal abnormality is the failure of the jejunal mucosa to adequately absorb digested substances, particularly nutrients. As a consequence, there is malabsorption of fat, carbohydrate, protein, vitamins, and minerals, resulting in general malnutrition. The basic symptoms of celiac disease are loss of weight, nausea and vomiting, abdominal pains, weakness, diarrhea consisting of pale, bulky, frothy, foul-smelling stools, and nutritional deficiency signs that develop from malabsorption, such as anemia, cheilosis, glossitis, peripheral edema, tetany, rickets, and hypoprothrombinemia with a tendency to bleed. The condition is completely relieved if gluten, derived chiefly from wheat, barley, oats, and rye is excluded from the diet. *Dietary management:* See *Diet, gluten-free*.

Cellobiose. Disaccharide formed by the partial hydrolysis of *cellulose*. It consists of two glucose units linked in a beta-1,4 configuration.

Cellulose. Polysaccharide that acts as a supporting structure for plant tissues. It yields glucose on complete hydrolysis; partial hydrolysis yields the disaccharide *cellobiose.* It is generally not digested by humans and merely provides bulk or roughage. The glucose units of cellulose are held together by beta-linkages which can be digested by the microorganisms that inhabit the alimentary tract of ruminants. The human gastrointestinal tract has no enzymes capable of hydrolyzing the beta-linkages.

Centers for Disease Control (CDC). Government agency in charge of developing the techniques of nutritional assessment for others to use. By using the same standard methodology, valid comparisons can be made and results from different segments of the population can be integrated.

Cephalin. Phosphatide (phospholipid) that, on hydrolysis, yields phosphoric acid, glycerol, a mixture of saturated and unsaturated fatty acids, and either ethanolamine or serine. It is found in the brain, in nerve tissues, and in the lipid portion of glandular organs. It participates in *blood clotting* as thromboplastin, a cephalin-protein complex, and in the manufacture of the protoplasm and the cell membrane.

Cephalosporin. A broad-spectrum antibiotic that resembles penicillin in its action. It may cause nausea, vomiting, diarrhea, dyspepsia, and glossitis. Prolonged use may cause hypokalemia and vitamin K deficiency. Some brand names are Ancef, Ceclor, Duricef, Keflex, and Ultracef.

Cerebral palsy. Variety of neurologic dysfunctions secondary to brain damage as a result of birth injury, cerebral hemorrhage, or prematurity. Two general types of motor disability are known: *athetosis,* which is characterized by constant, uncontrollable movements, and *spastic paralysis,* which is characterized by limited activity. The motor dysfunction varies in severity and distribution, affecting one or more extremities or the trunk, head, and neck. Descriptive terms such as monoplegia, hemiplegia, and paraplegia are used to specify the distribution of the dysfunction. *Dietary manage-ment:* special feeding devices are needed to ensure adequate food intake and prevent malnutrition. Avoid stringy, hard-to-chew foods. Provide extra fluids and fiber for normal bowel movement. Adjust calorie needs, reducing intake for spastic patients who tend to gain weight, and increasing intake for the athethoid type. Some of the latter patients need as much as 4,000 kcal/day. Tube feeding may be indicated when there is difficulty in swallowing. See also *Dysphagia.*

Cerebroside. A glycolipid that, on complete hydrolysis, yields one molecule each of fatty acid, 4-sphingenine, and galactose. It occurs in the brain and myelin sheaths of nerves.

Cerebrovascular accident (CVA). Commonly known as "stroke." Partial brain damage as a result of a constricted blood supply caused either by ruptures, clots, or blood vessel spasms. It may lead to impaired hearing, sight loss, or speech defects, depending on which brain hemisphere is affected. *Dietary management:* immediately restore fluid and electrolyte balances. Give pureed, ground, chopped, or soft foods if the patient has chewing and swallowing difficulties. Avoid milk if the patient is unable to clear salivary and mucus secretions. Tube feeding may be necessary if the gag reflex is lacking. Ensure adequate nutrition, especially calories, protein, and fluid. Monitor weekly weights and adjust caloric intake accordingly. Nutritional intervention after a stroke must address predisposing risk factors like obesity, hypertension, hyperlipoproteinemia, and diabetes mellitus. A reduction of cholesterol, sodium, and fat intake may be necessary.

Ceroid. An insoluble brown substance found in atheromatous plaques and in fat deposits of certain forms of liver disease. It is associated with disorders in lipid metabolism.

Ceruloplasmin. The transport form of plasma copper bound to alpha-globulin. It is important in the regulation of copper absorption by reversibly binding and releasing copper at various sites of the body. A low plasma ceruloplasmin concentration is associated with *Wilson's disease.*

CF. Abbreviation for *citrovorum factor* and *cystic fibrosis.*

CHD. Abbreviation for *coronary heart disease.*

Cheilosis. Cracks and fissures at the corners of the mouth characteristic of *riboflavin* deficiency. The lesions of the lips begin with redness and denudation along the line of closure or may appear as pale macerations at the angles of the mouth. The lips look dry and chapped, and shallow ulcerations or crusting may occur in severe deficiency. Nonnutritional factors such as cold and wind may also cause cheilosis. Patients receiving long-term antibiotic therapy, especially chloramphenicol, develop cheilosis, which responds readily to riboflavin supplementation.

Chemical dependency. Addiction to alcohol, nicotine, street drugs (marijuana, cocaine, and the like), and/or certain prescription drugs to the extent of jeopardizing general health and wellness. See *Alcoholism* and *Nutrition, chemical dependency.*

Chemical score. A measurement of protein quality. Calculated by the following ratio:

$$\frac{\text{mg of amino acid per gram of test protein} \times 100}{\text{mg of amino acid per gram of the reference protein}}$$

The reference protein established by the Food and Agriculture Organization contains the essential amino acids in an "ideal" protein pattern. The disadvantage of the chemical score method compared to the biologic value (BV) and the protein efficiency ratio (PER) is that it cannot exhibit any toxicity of the test protein, since the last two methods use animal (rat) feeding.

Child Nutrition Act. A legal measure enacted in 1966 that appropriated funds for schools to start and expand school lunch programs and to feed preschool children. A pilot school breakfast program was also initiated. It provides cash assistance to state educational agencies to help schools operate nonprofit breakfast programs that meet established nutritional standards.

Chinese restaurant syndrome. A disorder usually caused by a reaction to monosodium glutamate (MSG), characterized by a burning sensation, chest tightness, face flushing, and throbbing headaches. These symptoms may persist for about 20 minutes to an hour. *Dietary management:* avoid MSG in seasoning foods and in commercially prepared foods. Drink plenty of fluids.

Chloral hydrate. A sedative and hypnotic used principally in the treatment of insomnia. It may cause an unpleasant taste in the mouth, nausea, vomiting, gastritis, flatulence, and diarrhea. It is excreted in breast milk; infants must be observed for sedation. Brand names are Noctec, Aquachloral Supprettes, and Oradrate.

Chlorambucil. An antineoplastic agent used in the treatment of lymphocytic leukemia and malignant lymphomas. Adverse gastrointestinal effects, including nausea, vomiting, anorexia, diarrhea, and abdominal discomfort, are usually mild and last for less than 24 hours. However, nausea and weakness may persist for up to 7 days following a single high dose of the drug. The brand name is Leukeran.

Chloramphenicol. A broad-spectrum antibiotic used for the treatment of serious infections caused by susceptible strains of *Escherichia coli,* pneumococci, and other susceptible organisms. It inhibits protein synthesis and may increase the need for riboflavin, pyridoxine, folic acid, vitamin B_{12}, and iron. It may also cause nausea, diarrhea, glossitis, stomatitis, and impaired taste. Chloramphenicol is excreted in breast milk and can also affect infants adversely. Brand names are Chloromycetin and Mychel.

Chloride. An essential mineral found largely in the extracellular fluids. It is a constituent of gastric juice as hydrochloric acid and is essential in maintaining osmotic pressure and acid-base balance. Chloride ions readily pass into and out of red blood cells (chloride shift), which is important in buffering action and maintenance of blood pH. Dietary chloride is supplied mainly by table salt; meats, seafoods, milk, eggs, and processed foods are other sources. It is readily absorbed and is excreted in the urine and sweat. Chloride loss parallels the loss of sodium; hence, chloride is concurrently lost in conditions associated with sodium depletion, as in excessive sweating, chronic diarrhea, and persistent vomiting. Chloride deficiency is characterized by loss of appetite, muscle weakness, lethargy, and metabolic alkalosis.

Chloride shift. Exchange of chloride ion for bicarbonate ion in the intracellular fluid without a corresponding movement in cations. Bicarbonate ions diffuse into the plasma when its concentration of red blood cells is high. To maintain ionic equilibrium, chloride ions diffuse from the plasma into the red cells.

Chlorine (Cl). Element universally found in biologic tissues as the *chloride* ion. As free chlorine, it is a disinfecting, bleaching, and purifying agent. Chlorinated water contains 1 part chlorine per 1 million parts of water.

Chlorosis. Form of hypochromic microcytic anemia common in young women. It is characterized by a greenish tinge to the skin.

Chlorothiazide. A thiazide diuretic used in the treatment of edema and hypertension. It increases the excretion of riboflavin, potassium, magnesium, zinc, and sodium. It may also decrease carbohydrate tolerance and increase blood glucose, and may cause dry mouth, anorexia, gastric irritation, diarrhea, and constipation. It is excreted in milk. Brand names are Aldoclor, Diupres, and Diuril.

Chlorpromazine. A phenothiazine antipsychotic agent. It may induce riboflavin depletion, increase serum cholesterol, and alter glucose tolerance, causing hyper- or hypoglycemia. It may also cause fluid retention, with resultant weight gain. It is excreted in breast milk. Brand names are Thorazine, Chlorazine, Ormazine, and Promaz.

Chlorpropamide. A sulfonylurea antidiabetic agent used for the management of noninsulin-dependent diabetes mellitus. It acts by stimulating the release of insulin from the pancreas. It has a metallic taste. Adverse effects are dose related and may include nausea, vomiting, abdominal cramps, constipation, and diarrhea. Weight gain may occur due to fluid retention or increased appetite and food intake. There is a higher risk of severe hypoglycemia with this drug than with other oral hypoglycemic agents. Alcohol should be avoided; it may cause headache and a flushing reaction. It is excreted in the breast milk. Brand names are Diabenese and Glucamide.

CHO. Abbreviation for *carbohydrate*.

Cholecalciferol. Vitamin D_3, now called *calciol*. The form of vitamin D occurring in animal cells and produced by irradiation of the provitamin 7-dehydrocholesterol underneath the skin. See *Vitamin D*.

Cholecystitis. Acute or chronic inflammation of the gallbladder. It is commonly due to bacterial infection and obstruction of the cystic duct by stones, tumor, fibrosis, or adhesions. Acute cholecystitis is characterized by epigastric pain that radiates to the shoulder and lower abdominal region, nausea and vomiting, chills and fever, and jaundice. Sensitivity to fatty foods, colicky pain, belching, and flatulence are the general features of the chronic type. *Dietary management:* in acute cases, nothing is given orally for 24 hours or more. Then a clear liquid diet is given for 2 to 3 days. The diet progresses to a moderately low fat intake (about 50 to 60 gm/day) to promote the flow of bile and induce drainage of the biliary tract. Some patients may not tolerate spices and gas-forming vegetables. For chronic cholecystitis, provide a moderately low fat intake, as previously mentioned.

Cholecystokinin. Hormone that regulates the contraction of the gallbladder. It is secreted in the upper portion of the small intestine when fat enters the duodenum and is carried by the bloodstream to the gallbladder, causing it to contract.

Cholelithiasis. Formation of stones in the gallbladder; the stones are made of cholesterol, calcium and other inorganic salts, and bilirubin. An increased incidence of gallstones is associated with obesity, diabetes, use of oral contraceptives, hypercholesterolemia, and cholecystitis. *Dietary management:* in an acute gallstone attack, use a low-fat diet to decrease gallbladder contraction and lessen the pain. Unless fat induces symptoms, a low-fat diet is not necessary. If the gallbladder is sluggish, a moderate fat intake is desirable to stimulate its contraction and prevent stagnation of bile. A high fiber intake is also beneficial. It is unlikely that restriction of cholesterol in the diet has any appreciable effect on reducing cholesterol stones.

Cholestanol. Compound formed by the reduction of the double bond of cholesterol. It is a minor constituent of blood sterols and some tissues. It is found in greater concentration in the feces.

Cholestatic liver disease. This disorder disrupts excretion of bile salts, affecting the absorption of fats and fat-soluble vitamins. There is a deficiency in fat-soluble vitamins, as well as C and B complex vitamins, protein, and iron. *Dietary management:* supplement a low-fat diet (30 to 40 gm/day) with fat-soluble vitamins A, D, E, and K. Monitor malabsorption and adjust the diet according to the patient's food tolerance.

Cholesterol. A fatlike compound with a complex ring structure; the chief sterol in the body found in all tissues, especially the brain, nerves, adrenal cortex, and liver. It is synthesized in the liver and other organs (endogenous cholesterol) and is found only in animal products (exogenous source) such as egg yolk, liver and other glandular organs, brain, milk fat and butter, and meats. Biosynthesis of cholesterol is regulated by the amount in the body; as total body cholesterol increases, synthesis tends to decrease. Endogenous cholesterol is also influenced by caloric intake, certain hormones, bile acids, and the degree of saturation of fatty acids in the diet. The average American diet provides at least 450 mg cholesterol per day, but the recommended intake is 300 mg or less per day. The current interest in cholesterol is due to its role in cardiovascular diseases, particularly *atherosclerosis.* A plasma cholesterol level higher than 200 mg/dl is a risk factor associated with atherosclerotic disease. See *Hyperlipoproteinemia* and *Nutrition, heart disease.* For the cholesterol content of selected foods, see Appendix 34.

Cholestyramine. Antilipemic agent used as an adjunct to diet therapy to decrease elevated serum cholesterol and LDL levels in type II hyperlipoproteinemia and to reduce the risks of atherosclerotic artery disease and myocardial infarction. It has a gritty texture and an unpleasant taste. Long-term use may impair the absorption of fat-soluble vitamins, carotene, folic acid, vitamin B_{12}, iron, calcium, and potassium. It may also cause bloating, flatulence, steatorrhea, indigestion, and constipation. The brand name is Questran.

Choline. A methyl group donor that occurs in some phospholipids and is a component of sphingomyelin, lecithin (phosphatidylcholine), and the neurotransmitter acetylcholine. It is an essential nutrient for several animal species, including the dog, cat, and rat, but has not been shown to be a dietary essential for humans. Choline can be readily synthesized in the body from ethanolamine and methyl groups derived from methionine. It is found in a wide range of foods; eggs, liver, organ meats, milk, legumes, and nuts are good sources. Choline is not a typical vitamin and has no known coenzyme function. However, some authorities classify it with the B vitamins since it appears to be required in the diet under certain conditions. The demand for choline-containing compounds is high during growth and development and may exceed the synthetic capacity in the human newborn. Choline may also be deficient in certain neurologic diseases, especially in the elderly. Fatty liver is the most common manifestation of choline deficiency in experimental animals. Other manifestations of deficiency include liver cirrhosis and hemorrhagic degeneration of the kidneys, adrenals, heart, and lungs.

Cholinergic. Term applied to nerve fibers that liberate acetylcholine when a nerve impulse is transmitted.

Chondroitin. Mucopolysaccharide that, on hydrolysis, yields glucuronic acid and galactosamine. As chondroitin sulfate, it is found in small quantities in the eyes, skin, and connective tissues.

Chromium (Cr). An essential trace mineral occurring in minute amounts in the blood and various tissues. Chromium is required to maintain normal glucose metabolism and is a part of the glucose tolerance factor which potentiates the effect of insulin on peripheral tissues. It is also involved in amino acid transport and breakdown of glycogen and lipids. Chromium deficiency results in impaired glucose tolerance in the presence of normal concentrations of circulating insulin, impaired amino acid metabolism, and elevated serum cholesterol and triglycerides. The primary deficiency usually results from inadequate chromium supplementation in patients on long-term parenteral nutrition and with high intakes of fiber and phytate in a diet low or marginal in chromium. The average daily intake is about 60 to 90 mg/day, with less than 1% absorbed in the gastrointestinal tract. It is transported to the liver bound to transferrin and is distributed throughout the human body. Its concentration in various tissues declines with age, depending on the dietary intake. This decline may contribute to the glucose intolerance of the elderly. Good food sources are brewer's yeast, liver, meats, and whole grains. Trivalent chromium, the chemical form that occurs in foods, is not toxic in amounts normally consumed. Other chromium compounds, however, are known to be corrosive to the skin and mucous membranes of the respiratory and intestinal tracts. Chronic exposure and inhalation of chromium, as among mine workers, has been associated with an increased incidence of bronchial cancer. Excessive chromium results in allergic and eczematous dermatitis and in systematic effects on the liver and kidneys. See Appendix 2 for the estimated safe and adequate daily dietary intake of chromium.

Chronic obstructive pulmonary disease (COPD). A disorder that is usually a result of asthma, bronchitis, emphysema or heavy smoking, and air pollution. The bronchial air flow is blocked and the person suffering from COPD constantly feels weak, which adds to the problem of not getting enough to eat. *Dietary management:* the goal is to balance the need for oxygen and the elimination of carbon dioxide. Carbohydrate

metabolism results in more carbon dioxide production than fat or protein. Fat is a preferred energy source due to its lower respiratory quotient. Thus, carbohydrate should not supply more than 45% of total calories; fat intake should be maintained at about 40% and the rest in good-quality proteins, but not over 15% because excessive protein may increase the ventilatory drive in patients with limited alveolar reserve. Give six to eight small feedings of easily digested foods with supplemental vitamins and minerals. Monitor fluid intake since there is a tendency to retain water. For patients with *edema,* sodium restriction (2 to 3 gm/day) is indicated. Some patients may need enteral feedings or supplemental formulas for between-meal nourishments.

Chronic renal failure (CRF). Kidney disorder in which renal functions of excreting wastes, conserving electrolytes, and concentrating urine are impaired. CRF involves a permanent reduction of kidney functions and may be a result of many diseases, including a bout of *acute renal failure.* Other causes are nephrosclerosis, pyelonephritis, glomerulonephritis, malignant hypertension, ischemic disease, collagen disease, and diabetes mellitus. Clinical signs and symptoms are varied, depending on the severity or stage of the disorder (mild, moderate, or severe) and the causative factors. They include nausea, anorexia, thirst, fatigue, irritability, chest pain, dyspnea, peripheral neuropathy, failing vision, abdominal pains, pericarditis, anemia, and uremic convulsions. Uremia develops when the glomerular filtration rate (GFR) is 10 to 15 ml/min, creatinine clearance is below 20 ml/min, and blood urea nitrogen is 90 mg/dl and above. Treatment is divided into three categories: (1) use of dietary modifications and drug therapy, (2) renal dialysis, and (3) kidney transplantation. The overall goal is to avoid the last two categories; hence, nutritional assessment and intervention become crucial. *Dietary management:* protein needs are based on the GFR: at 5 to 10 ml/min, protein is restricted to 0.55 to 0.6 gm/kg/day. If the GFR is 11 to 15 ml/min, protein is restricted to 0.65 to 0.75 gm/kg/day. If the GFR is 16 to 20 ml/min, the protein allowance is 0.8 to 0.9 gm/kg/day. Sodium levels are restricted to 1 to 2 gm/day. The calorie level is specified, especially with diabetes mellitus. A quick method of calculating caloric needs is based on the GFR (in milliliters per minute) as follows: 40 kcal/kg body weight/day (GFR over 20), 45 kcal/kg body weight/day (GFR of 10 to 20), and 50 kcal/kg body weight/day if GFR is below 10. Potassium, calcium, phosphorus and fluid levels are also specified, depending on the medical problems. There are now several commercial supplements to meet the needs of persons on a high-carbohydrate, low-protein, low-electrolyte diet. Monitor also for the side effects of drug therapy.

Chyle. The milky white emulsion of fat globules formed in the small intestine and transported into the lymph.

Chylomicron. The largest and lightest (least dense) of the *blood lipids,* approximately 1 μ in diameter and consisting chiefly of triglyceride and smaller amounts of cholesterol, phospholipid, and protein. It is therefore classified as a lipoprotein. Chylomicrons are normally synthesized in the intestines and serve to transport absorbed dietary triglycerides to sites of utilization in the tissues passing through the lymphatic system and then into the bloodstream. They are responsible for the turbid, milky appearance of normal plasma after a fatty meal. About 90% of the triglycerides from absorbed fats are transported as chylomicrons. Their presence in the plasma 12 to 16 hours after eating is abnormal. In type I hyperlipidemia, the body cannot clear the chylomicrons at a normal rate. See *Hyperlipidemia* and *Lipoprotein.*

Chylothorax. An accumulation of chyle within the pleural/thoracic space; characterized by severe coughing, vomiting (usually after heavy meals), thoracic cage compression, or thoracic duct trauma. *Dietary management:* restore fat, protein, and other nutrients lost due to exudation. Maintain serum levels of vitamin A and zinc.

Chyme. Thick, semifluid mass into which food is converted after gastric digestion. It is in this form that food passes into the small intestine.

Chymotrypsin. Endopeptidase secreted by the pancreas as an inactive proenzyme, chymotrypsinogen. Administration of chymotrypsin has a marked therapeutic effect on the control of certain cases of insulin-resistant diabetes.

Cimetidine. A histamine H_2 inhibitor used for the treatment of confirmed duodenal ulcer. It reduces basal gastric acid secretion by 80% and meal-stimulated acid secretion by 50%. Cimetidine can induce vitamin B_{12} deficiency, especially if taken by vegans for an extended period (over 1 year), and can increase the risk of bleeding associated with warfarin-induced vitamin K deficiency. It has a bitter taste and may also cause iron malabsorption, constipation, and transient diarrhea. The brand name is Tagamet.

Cirrhosis. Chronic, progressive disease of the liver in which fibrous connective tissue replaces the functioning liver cells. There are many types of cirrhosis caused by a number of conditions, such as chronic alcoholism (alcoholic cirrhosis), various infections such as syphilis and malaria, obstruction of the bile duct, and nutritional deficiency. There is loss of appetite, polyneuritis, cheilosis, a low serum albumin level, and edema due to protein deficiency. In advanced cases, ascites and esophageal varices complicate the condition, often ending in liver failure and hepatic coma. *Dietary management:* a liberal calorie and protein diet (about 50% more than the recommended dietary allowance), with a moderate amount of fat, is recommended. The objectives of dietary treatment are to promote healing and regeneration of liver tissue and to prevent fat stasis and formation of fibrous tissues. Provide 1.5 to 2.0 gm protein/kg/day and 300 to 350 gm carbohydrate/day to spare protein. Protein should be immediately curtailed in impending coma. Restrict sodium to 500 mg/day if ascites and peripheral edema are present. Avoid fibrous and coarse foods in cases of esophageal varices. Alcohol is not allowed.

Cisplatin. A potent antineoplastic agent used for the treatment of metastatic tumors and other neoplasms. The drug is generally considered the most emetogenic of all the antineoplastic agents. It causes marked nausea, vomiting, and anorexia 1 to 6 hours after administration, which may persist for 5 to 10 days. It may also cause depletion of magnesium, calcium, potassium, zinc, and phosphate, which may result in low serum levels of these minerals. The brand name is Platinol.

Citric acid cycle. See *Krebs cycle.*

Citrotein. Brand name of a high-protein, low-fat, flavored supplement for oral feeding. It is made with egg white solids, sucrose, maltodextrin, and partially hydrogenated soy oil. It comes in powder form that readily dissolves in cold water and is appropriate for clear liquids. See also Appendix 39.

Citrovorum factor (CF). Growth factor for the organism *Leuconostoc citrovorum;* has been given the name *folinic acid,* a biologically active form of the vitamin folic acid.

Citrulline. An amino acid first isolated from watermelon, although it does not appear to be a constituent of common proteins. It is closely related to arginine and is involved in the *urea cycle.*

Citrullinemia. An inherited metabolic disorder of the urea cycle due to lack of the enzyme arginosuccinic acid synthetase. Characteristic symptoms are elevated levels of citrulline in the blood, urine, and cerebrospinal fluid, hyperammonemia, persistent vomiting, ataxia, seizures, and progressive mental retardation. Until recently, this disorder was fatal within a few weeks. Dietary treatment with protein restriction plus supplementation with the essential amino acid, arginine, and benzoic acid has led to some long-term survival with mental retardation.

Cl. Chemical symbol for chlorine.

Clearance test. Test for kidney function. It measures the excretory efficiency of the kidney in "clearing" blood of a substance over a given period of time. It may also be used as a test for liver function to determine the ability of the liver to remove a substance from the blood.

Clearing factor. A lipoprotein lipase present in various tissues, notably the heart, lungs, and adipose tissue. It appears in the plasma following a meal and "clears" the blood of its turbid, milky appearance by hydrolyzing the triglycerides present in the chylomicrons and in lipoproteins. It also mobilizes fatty acids from the fat depots. This enzyme is enhanced by *heparin* and activated by calcium and magnesium ions.

Cleft palate. Congenital deformity characterized by incomplete closure of the lateral halves of the palate or roof of the mouth. This presents feeding difficulties, as food passes through the roof of the mouth into the nasal cavity. *Dietary management:* inability to suck adequately presents a problem. Food may back up in the nose and can cause choking. In the newborn, a medicine dropper or a plastic bottle and a soft nipple with an enlarged hole may be used. Milk can be squeezed a little at a time in coordination with the infant's chewing motions. Pureed baby foods may be diluted with milk and spoon-fed. For young children, special feeding devices are needed. However, most patients with cleft palate usually undergo surgical repair, after which a normal diet is gradually introduced.

Clindamycin. An antibiotic used in the treatment of serious respiratory tract and skin infections caused by susceptible organisms. The drug has a persistent bitter taste. It may cause nausea, vomiting, bloating, esophagitis, anorexia, weight loss, and hypokalemia. In addition, nonspecific colitis characterized by severe diarrhea and abdominal cramps may develop 2 to 9 days after initiation of treatment or even several weeks after the drug has been discontinued. The brand name is Cleocin.

Clofibrate. An antilipemic drug used as an adjunct to diet in the management of type III hyperlipoproteinemia that does not respond to diet therapy alone. The drug has an unpleasant aftertaste and decreases taste acuity. It decreases the absorption of carotene, vitamin B_{12}, iron, and electrolytes, increases the urinary excretion of protein, and may decrease the activity of intestinal disaccharidases. Adverse gastrointestinal effects include nausea, dyspepsia, diarrhea, stomatitis, and gastritis. The brand name is Atromid-S.

Clonidine. An imidazole derivative antihypertensive agent. It may cause constipation, dry mouth, loss of appetite, and weight gain due to sodium and fluid retention. A mild sodium-restricted diet may be necessary. Brand names are Catapres and Combipres.

Clotting time. The time it takes for blood to clot or coagulate. Normally, it is 4½ minutes. A delay in blood clotting time indicates vitamin K deficiency.

CMP. Abbreviation for cytidine monophosphate. See *Cytidine phosphates.*

Co. Chemical symbol for cobalt.

Co I, Co II, Co III. Abbreviations for *coenzyme I, coenzyme II,* and *coenzyme III,* respectively.

CoA. Abbreviation for *coenzyme A.*

Coagulation. 1. Curdling or clotting; formation of a clot or coagulum, as in blood or milk. 2. In colloid chemistry, the solidification of a sol into a gelatinous mass. Coagulation is usually an irreversible process.

Cobalamin. Collective term given to the many forms in which vitamin B_{12} may appear in animal tissues, all of which contain cobalt as an integral part of the molecule. The predominant forms are methylcobalamin, adenosylcobalamin, and hydroxocobalamin. Cyanocobalamin is the commercially available form of vitamin B_{12}.

Cobalt (Co). A trace mineral normally present in animal tissues as an integral part of vitamin B_{12}. The need for cobalt other than its role in the synthesis of vitamin B_{12} is not known. Only 10% of the cobalt in the body is in vitamin form; inorganic cobalt is found in the plasma attached to albumin and deposited in the bone, muscle, and other tissues. Whether inorganic cobalt has a role in human metabolism has not been demonstrated. There are no documented cases of what might be considered cobalt deficiency. The average American consumes 5 to 10 mg/day cobalt, mainly as inorganic cobalt

from vegetables and whole grains and as cobalamin in animal foods. It is readily absorbed and is excreted mainly in the urine, with little body storage. Cobalt salts have been used pharmacologically in the treatment of anemias that are refractory to iron, folate, and vitamin B_{12}. When taken in large doses, cobalt can produce toxic effects, including goiter, hypothyroidism, hypotension, and heart failure. Toxicity from dietary intake has not been a problem.

Cobamide. Generic name given to vitamin B_{12}-containing coenzymes. The two cobamides active in human metabolism are methylcobalamin and 5-deoxyadenosylcobalamin.

Codex Alimentarius Commission. Committee created by the Food and Agriculture Organization and the World Health Organization to develop international food standards on a worldwide, regional, or group-of-countries basis and to publish these standards in a food code called *Codex Alimentarius.* These food standards aim at protecting consumers' health and ensuring fair practices in the food trade.

Coefficient of digestibility. Percentage portion of the ingested food constituent retained in the body and not excreted in the feces. The *average* coefficients of digestibility of foods are 98% for carbohydrate, 95% for fat, and 92% for protein.

Coenzyme. An organic dialyzable and heat stable enzyme cofactor. It is required for the activity of many enzymes. Coenzymes usually contain vitamins as part of their structure, and they function as acceptors of electrons and functional groups.

Coenzymes I and II (Co I and Co II). Hydrogen and electron transfer agents known to be a complex of nicotinamide, D-ribose, phosphoric acid, and adenine. They play a vital role in metabolism and participate in many forms of biologic oxidation. Their two major functions are the removal of hydrogen from certain substrates in cooperation with dehydrogenases and the transfer of hydrogen (or electrons) to another coenzyme in the hydrogen transport series. Coenzyme I is also called nicotinamide adenine dinucleotide (NAD) or diphospho-pyridine nucleotide (DPN). Coenzyme II is also called nicotinamide adenine dinucleotide phosphate (NADP) or triphosphopyridine nucleotide (TPN). It is a complex of nicotinamide, adenine, two molecules of D-ribose, and three molecules of phosphoric acid.

Coenzyme III (Co III). Cysteine sulfinic acid dehydrogenase, an enzyme that catalyzes the oxidation of cysteine sulfinic acid to cysteic acid. This dehydrogenase has been named coenzyme III because it requires as coenzyme a pyridine nucleotide similar in structure to *coenzymes I* and *II*. It is found in microorganisms and animal tissues, particularly in the liver, kidneys, and heart.

Coenzyme A (CoA). Pantothenic acid joined to adenosine phosphate by a pyrophosphate bridge and to beta-mercaptoethylamine by a peptide bridge. It functions in acetylation and acylation reactions, oxidation of ketoacids and fatty acids, formation of acetylcholine, and synthesis of triglycerides, phospholipids, steroids, and porphyrins.

Coenzyme Q (CoQ). A lipidlike substance, similar to vitamins K and E in its chemical makeup, that belongs to a group of compounds known as *ubiquinones*. It is found in practically all living cells and appears to be concentrated in the mitochondria. The form which appears to be biologically active has long carbon side chains (about 30 carbon atoms). It helps in the release of energy in the oxidation-reduction system and the respiratory chain.

Cofactor. General term given to the nonprotein fraction of an enzyme necessary for its full activation. Cofactors are divided loosely into three groups: a *prosthetic group,* which is firmly attached to the protein portion of the enzyme; a *coenzyme,* which is easily dissociated from the protein enzyme; and *metal activators,* which are mono- and divalent cations such as K, Mn, Mg, Ca, and Zn and which may be either firmly or loosely bound to enzyme protein. See also *Enzyme.*

Colchicine. Alkaloid from the root of a lily plant, *colchicum autumnale,* that is of value in the treatment of gout. It may decrease the absorption of vitamin B_{12}, fat, carotene, sodium, potassium, and iron and may decrease lactase activity. It may also cause nausea, vomiting, diarrhea, abdominal cramping, loss of appetite, and weight loss. Brand names are Colbenemid and Proben-C.

Colectomy. Surgical excision of the colon to treat cancer or severe ulcerative colitis. *Dietary management:* provide a low-residue diet several days before surgery. Postsurgical feeding is by parenteral means initially, followed by per os feeding with the same dietary modifications as for *rectal surgery.*

Colestipol. Basic anion-exchange resin that binds bile acids in the intestine, forming a nonabsorbable complex which is excreted in the feces. It is antilipemic and is used for the treatment of primary type IIa hyperlipoproteinemia. High long-term use causes folate deficiency and depletion of fat-soluble vitamins due to malabsorption, especially of vitamins A and E. It may also cause abdominal discomfort and distention, constipation, and occasionally fecal impaction. The brand name is Colestid.

Colic. 1. Pertaining to the colon. 2. Abdominal pain, a symptom of various conditions. See *Infantile colic.*

Colitis. Acute or chronic inflammation of the colon or large bowel due to one or more causes. *Mucous colitis* is characterized by abdominal distress, constipation or diarrhea, and the passage of mucous or membranous masses in the stools. *Spastic colitis,* also called irritable colon or "unstable colon," is associated with increased tonus or abnormal activity of the colon. *Ulcerative colitis* is a chronic condition characterized by an ulceration of the mucosa and passage of pus and blood in the stools. For dietary management, see *Crohn's disease.*

Collagen. An albuminoid; the insoluble protein of connective tissue, bones, tendons, and skin. It is resistant to animal digestive enzymes but is hydrolyzed to soluble gelatin by boiling in water, dilute acids, or alkalis. Collagen constitutes one-third of the body proteins and possesses remarkable qualities.

Colon. The large intestine, which extends from the cecum to the rectum. It has four parts: the ascending colon, transverse colon, descending colon, and sigmoid colon. For its function, see *Absorption, nutrients.*

Colostomy. Formation of an artificial outlet from the colon through the wall of the abdomen. The need arises when part of the colon becomes obstructed or has to be removed because of a diseased condition. *Dietary management:* start with a clear liquid diet and progress gradually to one low in residue. Then give a soft or low-fiber diet as tolerated. A liberal supply of calories and protein (at least 1.5 times the recommended dietary allowance) will speed up recovery and prevent weight loss.

Colostrum. First milk secreted by the mammary gland a few days after parturition. Compared to later milk secretion, it is higher in protein content and immunoglobulins that contain antibodies responsible for the immunity of the newborn. Colostrum is also higher in beta-carotene, riboflavin, and niacinamide content but has less fat and carbohydrate than later milk.

Community Nutrition Institute (CNI). A private, nonprofit organization that provides nutritional and technical assistance to individuals, groups, and programs. Its major activity is to publish the *CNI Weekly Report,* a newsletter that provides information on legislative and bureaucratic actions which affect all aspects of nutrition.

Compleat. Brand name of a ready-to-use, blenderized formula for tube feeding made with nonfat dry milk, pureed beef, green beans, peas, peach, orange juice, maltodextrins, and corn oil. Contains about 6 gm fiber per liter. Also available without lactose and in isotonic form (Compleat Modified). See also Appendix 39.

Comply. Brand name of a high-calorie, lactose-free nutritional supplement containing sodium and calcium caseinates, maltodextrin, sucrose, and corn oil. The former brand name was Fortical.

Congestive heart failure (CHF). Reduced efficiency of heart pumping, with less circulation of blood to the body tissues. It is caused by a coronary or other cardiac disease, lung disorder, or severe anemia. Clinical signs include edema, dyspnea, cachexia, and decreased renal flow. *Dietary management:* the overall objective is to supply nutrients adequately without overworking the cardiovascular and respiratory systems. Calorie intake is restricted if the patient is obese or overweight, and fluid intake is restricted to 0.5 to 0.7 ml per kcal per day. Sodium is restricted to 1 to 2 gm/day, with supplemental potassium given as needed. Feeding small meals and snacks six to eight times a day, consisting of non-gas-forming and easy-to-digest foods, is recommended. Alcohol and caffeine are not allowed. In serving foods, extremes of temperature are avoided. For severe CHF, enteral or parenteral feeding may be necessary before feeding by mouth is initiated.

Conjunctival xerosis. Condition characterized by dryness, thickening, pigmentation, lack of luster, and diminished transparency of the conjunctiva of the exposed part of the eyeball. It is due to keratinization of the epithelial cells of the conjunctiva and is seen in *vitamin A* deficiency.

Conservation of energy. Energy cannot be created or destroyed, although it can be changed from one form to another. Thus the sum of all forms of energy remains constant. For example, the amount of heat (or energy) obtained from food is equal to the amount of energy expended in the forms of heat, work done, and energy in waste products (assuming that there is no gain or loss of weight). Energy intake greater or less than its expenditure would result, respectively, in storage or utilization of potential energy in the form of depot fat.

Constipation. Infrequent or difficult bowel movement; retention of the feces in the colon beyond the normal length of emptying time. Chronic or habitual constipation often causes headache, a feeling of malaise, loss of the power to concentrate, foul breath, and dullness of special senses. There are two kinds of constipation: *atonic,* which indicates a lack of muscle tonus of the intestines, resulting in stasis of the colon, and *spastic,* which pertains to uncontrolled contractions of the intestines. *Dietary man-*

agement: diet is not a cure but provides relief or comfort to the patient. In atonic constipation, a high-fiber diet (35 to 40 gm/day) will stimulate peristalsis, provide bulk to the intestinal contents, and help retain water in the feces to facilitate bowel movement. Emphasis is placed on dietary fiber; rich sources are whole-grain cereals, raw fruits, legumes, and leafy vegetables. Increase fluid intake and encourage regular exercise. In spastic constipation, a low-fiber diet will prevent undue distention and stimulation of the bowel. See *Diet, fiber-modified.*

Continuous ambulatory peritoneal dialysis (CAPD). A method of home or self-dialysis therapy without a dialysis machine. See *Peritoneal dialysis.*

Continuous cyclic peritoneal dialysis (CCPD). A dialysis technique applied at home using automated devices for night therapy. See *Peritoneal dialysis.*

Controlyte. A high-calorie, protein-free, low-electrolyte dietary supplement for protein-restricted diets. It is a hydrolysate of cornstarch and vegetable oil; 1 teaspoon of powder gives approximately 50 kcal. It may be added to a variety of foods or mixed with water and served as a beverage.

Copper (Cu). Essential trace mineral in humans, all vertebrates, and some lower animal species. It is a component of several enzymes involved in various functions, including the release of energy in the cytochrome system, melanin production in skin, absorption and transport of iron, formation of hemoglobin and transferrin, production of catecholamine in the brain and adrenal, metabolism of glucose, cholesterol and phospholipid, synthesis of collagen and elastin, and detoxification of superoxide radicals. Copper deficiency in humans is not common but has been observed in long-term use of total parenteral nutrition inadequate in copper, and in association with hypoproteinemia, malabsorption syndromes, jejunoileal bypass, nephrotic syndrome, high zinc intake, and *Menke's disease,* a rare genetic disorder of copper metabolism. Excess loss of copper, as through kidney dialysis, can also cause a deficiency. Symptoms of deficiency include decreased serum copper and *ceruloplasmin,* anemia similar to that caused by iron deficiency, impaired glucose tolerance, poor wound healing, immune defects, and central nervous system and cardiovascular disorders. Copper is widely distributed in foods; good food sources are liver, shellfish, legumes, nuts, and whole grains. High intakes of zinc, ascorbic acid, iron, and fiber interfere with the bioavailability of copper. The body's copper content is homeostatically controlled, and there is little storage of the excess, except in certain disease states like *Wilson's disease.* Copper toxicity has been seen in renal dialysis in which an excess of copper was transferred from the dialysis bath to the patient or when copper tubing was used in hemodialysis machines. Acute copper poisoning has occurred from accidental ingestion of copper salts by children, soft drinks served from defective equipment, and consumption of foods and beverages cooked or stored in copper-lined vessels. Symptoms of acute poisoning are vomiting, dizziness, and diarrhea with bleeding, and, in severe cases, circulatory collapse, severe hemolysis, and liver and kidney failure.

CoQ. Abbreviation for *coenzyme Q.*

Cori cycle. Series of reactions that make possible the conversion of muscle glycogen to blood glucose. Muscle glycogen cannot contribute directly to blood glucose because of lack of glucose-6-phosphatase, which is present only in the liver. In the absence of oxygen, lactic acid formed in the muscles diffuses into the blood and is taken up by the liver, which is able to convert lactic acid to glucose and, eventually, to liver glycogen.

Corneal vascularization. Formation of fine capillary blood vessels on the periphery of the cornea due to congestion of the normal limbal plexus. It may be nonspecific and may occur in any inflammatory or irritating process affecting the cornea. It is also seen in *riboflavin deficiency.*

Corneal xerosis. Hazy, milky, or opaque appearance of the cornea, usually most marked in the lower central area. It is due in part to cellular infiltration of the corneal stroma; it is seen in *vitamin A deficiency.*

Coronary heart disease (CHD). Condition characterized by inadequate coronary circulation because of narrowing of the lumen or complete occlusion of the coronary arteries due to atherosclerosis, thrombus formation, or embolism. As a consequence, the heart is deprived of its oxygen and its nutrient supply. Epidemiologic and clinical investigations have identified several risk factors associated with susceptibility to coronary heart disease. These include high blood pressure, elevation in plasma lipids, especially cholesterol, obesity, physical inactivity, and heavy cigarette smoking. Hardness of water and iodine and sugar intake have also been implicated, although their exact relationship with the disease has not been exactly defined. *Dietary management:* weight reduction and/or maintenance of healthy weight by an appropriate combination of physical activity and caloric intake is recommended. Specific dietary advice varies with the nature of the blood lipid profile. For details, see the discussion of the dietary management of hyperlipoproteinemia. See also *Nutrition, heart disease.*

Cor pulmonale. A disorder due to hypertension of the pulmonary circulation; characterized by hypertrophy of the right ventricle of the heart. Symptoms and clinical signs include coughing, fatigue, cyanosis, and hypoxia. About 80% of patients with cor pulmonale have chronic obstructive pulmonary disease. *Dietary management:* give foods of high nutrient density in small, frequent feedings. Monitor fluid and potassium intake and restrict sodium if edema is present. See also *Chronic obstructive pulmonary disease.*

Corticosteroid. Term applied to the steroid hormones secreted by the adrenal cortex and other natural or synthetic compounds having the same activity as the *adrenocortical hormones.* These hormones are used for their anti-inflammatory and immunosuppressant properties. Cortisone, hydro-

cortisone, and prednisone are among the corticosteroids available. Long-term use of these drugs can cause generalized protein depletion and can have a variety of nutritional implications, including increased need for ascorbic acid, folic acid, vitamin B_6, and vitamin D; decreased wound healing; decreased bone formation; decreased absorption of calcium and phosphorus; and increased urinary excretion of ascorbic acid, potassium, zinc, and nitrogen. Some brand names are Decadron, Deltasone, Medrol, and Merticorten.

Corticosterone. Steroid hormone found in the adrenal cortex. It influences carbohydrate metabolism and electrolyte balance.

Cortisol. 17-Hydroxycorticosterone, the major adrenal cortical steroid influencing carbohydrate metabolism. It increases the release of glucose from the liver, stimulates gluconeogenesis from amino acids, and decreases the peripheral utilization of glucose. Cortisol is released into the blood and transported to the tissues in combination with a globulin as transcortin.

Coumarin. An anticoagulant with a hypoprothrombinemic effect, especially when the dietary intake of vitamin K is inadequate. Prescribed for treatment of embolism and thrombosis, but not in cases of hemorrhagic risks.

Cow's milk allergy. Syndrome of malabsorption, diarrhea, and vomiting associated with variable villus atrophy attributable to an allergy to cow's milk protein. Exclusion of cow's milk results in clinical and histologic remission, while challenge produces inflammatory changes and villus atrophy within 24 hours. Additional symptoms include urticaria, asthma, and anaphylaxis after milk intake. Some patients also exhibit a low-grade colitis that responds to elimination of cow's milk. It is a disease of neonates; after the age of 2 years, most children overcome their intolerance.

Cr. Chemical symbol for chromium.

C-Peptide. A part of the endogenous insulin, but not present in exogenous (manufactured) insulin. Its measurement indicates functional pancreatic beta cells. This helps in determining whether a person is Type I (insulin-dependent) or Type II (noninsulin-dependent) diabetic.

Creatine. Methyl guanidine derivative of acetic acid. As creatine phosphate, it acts as a source of *high-energy phosphate* and plays an essential part in the release of energy in muscular contraction. It is present in the muscle, brain, and blood; trace amounts are also normally present in the urine. It is excreted in abnormally large amounts in conditions accompanied by failure to burn carbohydrate (as in starvation, diabetes mellitus, and severe liver disease), in diseases of muscles (as in myasthenia gravis and muscular dystrophy), and in conditions accompanied by excessive tissue breakdown (as in fevers and wasting diseases).

Creatine index. Measure of the ability of the body to retain ingested creatine, as determined under standard conditions. The percentage retained is high in hypothyroidism and low in hyperthyroidism and other conditions accompanied by muscle wasting.

Creatinine. A waste product of *creatine,* formed largely in the muscles by irreversible nonenzymatic removal of water from creatine phosphate. It is excreted in the urine through the glomeruli of the kidney. The excretion of creatinine in the urine is constant from day to day for a given individual. Thus urinary creatinine is an index of muscle mass when kidney function is normal. It is increased in body protein breakdown (catabolism) and possibly by lack of carbohydrate and fat in the diet so that protein is used for energy needs. See *Creatinine-height index.* See also *Serum creatinine.*

Creatinine clearance test. Test for renal function based on the rate at which ingested creatinine is filtered through the glomeruli. Normally this is 70 to 130 ml/min. In severe renal disease, creatinine clearance may fall to 5 ml/min.

Creatinine coefficient. Amount of urinary creatinine excreted in 24 hours/kg body weight. Average excretion is 23 mg/kg body weight for men and 18 mg/kg body weight for women. When expressed in terms of body size, the creatinine excretion of different individuals of the same age and sex is constant from day to day. The creatinine coefficient may thus be regarded as an index of muscle mass. However, creatinine excretion decreases with age, and a consensus is lacking on the effect of exercise, stress, steroids, and amount of meat intake. Creatinine excretion can be expressed in terms of an expected value for body weight. See *Creatinine-height index.*

Creatinine-height index (CHI). An indirect measurement of somatic protein or lean body mass if renal function is normal and fluid intake is adequate. The amount of *creatinine* in a 24-hour urine output is measured, and the index is calculated from the following formula:

$$CHI = \frac{\text{actual 24-hour creatinine excretion (mg)}}{\text{expected 24-hour creatinine excretion (mg)}} \times 100$$

See Appendix 29.

Cretinism. Chronic condition occurring in fetal life or early infancy due to deficient thyroid activity. It is characterized by arrested physical and mental development, dry skin, chubby hands, large protruding tongue and abdomen, and low basal metabolic rate. See also *Myxedema.*

Criticare HN. Brand name of a monomeric (elemental) formula for oral or tube feeding; contains free amino acids, small peptides, maltodextrin, modified starch, and safflower oil. It is lactose-free, low in fat, and has minimum residue. See also Appendix 39.

Crohn's disease. Also known as "regional enteritis." A disorder, usually chronic and inflammatory, that affects the digestive tract. Ordinarily, it involves the colon and the ileum, but it may also affect areas anywhere from the mouth to the anus. Symptoms include ulcerative lesions, chronic diarrhea, and upper abdominal pain. Scarring and thickening of the intestinal wall result in intestinal obstruction and malabsorption. Of unknown cause, it has no effective medical treatment as yet, although corticosteroids and antibiotics are used to correct symptoms. Crohn's disease is confused with *ulcerative colitis,* which is another inflammatory bowel disease. *Dietary management:* protein-energy malnutrition (PEM) is a common problem. Increase caloric and protein intake about 50% more of required needs. Due to the occurrence of certain food intolerances and lack of appetite, the patient has reduced intake of vitamins and minerals, particularly vitamin A, B_1, B_2, B_6, B_{12}, folate, calcium, and iron. Supplemental multivitamins and minerals are therefore beneficial. Dietary fat should be limited (40 to 50 gm/day) if steatorrhea is evident. If hyperoxaluria is present, avoid grapefruit, tea, and cola drinks. For severe cases of Crohn's disease an elemental diet is given, progressing to a low-residue diet in small, frequent feedings.

Crude fat. The fat, lipids, and other fat-soluble materials in food that are extractable by fat solvents, such as petroleum ether, ethyl ether, chloroform, or benzene. In the *proximate analysis* of foods, this is sometimes referred to as ether extract or ether-soluble fraction.

Crude fiber. The ash-free, insoluble residue left after boiling a food sample first with dilute acid and then with dilute alkali to simulate gastric and intestinal digestion. It is commonly called "indigestible carbohydrate." See under *Fiber.*

Crude protein. Food nitrogen content, as derived from protein and nonprotein nitrogenous materials. Crude protein is obtained by multiplying the nitrogen content of foods (as determined by the Kjeldahl process) by the factor 6.25. See *Kjeldahl method.*

Cryptoxanthin. A yellow pigment belonging to the *carotenoid* group that can be converted into *vitamin A* in the body. It is one of the chief pigments in yellow corn, paprika, and oranges.

CT. Abbreviation for *calcitonin.*

CTP. Abbreviation for cytidine triphosphate. See *Cytidine phosphates.*

Cu. Chemical symbol for copper.

Curling's ulcers. Deep ulcers that usually develop in the duodenum of patients suffering from extensive burns, causing major bleeding. *Dietary management:* initially, total parenteral nutrition may be required, since the patient cannot be fed orally. When oral feeding can be resumed, follow dietary modifications for *burns.*

Cushing's syndrome. Condition due to hypersecretion of the adrenocortical hormones because of hyperplasia or tumor of the adrenal cortex, basophilic adenoma of the pituitary gland, or prolonged use of large doses of adrenocorticotropic hormone (ACTH). The chief features of the syndrome include obesity of the trunk, face, and buttocks, purplish striae over the abdomen, pigmentation of the skin, hypertension, hyperglycemia, excessive growth of hair, and loss of sexual function. *Dietary management:* correct *hyperglycemia, hypertension,* and *obesity.*

CVD. Abbreviation for *cardiovascular disease.*

Cyanocobalamin. Synthetic form of vitamin B_{12} used in vitamin pills and pharmaceuticals. It is a *cobalamin* with a cyanide group attached to the cobalt atom.

Cyclamate. An artificial, nonnutritive sweetener which is the sodium or calcium salt of cyclohexylsulfamic acid. It is 30 times sweeter than sucrose. Used widely in the 1960s, it was banned in 1970 for commercial use in the United States pending additional studies to resolve some problems regarding its safety for human consumption. On June 10, 1985, the National Academy of Sciences (NAS) panel of scientists reported that studies did not indicate any carcinogenicity of cyclamates in human beings. Petition for reapproval by the Food and Drug Administration (FDA) is pending, based on data from about 75 new studies in favor of cyclamate use. At least 40 other countries have approved the use of cyclamates.

Cyclophosphamide. An alkylating agent used alone or as a component of various chemotherapeutic regimens in the treatment of lymphomas and other malignant diseases. Anorexia, nausea, and vomiting occur commonly, especially at high doses. Occasionally, diarrhea, hemorrhagic colitis, mucosal irritation, and oral ulceration may occur. The agent is excreted in breast milk. The brand name is Cytoxan.

Cycloserine. An antibiotic used in the treatment of tuberculosis and urinary tract infections caused by susceptible bacteria. It acts as a pyridoxine antagonist and decreases protein synthesis. It may also decrease the absorption of calcium, magnesium, and folate. The brand name is Seromycin.

Cystathionine. An intermediate product in the conversion of methionine to cysteine.

Cystathioninuria. Inborn error of metabolism characterized by mental retardation and elevated *cystathionine* in blood and urine. It is probably a defect in the methionine-cysteine pathway. In some instances, the biochemical abnormality can be corrected by administration of pyridoxine.

Cysteine. Alpha-amino-beta-mercaptopropionic acid, a sulfur-containing amino acid formed by the reduction of cystine.

Cystic fibrosis (CF). Also called mucoviscoidosis due to the highly viscous secretions of the mucus-producing exocrine glands. It is a life-threatening congenital disease occurring in infants and young children. CF is characterized by generalized dysfunction of the exocrine glands involving the pancreas, respiratory system, salivary glands, gastrointestinal tract, biliary system, and paranasal glands. The sweat contains large amounts of sodium chloride and, to a lesser extent, potassium. Abnormal mucus secretion causes obstruction of mucus-producing cells or organ passages, resulting in asthma, recurrent pneumonia, and sinusitis as common symptoms of the disease. Lack of pancreatic enzymes interferes with the utilization of protein, fat, and carbohydrate. Vitamin deficiencies occur because of digestive defects, and death usually results from malnutrition or bronchopneumonia. *Dietary management:* provide a high-calorie, high-protein, liberal-fat, and high-sodium diet, supplemented with fat-soluble vitamins, considering the age and food tolerances of the child. Dietary intakes are increased to 120 to 150% of required needs for calories, 150 to 200% for protein, and 150% for other nutrients. An additional salt intake per day (½ to 1 teaspoon) is necessary when there is excessive loss during sweating. Besides sodium and chloride, other minerals that need monitoring are potassium, calcium, iron, zinc, and selenium. Fat restriction is not necessary if a pancreatic enzyme preparation (e.g., Pancreatin and Cotazym) is taken at each meal and with snacks. For infants with severe pulmonary problems, the conventional infant formula may be given together with pancreatic enzyme therapy. Infants who fail to gain weight in spite of adequate caloric intake need formulas containing casein hydrolysate and medium-chain triglycerides. Older children usually tolerate a regular diet without difficulty with pancreatic enzyme therapy. Younger children absorb only 50 to 60% of their food intake.

Cystine. A sulfur-containing nonessential amino acid found in large amounts in *keratins*. It is relatively insoluble at the pH of normal urine and can crystallize or precipitate to form cystine stones.

Cystinosis. A rare hereditary disorder characterized by accumulation of cystine in the lysosomes of many cells, including those of the bone marrow, cornea, and kidneys. Progressive accumulation of cystine leads to renal tubular damage, aminoaciduria, hypophosphatemic rickets, and potassium-wasting acidosis. Treatment includes adequate fluid intake, supplemented by potassium in the form of potassium citrate, to correct the acidosis and vitamin D with or without phosphate to correct the rickets.

Cystinuria. A hereditary disorder characterized by a defect in the transepithelial transport of cystine, lysine, ornithine, and arginine in the intestine and kidney. The renal tubules fail to reabsorb these acids, which pass in large amounts into the urine, where cystine, the least soluble amino acid, tends to precipitate out and form stones. The simplest therapeutic measure is to ensure a good flow of dilute urine by maintaining a high fluid intake (about 3 liters/day), especially during the night, when the most concentrated urine is produced. An alkaline-ash diet can help alkalinize the urine to prevent precipitation of cystine, although the use of alkalinizing agents and penicillamine is more effective. See *Diet, alkaline-ash.*

Cytabarine. A pyrimidine antagonist; an antimetabolite used with other chemotherapeutic agents for remission induction in nonlymphocytic leukemia. Adverse effects are dose-related and may cause severe nausea, vomiting, diarrhea, oral inflammation or ulceration, and anorexia. These may result in hypokalemia, hypocalcemia, protein-losing enteropathy, and weight loss. The brand name is Cytosar-U.

Cytidine phosphates. Mono-, di-, and triphosphoric esters of cytidine as cytidine monophosphate (CMP), cytidine diphosphate (CDP), and cytidine triphosphate (CTP). As cytidine phosphate derivatives, they are involved in the biosynthesis of lecithin and cephalins.

Cytochrome oxidase. An iron-containing oxidase that accepts electrons from the other *cytochromes* and passes them on to oxygen, which is the ultimate hydrogen acceptor.

Cytochromes. Group of oxidation-reduction enzymes that are primarily concerned with the transfer of electrons from flavoproteins and other substrates to oxygen or their electron acceptors.

D

Dactinomycin. An antineoplastic antibiotic; used as a component of various chemotherapeutic regimens in conjunction with surgery and/or radiation therapy. Nausea and vomiting occur within a few hours after administration and can last for up to 24 hours. The antibiotic also causes diarrhea, stomatitis, oral lesions, and anorexia, and may decrease the absorption of calcium, iron, and fat. The brand name is Cosmegan.

Dark adaptation. Speed with which the eye adjusts to a change in intensity of light. This depends on the amount of vitamin A in the body. In humans, maximal dark adaptation of the rods requires about 25 minutes; it is longer in vitamin A deficiency.

Daunorubicin. An anthracycline antibiotic that has cytotoxic and immunosuppressive effects; used for treatment of leukemia. Nausea and vomiting may occur soon after administration and last for 1 to 2 days. The drug may also cause stomatitis as early as 5 to 7 days after administration, which begins as a burning sensation with erythema of the oral mucosa, leading to ulceration. The brand name is Cerubidine.

DBW. Abbreviation for desirable body weight. See *Weight.*

DCH. Abbreviation for *delayed cutaneous hypersensitivity.*

Decalcification. Demineralization; the loss of calcium salts from bones and teeth. It may be due to a number of dietary or physiologic factors, including lack of calcium in the diet; deficiency of vitamin D, which is needed for the absorption of calcium from the intestines; loss of excessive dietary fats (steatorrhea) excreted as insoluble soaps with calcium; the presence of oxalates that bind dietary calcium; a low ratio of calcium to phosphorus (less than 1.0) in the blood; inadequate *parathormone;* and *immobilization,* as in bedridden persons.

Decubitus ulcer. Also called bed sore or pressure sore. An ulcer due to local interference with circulation, usually caused by lack of oxygen; common among patients who are bedridden or immobilized and those with circulatory disorders. The extent and depth of pressure ulcers are related to hydration status and undernutrition, especially hypoproteinemia. Wound drainage from the lesion contains about 400 mg nitrogen, corresponding to almost 2.5 gm protein, and up to 30 gm protein can be lost through drainage from a single large open wound in 24 hours. Closely related to protein is the level of ascorbic acid which is necessary for the synthesis and maintenance of collagen, the chief protein component of connective tissue. *Dietary management:* restore normal nutriture, especially protein status. Emphasize the importance of fluids, adequate calories, and high protein (1.5 gm/kg/day), vitamin C (100 to 200 mg/day), and zinc (15 to 20 mg/day) for the healing of tissues. Correct vitamin and mineral deficiencies, especially of iron if the patient is anemic.

Deficiency disease. Condition arising from a deficiency or lack of one or more of the essential nutrients because of *primary* or dietary inadequacy or as a result of *secondary* or conditioned inadequacy. The condition may be a progressive, continuous process that, if uncorrected, eventually leads to depletion of body nutrient reserves. Biochemical changes or "lesions" occur in selected tissues or in the body at large; these eventually result in functional changes such as loss of appetite, easy fatigability, and gastrointestinal disturbances. As the nutritional deficiency continues, anatomic lesions develop and gross clinical signs and symptoms like glossitis, cheilosis, and dermatitis become manifest. In summary, the development of a deficiency disease may be envisioned to occur in five stages: nutritional inadequacy, tissue depletion, biochemical changes, functional changes, and anatomic lesions. There are two categories of deficiency disease:

Primary. Also called dietary deficiency disease; a condition due to the failure to ingest an essential nutritional factor in amounts sufficient to meet existing requirements of the body. This may, in turn, be due to poor food habits, poverty, ignorance, lack of food, or excess consumption of highly refined foods.

Secondary. Also called conditioned deficiency disease; a condition due to failure to absorb or utilize an essential nutrient because of an environmental condition or a bodily state and not because of dietary lack or failure of ingestion. The conditioning factors may be grouped into six categories: interference with ingestion, interference with absorption, interference with utilization, increased nutrient requirement, increased nutrient destruction, and increased nutrient excretion.

Dehydration. 1. Drying; removal of water from food, tissue, or substrate. 2. Condition resulting from excessive loss of water, accompanied by losses of electrolytes, particularly sodium, potassium, and chloride ions. The person experiences thirst and reduced urinary volume. Dehydration may range from mild (water loss is about 2% of initial body weight) to extreme (20% weight loss, which could be fatal). For an adult, a reduction of a pound of body weight within 24 hours due to fluid losses is a manifestation of dehydration. Fever, acidosis, excessive sweating, diarrhea, and excessive vomiting are common causes of dehydration. *Dietary management:* rehydrate immediately with fluids and electrolyte solutions. It is safest to use solutions of lower osmolality than that of the plasma. Salty broths, fruit juices, and milk beverages are excellent fluid sources. Monitor fluid intake/output and serum electrolyte levels to assess whether rehydration is adequate. See also *Electrolyte balance* and *Water balance.*

Dehydroascorbic acid. Oxidized form of vitamin C; the reduced form is ascorbic acid. These two compounds are readily and reversibly oxidized and reduced. Both are biologically active, although dehydroascorbic acid is somewhat less stable than ascorbic acid.

7-Dehydrocholesterol. Cholesterol derivative in the skin that is converted to vitamin D by irradiation or exposure to ultraviolet light. See *Vitamin D.*

Dehydroretinol. Vitamin A$_2$; the form of vitamin A found in the retina and liver of freshwater fishes. It differs from retinol (vitamin A$_1$) in having one more conjugated double bond and has about one-third the biologic activity of retinol. See *Vitamin A.*

Delayed cutaneous hypersensitivity (DCH). A skin test used to assess immune function prior to and following institution of nutritional support. A negative reaction or induration less than 5 mm in diameter to the intradermal injection of three to five antigens is indicative of *anergy* or lack of immunocompetence. See *Hypersensitivity skin test.*

Denaturation. Any alteration in the structure of a native protein, giving rise to definite changes in chemical, physical, or biologic properties such as decrease in solubility at the isoelectric point, loss of biologic specificity, loss of ability to crystallize, increase in viscosity and digestibility, and changes in molecular shape. Denaturation may be brought about by heating, freezing, irradiation, pressure, and treatment with organic solvents.

Dental caries. Tooth decay; demineralization of the inorganic portion and dissolution of the organic substance of the teeth. Three factors are involved in the development of dental caries: the host's teeth, microflora, and the substrate in the mouth. Dental caries will not develop if the teeth are caries resistant and the mouth is kept clean and free of food particles that will sustain the growth of cariogenic bacteria. Evidence indicates that sucrose, especially if taken between meals, is the chief dietary component promoting dental caries. The production of acid from the bacterial fermentation of carbohydrates is the immediate cause of the breakdown of the enamel and dentin. Fluorine and other nutrients in foods can also accelerate or reduce the development of dental caries. The following are recommended dietary measures to prevent tooth decay: (1) fluoridation of drinking water where the supply is deficient in natural fluorine, (2) restricted consumption of sticky starches and sugary confections, (3) avoidance of between-meal consumption of sweets, and (4) eating a balanced diet and including starch and dietary fiber with meals. Raw fruits and vegetables have a cleansing effect if sticky starches and sweets are eaten with the meal. See also *Fluoride* and *Nutrition, dental health.*

Deoxycorticosterone (DOC). Also called "desoxycorticosterone"; a hormone produced by the adrenal cortex. It is corticosterone without the oxygen atom at carbon atom 11. Except for aldosterone, it has a greater electrolyte-regulating effect than the other corticoids. It is prepared synthetically as the acetate (DOCA) and is useful in the treatment of Addison's disease.

Deoxypyridoxine. Synthetic structural analog and antagonist of vitamin B_6; it competes for binding with pyridoxal phosphate-dependent enzymes but cannot function as a coenzyme. It is used in the experimental induction of vitamin B_6 deficiency.

Deoxyribonucleic acid (DNA). Also called deoxyribose nucleic acid; the main carrier of genetic information necessary for the synthesis of specific proteins. It is found in the nuclei of cells as part of the chromosome structure and consists of phosphoric acid, purines (adenine and guanine), pyrimidines (cytosine and thymine), and the sugar deoxyribose. The structure of DNA is envisioned as a double helix in which the purine and pyrimidine bases are inside the helix, with the sugar and phosphate backbone outside the helix. The chains are held together by hydrogen bonding.

Depression. An abnormal emotional state characterized by an excessive, unrealistic, inappropriate reaction to events (environmen-

tal changes) or inner (endogenous) conflicts. There are many factors leading to intrapsychic conflicts. Visible signs related to nutrition include mood swings in eating (lack of appetite or increased appetite and irregular mealtimes), poor choices of food, skipping meals, and weight control problems. *Dietary management:* adjust caloric intake and maintain optimum body weight. Assess eating habits and identify nutritional inadequacies; modify the diet accordingly. Consider the effects of certain drugs prescribed for depression on specific nutrients, i.e., observe dietary guidelines for drug-nutrient interactions.

Dermatitis. Inflammation of the skin. There are many forms and causes, e.g., prolonged exposure to the sun's rays, allergy, and infection. Dermatitis is also seen in association with deficiency states due to lack of biotin, niacin, vitamin B_6, and essential fatty acids. See also *Nutrition, dermatology.*

Detoxification. Also called detoxication; the chemical changes in the body that serve to convert toxic substances into forms that are less toxic and more readily excretable. The detoxification mechanism involves oxidation, reduction, hydrolysis, or conjugation with a compound occurring normally in the body, such as glycine, cysteine, or glutamine.

Deuterium. Heavy hydrogen; the *isotope* of hydrogen with an atomic weight of 2. It is used in tracer studies and body water determinations.

Dextran. Polysaccharide of glucose produced by the action of microorganisms on sugar. It is used in gel filtration chromatography and as a substitute for blood plasma in the treatment of severe burns and hemorrhagic shock.

Dextrimaltose. Preparation of dextrin and maltose; used as a carbohydrate modifier in infant milk formulas.

Dextroamphetamine. The dextrorotatory isomer of amphetamine; used as an anorexiant and for treatment of narcolepsy and hyperactivity. Its anorexigenic effect is temporary, lasting for only a few hours. When it is used for the treatment of obesity, a low-calorie diet is recommended. The drug has a metallic taste and may cause cramps, constipation, and a decreased tissue ascorbic acid level. Brand names are Dexedrine and Biphetamine.

Dextrose. Also called *glucose.*

Diabetes. Condition characterized by excessive thirst and urination. If used without qualification, the term refers to *diabetes mellitus.*

Diabetes insipidus. A condition due to lack of *vasopressin,* causing a secondary deficiency in *antidiuretic hormone.* Excessive fluid is lost through the kidneys, leading to dehydration. *Dietary management:* potassium supplementation may be needed. Alter nutrition with more sweetened beverages. In some patients, benzothiadiazine diuretics can be effective.

Diabetes mellitus (DM). A group of diseases characterized by abnormal glucose metabolism. Insulin is not manufactured by the pancreas or is produced in too small quantities, and, if present, is not utilized by the body. DM is classified as follows:

Gestational diabetes mellitus (GDM). Occurs during pregnancy, affecting approximately 2% of pregnancies. The cause is unknown, but it may be due to insulin resistance. After parturition, the blood glucose level reverts to normal. However, GDM increases the risk of developing diabetes later in life. For further details, see *Gestational diabetes mellitus.*

Impaired glucose tolerance (IGT). The oral glucose tolerance test is abnormal, especially during the postprandial period, while the fasting blood glucose level is normal or a little high. IGT patients are classified as either obese IGT, nonobese IGT, IGT with pancreatic disease, or IGT that may occur during administration of central parenteral nutrition. In some cases, IGT may be a developmental stage leading to IDDM or NIDDM; hence its former designations, "prediabetes" and "borderline DM," which are no longer used.

Insulin-dependent diabetes mellitus (IDDM). Or Type I; usually develops before the patient reaches 40 but may occur at any age. About 10 to 15% of diabetes mellitus cases are insulin-dependent. There is an obvious incapacity of the beta cells of the pancreas to produce insulin; thus, insulin injection is needed to utilize glucose, prevent ketosis, and sustain health. If the disease is uncontrolled, the immediate manifestations are fatigue, polyuria, polyphagia, polydipsia, and eventually ketoacidosis. While conventional insulin therapy may require one or two intermediate and/or regular insulin mixtures, intensive insulin therapy necessitates the use of a quick-acting regular insulin prior to taking meals, along with an injection of long-acting (ultralente) insulin once a day.

Noninsulin-dependent diabetes mellitus (NIDDM). Or Type II. Most cases (85 to 90%) of diabetes mellitus are of this type, which occurs in mid-adulthood, although there are also individuals who develop Type II DM under 40 years of age. Unlike Type I, which usually has a sudden onset, Type II is characterized by slow development, and the symptoms are less pronounced. No insulin injection is necessary since some pancreatic insulin is produced. Medication consists of oral hypoglycemic agents unless diet and exercise suffice, especially with obese persons. Persistent hyperglycemia may be corrected by combined therapy consisting of oral hypoglycemic agents and insulin. In periods of stress or in certain infections, slight ketosis may develop.

Secondary diabetes mellitus. The preferred designation is other types of DM since a number of disorders lead to the development of diabetes. These include pancreatic diseases (pancreatitis, pancreatic cancer, pancreatectomy, cystic fibrosis, hemochromatosis); certain genetic syndromes (hyperlipedemia, myotonic dystrophy, Prader-Willi syndrome); and hyperendocrinopathy and insulin receptor abnormalities. In such cases, dietary treatment should be consonant with therapy, either through a controlled diet or a combination of diet and insulin therapy.

Diabetes mellitus, complications. Classified as acute or chronic. For acute complications, see *Diabetic ketoacidosis, hyperglycemic, hyperosmolar, nonketotic syndrome, hyper-*

glycemia, and *hypoglycemia.* Chronic complications of DM usually occur over a period of years. The generally recognized ones are cardiovascular disease especially atherosclerosis and retinopathy, or disease of the eyes; nephropathy, or disease of the kidneys; neuropathy, or disease of the nervous system; and an increased incidence of infections, e.g., urinary tract infection (UTI) and cutaneous infections.

Diabetes mellitus, dietary management. Caloric intake is adjusted to bring about weight changes and maintain a healthy weight. The food exchange system is used, and a meal plan, with or without snacks, is calculated with the following dietary guidelines: (1) about 50 to 60% of kcal/day comes from carbohydrates, 12 to 20% from protein, and the rest from fats. Of the 30% of total calories provided by dietary fats, 10% comes from polyunsaturated fatty acids, 10 to 15% from monounsaturated fatty acids, and less than 10% from saturated fatty acids. (2) Distribute the nutrients throughout meals and snacks, with the goal of maintaining normal blood glucose levels. Sugars and concentrated sweets are avoided. Carbohydrates, protein, and fat are divided into the three meals or may include an evening snack with the following distribution: one-sixth, one-third, one-third, and one-sixth. (3) Timing and regularity of meals are important for diabetics, especially those with IDDM, to avoid swings in glycemic levels. The meal plan and spacing should consider the lifestyle and preferences of the individual and his or her medications (kind, dose, and time taken). For example, the carbohydrate distribution is based on the peak action and duration of insulin in IDDM. In rapid-acting insulin therapy, 25% of carbohydrate is given for breakfast, 10% for the midmorning snack, 30% at noon or for lunch, 25% for dinner, and 10% for bedtime snack. In slow-acting insulin therapy, carbohydrate is distributed as follows: 20% for breakfast, 25% at noon or for lunch, 35% for dinner, and 20% for bedtime snack. (4) Dietary fiber is emphasized; the recommended intake is 35 gm/day or 25 gm/1000 kcal/day for low-calorie diets. (5) Dietary cholesterol is also monitored and should not exceed 300 mg/day. (6) Bring about gradual weight loss in obese patients, especially those with Type II DM. See also *Weight control.*

Diabetic ketoacidosis (DKA). One of the acute complications of *diabetes mellitus.* It occurs when blood glucose cannot get into the body cells or when not enough insulin is available to utilize glucose. Instead, *ketones* are used to provide energy. The warning signs of DKA are: the appearance of ketones in the urine, especially when the blood glucose levels are 250 mg/dl or higher excessive thirst, polyuria, nausea, and vomiting, dehydration, and abdominal pain. Immediate treatment consisting of insulin, electrolytes, and fluids is essential. In severe ketoacidosis, fluid and electrolytes are administered intravenously. A 5% glucose solution is given as hyperglycemia and glycosuria subside. If there is no vomiting, clear broth and tea may be given, followed by fruit juices and other liquids. See also *Ketoacidosis* and *Ketone test.*

Dialysis. Process of separating substances in solution by selective diffusion through a semipermeable membrane. See *Renal dialysis.*

Diarrhea. Condition characterized by frequent passage of loose, watery, and unformed stools. Kinds of watery diarrhea are the passive movement of water and electrolytes, with increased hydrostatic pressure, as in inflammatory bowel disease, salmonellosis, and fungal infections; and the active movement of water into the mucosa, as in enterotoxic infections and excessive hydrochloric acid secretion in the stomach. Diarrhea may be functional or organic and may be due to a number of causes, e.g., intestinal infection, ingestion of poison, overeating, nervous disorder, endocrine disturbance, and food malabsorption and sensitivity. Diarrhea may also be associated with nutritional disorders such as pellagra and protein-calorie malnutrition.

Acute d. A diarrhea characterized by the sudden onset of watery stools at frequent intervals, accompanied by abdominal pain, weakness, fever, and cramps 24 to 48 hours after a precipitating event. It may also be symptomatic of a chronic gastrointestinal disease or infection.

Chronic d. A persistent diarrhea (lasting for 2 weeks or more). Nutritional deficiencies occur rapidly due to decreased absorption.

Dietary management: in severe diarrhea, food is withheld for 12 to 24 hours, and fluids and electrolytes are given to prevent dehydration. In infants, give a half-strength formula low in carbohydrate and fat. The addition of 5 to 10% apple powder, banana flakes, or a pectic-agar mixture may hasten the development of formed stools. In adults, start with simple foods low in residue and gradually build up to a normal diet as the condition improves. See also Appendix 38.

Diazepam. A benzodiazepine tranquilizer used primarily for relief of anxiety and agitation; also used as a muscle relaxant, as an anticonvulsant, and in the management of alcohol withdrawal. It can stimulate appetite, increasing food intake and weight, but when given in high doses it may cause dry mouth and reduced food intake. Brand names include Valium, Valrelease, and Q-pam.

Diazoxide. A rapid-acting hypotensive and hyperglycemic agent that is structurally related to the thiazide diuretics but has no diuretic activity; used in severe hypertension and hypoglycemia due to hyperinsulinism. Severe hyperglycemia may develop, especially in patients with renal disease and carbohydrate metabolic disorders; weight gain may also occur due to retention of sodium and water. Other side effects include nausea and vomiting, taste alteration, abdominal discomfort, anorexia, and constipation. Brand names are Hyperstat and Proglycem.

Dicumarol. Brand name of bishydroxycoumarin; an anticoagulant present in spoiled sweet clover that is structurally similar to vitamin K. It counteracts the formation of clotting factors, notably prothrombin, whose production requires the presence of vitamin K. Dicumarol and its various derivatives are prepared synthetically and used in the treatment of thrombosis.

Diet. 1. The usual foods and drinks regularly consumed. 2. To take food according to a regimen. 3. Food prescribed, regulated, or restricted in kind and amount for therapeutic or other purposes. Dietary guidelines for all healthy Americans over 2 years old are as follows: eat a variety of foods; achieve and maintain a healthy weight; choose a diet low in fat, saturated fat, and cholesterol; choose a diet with plenty of vegetables, fruits, and grain products; use sugars in moderation; use salt and sodium in moderation; and if you drink alcoholic beverages, do so in moderation.

Diet, adequate. Diet that meets all the nutritional needs of an individual. A dietary pattern based on the *basic four food groups* is a practical way of planning for dietary adequacy to meet the recommended dietary allowances for specific nutrients. See Appendices 1 and 5.

Diet, antiesophageal. See *Reflux esophagitis.*

Diet, ash. The mineral elements in foods (ash) form a residue that is excreted in the urine. Foods are said to be acid-ash (acid-forming) or alkaline-ash (basic-forming) on the basis of their influence on the pH of the urine. The acid-forming elements in foods, such as sulfur, phosphorus, and chloride, decrease the pH of the urine; the alkaline-forming elements, such as sodium, potassium, magnesium, and calcium, increase the pH of the urine. Foods that have no effect on urine pH are neutral-ash foods. Thus, by changing the composition of the diet, the urine may be made either acidic or alkaline. In general, cereals and protein-rich foods have a predominance of the acid-forming elements. Fats, oils, and sugars give a neutral ash.

Acid-ash d. Diet emphasizing the use of large amounts of acid-forming foods while restricting the intake of alkaline-forming foods such as fruits, vegetables, and milk. An acid urine favors the excretion of kidney stones consisting of calcium and magnesium phosphates, carbonates, and oxalates;

it also enhances the effect of some medications used for urinary tract infection.

Alkaline-ash d. Diet emphasizing the intake of large amounts of alkaline-forming foods such as fruits, vegetables, and milk while limiting the intake of acid-forming foods such as meat, fish, eggs, and cereals. The diet is prescribed for patients with uric acid cystine stones in the kidneys. An alkaline urine is beneficial in keeping these stones in solution.

Diet, balanced. Diet containing all the required nutrients in *proper proportion* with respect to one another for optimum nutrition. A more appropriate term to use is "adequate diet," since a diet that is quantitatively balanced for optimum nutrition is rather difficult to attain.

Diet, basic-ash. See *Alkaline-ash d* under *Diet, ash.*

Diet, bland. Diet used in treating gastric ulcers; eliminates or restricts the intake of substances known to cause gastric irritation and excessive gastric acid secretion. These substances include black pepper, chili powder, and red pepper; coffee, both regular and decaffeinated; alcohol; soft drinks with caffeine; and any food that is not tolerated. The diet is highly individualized and restricts only those foods that cause discomfort. The traditional diet, with progressive levels of food intake previously prescribed for peptic ulcer, was bland and smooth in texture and was given in six small feedings. Milk was an important part of the diet because it was believed to buffer gastric contents, and rough or coarse foods were excluded on the presumption that they irritate the gastric mucosa. When used in conjunction with H_2 blockers and antacids, the traditional bland diet was found to be no more effective than a general unrestricted diet in speeding the rate of healing of an ulcer and in reducing gastric acid secretion. The current dietary recommendation is to encourage the patient to eat anything that does not produce symptoms, to avoid foods that do, and to have three well-balanced meals a day but no late-evening snack, since it stimulates nocturnal secretion of acid.

Avoidance of coffee and caffeinated soft drinks that induce acid secretion may prevent heartburn and discomfort due to reflux.

Diet, brat. Diet consisting of banana, rice, unsweetened applesauce, and toast. It is prescribed for diarrhea in infants and children but is not recommended for the treatment of diarrheal illness. The beneficial effect of this diet is not supported by controlled scientific studies. Its use should be limited to 1 day when prescribed. The diet is nutritionally inadequate.

Diet, calcium-modified. Calcium intake varies widely among individuals, depending upon the consumption of dairy products. The calcium content of a diet that includes a variety of foods, but no milk and milk products, can be estimated as approximately 200 mg/1,000 kcal/day. For most individuals, this is equivalent to 300 to 500 mg of calcium per day. The intake of milk (300 mg calcium per cup), cheese, and other milk products (average of 150 to 200 mg calcium per serving) contributes more than 55% of the total daily calcium intake.

High-calcium d. Diet offered to meet the calcium needs of persons depleted by disease, traumatic stresses, or prior dietary inadequacies. The diet is basically a well-balanced regular diet supplemented with additional high-calcium foods (about 400 to 600 mg Ca/day), derived from milk and dairy products, protein foods, fruits and vegetables, and grain products.

Low-calcium d. Diet that generally restricts the intake of milk, milk beverages, cheese, yogurt, and ice cream. It usually consists of 500 to 600 mg calcium, but the diet should be supplemented with multivitamins and minerals if the regimen is to be continued for an extended period of time. A low-calcium diet is recommended for patients with renal hypercalciuria and absorptive hypercalciuria.

Diet, calcium-phosphorus-restricted. Diet prescribed in the treatment of calcium phosphate stones. It restricts the intake of calcium and phosphorus to minimal levels while maintaining nutritional adequacy. Foods high in these minerals (such as milk and milk products, whole-grain cereals, organ meats, sardines, leafy green vegetables, legumes, nuts, and cocoa) are either restricted or omitted from the diet, depending on the level of intake prescribed by the physician. A strict to moderate restriction ranges from 200 to 400 mg calcium and 700 to 1000 mg phosphorus.

Diet, calcium test. A calculated diet used in the study of calcium metabolism under conditions of minimum intake. Calcium in the diet is limited to 200 mg or less, and phosphorus is limited to 600 mg. Fats and sugars are used to maintain caloric intake. The calcium content of drinking water should be checked; if it is unusually high, distilled water should be used for cooking and drinking.

Diet, calorie-modified. Diet in which the total intake of calories is either increased or decreased from normal to allow for a gain or loss in body weight.

Low-calorie d. Diet planned to permit loss of weight while maintaining health. A reduction of 500 kcal/day from the usual intake, while keeping activity constant, should bring about a loss in body weight of about 1 lb/week. It is best to arrive at a caloric allowance that is tolerable to the patient. A weekly weight loss of ½ to 1 lb is considered satisfactory. Weight loss of more than 2 lb/week is not advisable except under the close supervision of a physician. Care should be observed in planning the diet; caloric levels below 1200 are marginal in nutrient content and may necessitate vitamin supplementation. A liberal protein intake is essential for its satiety value and to prevent negative nitrogen balance; carbohydrate and fat are restricted to the caloric level desired. Foods to avoid include sauces, gravies, nuts, sweets, desserts, and fried foods.

High-calorie d. Diet with a prescribed caloric intake above normal to meet increased energy requirements and to provide weight gain. It is indicated in febrile conditions, hyperthyroidism, athetosis, undernutrition, and other conditions that result in loss of weight. The caloric increase may vary from 30 to 100% above the usual intake. It is best to individualize the diet. Observations with patients of both sexes and different ages show that men seem to prefer ingesting the additional calories through extra portions of the usual foods served at meals, children and adolescents prefer between-meal nourishment, and women seem to favor more concentrated foods.

Very-low-calorie d. (VLCD). Reducing diet that severely limits calories to fewer than 800 kcal/day to promote a large, rapid weight loss averaging 2 to 4 lb/week for women and 3 to 5 lb/week for men. The diet is very high in protein and low in carbohydrate, which is usually 30 to 50 gm/day; fat is restricted to that present in the protein source. Supplementation with vitamins and minerals up to 100% of the recommended dietary allowance is recommended. A VLCD is safe when administered properly under medical supervision. It is indicated for individuals who are at least 30% overweight and have a minimum *body mass index* of 32. Because of the potentially life-threatening side effects of the diet, it is contraindicated in certain conditions: pregnancy and lactation, cardiac dysfunction, renal failure, hepatic disease, protein-wasting diseases, and severe psychologic disturbances. A VLCD may be planned with conventional foods or with the use of semisynthetic formula preparations. The formula is either a liquid or a powder to be mixed with liquid. Some formulas contain soluble fiber. Generally, the dieter is limited to the formula alone or with very limited quantities of low-calorie foods. The diet is usually preceded by 2 to 4 weeks on a well-balanced 1200-kcal diet to allow the body to adjust to the very low calorie level and to promote gradual diuresis, instead of the rapid sodium and water loss seen with abrupt introduction of the VLCD. At the end of the weight loss period of about 12 weeks, a period of gradual refeeding follows. The VLCD is the basis of commercial weight-reduction programs like Optifast, Medifast, Medibase, and the HMR Fasting Program. Throughout the weight reduction program, sessions are held on behavior modification, nutrition education, and exercise.

Diet, carbohydrate-modified. Diet that provides a specified level of carbohydrate or is restricted in the amount of a particular type of carbohydrate such as glucose, sucrose, fructose, galactose, or lactose.

High-carbohydrate d. Diet high in available carbohydrate to allow for glycogen formation, to ensure sufficient calories to meet needs, to spare protein, and to minimize tissue catabolism. It is indicated in liver diseases, Addison's disease, fasting hypoglycemia, acute glomerulonephritis, uremia, pernicious vomiting, and toxemias of pregnancy. The diet is modified in consistency or other nutrient content to suit specific disease conditions. Emphasis is placed on easily available carbohydrates such as sugar, syrups, jellies, and jams.

Restricted-carbohydrate d. Diet limited in carbohydrate content to reduce available glucose when carbohydrate metabolism is impaired, as in spontaneous hypoglycemia. It is also indicated for the dumping syndrome, epilepsy, and obesity. Restriction of specific types of carbohydrate, such as sucrose, lactose, maltose, and galactose, is also indicated in cases of intolerance of these sugars. See *Diet, galactose-restricted; Diet, lactose-restricted; Diet, maltose-restricted;* and *Diet, sucrose-restricted.*

Diet, chemically defined. See *Diet, elemental.*

Diet, cholesterol-restricted. Diet in which the intake of dietary cholesterol is restricted to a prescribed level. It is indicated for hypercholesterolemia, atherosclerosis, and gallbladder stones with cholesterol esters. Individuals who eat one or more eggs a day and use organ meats at regular intervals ingest 1000 mg/day or more of cholesterol. Omission of eggs and organ meats will bring down the intake of cholesterol to 300 mg/day. This amount can be further reduced if butter is not used and if skim milk and dairy products made from skim milk are substi-

tuted for whole milk. See Appendix 34 for the cholesterol content of foods.

Diet, cholesterol-restricted, fat-controlled. Diet designed to lower the blood cholesterol level by restricting the intake of foods high in cholesterol and saturated fats and by increasing the use of vegetable oils and special margarines high in unsaturated fats. This may be accomplished by limiting the intake of meat, fish, and poultry to two average servings per day (2 to 3 oz per serving); restricting the intake of eggs (i.e., egg yolk) to three per week; limiting the intake of cheese, shellfish, and organ meats (liver, kidney, sweetbreads, and heart) to a 2-oz portion as a substitute for an egg; restricting the intake of saturated fats by trimming visible fat and using only lean cuts of meat; using only liquid vegetable oils rich in MUFA and PUFA such as corn, cottonseed, soybean, safflower, and olive oils; avoiding commercially prepared, packaged foods containing whole egg, whole milk, and saturated fats; and eliminating cholesterol-rich foods such as fish roe, caviar, and brain. This dietary regimen restricts the intake of cholesterol to about half the normal intake of cholesterol, to not over 300 mg/day. Fat intake is restricted to less than 30% of total caloric needs, distributed as follows: less than 10% from saturated fatty acids, 10 to 15% from monounsaturated fatty acids, and close to 10% from polyunsaturated fatty acids. See Appendix 34.

Diet, copper-restricted. Diet prescribed in conjunction with oral administration of copper chelating agents used in the treatment of Wilson's disease and other disorders associated with elevated copper storage in the liver. Large quantities of food rich in copper are avoided. These include liver and organ meats, shellfish, mushrooms, nuts, oysters, dried beans, lentils and peas, and chocolate. At the discretion of the physician, low to moderate amounts of these foods may be allowed.

Diet, dental soft. See *Diet, mechanical soft.*

Diet, desensitizing. Diet aimed at decreasing the sensitivity of a person to a given food allergen. The food allergen is first excluded from the diet for an indefinite period. Then it is gradually added to the diet in small amounts until an average portion is tolerated.

Diet, diabetic. This diet follows the pattern of a normal diet for maintenance of good health and normal activity. Except for simple sugars that are rapidly absorbed and can produce hyperglycemia peaks, a diabetic can have more variety in his or her choice of foods. However, individualization is the rule; the dietary requirements of diabetics differ with the severity of the disease, the type and extent of insulin therapy received, and the amount of activity performed. The most important consideration is adjustment of total caloric intake to attain and maintain a healthy body weight. For further details, see *Diabetes mellitus, dietary management.*

Diet, dysphagia. Diet for individuals with difficulty in swallowing. To aid in the feeding of patients with dysphagia, four levels of dysphagic diets are available: level 1. pureed foods with thick liquids; level 2. lumpy pureed foods with thick liquids; level 3. finely chopped meats and vegetables; level 4. regular chopped (bite-size) foods with thin liquids.

Diet, elemental. Also called chemically defined formula diet; a mixture of basic nutrients of known quantitative composition. It consists of either hydrolyzed protein or synthetic L-amino acids, simple sugars, essential fatty acids, and all known required nutrients. It requires very little digestion, is almost completely absorbed by the upper small intestine, and is very low in residue. Elemental diets are indicated in inflammatory bowel disease, short bowel syndrome, malabsorption, pancreatitis, and preoperative nutrition.

Diet, elimination. A normal diet that excludes the intake of a specific food or food group known to produce allergic manifestations. Attention should be given to commercially processed or packaged foods that may contain the offending substance in disguised form. It is important to read the list of ingredients on all labels and packages.

Diet, elimination test. A series of allergy test diets beginning with a basic diet that consists of a few carefully selected foods least likely to cause allergic reactions. If the person on the basic diet is asymptomatic for 2 weeks, other foods are gradually added at 4-day intervals. Milk, eggs, and wheat are added last because these items are the most notorious food allergens. If relief of symptoms is not obtained even on the basic diet, it is probable that an agent other than food is the offending allergen. The most widely used test diet is the one designed by Rowe. See *Diet, Rowe's elimination.*

Diet, faddist. A craze diet based on the purported "magic quality" in a particular kind of food to treat or cure certain conditions. Common fad diets are the *Zen macrobiotic diet,* molasses diet, fruit diet, and various formula diets that have caught the fancy of overweight persons.

Diet, fat-modified. Diet that prescribes a specified level of fat in the diet, fatty acids ratio, or percentage of calories from fat. Modifications in the fat content of the diet are necessary in weight reduction; in diseases of the gallbladder, pancreas, and cardiovascular system; and in disturbances in fat absorption in association with such diseases as sprue, cystic fibrosis, and pancreatitis.

Fat-controlled d. Also called proportioned-fat diet; both the *amount* and the *kind* of fat are regulated. The diet is generally planned to provide 30% of the total calories/day from fat. The total amount of fat is then "controlled" or proportioned into less than 10% from saturated fatty acids, 10 to 15% from monounsaturated fatty acids, and up to 10% from polyunsaturated fatty acids. The objective of the diet is to increase the intake of the unsaturated fatty acids and reduce the intake of saturated fatty acids to bring about a decrease in serum cholesterol triglycerides. Polyunsaturated fatty acids are supplied by such oils as corn, soybean, cottonseed, and safflower oils. Animal products, palm oil, and hydrogenated fats are high in saturated fatty acids. Monounsaturated fatty acids are present in most vegetable oils, particularly olive oil and canola oil. It is recommended that people trim visible fats from meats and use lean meats and poultry without the skin, skim milk, and low-fat or nonfat yogurt and non-dairy creamers.

Liberal-fat d. A liberal fat allowance is about 40% of caloric intake, or approximately 100 to 130 gm/day of fat. A liberal fat intake often accompanies a high-protein, high-calorie diet prescribed for certain conditions that do not require any restriction in the fat content of the diet, such as undernutrition, burns, nephrosis, and ulcerative colitis. A high-fat diet is indicated in conditions that restrict the intake of carbohydrate and/or protein, as in dumping syndrome, functional hyperinsulinism, and uremia. In such cases, it is best to supply fat in the form of butter, margarine, cream, salad dressing, and vegetable oils.

Low-fat d. Reduction in the fat content of the diet to supply about 10 to 15% of caloric intake, or approximately 30 gm/day of fat. Indicated for acute attacks of pancreatitis and cholecystitis. This amount of fat is supplied by about 8 to 9 oz of lean meat, poultry, or fish per day. No foods rich in fat are allowed. Visible fats are trimmed from meat, and foods are prepared simply by broiling, baking, or boiling. The use of sugar, sweets, fruits, cereals, and starchy vegetables will increase caloric intake, and protein may be increased through the use of skim milk, egg white, and gelatin.

MCT fat d. Diet in which MCT oil is used in place of ordinary cooking fats and oils. MCT is a unique oil containing triglycerides of medium-chain fatty acids, which are more easily hydrolyzed and absorbed than the long-chain triglycerides present in conventional dietary fats. The diet is indicated for conditions in which ordinary dietary fats are poorly digested and absorbed, such as pancreatitis, cystic fibrosis, chyluria, sprue, intestinal resection, pancreatic insufficiency, deficient bile secretion, and biliary obstruction. Three to four tablespoons MCT oil (about 40 to 55 gm fat) or an amount recommended by the physician may be used in cooking, in salad dressings, sauces, or marinades for meats and vegetables, or simply mixed with fruit juices. The oil is colorless, odorless, and tasteless and mixes well with liquids.

Moderate-fat d. Diet with a fat allowance of 20 to 30% of caloric intake or about 50 to 70 gm/day of fat. A moderate fat intake is indicated in hepatitis, cirrhosis of the liver, and chronic gallbladder and pancreatic diseases. It is also recommended in weight reduction to lend palatability and satiety value to the diet. Fried foods, nuts, sauces, gravies, and other fatty foods should be avoided. It is best to get the fat allowance from lean meats, eggs, milk, butter, and other highly emulsified fats. Whenever necessary, additional calories may be supplied by sugar, sweets, and other carbohydrate-rich foods.

Very-high-fat d. One in which fat is approximately 80% or more of caloric intake. Carbohydrate intake is severely restricted to no more than 30 gm/day, and the protein allowance is slightly below normal levels. The aim of the diet is to maintain a ketogenic/antiketogenic ratio that will produce a state of ketosis. See *Diet, ketogenic.*

Diet, fat test. Two test diets are used in the diagnosis of gallbladder disease and the determination of fat absorption.

Fat-free test d. A test meal given the night before a radiologic examination of the gallbladder. The meal may consist of fat-free broth, fruits, plain gelatin, skim milk, and black coffee or tea. Nothing is given orally after midnight, and breakfast is withheld until after the examination is made. In some cases the examination is repeated after a *fatty meal,* which may consist of two fried eggs, buttered toast, whole milk, and coffee with cream.

High-fat test d. Calculated 100-gm fat test diet used to diagnose steatorrhea. It is usually given for 3 days unless otherwise indicated. The fat allowance should come mainly from eggs, meats, whole milk, and highly emulsified fats such as butter and cream. It is important to choose foods that are simply prepared to facilitate the fat intake calculation. The amount of fecal fat is analyzed after the high-fat diet is ingested. See *Fecal fat test.*

Diet, fiber-modified. Diet in which the amount of *dietary fiber* is higher or lower than the normal intake of about 25 gm/day.

High-fiber d. Diet providing more than 35 gm dietary fiber per day. Excellent sources are whole grain cereals and unrefined breads, high-fiber vegetables, raw fruits, and legumes. See Appendix 32. A high-fiber diet is a regular diet with an additional two to three servings of foods high in dietary fiber. It is indicated in atonic constipation and diverticular disease.

Low-fiber d. Diet that contains a minimal amount of indigestible carbohydrates or dietary fiber. The fiber content of the diet may be reduced by removing gristle and tough connective tissue in meats, removing seeds and skins from fruits and vegetables, omitting high-fiber foods, and using refined cereals and breads. It is indicated in narrowing of the intestine.

Diet, Feingold. Diet postulated to improve behavior and reduce hyperkinetic activity by eliminating foods containing salicylates, artificial colors (especially FD&C yellow no. 5), and the preservatives butylated hydroxyanisole (BHA) and butylated hydroxytoluene (BHT), monosodium glutamate (MSG), and sodium benzoate. No convincing experiments have been done to confirm the effectiveness of the diet.

Diet, fructose-restricted. Diet that restricts the intake of fructose from fruits and other foods high in sucrose content (on hydrolysis, sucrose yields glucose and fructose). It is prescribed for fructose intolerance. The degree of fructose restriction is highly individualized to fit the tolerance level. Table sugar, syrups, honey, sweets, and processed foods with added sugar are avoided or restricted. Fructose is found in all fruits; it is also present in sugar beets, green peas, and sweet potatoes.

Diet, full hospital. Also called regular diet or general diet. See *Diet, regular.*

Diet, galactose-restricted. Diet that eliminates foods containing galactose and lactose for the treatment of galactosemia. Milk and all products made with milk are not allowed since galactose is a component of lactose in milk. If a galactose-free diet is required, liver, pancreas, brain, and other organ meats that store galactose are also not alllowed. Package labels of commercially prepared products should be carefully checked. Those with added milk, lactose, casein, whey, dry milk solids, and curd should be avoided. Lactose is also used as a filler in certain artificial sweeteners and in the pharmaceutical industry. Some liberalization of the diet at about 12 years of age has been recommended, but this may not be wise because of the damaging effects of accumulated galactitol in the lens, liver, and kidney. Proprietary formulas low in galactose for infant feeding include Nutramigen, Isomil, Prosobee, and Pregestimil. See Appendix 39 for lactose-free formulas for children and adults.

Diet, general. See *Diet, regular.*

Diet, gliadin-restricted. More commonly called gluten-restricted diet; it excludes gliadin, which is a component of gluten found in wheat and other cereals. See *Diet, gluten-free.*

Diet, glucose-restricted. Diet prescribed in rare cases of glucose intolerance. This diet is difficult to plan, as glucose is present, either as free glucose or as a disaccharide component in milk, fruits, vegetables, and cereals. Newborn infants require a special proprietary formula based on calcium caseinate, fructose, and vegetable oil, with added vitamins and minerals. This regimen is usually followed until 6 months of age. Semisolid foods low in starch content are gradually introduced by the seventh month. At the age of 1 year, the infant should be taking egg, fish, meat, and restricted amounts of fruits and vegetables. Milk and starchy foods are not introduced until about 2 to 3 years of age.

Diet, glucose tolerance test. A preparatory diet given before a *glucose tolerance test* when the carbohydrate intake is known to be inadequate or if the person is on a weight reduction diet. A high-carbohydrate diet of at least 300 gm/day is given for 3 days prior to the test. The diet is not necessary if the person has been consuming an adequate diet prior to the test.

Diet, gluten-free. Also called gliadin-free diet; used in the treatment of gluten-sensitive enteropathy (celiac disease or nontropical sprue). The diet eliminates wheat, oats, rye, and barley and products containing these cereals. Rice, corn, and buckwheat contain a smaller amount of gluten, but they are usually tolerated. Milk and dairy products, meat, fish, poultry, eggs, fruits, vegetables, potato, yam, soybeans, fats, sweets, and gluten-free wheat starch can be taken as desired. It is important to read labels carefully, as many processed foods contain the restricted cereals in disguised form, as in fillers, stabilizers, or emulsifiers. Examples of such foods are malted milk, Ovaltine, hot cocoa mixes, cold cuts, and textured vegetable protein.

Diet, high-altitude. High-carbohydrate (65%), low-fat (20%) liquid diet recommended prior to rapid ascent to high altitudes. This diet has been found beneficial in reducing the clinical symptoms observed at high altitudes.

Diet, hospital. Diet used for hospital patients. The routine hospital diets are the *regular, soft,* and *liquid* diets. These may be modified to suit individual requirements for certain therapeutic purposes.

Diet, house. See *Diet, regular.*

Diet, 5-hydroxyindole acetic acid (5-HIAA) test. See *Diet, serotonin test.*

Diet, hydroxyproline test. Test diet eliminating meat and meat products, fish, gelatin, ice cream, marshmallows, salad dressings, and puddings. Used during the test period for urinary excretion of hydroxyproline to study bone collagen turnover in hyperparathyroidism and Paget's disease.

Diet, hyperlipoproteinemia. See *Hyperlipoproteinemia.*

Diet, ketogenic. Diet that is very high in fat and severely restricted in carbohydrates; it is prescribed to control epilepsy if drugs prove ineffective. The diet is calculated to have a fatty acid/available glucose ratio exceeding 2:1. Such a ratio causes the accumulation of ketones (produced from fat oxidation) and the inhibition of convulsive seizures. Foods high in carbohydrate such as breads, cereals, fruits, desserts, sweets, and beverages containing sugar are excluded from the diet; concentrated fat sources such as butter, cream, bacon, mayonnaise, salad dressings, and oils are taken in generous amounts. The use of medium-chain triglycerides in place of the usual dietary fats makes the diet more effective in inducing ketosis. It also allows more carbohydrate, making the diet more palatable.

Diet, lactose-restricted. Diet designed to limit the intake of lactose to the tolerance level in individuals who experience bloating, cramping, and diarrhea after the ingestion of products containing lactose. The restriction is highly individualized. Many lactose-intolerant individuals usually have no difficulty with small amounts of lactose. Most can manage 4 to 8 oz/day of milk if it is taken with meals, while others need to eliminate milk as a beverage. Cottage cheese, aged cheddar cheese, and fermented milk products like yogurt are tolerated by most persons. A few individuals highly intolerant of even a small amount of lactose may have to eliminate all products containing milk and lactose. It is important to examine labels carefully to detect hidden lactose. For example, lactose is added to some nondairy creamers, artificial sweeteners, and even some pharmaceutical products as a filler. The diet may be low in calcium, riboflavin, and vitamin D, depending upon the degree of milk restriction. Calcium supplementation may be indicated, especially in growing children, postmenopausal women, and women at risk for developing osteoporosis. A commercial lactase enzyme, when added to milk or taken with meals, can sufficiently hydrolyze lactose to allow the use of milk in the diet. Many lactose-free enteral products are also available as a substitute for milk. See Appendix 39.

Diet, leucine-restricted. Diet restricting the intake of leucine to the minimum requirement of 150 to 230 mg/kg body weight. For infants, a proprietary product low in leucine is available (MSUD Diet Powder). Protein-rich foods, particularly milk and eggs, are restricted until tolerance to these foods is established. Fruits and vegetables are added to the diet according to the infant's normal feeding schedule. Small amounts of carbohydrate feeding, equivalent to 10 gm, are given 30 to 40 minutes after each meal to help counteract the hypoglycemic effect of leucine. The child is usually able to tolerate a normal diet by the age of 5 to 6 years.

Diet, light. Diet that consists of foods that are easily digested and readily emptied from the stomach. It is often prescribed prior to surgery or gastric analysis; it is also indicated for patients, especially older ones, who are quite sick and cannot tolerate rich and heavy foods. The diet is given in three small meals, with between-meal feedings. Foods are prepared simply; fatty foods, rich pastries, concentrated desserts, and fibrous fruits and vegetables are restricted or given as tolerated.

Diet, liquid. Diet consisting of a variety of foods that are liquid, can be liquefied, or can easily melt in the mouth or at body temperature.

Clear liquid d. Diet of clear liquids that leaves little or no residue. It is used in pre- and postoperative patients, food intolerance, acute infections, and acute inflammatory conditions of the gastrointestinal tract. The primary purpose of the diet is to relieve thirst and help maintain water balance. Plain tea, black coffee, fat-free broth, ginger ale, plain gelatin, and glucose solution are the usual liquids given. Other liquids, such as Popsicles, fruit ices, fruit drinks, carbonated beverages, and clear fruit juices such as apple, grape, and cranberry, are often allowed to contribute additional calories. The diet is nutritionally inadequate and must not be used for more than 2 days. The use of commercially prepared low-residue liquid formulas should be considered if needed longer to provide more calories, protein, and other nutrients.

Cold semiliquid d. Diet prescribed after tonsillectomy and other mouth and throat surgery. Only cold liquids and cold soft, bland foods are given to avoid irritation and to prevent bleeding. Foods included are gingerale and other flavored drinks, iced tea, plain flavored gelatin, popsicles, plain yogurt, soft custard and pudding, fruit purees, and other cold foods tolerated. Chocolate products and red-colored beverages are not given because they may mask bleeding; milk beverages are omitted or restricted if excessive mucus is produced; acidic fruit juices may be irritating and should be avoided.

Full liquid d. Diet consisting of foods that are liquid or easily become liquid in the mouth or at body temperature. This diet bridges the gap between the clear liquid diet and the soft diet. It is used in acute conditions, for patients with fractured jaws, after oral and other types of surgery, and for patients too ill to eat solid foods. When properly planned, the diet can be made nutritionally adequate and can be used for relatively long periods of time. Six or more feedings per day are recommended. All liquids and foods that easily become liquid, such as plain ice cream, plain gelatin, strained cream soups, strained cereal gruel, soft custard, and puddings, are allowed in the diet.

Restricted liquid d. The diet order specifies the volume of liquid allowed in 24 hours, such as 500, 1000, 1200, or 1500 cc. The total fluid intake used by the nursing service for medication should be added to the total daily fluid intake. In addition to the usual liquid beverages, there are semisolid foods or foods that liquefy in the mouth which should be counted for fluid equivalents. For example, ½ cup gelatin yields 60 cc liquid; ½ cup ice cream or sherbet has 90 cc liquid; and thin cooked cereals have 50 % fluid.

Diet, macrobiotic. See *Diet, Zen macrobiotic.*

Diet, maltose-restricted. Diet that eliminates foods containing maltose or available maltose; prescribed for maltose intolerance. Excluded from the diet are corn syrup, corn sugar, beets, malted cereals, and other malted products. Since maltose is an intermediate product of starch digestion, the intake of starchy foods such as wheat, rice, corn, potato, and sweet potato is limited.

Diet, MCT. See under *Diet, fat-modified.*

Diet, meat-free test. Diet used to determine the presence of gastrointestinal bleeding. Meat, fish, and poultry are not given for 3 days prior to the test. These foods contain hemoglobin and myoglobin, which can give a false positive result, while vitamin C in excess of 500 mg/day can cause a false-negative reaction.

Diet, mechanical soft. Also called the "dental soft diet." It is used for patients who have difficulty in chewing due to poor dental condition or lack of teeth, or to the presence of sores and lesions in the mouth, following head and neck surgery, and for those who are debilitated and are too ill to eat the regular diet. It consists of foods that are soft, well cooked and easy to chew, and, if necessary, chopped, ground, or minced. Foods are best served moist, as in casseroles, or with gravy or sauce. The diet must be highly individualized according to each patient's chewing tolerance. All beverages are allowed, although patients with lesions in the mouth may not be able to take tart fruit juices.

Diet, methionine-restricted. Diet prescribed for homocystinuria. Products low in methionine and methionine-free chemically defined formulas are commercially available for infant feeding (e.g., Low Methionine Diet Powder, Product 3200K). The methionine level is controlled by adding specified amounts of milk or proprietary infant formula to these products. Small amounts of solid foods are introduced at the usual ages. Considerations in planning the diet are similar to those in phenylketonuria. This involves calculating the amount of formula needed to meet protein and calorie requirements and then determining the amounts of other foods permitted. As an adjunct to this diet, supplementary betaine or choline may be given to promote remethylation of homocysteine.

Diet, modified. A *regular diet* altered to meet specific body requirements under different conditions of health or disease. The diet may be modified in consistency, content (calories, carbohydrates, protein, fat, or specific nutrient), flavor, methods of preparation or service, and frequency of feeding.

Diet, motor test meal. Test diet to determine the emptying time of the stomach. It consists of rice and raisins or berries with seeds, or a meat sandwich with 2 tablespoons of raisins, or a meal with stewed prunes given 12 hours before gastric analysis. The presence of fibers in the gastric contents indicates decreased stomach motility.

Diet, neutropenic. Diet that is prepared and served under strict sanitary conditions to minimize the microbial count, especially pathogens. Useful for immunocompromised patients who have neutrophil counts of less than 500/mm^3. The following measures in handling and serving foods are observed: restrict or avoid fresh fruits and vegetables; cook foods adequately; cover all food items properly; serve immediately after preparation; keep hot foods hot and cold foods cold, observing recommended temperatures for food safety; avoid cross-contamination; thaw fish, meat, and poultry in the refrigerator and cook thoroughly.

Diet, normal. Diet that supplies all the nutritional needs of a normal, healthy individual, with due consideration for age, sex, activity, and physiologic needs. It contains enough calories for energy, adequate protein for growth, and sufficient minerals, vitamins, and water for the proper functioning of the body.

Diet, no sugars and concentrated sweets. A liberalized diabetic diet prescribed for individuals with mildly impaired glucose tolerance who are maintaining an acceptable weight; those who need a diabetic diet but have poor intake; and diabetics who cannot or will not follow the food exchange system. Sugar and foods high in sugar are avoided. The diet does not use measurements or food exchanges.

Diet, optimal. The *best possible* diet that will supply all the essential nutrients at the *highest possible* level to achieve the *ultimate* goal of nutritional intake. The optimal diet is difficult to define in precise quantitative terms, as the optimum intake for each nutrient for every individual has not yet been established.

Diet, oxalate-restricted. Diet prescribed for urinary calcium oxalate stones. Foods high in oxalic acid such as spinach, rhubarb, endive, beets, green beans, sweet potato, swiss chard, collard, plums, all types of berries, nuts, tea, and cocoa are avoided. Plenty of fluids (3 to 4 liters) should be taken throughout the day to ensure a constantly high and diluted urine output.

Diet, phenylalanine-restricted. Diet restricting the intake of phenylalanine to approximately 15 to 25 mg/kg body weight, depending on the tolerance of amino acid and the age of the patient. Since natural protein foods contain about 5% phenylalanine, high-quality protein foods such as meats, fish, poultry, milk and milk products, and eggs are not allowed. The diet for infants consists of a special formula low in phenylalanine (e.g., Lofenalac and Phenyl-free). Controlled amounts of phenylalanine and low-protein foods like fruits, vegetables, and starches are gradually added as the child grows older. Phenylalanine restriction is usually continued until the age of 5 years or later, although there is no safe age when dietary restrictions can be discontinued. Cautious progression to a more normal diet later in life should be done, with frequent monitoring of blood phenylalanine levels maintained between 2 and 10 mg/dl.

Diet, phosphorus-restricted. Diet restricting the phosphorus intake to the minimal level. The intake of foods rich in phosphorus is limited. These include milk and milk products, legumes, fish, meat, leafy green vegetables, nuts, and whole-grain cereals. Calcium intake is also limited if the diet is prescribed for urinary calcium phosphate stones.

Diet, phytanic acid-restricted. Diet restricting the intake of phytanic acid and phytol, which are found in a wide variety of foods. Eliminated are rich sources of phytanic acid (primarily milk and dairy products) and phytol (primarily green vegetables, nuts, and legumes). The diet is prescribed for Refsum's disease.

Diet, potassium-free. Essentially a protein-free diet, since all foods except sugar and fat naturally contain potassium. Only butter soup, butter balls, hard candies, and *Controlyte* powder in potassium-free beverages (such as ginger ale, root beer, and Kool-Aid) are allowed in the diet. Foods with a negligible potassium content such as Popsicles, ice sherbet, cranberry juice, and gelatin may be given to lend variety to the diet.

Diet, potassium-restricted. Diet prescribed in hyperkalemia restricting potassium intake to 1500 to 2000 mg/day (37 to 50 mEq potassium), which is about half the average potassium content of a regular mixed diet. Since potassium is widely distributed in foods, its restriction also limits the intake of other essential nutrients, particularly protein and vitamins. Milk, meats, legumes, whole grains, leafy vegetables, and some fruits (bananas, prunes, melons, and citrus fruits) supply considerable amounts of potassium. Many other foods are supplementary sources. The diet thus requires careful planning and selection of foods.

Diet, protein modified. Diet that prescribes a specified level of protein or restricts the amount of a protein fraction or amino acid. An increase in protein intake is necessary in any of the following conditions: excessive metabolism of protein, as in fevers and hyperthyroidism; loss of protein from the body, as in severe burns and nephritis; failure of protein synthesis, as in liver disease; failure of protein absorption, as in sprue and celiac disease; and inadequate intake of protein, as in starvation and kwashiorkor. A reduction in protein intake is necessary whenever the body's ability to excrete waste products of protein metabolism is impaired, as in hepatic coma and acute glomerulonephritis. Restriction of a specific amino acid is called for in certain conditions, such as phenylketonuria and other inborn errors of amino acid metabolism. The suggested terminology for the different levels in protein content of the diet is listed below. See also *Diet, gluten-free; Diet, phenylalanine-restricted;* and *Diet, taurine-restricted.*

High-protein d. An allowance of 1.5 to 2.0 gm/kg protein for adults. Indicated in severe stress, depleted protein stores, hepatitis, and long bone fractures.

Liberal-protein d. A protein allowance of 1.2 to 1.4 gm/kg body weight or about 75 to 100 gm/day. A liberal protein intake is indicated in moderate stress, surgery, chronic obstructive pulmonary disease, and peritoneal dialysis.

Low-protein d. A protein allowance of 0.5 to 0.7 gm/kg/day for adults, but at least 40 gm/day. Indicated in chronic glomerulonephritis and chronic uremia. The protein in the diet is supplied by 1 egg, ½ cup of milk, 2 oz meat, 3 slices of bread or the equivalent, fruits, and low-protein vegetables. Additional calories are supplied by sugar and other sweets, fats, carbonated beverages, and baked products made from low-protein wheat starches.

Minimal-protein d. A protein allowance of 0.2 to 0.3 gm/kg or approximately 20 to 25 gm/day. It is prescribed for patients with acute renal failure, acute glomerulonephritis, and hepatic coma. The protein allowance is supplied by 1 egg, ½ cup of milk, 3 slices of bread or substitute, fruits, and low-protein vegetables. Extra calories are provided by liberal use of sugars, fat-rich foods, and protein-free starches. This dietary regimen will supply the essential amino acids for tissue synthesis; intake of nonessential amino acids is minimized. Because of their relatively greater content of nonessential amino acids in comparison with egg and milk proteins, meat, fish, and poultry are not recommended at this low level of protein intake.

Normal-protein d. A protein allowance of 0.8 to 1.0 gm/kg/day or about 50 to 65 gm/day for adults. Higher protein allowances are required during pregnancy, lactation, and growth periods, which may range from 1.5 to 2.0 gm/kg body weight.

Protein-free d. This diet permits no choice of food since even fruits and fruit juices contain small amounts of protein. A strict protein-free diet allows only sugar, fat, and carbonated beverages. Several commercial mixes for low-protein bread are available. The protein-free diet is prescribed when the kidney is unable to remove nitrogenous waste products from the blood, as in acute anuria, or when the liver is unable to convert blood ammonia to urea, as in hepatic coma.

Very-high-protein d. A protein allowance of 2.5 to 3.0 gm/kg/day for adults. Indicated for severe burns, severe sepsis, multiple fractures, and head injury. It is also prescribed for celiac disease and premature infants. Eggs, milk, cheese, meat, fish, and poultry are excellent protein sources of high biologic value. It is best to divide the protein allowance into three meals and three between-meal feedings.

SUGGESTED TERMINOLOGY	ALLOWANCE (gm/kg body weight)	APPROX. LEVEL (gm/day)
Protein free	0	0–5
Minimal protein	0.2–0.3	20–25
Low protein	0.5–0.7	30–40
Normal protein	0.8–1.0	50–65
Liberal protein	1.2–1.4	75–85
High protein	1.5–2.0	90–110
Very high protein	2.5–3.0	120–150

Diet, provocative. Allergy test diet containing the most allergenic foods, such as milk, egg, and wheat, unless the patient's history definitely contraindicates their use. If an allergy is due to food, some manifestations will show up within a week; otherwise, the allergy is due to a nonfood allergen.

Diet, prudent. Diet recommended by the American Heart Association for coronary heart disease (CHD). The general guidelines are as follows: reduce the amount of fat from the current 40% to less than 30%, with up to 10% polyunsaturated fatty acids, 10 to 15% monounsaturated fats, and saturated fats not exceeding 10% of the total kcal/day intake. Choose margarines made from liquid vegetable oils and salad dressings made with oils high in linoleic acid. Limit cholesterol intake to no more than 300 mg/day. Egg consumption should not exceed three per week for adults and four to six per week for children. Limit low-fat milk to 2 cups, include 1 oz of hard cheese (as a substitute for 2 oz of lean meat), and limit portion sizes to 2 or 3 oz of cooked lean meat, poultry, and fish twice a day. Increase carbohydrate intake to 55 to 60% of the total calories/day, including one or more whole grain breads, cereals, rice, oats, pasta, dried beans, and other legumes in each meal. Include at least four servings per day with as many fresh fruits and vegetables as possible to provide more fiber, vitamins (especially A and C), and other nutrients. Limit the use of refined sugar, salt, coffee, and alcohol. Combine foods to achieve the lowest cholesterol/saturated-fat index (CSI) possible.

Diet, pureed. Also called the "blenderized diet"; consists of a normal variety of foods that have been strained or put in a blender or osterizer. It is indicated for patients who have difficulty in chewing and/or swallowing, as in cases of stroke, neurologic disorders, jaw wiring, and oral surgery. Liquids may be added to achieve the desired consistency. Some individuals may need a pureed diet thinned in order to be fed via a straw or syringe; others may need a thicker consistency that will form a bolus or not break apart in the mouth. Use milk, cream, fruit and vegetable juices, broth, gravies, and sauces to enhance the flavor and nutrient value. The addition of butter or margarine, sugars, powdered milk, and grated cheese will provide extra calories and protein.

Diet, purine-restricted. Diet restricting the daily intake of purine to approximately 120 to 150 mg compared to a normal intake of 600 to 1000 mg/day. The diet is prescribed as an adjunct to drug therapy for gout and other disorders affecting purine metabolism; it is designed to lower the uric acid level in the body. Good food sources of purine such as liver and glandular organs, anchovies, sardines, and meat extractives are excluded from the diet. Moderate purine sources like fish and seafoods, meats, fowl, beans, peas, asparagus, mushrooms, cauliflower, and spinach are restricted, depending on the patient's condition. These foods are not allowed during acute gouty attacks. A 2-oz portion is permitted when the acute stage subsides, and two moderate servings per day may be taken in chronic conditions. Foods that are essentially free of purines may be taken as desired. These include breads and cereals, milk and milk products, eggs, fruits, vegetables (except those previously listed), sugars and other sweets, and beverages, except for alcohol which should be taken only in moderation. Encourage liberal fluid intake (2 to 3 liters/day) to dilute the urine and to promote uric acid excretion.

Diet, reducing. Low-calorie diet designed to reduce weight. The amount of caloric reduction from the normal intake varies, depending on the rate at which one expects to lose weight. Ideally, this should be about ½ to 1 lb/week, although a greater reduction in weight is necessary in extremely obese individuals. Reducing the number of calories from the normal intake by 3500 kcal/week or 500 kcal/day would theoretically reduce body weight by 1 lb/week. Several reducing regimens have been proposed, ranging from starvation diets to nibbling and from formula diets to calculated food intake. In order to be effective, a reducing diet must be nutritionally adequate (except for calories), acceptable to the patient, compatible with the food pattern to which the patient is accustomed, economically feasible, palatable, varied, and capable of providing a sense of well-being. Common types of reducing diets are a low-carbohydrate diet (reduction in total carbohydrate intake, both sugar and complex carbohydrates); a low-carbohydrate, high-protein, high-fat diet (high fat content risks increasing the serum cholesterol, high protein aggravates any kidney disorder, and vitamin B deficiency may develop if diet is prolonged); low-carbohydrate, limited-fat, limited-cholesterol diet (attempts to prevent an increase in serum cholesterol); a high-fat diet (high fat intake leads to atherosclerosis; fatigue and lassitude may occur); and a high-carbohydrate, low-fat, low-cholesterol, high-fiber diet (an increased intake of complex carbohydrates and vegetables, with limited intake of meat, refined sugar, and processed foods, is difficult to follow for prolonged periods). See also *Diet, calorie-restricted.*

Diet, regular. Also called "general," "house," or "full hospital diet"; it is a normal diet planned to provide the recommended daily allowances for essential nutrients but designed to meet the caloric needs of a bedridden or ambulatory patient whose condition does not require any dietary modification for therapeutic purposes. It also serves as a basis for the modification of therapeutic diets in the hospital. While there is no restriction as to the amounts and type of foods allowed, the diet calls for careful planning of menus, wise selection and proper preparation of foods, and attractive service so that it will appeal to patients with relatively poor appetites.

Diet, residue-modified. Diet that limits or eliminates the intake of foods that leave a high amount of residue in the colon. Foods with decreasing amounts of residue are carbohydrates with indigestible material, digestible carbohydrates, milk, fats, and protein.

Low-residue d. Diet often prescribed in the treatment of diarrhea and diseases involving the bowel, particularly in association with obstruction, distention, edema, and inflammation. A diet low in residue is desirable in these conditions, where the presence of bulky fecal masses would strain the colon. Foods recommended are fish, tender cuts of meat, chicken, hard-cooked egg, liver, gelatin, refined cereals, and nonfibrous cooked or canned fruits and vegetables. Limit milk and milk products to 2 cups/day. For lactose intolerance, see *Diet, lactose-restricted.*

Minimal-residue d. Diet designed to leave the least amount of residue in the lower bowel after digestion and absorption have taken place proximally. The diet is indicated prior to and following intestinal surgery, particularly of the colon, and during radiation therapy of the pelvic area. It may also be used initially during the acute stage of diarrhea, ileitis, colitis, and diverticulitis. Eliminated are milk, tough cuts of meat,

fish or poultry with skin, fibrous fruits and vegetables unless canned or cooked and strained, excessive fats, excessive sweets, spices, and condiments. As a substitute for milk, use a lactose-free, low-residue enteral product; several are commercially available. An elemental formula may be indicated during the acute stage of inflammatory bowel disease. See Appendix 39.

Diet, rotation. Series of meal plans for 4 to 5 days to test for relief from food allergies. These are modifications of Rinkel's rotary diversified diets, in which the foods are rotated rather than completely eliminating the suspected allergens.

Diet, routine hospital. Term referring to the *regular, soft,* and *liquid* diets commonly used in hospitals. They differ in the consistency and type of foods allowed.

Diet, Rowe's elimination. Series of four test diets for the diagnosis of food allergy. Each of the first three diets contains a cereal or a starch, one or two meats, a group of fruits and vegetables, and condiments and seasonings. The fourth diet consists only of milk, tapioca, and sugar. The patient is placed on each diet for a period of 1 week unless relief of symptoms is obtained. If the patient shows no improvement on any of the diets, the allergy is probably not caused by food.

Diet, salicylate-restricted. Diet recommended for some individuals who are sensitive to salicylates and develop urticaria (hives), itching, angioedema, and rhinitis or bronchial asthma after ingestion of aspirin or foods containing salicylate, such as apples, apricots, berries, cherries, currants, grapefruit, grapes, lemons, melons, nectarines, oranges, peaches, plums, prunes, raisins, cucumbers, green peppers, potatoes, tomatoes, and almonds.

Diet, serotonin test. Also called the "5-hydroxyindoleacetic acid (5-HIAA) test diet." Foods high in serotonin are eliminated from the diet 3 days prior to and during the urinary collection for the diagnosis of carcinoid tumors of the intestinal tract. These tumors produce excessive serotonin, which is metabolized and excreted in the urine as

5-HIAA. Intake of foods rich in serotonin alters the result of the test. Foods excluded are bananas, plantains, avocados, pineapples, passion fruit, plums, tomatoes, walnuts, eggplants, and vanilla.

Diet, sodium-restricted. Diet in which the sodium content is limited to a specified level, which may range from mild restriction to severe restriction. Sodium restriction is used primarily for the elimination, control, and prevention of edema accompanying congestive heart failure, cirrhosis of the liver, nephritis, nephrosis, toxemias of pregnancy, and adrenocorticotropic hormone therapy. It is also beneficial in the treatment of some cases of hypertension. Retention of sodium in the body requires retention of water to keep the sodium concentration of the fluid constant. As a consequence, edema or swelling of tissues results. The average American diet contains approximately 4 to 6 gm sodium (about 10 to 15 gm salt, or sodium chloride) per day. Sodium in the diet comes from two sources: sodium *naturally* present in foods and sodium *added* during cooking and food processing. Foods differ widely in their natural sodium content. In general, animal foods are relatively high in sodium; plant foods are generally low in sodium. Most of the sodium added to foods comes from table salt (or sodium chloride) and monosodium glutamate. The other forms of sodium commonly used in food processing are sodium bicarbonate, sodium citrate, sodium alginate, sodium benzoate, sodium hydroxide, and sodium sulfite. In addition, there is sodium in water and in some medicines.

3000 to 4000 mg sodium d. (130 to 175 mEq sodium). Also called "no added salt" diet (N.A.S. diet). The preferred name is "no extra salt" diet. It is essentially a normal diet with moderate use of salt in cooking. No additional (extra) salt or salty condiments is allowed at the table.

2000 to 3000 mg sodium d. (87 to 130 mEq sodium). Mild sodium restriction. A small amount of salt is allowed during cooking. No further addition of salt or salty condiments is allowed at the table. Foods extremely high in sodium, such as bacon, ham, salted crackers, and olives, are not allowed.

1000 to 1500 mg sodium d. (43 to 65 mEq sodium). Moderate sodium restriction. Foods are prepared without added salt or sodium compound, and no processed foods high in sodium are allowed. Up to 4 servings regular bread, 3 cups regular milk, and 7 oz unsalted meat or substitute are allowed.

500 mg sodium d. (22 mEq sodium). Strict sodium restriction. It restricts the intake of foods naturally high in sodium content, such as meat, fish, eggs, milk, and vegetables high in sodium (i.e., beets, carrots, celery, and spinach). Prepared foods with added salt are not allowed. The diet thus requires the use of unsalted bread, unsalted butter, and other low-sodium dietetic foods. Regular milk is limited to 2 cups/day; unsalted meats are limited to 6 oz/day.

250 mg sodium d. (11 mEq sodium). Lowest level of sodium restriction prescribed for the acutely ill patient. At this level of sodium restriction, the intake of meats is limited to 5 oz/day and low-sodium milk is substituted for regular milk. Only those foods low in natural sodium content are allowed. The diet is therefore unpalatable and monotonous. This severely restricted sodium diet is seldom prescribed now because of available drug therapy.

Diet, soft. Diet consisting of foods that are soft in texture, easily digested, without any harsh or coarse fibers, and prepared simply and not highly seasoned. Foods generally included are milk and dairy products; eggs, tender cooked meat, fish, and poultry; well-cooked vegetables; crisp lettuce and salad tomatoes; cooked or canned fruits; bananas and citrus sections; whole-grain or enriched breads and cereals; plain desserts; all beverages; and other foods as tolerated. The soft diet is traditionally used as a progression from the *full liquid* to a *regular* diet after surgery, although it has no proven physiologic advantage over the regular diet. Smaller but more frequent feedings might be better tolerated by patients who are still unable to handle all the foods on the regular diet served in three meals.

Diet, space. Bulk-free diet designed for the use of astronauts in space travel. It requires little or no digestion and supplies calories and other nutritional requirements. Foods developed for space travel must conform to weight and volume restrictions and must be protected against chemical and biological deterioration. Freeze-dried finger foods and beverage powders that easily rehydrate have been developed.

Diet, starch-restricted. Diet limiting the intake of starch from bread, cereals, cereal products, and root crops. It is prescribed in cases of starch intolerance due to lack of pancreatic amylase. Foods allowed are milk, eggs, meats, fruits, and vegetables low in starch content. Carbohydrate in the diet is obtained from sugar, syrups, sweets, fruits, and enzymatically hydrolyzed malted starches like dextrimaltose and glucose polymers.

Diet, starvation. Calorie-free diet designated to effect rapid weight reduction in a short period of time. Vitamin supplements are given to meet specific nutrient requirements, and water intake is liberal to prevent dehydration. Weight loss of 4 to 8 lb/day in the early days of starvation is not rare. How long one should stay on this diet depends on several factors. Since severe complications may develop, starvation or fasting as a treatment for extreme obesity should be done in a hospital under strict medical supervision. With fat loss, the individual also loses nitrogen. No method has been successful in losing fat without losing some nitrogen. See also *Nutrition, starvation.*

Diet, sucrose-restricted. Diet that limits the intake of sucrose because of intolerance to this disaccharide. All forms of sucrose are excluded, such as table sugar, jellies, jams, marmalades, preserves, corn syrup, maple syrup, other syrups, sweetened condensed milk, and other foods with added sugar and sorbitol. Most fruits, except for berries, lemons, and grapes, contain sucrose and are given in limited amounts. Vegetables high in sucrose content, such as beets, green peas, sweet potatoes, navy beans, and soybeans, are also restricted. Cereals, milk, eggs, meat, fish poultry, and vegetables low in sucrose are allowed in normal amounts.

Diet, supraglottic. Diet prescribed for patients with difficulty in swallowing even liquids. Thin liquids are usually more difficult to swallow without aspirating or spilling into the laryngeal inlet, as compared to thick liquids and semisolid foods that form a cohesive bolus. *Dietary management:* provide smooth, moist, blenderized foods to facilitate swallowing. These include mashed potatoes with gravy and cereals of medium consistency such as oatmeal. Give puddings, custards, solid ice cream, and milkshakes. For fruits, bananas, pureed apples, and strained pears are recommended. Finely chopped meats with large amounts of gravy or egg salad with mayonnaise should be considered.

Diet, synthetic. Diet used for the diagnosis of food allergy. It contains amino acids, sugar, water, vitamin concentrates, salt mixtures, and sometimes emulsified fats. The mixture is given orally or by tube feeding. Persons who are allergic to food should show marked improvement with the synthetic diet; those who are allergic to substances other than food do not show any relief of symptoms. If allergy to food is ascertained, other foods may be added to the synthetic diet to determine which ones are allergenic.

Diet, taurine-restricted. Protein-modified diet prescribed for the treatment of psoriasis. Certain high-protein foods are entirely eliminated; others are restricted as to amounts allowed per day. The daily food intake should not exceed ½ to 1 can evaporated milk diluted with an equal amount of water, 3 oz chicken, turkey, beef, or veal, and ½ cup cottage cheese or 1 slice American or Swiss cheese. Fruits, vegetables, fats, sugars, and breads may be taken as desired. Foods that are to be avoided are eggs and dishes containing eggs, pasteurized and homogenized milk, ice cream, fish, cold cuts, organ meats, meat extractives, meat gravies, soups, and broths.

Diet, therapeutic. A normal diet adapted or modified to suit specific disease conditions; one designed to treat or cure diseases. See *Diet, modified.*

Diet therapy. The branch of dietetics that is concerned with the use of food for therapeutic purposes. Its goals are to maintain good nutritional status, correct deficiencies that may have occurred, afford rest to the whole body or to certain organs that may be affected by disease, adjust the food intake to the body's ability to metabolize the nutrients, and bring about changes in body weight whenever necessary. A therapeutic diet is planned on the basis of a normal or regular diet, with amounts of nutrients adjusted to meet the requirements imposed by disease or injury; essential nutrients should be provided as generously as the limitation of the diet allows. The diet must be flexible and adapted to the patient's food preferences, eating habits, economic status, religious beliefs, and social customs. Foods included should be acceptable to the patient and should emphasize natural and commonly used items that are available and easily prepared at home. A correctly planned diet is successful only if the food is eaten.

Diet, tyramine-restricted. Diet eliminating the intake of foods containing high amounts of tyramine. It is prescribed for patients receiving monoamine oxidase (MAO) inhibitory drugs in order to prevent a sudden hypertensive reaction to the amine. Foods with high tyramine content are alcoholic beverages such as ale, beer, liqueurs, and red wines like burgundy, Chianti, sherry, sauterne, and vermouth; caviar; aged and processed cheeses; pickled herring and salted dried fish; dry and fermented sausages like salami, pepperoni, bologna, and corned beef; broad beans, lima beans, lentils, snow peas, and soybeans; liver; meat extracts; brewer's yeast; and soy sauce in large amounts.

Diet, vegetarian. See *Vegetarian.*

Diet, VMA test. Diet given 3 days before and during the urinary collection for vanillylmandelic acid (VMA) to diagnose pheochromocytoma in persons with unexplained hypertension. Foods that give rise to phenoxy acid in the urine and give false-positive results are restricted. These include banana, pineapple, orange, cheese, nuts, chocolate, coffee, tea, and foods containing vanilla extract. (Newer test procedures, such as urinary metanephrine measurement, do not require any dietary restriction.)

Diet, wheat-oat-rye-barley-free. See *Diet, gluten-free.*

Diet, Zen macrobiotic. Diet based on the belief that one's health and happiness depend on a proper balance between the "ying" and "yang" foods. The macrobiotic dietary pattern progresses in ten stages; eliminates desserts, fruits and salads, animal foods, soup, and vegetables, in that order; and replaces these with increasing amounts of cereal grains. The highest stage contains 100% cereals. All dietary stages encourage the restriction of fluid intake.

Dietary allowances. See *Recommended dietary allowances.*

Dietary counseling. Process of providing individualized professional guidance to assist persons in adjusting their daily food consumption to meet their health needs. Success in dietary counseling depends on the dietitian's ability to explain scientific details in the simplest language, considering the patient's background, socioeconomic needs, and personal preferences.

Dietary fiber. See under *Fiber.*

Dietary history. Dietary study method used in evaluating or assessing the dietary intakes of individuals. It is taken by 24-hour recall or repeated food records to provide information on the subject's past and present dietary habits, food likes and dislikes, usual food pattern, and type of meals normally eaten over a relatively long period of time. The dietary history is useful in food habit studies and furnishes data for classifying individuals into certain groups. See also *Dietary study.*

Dietary requirement. Minimum amount of a specific nutrient that is needed by the body to attain a specified state of health. Unlike the *recommended dietary allowance*, it has no added margin of safety and is stated for *definite* (not average) conditions of age, weight, activity, and food intake, as well as physiologic status and pathologic state. There is variability and lack of precision in the assessment of nutritional requirements for different nutrients. For this reason, the *minimum daily requirements* for certain nutrients are often stated as ranges, and average minimum dietary requirements should be considered only as close approximates and should not be interpreted as final and accurate.

Dietary standard. Quantitative summary or compilation of nutrient allowances or requirements for various groups of people. It is used to formulate and evaluate food intakes of large population groups; it also serves as a rationale or yardstick for planning adequate nutrition and scheduling agricultural production. The establishment of a dietary standard is not easy because of the lack of available information about certain nutrients, the wide range of individual variation in nutrient requirements, and the lack of agreement among authorities setting the standard. The nutrients included in the standard are those that are apt to be absent from or inadequate in the usual diet. Other nutrients, although required by the body, are not included in the tabulation. Either they are present in adequate amounts in the usual diet, or they are trace elements or vitamins for which there are insufficient data to serve as a basis for recommendation. Several countries have established dietary standards for their populations. One must recognize the philosophy behind the standard set in each country and must distinguish carefully between the use of such terms as "standard," "requirement," and "allowance" in the interpretation for purposes of comparison or evaluation. See Appendices 1 and 4.

Dietary study (survey). Method of determining or evaluating the dietary intake of an individual, group, or population. The adequacy of a given diet is determined by *qualitative* comparison with the basic food groups or by *quantitative* comparison with the recommended dietary standard of a particular country. A dietary study is used to detect the adequacy or inadequacy of diets in order to give valuable information concerning food habits, menu preparation, and food procurement, availability, and distribution. See also *Nutritional assessment.*

Dietary study, methodology. There are several methods of obtaining dietary information. These are generally classified into those applicable to individuals and those applicable to groups. Methods applicable to individuals include *estimation by recall,* with the subject or food provider for the subject recalling the food intake of the previous 24 hours or longer; the *food intake record,* which is a listing of all foods eaten (including between-meal intakes) for varying lengths of time, usually 3 to 7 days; the *dietary history* taken by recall, repeated food records, or both to discover the usual food pattern over relatively long periods of time; and the *weighed food intake* of subject taken by a trained person, a parent of the subject, or the subject personally. Methods applicable to groups include a *food account* or running reports of foods purchased or produced for household use; a *food list* or recall of estimated amounts of various foods consumed during a previous period, usually the past 7 days; and a *food record* or weighed inventory of foods at the beginning and end of the study, with or without records of kitchen and plate wastes.

Dietetic foods. Processed foods for therapeutic purposes. In the United States, a wide array of dietetic foods are commercially available. The most common are products containing nonnutritive (artificial) sweeteners such as low-calorie soft drinks, canned fruits and juices, puddings and gelatin desserts, confectionery, and baked goods. Other dietetic foods are labeled, e.g., "diabetic" foods; low-sodium products marked with the phrase "no salt added"; and products marked with the phrase "no fat or oil added." See also *Food labeling* and *Nutritional labeling.*

Dietetics. Combined science and art of regulating the planning, preparing, and serving of meals to individuals or groups under *various conditions of health and disease* according to the principles of nutrition and management, with due consideration for economic, social, cultural, and psychologic factors. The science consists of knowledge of nutrition, food, and the dietary constituents needed in different states of health and disease. The art consists of knowledge of the practical planning and preparation of meals at various economic levels, as well as attractive and pleasing service of food so that an individual, well or ill, will be encouraged to eat the food and adhere to the diet.

Dietetic technician. An individual specially trained in the areas of food and nutrition; a member of the food service or health care team under the supervision of a *dietitian.* This individual must have completed a combination of academic preparation and supervised practice with an associate degree from an accredited U.S. institution that sponsors an American Dietetic Association-approved program.

Dietitian. A professional trained to be a nutrition expert, i.e., to assist and educate individuals to improve their quality of life by eating the right kind and amount of food in health and disease. A registered dietitian (RD), to practice in the United States, must have earned a baccalaureate degree in college and must have completed 900 hours of supervised professional practice, after which an American Dietetic Association-developed and -monitored national examination must be passed. The institution that offers the undergraduate program, as well as the sites for the practical experiences, should be accredited by the American Dietetic Association. To maintain the RD status, 75 hours of approved continuing education must be completed every 5 years.

Diffusion. Redistribution of material by random movement; spreading out. *Simple diffusion* is movement of solutes from higher to lower concentration. *Facilitated diffusion* is carrier-mediated movement of solutes down their electrochemical potential, but the rate of movement is faster than can be accounted for by simple diffusion.

Diflunisal. A nonsteroidal anti-inflammatory agent used for relief of pain and inflammatory diseases; a derivative of salicylic acid. It imposes a risk of gastrointestinal blood loss leading to anemia; it may also cause gastric ulceration, stomatitis, dyspepsia, anorexia, nausea, and vomiting. The brand name is Dolobid.

Digestibility. Extent to which a foodstuff is digested and absorbed from the digestive tract and not excreted in the feces. The fecal residue excreted is primarily indigestible materials, secretions, linings shed from the digestive tract, and microoganisms with their end products.

   Apparent d. Measure of the difference between food intake and output in the feces, without consideration of fecal excretion not due to food eaten.

   True d. Measure of the difference between food intake and fecal output, with allowances for linings shed from the intestinal tract, bacteria, and residues of digestive juices that are not part of indigestible food fecal output.

Digestion. The mechanical and chemical breakdown of complex substances into their constituent parts; the conversion of food into smaller and simpler units that can be absorbed by the body. See Appendix 11.

Digoxin. A cardiac glycoside obtained from the leaves of *Digitalis lanata;* used in the treatment of congestive heart failure. Low body potassium causes increased levels of digoxin in the myocardium and potential toxicity; ensure a high potassium intake, especially if digoxin is taken with a potassium-wasting diuretic. Digoxin may increase urinary excretion of calcium, magnesium, and potassium; it may also cause anorexia, nausea, and vomiting. Brand names are Lanoxin and Lanoxicap.

Dihydroxyacetone. A ketotriose derivable from glycerol or glucose. As dihydroxyacetone phosphate, it is produced in the splitting of fructose-1,6-diphosphate by the enzyme aldolase during the anaerobic metabolism of glycogen.

1,25-Dihydroxycholecalciferol. Also called "calcitriol" and "calcifetriol." It is the active form of vitamin D in humans; it is a steroid derivative made by the combined action of the skin, liver, and kidneys. See *Vitamin D.*

Diose. Glycolic aldehyde; the simplest monosaccharide, containing only two carbon atoms.

Diphenoxylate. A synthetic narcotic used in the management of diarrhea. It may cause abdominal pain, distention, dry mouth, nausea, and vomiting, when taken in large amounts. Brand names are Clonil, Lomotil, Diphenatol, Lomenate, Lofene, Logen, and Lonox.

Diphosphopyridine nucleotide (DPN). See *Coenzymes I* and *II.*

Disaccharide. Sugar containing two monosaccharides joined in glycosidic linkage, with the elimination of a molecule of water. The most common are *lactose, maltose,* and *sucrose.*

Disaccharide intolerance. Inability to absorb certain disaccharides because of lack of certain specific disaccharidases, such as maltase, lactase, sucrase, and isomaltase. The condition may also be acquired from secondary surgical operations, infectious enteropathies, celiac disease, and other malabsorption states. Diarrhea is the principal symptom. Other clinical features include flatulence, abdominal pain, vomiting, and excretion of large amounts of volatile fatty acids. *Dietary management:* exclusion of the poorly tolerated disaccharide from the diet results in disappearance of symptoms. Replace it with utilizable carbohydrate. The deficiency of the deficient enzyme is apparently compensated for in later years. See *Diet, lactose-restricted; Diet, maltose-restricted;* and *Diet, sucrose-restricted.*

Disaster feeding. See *Emergency feeding.*

Diverticula. Herniations or outpouchings of the mucous membrane through gaps or weak spots in the circular muscle of the colon. Diverticula may be single or multiple and occur most frequently in the distal descending portion of the colon. They are formed because of unusually high intraluminal colonic pressures. *Dietary management:* the main therapeutic goal is to increase the caliber of the stools and distend the bowel wall by increasing dietary fiber. A low-residue diet is not recommended, except during acute phases of diverticulitis, ulcerative colitis, or infectious enterocolitis when the bowel is markedly inflamed. At that time, clear liquids or an elemental diet may be given. The diet may gradually progress to a regular diet. However, it is still advisable to avoid excessive intake of raw fruits and vegetables which are laxative to the patient. Excessive intake of spices such as pepper and chili pepper should also be avoided. A bulk-forming agent such as methylcellulose is beneficial in initiating normal colonic function and regular bowel action.

Diverticulitis. Inflammatory condition of a diverticulum (or diverticula) characterized by nausea, vomiting, fever, abdominal tenderness, distention, pain, and intestinal spasm. The inflammatory process may eventually lead to intestinal obstruction or perforation, necessitating surgery. *Dietary management:* increase the intake of dietary fiber, such as by using breads made with 100% whole-wheat flour and fruits and vegetables rich in fiber. See *Diet, fiber-modified.*

Diverticulosis. This condition is characterized by many small mucosal sacs, called *diverticula,* protruding through the intestinal wall. It occurs mostly in the sigmoid colon but is also evident in the gastrointestinal tract. There is apparently a defect in the muscle layers of the sigmoid colon, causing the lumen to narrow and the intraluminal pressure to increase. *Dietary management:* see *Diverticula.*

DMF. Refers to the total number of decayed, missing, and filled teeth. It is often used in surveys to determine the amount of *dental caries* present in a community or given population. Teeth, however, may be missing for other reasons, including removal because of local custom.

DNA. Abbreviation for *deoxyribonucleic acid.*

D/N ratio. Abbreviation for dextrose/nitrogen ratio. See *Glucose/nitrogen ratio.*

DOPA. 3,4-Dihydroxyphenylalanine, an intermediate product in the formation of *melanin,* ephinephrine, and norepinephrine from tyrosine. Used in the treatment of Parkinson's disease.

Dopamine. 3,4-dihydroxyphenylethylamine, an intermediate product in tyrosine metabolism and the precursor of norepinephrine and epinephrine. It is present in the central nervous system and is localized in the basal ganglia.

Down's syndrome (mongolism). Children suffering from this congenital defect are usually short and overweight, with signs of mental retardation. The condition is caused by trisomy of chromosome 21, directly correlated with the age of the mothers. *Dietary management:* aided feeding is obviously required to ensure increased intake and nutritional balance. Monitor the caloric level to avoid weight gain. Give a liberal protein intake and supplement the diet with vitamins and minerals, particularly vitamins A, B$_6$, and C.

Doxepin. A tricyclic antidepressant used for the treatment of depression. It may cause altered taste acuity, anorexia, and weight loss, as well as nausea, vomiting, diarrhea, and stomatitis. Brand names are Adapin and Sinequan.

Doxorubicin. An antineoplastic antibiotic used for the treatment of tumors, including breast and ovarian carcinomas. It causes nausea and vomiting on the day of therapy, which can be severe. Stomatitis and esophagitis may occur, especially if doxorubicin is administered daily for several days; stomatitis usually begins with a burning sensation, accompanied by erythema of the oral mucosa, and in 2 to 3 days may progress to ulceration which is sometimes severe enough to result in difficulty in swallowing. The anorexia and reduced food intake may cause weight loss. The brand name is Adriamycin.

DPN. Abbreviation for diphosphopyridine nucleotide. See *Coenzyme I* under *Coenzymes I* and *II.*

Dulcin. Nonnutritive sweetening agent 250 times as sweet as sugar. Not approved for food use in the United States but permitted in some European countries. Also called Sucrol and Valzin.

Dumping syndrome. A gastrointestinal disorder characterized by physical signs that develop when the stomach contents are emptied into the jejunum at an abnormally fast rate. Symptoms include nausea, vomiting, weakness, syncope, and diarrhea. See *Gastrectomy.*

Dynamic state. Continuous metabolism or turnover (i.e., synthesis, degradation, and replacement) of body constituents even at constant composition; a state of flux.

Dysgeusia. Taste perversion associated with a generalized decrease in taste acuity. This is a common complaint of cancer patients whose decreased appetite is partly due to dysgeusia, directly causing weight loss. One way to diminish this problem is to let the patients eat foods they like before chemotherapy. Taste acuity is also affected by drugs such as phenytoin, potassium chloride, lincomycin, antilipemics, and digoxin.

Dyspepsia. Gastric indigestion; a wide variety of complaints referable to the upper gastrointestinal tract following the ingestion of food. Typical symptoms are heartburn, nausea, epigastric pain, abdominal discomfort, belching, distention, and flatulence. It may be the result of an organic disease of the gastrointestinal tract, such as esophagitis, gastritis, or peptic ulcer, or it may be functional in nature and occur in the absence of any demonstrable organic lesion. Dyspepsia is also due to rapid eating, inadequate chewing, swallowing of air, or emotional stress. *Dietary management:* no simple dietary rule can be set down. Foods should be adequate, well cooked, not too spicy, and served in a relaxed atmosphere. It is best to eat small meals. In the majority of cases, dyspepsia is of nervous origin and disappears once the psychoneurotic cause is removed. If it is due to organic causes, a soft diet low in fat may be beneficial.

Dysphagia. Difficulty in swallowing. This disturbance in transferring food from the oral cavity to the stomach may result in aspiration if food enters the respiratory tract below the level of the true vocal cords. Either the stricture should be dilated or its cause removed. *Dietary management:* include flavorful, aromatic foods to stimulate swallowing. Some foods should be finely chopped, diced, well cooked, and soft, although semisolids can form a cohesive bolus. Caution should be exercised with liquids, since they may spill into the pharynx. See also *Diet, dysphagia.*

Dyssebacia. Disorder of the sebaceous follicles; plugging of the sebaceous glands. Nasolabial dyssebacia (seborrhea) is often seen in *riboflavin* deficiency. It is characterized by the appearance of enlarged follicles around the sides of the nose which may extend over the cheeks and forehead. The follicles are plugged with dry sebaceous material which often has a yellow color.

E

EAA. Abbreviation for *essential amino acid.*

Eating disorder. Collective term for anorexia nervosa, bulimia, bulimarexia, and compulsive eating. Basically, these are emotional disorders: anorexia is compulsive self-starvation with extreme fear of weight gain, resulting in 25% or more body weight loss; bulimia is compulsive binging, eating up to 10,000 kcal in 8 hours, and then purging by forced vomiting. About half of anorexics are also bulimics, hence the coined term "bulimarexia." The health risks of these eating disorders include malnutrition, osteoporosis, menstrual cycle shutdown, heart problems with dangerously low blood pressure, circulatory collapse, and cardiac arrest in the advanced stage. Behavioral problems include depression, lack of self-esteem, suicidal tendencies, impulsiveness, and inability to cope with problems, especially family relationships. Compulsive eating is the consumption of abnormally large amounts of food, possibly caused by psychologic factors, leading to *obesity.* Compulsive eaters respond more readily to external cues than to internal factors that control appetite. See *Anorexia, Bulimia, Bulimarexia,* and *Nutrition, weight control.*

Eclampsia. See *Pregnancy-induced hypertension.*

Edema. Presence of an abnormally large amount of fluid in the tissue spaces of the body due to a disturbance in the mechanisms involved in fluid exchange. Factors that tend to increase the volume of interstitial fluid include reduction in plasma osmotic pressure, rise in capillary blood pressure, increase in permeability of the capillary membrane, and obstruction of the lymph channels. Edema is seen in congestive heart failure, nephrotic syndrome, cirrhosis, and idiopathic edema. It is also seen in association with malnutrition, such as in beriberi, protein deficiency, and chronic starvation. Hypoalbuminemia is a major factor in the production of edema in patients with hepatic cirrhosis and nephrotic syndrome. Edema observed in burns is due to loss of plasma proteins and increased capillary permeability. *Dietary management:* depending on the cause of the edematous condition, protein, fluid, and/or electrolyte intakes are modified. Fluid retention is relieved with sodium restriction and increased potassium intake. Since edema is a sign of a disease or disorder, refer to the nutritional modifications for a particular disease for further details on dietary guidelines.

EFA. Abbreviation for *essential fatty acid.*

EFAD. Abbreviation for *European Federation of the Associations of Dietitians.*

EFNEP. Abbreviation for *Expanded Food and Nutrition Education Program.*

Egg white injury. Condition characterized by exfoliative dermatitis, muscle pains, anorexia, and emaciation as a result of prolonged, excessive intake of raw egg white. This is actually a *biotin* deficiency caused by the presence of *avidin* in raw egg white, which combines with biotin, rendering it unavailable for use. Cooking the egg destroys avidin. Biotin deficiency can be produced by eating abnormally large amounts of raw egg whites for a long time.

Eicosanoic acid. A fatty acid with 20 carbons in its straight chain. An example is arachidic acid, found in butter, peanut oil, and other fats.

Eicosanoids. Hormonelike compounds synthesized from polyunsaturated fatty acids. Examples are leukotrienes, prostaglandins, and thromboxanes.

Eicosapentaenoic acid (EPA). An omega-3 fatty acid with 20 carbons in its chain and five double bonds; the first double bond is found between carbon atoms 3 and 4, counting from the CH3— end. Fish oils are rich sources of EPA.

Elastin. An albuminoid, the characteristic protein of yellow elastic fibers abundant in ligaments, lung matrix, and blood vessel walls.

Electrolyte balance. Condition of electroneutrality in the body: the number of positively charged ions equals the number of negatively charged ions. Compensating shifts and losses/gains occur biochemically to maintain electrolyte balance. Electrolytes regulate water balance in the body. Failure to maintain the proper kind and amount of fluid in body compartments, i.e., fluid and electrolyte imbalance, is a medical problem. A typical electrolyte balance of cations and anions in the body fluids is as follows:

INTRACELLULAR FLUID (ICF) (mEq/liter)		EXTRACELLULAR FLUID (ECF) (mEq/liter)	
Na^+	35	Na^+	142
K^+	123	K^+	5
Ca^{++}	15	Ca^{++}	5
Mg^{++}	2	Mg^{++}	3
	175		155
Cl^-	5	Cl^-	104
$HPO_4^=$	80	$HPO_4^=$	2
$SO_4^=$	10	$SO_4^=$	1
Protein	70	Protein	16
HCO_3^-	10	HCO_3^-	27
	175	Organic acids	5
			155

The principal cation in the plasma and interstitial fluids is sodium, and the principal anion is chloride. In the intracellular fluid, the principal cation is potassium and the main anion is phosphate. The electrolytes, particularly Na^+ and K^+ ions, control the amount of water in the body compartments. Chloride (Cl^-), which is the main anion in the ECF, is the "balancer" for sodium: phosphate ion ($HPO_4^=$) is the main anion in the ICF. There is a larger concentration of protein in the blood plasma than in the interstitial fluid. If body water is decreased, serum electrolytes will be

increased. Water can move freely across cell membranes, but salts cannot. *Osmotic pressure* moves water from one side of the semipermeable membrane consisting of a dilute solution to the other side of a strong solution. When water in the cell is lost due to hypertonicity of the surrounding ECF, this is designated as *hypertonic dehydration*. When water in the cell is increased due to decreased solutes (hence, decreased osmotic pressure), this results in *hypotonic dehydration*, which causes reduced blood volume. Cellular edema occurs, and renal blood flow is impaired. Clinically, dehydration is a loss of both water and electrolytes. See also *Water balance*.

Emaciation. Extreme leanness; wasting away of body flesh.

Emergency feeding. Also called disaster feeding. Consideration of feeding in times of disaster, either natural or man-made (e.g., earthquake, flood, fire, volcanic eruption, or war). The first concern is to allay hunger and maintain morale. Problems such as lack of water, electricity, and cooking and refrigeration facilities must be considered. Canned and ready-to-eat packaged foods, which include instant powdered milk and other beverages, must be provided. This is especially important after a nuclear attack to avoid the hazards of radioactive contamination of food and drink. When an emergency is of more than a few days' duration, meeting nutritional needs must be considered. Health care facilities, as well as homes, must be prepared for disaster feeding, including not only food and water reserves but also fuel sources like charcoal and wood, a lighter or matches, disposable plates, cups, spoons and forks, and paper supplies, sanitary garbage disposal, manual can openers, etc.

Emphysema. Abnormal presence of air or gas in the body tissues or overdistention of air spaces in the lungs due to rupture of the pulmonary alveoli. May be caused by respiratory infections or air pollution. Characterized by labored breathing with wheezing and chronic cough. Dyspnea and fatigue are accentuated if the patient is obese.

Dietary management: because of the shortness of breath, the patient frequently does not eat enough and finds it difficult to chew and swallow. A soft diet high in nutrient density should be given in small, frequent feedings. Provide high-protein supplements for snacks to correct any tissue wasting. See also *Chronic obstructive pulmonary disease.*

"Empty" calories. Refers to carbohydrate-rich foods such as sugars, syrups, jellies, and other sweets that contribute mainly calories, with either no or insignificant amounts of the other nutrients. See also *Junk food.*

Emulsification. Process of lowering surface tension or breaking up large particles of an immiscible liquid into smaller ones that remain suspended in another liquid. An agent that has this ability is called an emulsifier, e.g., bile salts and lecithin. Emulsification of fat by the action of bile salts facilitates its digestion.

Enalapril. An angiotensin-converting enzyme inhibitor used in the management of hypertension. It may cause loss of taste perception, dry mouth, anorexia, and gastritis; it may also cause hypoalbuminemia and hyperkalemia. Brand names are Vasotec and Vaseretic.

Encephalomyelitis. Inflammation of the brain and spinal cord; characterized by fever; head, neck, and back pains; and nausea and vomiting. Depending on the extent of the damage to the central nervous system, more serious manifestations include personality changes, seizures, paralysis, coma, and even death. *Dietary management:* feeding problems are related to symptoms like fever, nausea and vomiting, and paralysis, which vary with each case. The ability to eat and swallow, self-feeding problems, loss of appetite, and reduced digestive processes need individualized monitoring. Enteral tube feeding is used for comatose patients whose gastrointestinal tract is functional.

Endemic. Prevalent in a particular region or locality. An endemic disease is one that has a low incidence but is more or less constantly present in a given population, e.g., endemic goiter.

Endergonic reaction. Reaction requiring an input or supply of energy to push the reaction; usually associated with anabolism.

Endocarditis. Acute or chronic inflammation of the inner lining of the heart and its valves. See *Carditis.*

Endocrine. Secreting internally or into the bloodstream. The *endocrine glands* are ductless glands producing internal secretions called "hormones" that are discharged directly into the bloodstream. These glands include the adrenals, thyroid, parathyroid, pituitary, gonads, pancreas, pineal gland, and thymus. The last gland is now classified as part of the lymphatic system. The endocrine system affects growth and development, digestion and metabolism, water and electrolyte balance, and many other vital processes in the body. See also *Hormone.*

Endogastritis. Inflammation of the mucous membrane of the stomach. See *Gastritis.*

Endogenous. Originating or coming from within or inside the cell or tissue.

Endopeptidase. Proteolytic enzyme that splits centrally located peptide bonds of protein. Examples are pepsin, trypsin, and chymotrypsin.

Endothermic. Chemical reaction requiring the uptake or absorption of heat.

End-stage renal disease (ESRD). The last phase of renal failure; when medical measures have been exhausted, renal *dialysis* or *kidney transplantation* may be considered. See also *Acute renal failure* and *Chronic renal failure.*

Energy. Capacity to do work. It exists in six forms: kinetic, potential, thermal, nuclear, radiant or solar, and chemical. Chemical energy in the human body is released by the metabolism of foods. Carbohydrates, fats, proteins, and alcohol are chemical sources of energy. Energy is needed by the body for muscular activity, to maintain body temperature, and to carry out metabolic processes. Energy comes from the oxidation of foods and is measured in terms of *calories* or *joules.* See *Basal metabolism; Food, energy value;* and *Metabolizable energy.* See also *Energy balance, Energy requirement,* and Appendix 15.

Energy balance. Also called caloric balance; the equilibrium between energy intake and energy output. When energy intake exceeds energy needs, the extra energy is stored, leading to an increase in body weight (positive balance). When energy intake is less than energy needs, the body utilizes its own reserves, resulting in loss of weight (negative energy balance). See *Nutrition, weight control.*

Energy measurement. The potential energy available in a food is measured directly by using a bomb calorimeter or indirectly by calculation using these values: 4 kcal/gm carbohydrate, 4 kcal/gm protein, 9 kcal/gm fat, and 7 kcal/gm alcohol. For dextrose, 3.4 kcal/gm is used. Energy values in foods and beverages as reported in food composition tables and the food exchange lists use these physiologic fuel values expressed in kcal or Calories. For measuring energy expenditures of the body, see under *Calorimetry.*

Energy requirement. For a normal adult, the energy needs are estimated by adding the resting energy expenditure (REE), plus the energy used for physical activity (PA), plus the thermal effect of food, formerly called "specific dynamic action of food (SDA)." The thermal effect of food is usually only 5 to 10% of total energy needs, and for practical purposes, some practitioners do not add this factor. Energy needs vary among individuals due to the effects of factors like age, body composition and size, genetic makeup, growth, lactation, pregnancy, nutritional status, and climate or environmental temperature. In certain pathologic conditions or disorders (e.g., endocrine abnormalities, fevers, infections, burns, trauma), energy requirements are altered. For details in calculating energy requirements in various conditions, see Appendix 24. Recommended dietary allowances (RDA) for energy are average values for groups of individuals according to age, sex, and physiologic state, as given in Appendix 1. See also *Basal metabolism, Nutrition, weight control,* and *Resting energy expenditure.*

Enfamil. Brand name of a milk formula for routine infant feeding; made of nonfat cow's milk, lactose, soy oil, and coconut oil. Provides 20 kcal/oz and is also available in 13 kcal/oz and 24 kcal/oz formulations, with or without iron. Enfamil Premature is a modified formula for premature infants with a limited intake or for infants recovering from illness with increased needs. See also Appendix 37.

Enrich. Brand name of a polymeric, lactose-free formula with fiber for oral or tube feeding; made of sodium and calcium caseinates, soy protein isolate, hydrolyzed cornstarch, sucrose, soy polysaccharide, and corn oil. Contains 13.6 gm fiber/liter. See Appendix 39.

Enrichment. 1. Addition of vitamins and minerals (thiamin, niacin, riboflavin, and iron) to flours and cereal products to restore those lost in milling and processing. Minimum and maximum levels for addition have been set. 2. In countries other than the United States, this refers to the addition of vitamins, minerals, amino acids, or protein concentrates to foods to improve their nutrient content. See *Fortification.*

Ensure. Brand name of a polymeric, lactose-free low-residue product for tube feeding or oral supplementation; made of calcium and sodium caseinates, soy protein isolates, corn syrup solids, sucrose, and corn oil. Also available in higher-nitrogen (Ensure HN), high-calorie (Ensure Plus), and high-calorie, high-nitrogen (Ensure Plus HN) formulas. See also Appendix 39.

Enteral nutrition. Ingestion of food by mouth or by means of a tube via the gastrointestional tract. Enteral nutrition products may be administered orally, via nasogastric tube, gastrostomy tube, or needle catheter jejunostomy. Enteral products may be *monomeric* or *oligomeric* (i.e., chemically defined formula made up of amino acids or short peptides and simple carbohydrates) or *polymeric* (i.e., more complex protein and carbohydrate sources) in composition. *Modular* supplements are used for individual supplementation of protein, carbohydrate, or fat when formulas do not offer sufficient flexibility. *Specialized* formulas are indicated for specific disease states, such as hepatic encephalopathy, renal failure, and trauma or high stress. Formulas for hepatic failure contain high concentrations of branched-chain amino acids (BCAA) and low concentrations of aromatic amino acids (AAA); formulas for renal failure contain only essential amino acids as the source of protein; and formulas for high stress and trauma contain high concentrations of BCAA but, unlike the hepatic products, are not restricted in the amount of AAA. See Appendix 39.

Enteric. Pertaining to the intestines.

Enteritis. Acute or chronic inflammation or irritation of the intestinal mucosa, chiefly the small intestine. It may result from overeating, food or chemical poisoning, ingestion of irritants, or bacterial or protozoan invasion. Often accompanied by diarrhea and abdominal pain. *Dietary management:* see *Gastritis.*

Enterocolitis. Inflammation of the small intestine and colon. *Dietary management:* monitor the ability to digest food, giving foods tolerated by the patient. As the condition improves, give a diet low in fiber and moderately restricted in fats to 25% of the total caloric needs. See also *Enteritis.*

Enterocrinin. Hormone produced by the intestinal mucosa that stimulates the glands of the small intestine to secrete digestive fluid.

Enterogastrone. Hormone produced by the duodenum stimulated by the ingestion of fat. It inhibits gastric secretion and motility.

Enterostomies. Term for tube placement, usually by a surgical procedure, for the purpose of delivering nutrient formulas for enteric feeding via the pharynx, cervical esophagus, stomach, or jejunum. See also *Gastrostomy, Jejunostomy,* and *Ostomy.*

Entralife. Brand name of lactose-free liquid supplement for oral feeding available in different flavors; contains whey protein concentrate and soy protein, hydrolyzed corn starch, sucrose, corn oil (70%), and MCT oil (30%). See also Appendix 39.

Entrition. Brand name of a tube feeding formula that is low in residue, lactose-free, and isotonic; contains sodium and calcium caseinates, maltodextrin, and corn oil. Also available in higher nitrogen content (Entrition HN) and as prefilled, ready-to-use EntriPak with an Entrition pouch closed system for enteral delivery. See also Appendix 39.

Enzyme. Organic catalyst produced by living cells that is responsible for most of the chemical reactions and energy transformation in both plants and animals. Many enzymes are simple proteins, often existing as inactive *proenzymes or zymogens;* other enzymes require, in addition to the protein molecule, another factor in order to exhibit full activity. This *cofactor* may be an inorganic element such as zinc, or it may be an organic molecule such as a vitamin or its derivative. Some enzymes are thus described in terms of their protein portion, or *apoenzyme,* and their cofactor portion is designated a *coenzyme, prosthetic group,* or *activator.*

Eosinophil. Type of white blood cell that has an affinity for a red-staining dye known as *eosin.* Under the microscope, such white cells are seen to contain many red grains. The normal eosinophil count ranges from 0.5 to 4% of the total number of leukocytes in 1 mm^3 of blood.

Epilepsy. Nervous disorder characterized by episodes of motor, sensory, or psychic dysfunction, with or without unconsciousness and/or convulsions. The most common episodes are *grand mal, Jacksonian, petit mal* and *psychomotor epilepsy. Dietary management:* a regular diet is sufficient for those who respond to drug therapy. Monitor the side effects of anticonvulsant drugs, especially those that interfere with vitamin D and the B complex. Some drugs cause gastric irritation and weight loss. If drug therapy is not effective, ketogenic diets could be beneficial. See *Diet, ketogenic.*

Epinephrine. Adrenaline, the major hormone of the adrenal medulla. It is secreted in response to stimulation of nerve fibers by a variety of factors, including fear, anger, pain, hypoglycemia, hemorrhage, muscular activity, and anesthetic drugs. Its action is varied, causing dilatation of the skeletal muscles as well as coronary and visceral vessels and resulting in *increased* blood flow in these regions, *constriction* of the capillaries of the skin and arterioles of the kidney, elevation of the respiratory quotient with an increase in oxygen consumption and carbon dioxide production, and acceleration of glycogenolysis with formation of glucose in the liver and lactic acid in the muscles. See also *Norepinephrine.*

Epithelium. Covering of the skin and internal mucous membrane lining the body cavities, including vessels and passages. It consists of cells joined by small amounts of cementing substances. See *Nutrition, dermatology.*

Ercalcidiol. New name for 25-hydroxyvitamin D_2, also known as "25-hydroxyergocalciferol." See *Vitamin D.*

Ercalciol. New name for ergocalciferol; vitamin D_2 or irradiated ergosterol. A compound that has vitamin D activity and that is obtained by ultraviolet irradiation of ergosterol.

Ercalcitriol. New name for 1,25-hydroxy vitamin D_2, also known as 1,25-hydroxyergocalciferol. See *Vitamin D.*

Ergocalciferol. Also called ercalciol; irradiated ergosterol or vitamin D_2. Formerly called calciferol or viosterol. See *Vitamin D.*

Ergosterol. Provitamin D_2, a sterol found chiefly in yeasts and widely distributed in plants. See *Vitamin D.*

Erucic acid. *Monounsaturated fatty acid* containing 22 carbon atoms; found in rape seed, and other vegetable seed oils.

Erythrobic acid. D-Ascorbic acid, a form not utilized by humans to any appreciable extent. It is used as a meat preservative.

Erythrocuprein. A copper-containing protein found in the red blood cells. It contains two atoms of copper per mole and accounts for most, if not all, of the copper in the red blood cells.

Erythrocyte. Or red blood cell (RBC). The pigmented biconcave and nonnucleated cell that transports oxygen to the tissues. See *Hemoglobin* and Appendix 30.

Erythromycin. A broad-spectrum antibiotic effective against a wide variety of organisms, including gram-negative and gram-positive bacteria. Gastric acidity inactivates the drug, and the rate of drug absorption is decreased when given with food; it should not be taken with fruit juice or other acidic juices. Gastrointestinal side effects are dose-related. Abdominal pain and cramping occur frequently; nausea, vomiting, and diarrhea may also occur. Brand names are E-Mycin, Erythrocin, Ilosone, and Pediamycin.

Erythropoiesis. Formation or development of erythrocytes from the primitive cells to the mature erythrocytes. See *Hemopoiesis.*

Erythropoietin. Hormone produced by the kidney that stimulates the production of red blood cells. See *Hemopoiesis.*

ESADDI. Abbreviation for *estimated safe and adequate daily dietary intake.*

Esophageal cancer. A neoplastic disease usually affecting the middle or lower third of the esophagus; causative factors are prolonged, heavy smoking and alcohol consumption, achalasia, hiatal hernia, aflatoxins, and betel-nut chewing seen in some Asian and African regions. Symptoms include anorexia, weight loss, persistent coughing, dysphagia, anemia, dehydration, malnutrition, and general malaise. In advanced cases, there is vocal cord paralysis and hemoptysis. *Dietary management:* in the early stages when oral feeding is still adequate, provide a liberal intake of calories and protein in small, frequent feedings. MCT source are helpful in malabsorption cases, especially when esophageal resection has been done. In advanced stages when per os feeding is not sufficient to correct weight loss and malnutrition, or dysphagia has worsened, specialized nutrition support is provided with gastrostomy feeding or total parenteral nutrition.

Esophageal reflux. See *Reflux esophagitis.*

Esophagitis. Inflammation of the mucosal lining of the esophagus. May be due to irritations, infections, or backflow of gastric contents from the stomach, as in gastroesophageal reflux. Drug therapy is the treatment of choice to neutralize acidity. *Dietary management:* a soft diet, as tolerated by the patient, is recommended to prevent irritation of the esophagus. Many patients avoid acidic fruits and juices. Some find fatty and spicy meals irritating.

Esophagus. A hollow muscular tube measuring about 2 cm in diameter and 25 to 30 cm in length extending from the pharynx to the stomach. See *Digestion.*

ESRD. Abbreviation for *end-stage renal disease.*

Essential amino acid (EAA). See under *Amino acid.*

Essential fatty acid (EFA). See under *Fatty acid.*

Estimated safe and adequate daily dietary intake (ESADDI). Amount recommended for a nutrient listed as tentative by the Food and Nutrition Board, but the given value or range is considered safe and adequate until more information is gathered to establish the recommended dietary allowance (RDA). Upper levels in the "safe and adequate range" should not be habitually exceeded because of the toxic levels of many trace elements. See Appendix 2.

Estrogen. Collective term for the natural or synthetic female sex hormones. The naturally occurring estrogens, like estradiol, estrone, and estriol, are produced principally by the maturing follicles in the ovary, although they are also formed in the placenta and adrenal cortex. Two synthetic estrogenic compounds of therapeutic importance are ethynylestradiol and diethylstilbestrol (DES). The estrogens are responsible for the development of the female sex organs, growth of the genitalia and mammary glands, and development of secondary sex characteristics; they also affect calcium and phosphorus metabolism and probably are related to bone metabolism, lipid metabolism, and skin or related structures. Synthetic estrogens are used in treating a variety of conditions associated with a deficiency of estrogenic hormones. A high dose impairs folate absorption and may cause folate deficiency; it may also increase serum triglycerides, decrease glucose tolerance, and increase weight due to salt and fluid retention. Estrogen is excreted in breast milk. Brand names are Estrace, Estrone, Estratab, and Premarin.

Ethacrynic acid. A loop diuretic used in the treatment of hypertension and edema associated with congestive heart failure. Diuresis results in increased excretion of potassium, sodium, chloride, calcium, magnesium, and zinc. Potassium depletion occurs frequently, and dehydration is most likely to occur in geriatric patients and those on restricted salt intake. Other side effects may cause carbohydrate intolerance, anorexia, dysphagia, and abdominal discomfort. The brand name is Edecrin.

Ethanol. Ethyl alcohol, the form of alcohol that is ingested in alcoholic drinks. See *Alcohol* and Appendix 33.

Ethanolamine. Beta-aminoethyl alcohol, a basic component of certain cephalins. It may be formed by reduction of glycine or decarboxylation of serine and forms choline when methylated by methionine. A lipotropic agent, it can prevent the formation of fatty livers.

European Federation of the Associations of Dietitians (EFAD). An organization of national dietetic associations in European countries. Membership is approved if the national dietetic association has more than 50% legally qualified dietitians. The aims of the federation are to encourage a better nutritional status for the populations of the member countries of the Council of Europe; to develop dietetics on a scientific and professional level; to promote the development of the dietetic profession; to improve the teaching of dietetics; and to pursue these objectives with the help of international organizations.

Exceed. Brand name of a fluid replacement and energy drink; provides 460 kcal/16 oz from 100% carbohydrate calories.

Exchange list. Grouping of foods based on similarity in nutrient composition. Each food within the list has approximately the same food value and may be used interchangeably.

Exergonic reaction. Reaction accompanied by a release of energy; usually associated with catabolism.

Exogenous. Coming or originating from the outside; not from within; due to an external cause.

Exophthalmic goiter. Goiter characterized by protruding eyeballs. See *Goiter.*

Expanded Food and Nutrition Education Program (EFNEP). A program designed by the U.S. Department of Agriculture to teach low-income families, particularly those with small children, the skills to develop and consume nutritionally adequate meals. Trained nutrition aides, who are often members of the local communities, work on a one-to-one basis in the homes of the low-income homemakers, using demonstration techniques reinforced with newsletters and printed educational handouts.

Extension, USDA. Also called the Cooperative Extension Service. Established to teach nutrition directly to rural residents in the United States. Extension nutrition program activities include the Expanded Food and Nutrition Education Program (EFNEP), group meetings with youth clubs, homemakers' clubs, agricultural producers, and other special interest groups in both urban and rural areas.

Extrinsic factor. Literally, a substance originating from the outside. In nutrition, this refers to the extrinsic factor discovered by Castle or vitamin B_{12} obtained from food. See *Vitamin B_{12}.*

F

F. Chemical symbol for fluorine. See also *Fl.*

Factor. Any constituent that tends to produce a result. In nutrition, it refers to an essential or desirable element in the diet that has some effect on the growth, reproduction, or health of organisms. It may be a vitamin, a mineral, or any other nutrient. The structure of the factor may be identified or it may remain unidentified.

FAD. Abbreviation for flavin adenine dinucleotide. See *Flavin nucleotide.*

Failure to thrive. Also called "failure to grow"; infants and toddlers fail to grow and develop normally because of inadequate intake of food; unusually high energy requirements; excessive losses, as in diarrhea and excessive vomiting; or a combination of two or more of these factors. Most patients have no medical or organic problem. Usually the cause is parental neglect or ignorance. Failure to thrive frequently affects the child who has been deprived of adequate maternal love and attention. *Dietary management:* if the disorder is a result of inadequate mother-child bonding, therapy is directed to solving the psychosocial problems because they affect the appetite of the child, who may even refuse to eat. Nutrition education is needed for mothers who provide inadequate foods and do not follow proper timing and spacing in feeding the child. Nutrient intakes, particularly for calories and protein, should be assessed.

Fair Packaging and Labeling Act. This act, passed in 1966, set regulations for labeling and packaging consumer commodities such as foods, drugs, medical devices, and cosmetics as defined in the Food, Drug, and Cosmetic Act. Meat products, poultry, poultry products that are not canned, and prescription drugs do not come under this law. See *Nutritional labeling.*

Famotidine. A histamine H_2-receptor antagonist effective in reducing gastric acid secretion; used for the short-term management of confirmed active ulcer. There is a risk of vitamin B_{12} depletion with famotidine; it may be excreted in breast milk and may also cause anorexia, dry mouth, dysgeusia, and abdominal discomfort. The brand name is Pepcid.

Fanconi syndrome. Condition characterized by a low renal threshold for amino acids. A generalized aminoaciduria occurs even with normal levels of amino acids in the blood; there is also loss of glucose and phosphates in the urine. This leads to withdrawal of calcium from the bones to neutralize the acids. As a result, conditioned rickets or osteomalacia may occur. Diet therapy is aimed at replacing losses; infants may require vitamin D therapy and neutral phosphates.

FAO. Abbreviation for *Food and Agriculture Organization.*

Farnoquinone. Vitamin K_2, a naphthoquinone derivative. Originally isolated from putrid fish meal; it is synthesized by a large number of intestinal bacteria. See *Vitamin K.*

Fast foods. Foods commercially prepared and served by franchised food chains, restaurants, and other food service facilities which consumers find convenient, time-saving, and relatively economical. Many food companies have nutritional data for the products they serve. Several current reference books on nutrition and diet therapy have compiled food composition data from the more popularly known fast food chains.

Fat. In the strictest sense, the term means *neutral* or *true fat.* It is a *triglyceride,* which is an organic ester of three molecules of fatty acid combined with one molecule of glycerol. This is the form in which fats occur chiefly in foodstuffs and in fat depots of most animals. Neutral fat may be *soft* or *hard,* depending on the length of the fatty acid chain; or it may be *liquid* or *solid,* depending on the degree of saturation or unsaturation of the fatty acids. See also *Fatty acid* and *Lipid.*

Fat, body. There are two types of body fat: protoplasmic and depot fat. Protoplasmic fat is part of the essential structure of cells. In addition to neutral fat, it contains other lipids, such as phospholipid, cholesterol, and cerebroside. Protoplasmic fat is of constant composition and is not altered by variations in food intake; hence it is not reduced during starvation. Depot fat or *adipose tissue* is the fuel store of the body, and is found mainly in the subcutaneous tissue and around visceral organs. This fat store is either filled up or depleted, depending on the balance between the energy value of food eaten and expended. The adipose cell can store as much as 50 times its weight, and if filled up to its maximum, new adipose cells can be formed; hence the body has a very large capacity for storing fats. See also *Obesity.*

Fat functions. Fat is a concentrated source of energy, yielding about 9 calories/gm. It is a carrier of fat-soluble vitamins, adds palatability and satiety value to the diet, and has protein-sparing action. In addition, fat acts as a shock absorber, serves as a padding around vital organs, and insulates the body against the loss of heat. It stores energy efficiently, using the least amount of water among the fuel nutrients. When the person is at rest or engaging in light activities, about 40% of the energy needed by the body comes from fatty acids.

Fat intake, recommended. A satisfactory fat intake is 30% of the total caloric needs per day. For example, an adult requiring 1800 kcal/day needs 60 gm fat (540 kcal from fat). Fatty acid intake should be proportioned as follows: 10% of calorie needs from polyunsaturated fatty acids, 10% from monounsaturated fatty acids, and 10% from other fatty acids. Linoleic acid at a level of 1 to 2% of the total kcal/day is recommended to prevent essential fatty acid deficiency. Infants consuming 100 kcal/kg body weight per day need 0.2 gm of dietary linoleic acid per kilogram of body weight. An adequate linoleic acid intake for adults is 3 to 6 gm/day.

Fat-soluble. Generally refers to substances that cannot be dissolved in water but can be dissolved in fats and oils or in fat solvents such as ether and chloroform. The fat-soluble vitamins are vitamins A, D, E, and K.

Fatty acid (FA). An organic acid containing carbon, hydrogen, and oxygen; generally consists of a carbon chain that terminates in a —COOH group. It is found abundantly in ester linkage in several lipid compounds, or it may exist as a free or nonesterified fatty acid. With a few exceptions, fatty acids occurring in natural fats contain an even number of carbon atoms (4 to 24). Fatty acids are generally classified according to dietary essentiality, the number of carbon atoms, or the degree of saturation between the carbon atoms. See Appendix 10.

Essential FA (EFA). Polyunsaturated fatty acids that are necessary for growth, reproduction, health of the skin, and proper utilization of fats. According to this definition, three FA may be considered *physiologically essential:* linoleic, linolenic, and arachidonic acids. Linoleic acid and alpha-linolenic acid must be present in the diet. Linoleic acid serves as a precursor for the biosynthesis of arachidonic acid. EFA are important for membrane structure and transport processes. Clinical symptoms of EFA deficiency include mild diarrhea; dryness, thickening, and desquamation of the skin; coarsening of the hair and hair loss; impaired wound healing; and brittle and osteoporotic bones. Blood changes include decreased cholesterol levels, increased red blood cell fragility and anemia, and increased capillary permeability. Hepatomegaly, increased serum glutamic-oxaloacetic transaminase, serum glutamic-pyruvic transaminase, and lactic dehydrogenase, and fatty liver have been reported after 4 to 6 weeks of fat-free parenteral nutrition.

Free FA (FFA). Also called "nonesterified fatty acid"; plasma FFA, such as oleic, palmitic, stearic, and linoleic acids, are bound to serum albumin as part of the lipoproteins. They are believed to aid in the transport of fat, both from alimentary sources and from fat depots, to be oxidized in various tissues. During fasting, FFA from depot fat increases, whereas glucose and insulin administration decrease the movement of depot fatty acids to plasma FFA. In fats and oils, the amount of free FA is a measure of the degree of hydrolytic rancidity.

Long-chain FA (LCFA). Those containing 12 to 22 carbon atoms. The most prevalent one in foods is stearic acid (18 carbon atoms).

Medium-chain FA (MCFA). Those containing 6 to 10 carbon atoms. Although not prevalent in foods, MCFA are more readily absorbed than LCFA. Examples are caprylic acid (8 carbon atoms) and capric acid (10 carbon atoms). Commercial preparations of triglycerides made from these FA (MCT) are used to treat patients with gastrointestinal tract disorders.

Monounsaturated FA (MUFA). Also called monoenoic fatty acids; those with only one unsaturated linkage or double bond, having two hydrogen atoms fewer than the saturated form. The most abundant monounsaturated FA in fats and oils are oleic and palmitoleic acids. Olive oil and canola oil are excellent sources of monounsaturated FA. Of animal fats, lard, beef suet, and chicken fat have about 40 to 45% of total FA as monounsaturates.

Nonesterified FA (NEFA). See *Free FA* under *Fatty acid.*

Omega FA (OFA). FA designated by the position of the double bond starting from the omega end or the methyl (CH3−) carbon. The symbol ω for omega is used, followed by a number indicating the location of the nearest double bond. The three classes of omega FA of dietary significance are omega-3 (ω3) such as *linolenic acid, eicosapentaenoic acid,* and *docosahexaenoic acid;* omega-6 (ω6) such as *linoleic acid* and *arachidonic acid;* and omega-9 (ω9) such as *oleic acid.* The omega-3 FA are abundant in fish oils.

Recent studies support the role of omega-3 FA in reducing the risk of heart attack. Omega-3 FA and omega-6 FA strengthen the immune system of the body and produce *eicosanoids.*

Polyunsaturated FA (PUFA). Those having two or more unsaturated linkages or double bonds and classed as dienoic, trienoic, and tetraenoic. Of greatest interest are linoleic acid (two double bonds), linolenic acid (three double bonds), and arachidonic acid (four double bonds). See also *Essential FA* and *Omega FA* under *Fatty acid.*

Saturated FA (SFA). Those having all the carbon atoms of the molecule linked to hydrogen so that only single bonds exist. Saturation of FA accounts for the firmness of fats at room temperature. The most common ones in animal fats are palmitic and stearic acids.

Short-chain FA (SCFA). Those containing fewer than 6 carbon atoms. These are not abundant in food fats and yield only about 5 calories/gm compared to 9 calories/gm from the LCFA. Examples are caproic acid (6 carbon atoms) and butyric acid (4 carbon atoms).

Unsaturated FA (UFA). Those containing one or more double bonds between one or more of the carbon atoms in the chain. Unsaturation alters certain properties of FA. In general, the melting point is greatly lowered and the solubility in nonpolar solvents is enhanced. All the common UFA in nature are liquid at room temperature. They are abundant in vegetable oils such as olive oil, corn oil, cottonseed oil, and soybean oil. See also *Monounsaturated FA* and *Polyunsaturated FA* under *Fatty acid.*

Very-long-chain FA (VLFA). FA with a carbon chain consisting of 24 or more carbon atoms. An example is hexacosanoic FA (C26:0), which is associated with *adrenoleukodystrophy.*

Fatty liver. Accumulation of fatty deposits rich in cholesterol esters in the liver. This may be the result of a number of causes, including lack of *lipotropic factors;* liver poisoning by phosphorus, chloroform, and other chlorinated compounds; and following chronic infectious diseases such as tuberculosis, metabolic disorders such as diabetes, or various nutritional disorders such as kwashiorkor, chronic alcoholism, and vitamin E deficiency. *Dietary management:* restrict fats to 50 gm/day and cholesterol to 200 mg/day. Use of *MCT* is beneficial.

Favism. An inherited metabolic disorder characterized by vomiting, dizziness, prostration, jaundice, and hemolytic anemia (which is sometimes fatal in children) following the ingestion of fava beans or even the inhalation of its pollens by susceptible individuals. It is due to deficiency of the enzyme glucose-6-phosphate dehydrogenase. Children are more prone to hemolytic episodes than adults. A singular feature of favism is the increasing tolerance to fava beans with age in affected individuals.

FDA. Abbreviation for *Food and Drug Administration.*

Fe. Chemical symbol for iron.

Fecal fat test. Diagnostic test for malabsorption or cystic fibrosis by determining the amount of fat in the stools. A diet containing at least 100 gm/day fat is given for 3 days before the stool specimen is collected. An example of a day's intake for 100 gm fat may consist of 2 cups (16 oz) of whole milk, 3 servings (9 oz) of lean meat, 1 egg, 4 servings of fruits and vegetables, 6 slices of bread or equivalent, and 10 pats (10 teaspoons) of butter or margarine.

Federal Trade Commission (FTC). Federal agency of the U.S. government that protects the consumer from false advertising and unfair and deceptive trade practices.

Fenoprofen. A nonsteroidal anti-inflammatory agent used for treatment of rheumatoid arthritis and osteoarthritis; it also has analgesic and antipyretic activity. It has a metallic taste and can cause gastric mucosal damage, which may result in ulceration and/or bleeding. It can also induce fluid retention and weight gain, and may cause dyspepsia, dry mouth, aphthous lesions, and abdominal discomfort. Brand names are Fenoprofen and Nalfon.

Fermentation. Also called glycolysis; the enzymatic oxidation of carbohydrate under anaerobic or partially anaerobic conditions.

Ferriprotoporphyrin. See *Hemin.*

Ferritin. An iron-protein complex found chiefly in the liver, spleen, bone marrow, and reticuloendothelial cells; it contains 23% iron. Ferritin functions in the absorption of iron through the intestinal mucosa and serves as a storage form of iron in the body. When the storage capacity of ferritin is exceeded, iron accumulates in the liver as *hemosiderin.* See also *Hemosiderosis.*

Ferroprotoporphyrin. See *Heme.*

Fetal alcohol syndrome (FAS). Congenital defect in an infant delivered by an alcoholic mother who consumed at least 3 oz alcohol per day during pregnancy. It has also been observed that ingestion of alcohol even occasionally during the gestation period may be harmful. It is best to educate and warn expectant mothers of the serious consequences of alcohol on the fetus. Clinical signs seen in the infant are low birth weight, limb and facial/head malformations, cardiovascular defects, retarded physical growth and mental development. *Dietary management:* in serious cases, tube feeding or total parenteral nutrition may be needed. Oral formulas are resumed as soon as possible. See nutritional principles for *Low-birth-weight infants.*

Fever. 1. Elevation in body temperature above normal (98.6°F or 37°C); pyrexia. 2. Any disease characterized by a marked increase in temperature, acceleration of basal metabolism, increase in tissue destruction, and loss of body water, sodium, and potassium. Fevers may be *acute,* as in influenza, chickenpox, and pneumonia; *chronic,* as in tuberculosis; or *intermittent,* as in malaria. When fever rises sharply, it may cause convulsions and delirium. *Dietary management:* The diet should be high in calories (150% of the resting energy expenditure) due to the elevated metabolic rate, which increases 7% for every 1°F (13% for every

1°C) rise in body temperature. Protein is increased (1.3 to 1.5 gm/kg/day) to replace nitrogen losses from tissue destruction characteristic of febrile conditions. A liberal supply of carbohydrates will spare protein and replenish glycogen stores. Fluid intake will depend on losses from excretion (urination, perspiration, insensible losses, etc.), which may be as much as 2.5 to 4 liters/day. Severe dehydration may require intravenous treatment. For oral liquids, salty broths, nourishing drinks like milk, vitamin C-rich beverages, and nutrient-dense liquids are preferred. In acute fevers, at least eight feedings are provided, progressing from a full liquid diet to a soft diet. Eventually, a regular regimen is resumed as tolerated. If fever is a symptom of a disorder that requires other dietary modifications, follow the guidelines as needed for the primary cause of the febrile condition.

FFA. Abbreviation for *free fatty acid.*

FH₄. Abbreviation for *tetrahydrofolic acid.*

Fiber. 1. Threadlike, elongated structure of organic tissue such as muscle fiber or nerve fiber. 2. In nutrition and diet therapy, fiber consists of nondigestible materials which include *plant fibers:* mostly cellulose, hemicellulose, lignin, agar, pectins, gums, and mucilages; animal tissues like ligaments and gristle in meats; and undigested pharmaceutical products. Formerly called bulk or roughage. The term *dietary fiber* is now used in dietetics.

Crude fiber. Complex polysaccharide that cannot be hydrolyzed by human digestion or by acids and alkalis in the laboratory. Earlier food composition tables that reported *fiber* referred to crude fiber, which is mainly cellulose. Newer chemical techniques now differentiate food fibers as soluble or insoluble dietary fibers.

Dietary fibers. Complex polysaccharides that are not digested in the human intestine. These include the *insoluble* dietary fibers: cellulose, hemicellulose, and lignin, which do not dissolve in water but instead absorb water, contributing bulk to the stools and preventing constipation and diverticulosis;

and the *soluble* dietary fibers: pectins, gums, mucilages, and algal substances. Soluble dietary fibers are useful in lowering blood cholesterol, managing obesity, cardiovascular disease, and diabetes mellitus, and preventing colon cancer. Recommended daily intake of dietary fiber is 25 to 35 gm/day for adults. Too much fiber may cause diarrhea in persons not accustomed to a high fiber intake. See also Appendix 32.

Fibrin. A colorless, insoluble protein mainly responsible for blood clots. It is formed from the interaction between a soluble precursor, *fibrinogen,* and an enzyme, *thrombin.* Fibrin serves as the essential network in which blood cells are enmeshed to form the clot. Dissolution of fibrin by enzyme action is called *fibrinolysis.*

Fibronectin. A plasma glycoprotein and *opsonin* of the reticuloendothelial system. It is not synthesized in the liver and has a short half-life (less than 1 day). As a nutritional marker, plasma fibronectin is sensitive to starvation and repletion; a decrease in plasma concentration is seen in burns, sepsis, surgery, and shock. The normal plasma fibronectin level is 2.92 ± 0.2 gm/dl.

Fibrosis. Formation of tough, fibrous connective tissue in an organ beyond the amount normally present.

FIGLU. Abbreviation for *formiminoglutamic acid.*

Fish skin. Dry skin that comes off in fine or rough scales. See *Xeroderma.*

Fistula. 1. Deep ulcer, often leading to an internal hollow organ, as a result of incomplete healing of a wound, an abscess, or other disease conditions. 2. An abnormal passage or communication between two organs, often from an internal organ to the surface of the body. Most bowel fistulas occur secondary to abdominal surgery; other causes include inflammatory bowel disease, cancer, radiation therapy, and trauma. Patients become malnourished because of loss of nutrients, especially albumin, through drainage, increased metabolism associated with infection, and poor nutritional intake secondary to decreased appetite and mechanical obstruction. *Dietary management:* provide a high-calorie (up to twice the basal energy expenditure) and high-protein (1.5 to 2.0 gm/kg) diet via nasogastric tube feeding of a chemically defined or polymeric product or by total parenteral nutrition. When giving a nasogastric tube feeding, the tube should be passed 40 cm beyond the fistula to avoid reflux of food through the fistula. Total parenteral nutrition should be reserved for patients with high-output (drainage) fistulas in the upper small intestine and with distal ileal or colonic fistulas.

Fl. *Fluoride* ion.

Flaky-paint dermatosis. Also called crazy-pavement dermatosis: extensive, often bilateral hyperpigmentation of the skin that peels off, leaving a hypopigmented skin with superficial ulceration. It is characteristic of protein-energy malnutrition (PEM), which occurs in patches, usually on the buttocks, thighs, and arms.

Flatulence. Gastrointestinal discomfort, with or without pain, due to the presence of excessive amounts of air or gas in the stomach and intestinal tract. The gases in these organs are nitrogen, hydrogen, oxygen, carbon dioxide, methane, and traces of others. They are produced in the gastrointestinal tract or are swallowed. Ingested air accounts for most of the gas in the esophagus and stomach, which may escape by belching. Hydrogen, carbon dioxide, and methane are produced in the intestine and constitute the bulk of the flatus, most of which passes through the rectum. Complaints of "too much gas" by patients may be due to an abnormality of intestinal motility associated with some diseases. *Dietary management:* flatulence among individuals varies according to the foods they eat and their swallowing and eating habits. Flatulence can be relieved by avoiding foods that an individual finds "gassy." The foods usually implicated are legumes, the cabbage family, onions, prunes, raisins, bananas, sugar alcohols, bran and high-fiber grains, rich sauces and gravies, lactose in milk and ice cream, fermented foods, and carbonated beverages. Eating practices that are conducive to swallowing air include eating rapidly, drawing on straws, repetitive swallowing as in chewing gum and tobacco, sucking candies, and sipping liquids. Lack of exercise and stress factors may cause gas retention.

Flavin. Any one of a group of yellow pigments widely distributed in plants and animals, including *riboflavin.* They have an intense green fluorescence.

Flavin nucleotide. Derivative of the vitamin *riboflavin* that participates as a coenzyme in many oxidation-reduction reactions.

Flavin adenine dinucleotide (FAD). Riboflavin-5-phosphate attached to adenosine monophosphate. It forms the prosthetic group of certain enzymes and is important in electron transport mitochondria.

Flavin mononucleotide (FMN). Riboflavin-5-phosphate; it arises from riboflavin by reaction with adenosine triphosphate and the enzyme *flavokinase.* FMN acts as a coenzyme for a number of oxidative enzymes.

Flavonoids. More commonly called *bioflavonoids* to indicate having biologic activity; a large group of flavone derivatives, including hesperidin, rutin, and quercitin, that are widely distributed in plants and concentrated in the skin, peel, and outer layers of fruits and vegetables, as well as in tea, coffee, wine, and beer.

Flavoprotein. Flavin-containing protein that constitutes the *yellow enzyme;* has as a prosthetic group either a phosphoric acid ester of riboflavin (flavin mononucleotide, or FMN) or the latter combined with adenylic acid (flavin adenine dinucleotide, or FAD).

Fletcherism. System advocating thorough chewing of food (as many as 30 times) to obtain greater satisfaction from food flavors, to induce more effective secretion of digestive juices, and hence to enhance digestion and utilization of food. It is also claimed that chewing for a long time satisfies the appetite with much less food, thus reducing the total amount of food ingested.

Floxuridine. A pyrimidine antagonist used as an antiviral and antineoplastic agent. Among its adverse effects are nausea, vomiting, anorexia, glossitis, stomatitis, diarrhea, enteritis, and gastric ulceration. The brand name is FUDR.

Fluid balance. A state of equilibrium in which the amount of liquids ingested equals the amount lost from the body via the urine, feces, perspiration, lungs, etc. See also *Water balance* and *Water requirement.*

Fluoridation. Addition of small amounts of fluoride in public water supplies wherever natural fluoride concentrations are low; an effective and practical means of reducing dental caries. Recommendations approved by national and international organizations call for fluoride concentrations between 0.7 and 1.2 mg/liter. In the United States, the Food and Nutrition Board recommends that water supplies be fluoridated at a level of 1 ppm (1 mg/liter) to provide 1.5 to 4 mg fluoride for adults. This level is considered safe and does not present any known health risk. The topical application of stannous fluoride and the addition of fluoride to mouth rinse and toothpaste are other ways of preventing tooth decay. See also *Dental caries.*

Fluoride. A binary compound of fluorine; found in trace amounts in human tissues, particularly in the teeth, bones, thyroid gland, and skin. There is controversy regarding the status of fluoride as a dietary essential nutrient. However, the beneficial effect of fluoride in preventing dental caries in the teeth of growing children is well established. Fluoride is retained in the teeth and bones, where it forms fluoroapatite, which is important for hardening tooth enamel and contributes to the stability of bone mineral matrix. Fluoride intake in the United States from food, beverages, and water is about 0.9 to 1.7 mg/day. It is present in small but varying concentrations in all soils, water supplies, plants, and animals; it is therefore a constituent of all diets. The chief source is drinking water; tea, seafoods, and marine fish are also good sources. It is readily absorbed (about 90%), and excretion is mainly in the urine. The potential for toxicity is high when it is consumed in exces-

sive amounts. Of all the elements, fluoride has the narrowest range of safe and adequate intake. Mottling of the tooth enamel results from slight exposure of about three to four times the intake necessary to prevent caries. Chronic toxicity, called *fluorosis,* occurs after years of daily exposure. An acute toxicity, resulting in death, has been reported with the ingestion of one dose of 5 to 10 gm sodium fluoride. See Appendix 2.

Fluorine (F). A nonmetallic gaseous element belonging to the halogen group. Fluorine, in the form of *fluoride,* is incorporated into the structure of bones and teeth and provides protection against dental caries.

FMN. Abbreviation for flavin mononucleotide. See under *Flavin nucleotide.*

Folacin. Generic descriptor for all *folates* and related compounds that exhibit qualitatively the biological activity of tetrahydropteroylglutamic acid or *folic acid.*

Folic acid. Pteroylglutamic acid (PGA), a water-soluble vitamin; alternative names are folacin and folate. The generic name "folic acid" was originally applied to a number of compounds having the same biologic property as PGA. This vitamin was first recognized as a factor necessary for normal growth and hemopoiesis of certain microorganisms and animals and has been given various names such as vitamin M, vitamin B_c, vitamin B_{10} and B_{11}, rhizopterin, citrovorum factor, *Lactobacillus casei* factor, norite eluate factor, and factor SLR. When the substance was finally isolated from spinach, it was called folic acid because of its great abundance in dark green leaves (foliage). As a coenzyme, folic acid is involved in single carbon metabolism, which is an important cellular synthetic mechanism. It also plays a role in the synthesis of purines, citrulline and aspartic acid, metabolism of fatty acids, and carboxylation and decarboxylation reactions. Folic acid is widely distributed in plant and animal tissues. Good food sources are liver, beef, leafy vegetables, legumes, and whole grains. Folate is absorbed as mono- and polyglutamate in the proximal part of the intestine, and then converted in the liver to tetrahydrofolic acid (folinic acid) which is the active metabolite. This conversion is enhanced by ascorbic acid. Folate deficiency may occur either as a result of inadequate intake, increased requirement (infancy, pregnancy, hyperthyroidism), deficient absorption (malabsorption syndromes, bowel resection, genetic disorders), increased losses (kidney dialysis, liver disease), or drug interference (anticonvulsant, antimalarial, barbiturate, cholestyramine, methotrexate, pyrimethamine, triamterene, trimethoprim, etc). Manifestations of deficiency resemble those of vitamin B_{12} but does not lead to degeneration of the cord; symptoms include glossitis and other oral lesions, gastrointestinal disturbances, and megaloblastic anemia. There have been rare reports of gastrointestinal disturbances with high doses of folic acid. An excessive intake is not recommended because it can mask a diagnosis for pernicious anemia and may have potential for toxicity. In laboratory animals, large doses of folic acid given parenterally precipitated in the kidney and produced kidney damage. For Recommended Dietary Allowances, see Appendix 1.

Folinic acid. Also called citrovorum factor and leucovorin; a reduced and formylated derivative of folic acid that is more stable to air oxidation than the parent compound. It is the name given to citrovorum factor, a substance in the liver required for the growth of *Leuconostoc citrovorum*. The calcium salt (leucovorin calcium) is used to treat folic acid deficiency and as an antidote to folic acid antagonists.

Follicular keratosis. Also called "follicular hyperkeratosis"; a skin condition seen in vitamin A deficiency. The skin becomes rough, dry, and scaly, and the hair follicles are blocked with plugs of keratin, which appear as prominent projections along the upper forearms and thighs, and also along the shoulders, back, abdomen, and buttocks.

Folliculosis. Condition characterized by dry, rough skin, especially in the area of the shoulder and back of the arm. The follicles are raised above the surface, giving the superficial appearance of chronic gooseflesh.

The condition is seen in vitamin A deficiency but should not be confused with *follicular keratosis,* as no horny plugs project from the follicular orifices.

Food. Anything that, when taken into the body, serves to nourish, build, and repair tissues, supply energy, or regulate body processes. Aside from its nutritional function, food is valued for its palatability and satiety effect, as well as for the varied meanings attached to it (emotional, social, religious, cultural, etc.) by different individuals, groups, or races. The so-called ethnic foods reflect the cultural differences of food habits.

Food account. Method used in dietary studies and surveys involving groups or the population at large. It consists of running reports of foods purchased (or produced) for household use. It is useful in checking trends in purchasing certain foods or food groups.

Food additive. Any substance, other than the basic foodstuff but not including chance contaminants, present in food as a result of any aspect of food production, processing, storage, or packaging. Generally classified as *intentional additives* (those added to perform a specific function, such as improvement in nutrient value, flavor, color, etc.) and *accidental additives* (those which unavoidably become part of the product through some phase of production, processing, or packaging).

Food adulterant. Any substance, such as a toxic organism, filth, pesticide residue, or poisonous substance, found in foods that is harmful to health or any substance added to increase the bulk or weight of a product.

Food allergen. Food that produces allergic manifestations. The most common food allergens are wheat, milk, egg, shellfish, chocolate, nuts, and onion. Food allergy, however, may develop with any kind of food. The adverse immunologic reaction to allergen(s) in an individual may be harmless to most persons in similar amounts. Allergic symptoms may appear within a few minutes, a few hours, or 1 to 3 days after ingestion of the food allergen. Symptoms are varied, generally affecting the nasobronchial and cutaneous tissues. Gastrointestinal disturbances include diarrhea, nausea and vomiting, and abdominal pain. *Dietary management:* the initial treatment is to identify the food allergen and avoid it entirely. A food history is taken, and food records are kept. If symptoms have disappeared when the suspected food allergen has been eliminated for at least 6 weeks, that food is reintroduced and reactions are observed again. Sometimes more than one item is implicated and a series of elimination diets can be useful. See *Diet, Rowe's elimination.* During the test period, monitor nutritional adequacy, giving supplementary vitamins and minerals if necessary.

Food analysis. Quantitative or qualitative determination of food components using different techniques. The general method of food analysis is by proximate determination of water, nitrogen (protein), ether extract (fat), ash, and carbohydrate (by difference). Specific mineral and vitamin components are determined by different methods. The *Official Methods of Analysis* published by the *Association of Official Agricultural Chemists* is a good reference for accepted methods. See also *Proximate analysis.*

Food and Agriculture Organization (FAO). International organization of the United Nations directly concerned with the production, distribution, and consumption of foods to improve nutrition and raise the standard of living of the people of all countries. It provides technical assistance through five divisions: agriculture, economics, fisheries, forestry, and nutrition.

Food and Drug Administration (FDA). Agency of the U.S. Department of Health and Human Services that enforces legislation concerning food, drugs, and cosmetics. It safeguards the food supply to ensure that it is fit for human consumption; some of its main activities are to monitor food and nutrition labeling, food additives, and food-drug interactions.

Food and Nutrition Board (FNB). Board of the National Academy of Sciences/National Research Council that was established in 1940 to serve as an advisory group on nutrition to U.S. agencies. It promotes needed research and helps interpret nutritional sci-

ence in the interest of public welfare. Specific activities are carried on by committees composed of experts in each field.

Food and Nutrition Information Center (FNIC). A branch of the U.S. Department of Agriculture that provides serials, monograms and audiovisual materials including computer information to nutritionists, dietitians, food service managers, and others. It also prepares bibliographies on specific food and nutrition topics, which are also available to consumers, educators, and other professionals.

Food and Nutrition Service (FNS). A branch of the Food and Consumer Services, U.S. Department of Agriculture, responsible for programs that provide food for needy persons, such as the Family Nutrition Program, Food Stamp Program, National School Lunch Program, and Special Milk Program for Children.

Food balance sheet. Measure of the food available per person. It is calculated by dividing the total food for the year by the number of people in the country.

Food-borne disease. Disease caused by the ingestion of food that contains bacteria, parasites, naturally occurring toxicants, chemical poisons, or radioactive fallout. See *Food poisoning.*

Food composition tables. Tabulated data on quantities of different nutrients per 100 gm or per serving portion of a food item. Most commonly used in the United States is Handbook Number 8, *Composition of Foods— Raw, Processed and Prepared,* published by the U.S. Department of Agriculture; originally issued in 1950 and revised in 1963, it has been constantly updated starting in the 1970s. As more food products have been processed and sold commercially, analyses of nutrients for these products have been included. The food composition tables are constantly being updated. Presently, there are 16 volumes covering different food items. Food values are given in terms of a 100-gm edible portion (EP) and 1 lb as purchased (AP) of the foods. Information is given about the energy value and nutrient content of various food items, including water, protein, fat, saturated fatty acids, unsaturated fatty acids (oleic acid and linoleic acid), carbohydrate, calcium, phosphorus, magnesium, iron, sodium, potassium, copper, zinc, manganese, vitamin A, thiamin, riboflavin, niacin, vitamin B_6, folacin, vitamin B_{12}, pantothenic acid, ascorbic acid, and others. There are other food composition tables compiled by others (e.g., Pennington, Bowes and Church, etc.) using U.S. Department of Agriculture data, food industry analyses, university laboratories, and so on that are also useful references, some of which deal with special dietary components like alcohol, cholesterol, and caffeine. Currently, the use of computer software for food composition data is an important tool for practitioners and researchers.

Food, Drug, and Cosmetic Act. Law passed in 1938 to provide for safe, effective drugs and cosmetics, pure wholesome foods, and honest labeling and packaging. Recent amendments are concerned with pesticides, food additives, and color additives. The Food and Drug Administration enforces this act and its amendments.

Food, energy value. Also called "fuel value of food"; oxidation of foodstuffs in the *bomb calorimeter* yields on the average, 4.15, 9.40, and 5.65 calories/gm of pure carbohydrate, fat, and protein, respectively. However, the *physiologic fuel* values of foods when burned by the body are somewhat lower because of incomplete digestion of the three nutrients and incomplete oxidation of protein. Experiments conducted by Atwater on typical American mixed diets showed that the digestibility of carbohydrate was 98%, protein 92%, and fat 95%, and that the urinary energy loss for incomplete oxidation of protein was 1.25 calories/gm protein. On the basis of these observations, the Atwater values for the available energy of the three foodstuffs were derived. Later experiments showed that each food has a specific coefficient of digestibility, making the fuel value specific for each type of food. The Nutrition Division of the Food and Agricultural Organization therefore proposed the use of *specific fuel factors* for estimating the ca-

loric value of foods. See *Atwater values* and *Specific fuel factor (value)*.

Food fad. Idea associated with food that becomes fashionable for a time to meet the needs of a current trend, usually at the sacrifice of important nutrients. A food fad may be an exaggerated truth about a food or a claim that it is a cure-all. Food fads are usually short-lived and remain popular only until they are replaced by another fad. Many diets for weight reduction are currently based on common fads.

Food fallacy. False belief about food; misrepresentation, misinterpretation, or misinformation about a food fact. A *fact* implies a scientific basis, and facts about food are the result of research.

Food group. Classification of various foods into groups on the basis of similarity in nutrient content of the members of each group. It is a practical guide in planning diets that will satisfy nutrient allowances by merely defining the number of servings to eat from each group. See Appendices 5 and 6.

Food intolerance. Collective term for a wide variety of adverse reactions to foods which includes *food allergies* (e.g., milk, egg, or seafood allergies), malabsorption syndrome, enzyme defect as in inborn errors of metabolism, and many others. A systematic classification of food intolerances groups them as protein-induced, carbohydrate-induced or lipid-induced reactions.

Food inventory. Method of recording the food intake of a group or family. It consists of a weighed inventory of foods at the beginning and end of the study together with day-to-day records, with or without records of kitchen and plate wastes. Nutrients are calculated from food tables or by laboratory analysis of the foods.

Food labeling. A format on packaged foods that gives nutrition information and a list of ingredients, as required by law. The Food and Drug Administration (FDA) regulates the labeling of most food products, except alcoholic beverages, which are regulated by the Bureau of Alcohol, Tobacco and Firearms. Produce like fresh fruits and vegetables, and some products with Standards of Identity filed with the FDA, need not comply with the food and nutrition labeling requirements. Food labels must state the product's name, manufacturer, and address, the amount of the contents, and the ingredients in descending order by weight. If a manufacturer adds a nutrient to the product or makes some claim about its nutritional value, it must be so stated on its *nutritional labeling.* Currently, the Nutrition Labeling and Education Act of 1989 is under study by the U.S. Congress. A federal regulation states that food labeling regulations announced in 1990 should be implemented as soon as possible and that the deadline for compliance by food manufacturers is January 1, 1993.

Food list. Method used in dietary studies applicable to groups. The subject reports an estimated quantity (by weight, retail unit, or household measure) of various foods consumed during a previous period, usually the past 7 days. A list of foods may be used to aid recall.

Food poisoning. Toxic effects due to ingestion of contaminated or poisonous foods resulting in gastrointestinal disturbances like vomiting, diarrhea, and abdominal cramps. The affected person usually has fever, headaches, and double vision, and is dehydrated and weak. Infants, young children, the elderly, and individuals with poor health and nutriture are more at risk than others. The common food-poisoning agents are *Salmonella, Staphylococcus aureus, Clostridium botulinum, Clostridium perfringens, Campylobacter jejuni,* and *Listeria monocytogenes. Dietary management:* depending on the severity of the gastrointestinal disturbances and dehydration, intravenous glucose and electrolytes are immediately administered. As the patient improves, the diet order progresses from full liquid to soft and regular foods.

Food record. Method used in dietary studies. It consists of taking records of foods (including between-meal snacks) for varying periods of time, usually 3 to 7 days. The accuracy of the method depends on the ability of the subjects to estimate quantities of foods and the correct application of food tables to calculate the nutrient content.

Food Research and Action Center (FRAC). A nonprofit national organization which aims to alleviate hunger and malnutrition in the United States. It publishes a bimonthly newsletter, *Foodlines.*

Food Stamp Program. The primary purpose of this nationwide program is to alleviate hunger and malnutrition among the indigent. It enables households with incomes below the poverty line to receive a specified number of stamps without money transactions, which can be used to purchase food items in normal food outlets. There are restrictions on the food items to be purchased (e.g., no gourmet items or alcoholic beverages) to encourage the purchase of more nutritious foods.

Foot drop. Condition in which the foot hangs or falls down due to paralysis of the lower limbs, as seen in polyneuropathy of *beriberi.*

Formiminoglutamic acid (FIGLU). A metabolite of histidine seen in the urine of individuals deficient in folic acid. It is also seen in patients with acute leukemia who are receiving folic acid antagonist therapy such as methotrexate and aminopterin.

Fortification. Addition of one or more nutrients such as vitamins, minerals, amino acids, or protein concentrates to food so that it contains more of the nutrients than were originally present. Examples include the addition of vitamin A to margarine, vitamin D to milk, lysine to bread, and iodine to salt.

FreAmine. Brand name of an amino acid solution with electrolytes for total parenteral nutrition; available in 3%, 8.5%, and 10% amino acid concentration. Also available as 6.9% FreAmine HBC, with high branched-chain amino acids. See Appendix 40.

Free fatty acid (FFA). Unesterified fatty acid. See *Fatty acid.*

Fröhlich's syndrome. Disturbance in fat deposition usually occurring in children before puberty; characterized by the presence of superficial fat in the body and the external genitalia. It may be the result of an inherent defect in the pituitary gland or atrophy of the secretory cells by tumor injury or infectious disease.

Fructose. Levulose or fruit sugar. A 6-carbon monosaccharide found in fruits and honey and obtained from hydrolysis of sucrose to glucose and fructose. It is an essential intermediate in carbohydrate metabolism. Much sweeter than sugar, it is sometimes used as a sweetener in foods. Its use in large amounts can cause osmotic diarrhea and high blood triglycerides.

Fructose intolerance. A genetically inherited metabolic defect due to a deficiency of the enzyme fructose-1-phosphoaldolase, which results in hypoglycemia and hypophosphatemia with associated vomiting, lethargy, and coma; the long-term effect may lead to jaundice and enlargement of the liver. Another disorder in enzyme deficiency, fructose 1,6-diphosphatase, also results in hypoglycemia with hyperventilation, shock, and convulsions. The essential treatment for hereditary fructose intolerance is immediate and lifelong removal of all sources of fructose from the diet, with frequent meals and avoidance of long fasts. The management of crises with severe hypoglycemia and acidosis may require the administration of glucose and bicarbonate. See also *Diet, fructose-restricted.*

Fructosuria. Presence of fructose in the urine; a genetically inherited metabolic defect due to a deficiency of the enzyme fructokinase.

The disorder does not cause any clinical symptoms and is usually found incidentally when urine is tested as a screen for diabetes. It does not require any dietary modification.

Fruitarian. Person whose diet consists chiefly of fruits. See also *Vegetarian.*

Fuel factors. Energy values per gram of carbohydrate, protein, and fat. See *Atwater values; Food, energy value;* and *Specific fuel factor (value).*

Fumaric acid. Transethylene dicarboxylic acid, an intermediate product in carbohydrate metabolism.

Fundus. Base or part of an organ farthest from the mouth or opening, such as the fundus of the stomach.

Furanose. Cyclic structural formula of a sugar in which the oxygen ring bridges carbon atoms 1 and 4 in aldoses or carbon atoms 2 and 4 in ketoses.

Furosemide. A powerful diuretic used in the management of edema associated with congestive heart failure and hypertension. It acts by inhibiting reabsorption in the ascending loop of Henle in the kidney (hence, is a loop diuretic), thus causing diuresis and increased excretion of potassium, sodium, chloride, magnesium, and calcium. It may cause low blood levels of these electrolytes if dietary intake is inadequate. Furosemide is excreted in breast milk. Its side effects include anorexia, dry mouth, constipation, and stomach distress. Brand names are Lasix, Furomide, Lo-Aqua, and Myrosemide.

G

GABA. Abbreviation for gamma-amino butyric acid. Important neurotransmitter synthesized from glutamic acid.

Galactan. Also called "galactosan"; a polysaccharide that yields galactose on hydrolysis.

Galactoflavin. An analog of riboflavin that is a potent inhibitor; D-galactose replaces D-ribose in the molecule.

Galactokinase. Enzyme that catalyzes the phosphorylation of galactose to galactose-1-phosphate.

Galactosamine. An amino sugar; galactose containing an amino group in carbon atom 2. It is found in the polysaccharide of cartilage, in chondroitin (as chondrosamine), and in the structural material of the skeletons of arthropods.

Galactose. A 6-carbon monosaccharide differing from glucose only in the position of the hydroxyl group on carbon atom 4. It is seldom found free in nature; it occurs mainly linked with glucose to form lactose (milk sugar). It is also a constituent of cerebrosides, gangliosides, and certain polysaccharides such as agar and flaxseed.

Galactosemia. 1. Presence of galactose in the blood. 2. An inborn error of metabolism characterized by the inability to metabolize galactose due to a deficiency in one of three enzymes: galactokinase, galactose-1-phosphate uridyl transferase, and uridine diphosphate galactose-4-epimerase. Galactose accumulates in the blood and is excreted in the urine; the clinical symptoms are varied and include jaundice, enlarged liver and spleen, anorexia, weight loss, vomiting, diarrhea, ataxia, mental retardation, and cataract formation. The key element in the treatment of galactosemia is a diet as low as possible in galactose. See *Diet, galactose-restricted.*

Galactose tolerance test. A liver function test that measures the ability of the liver to remove galactose from the bloodstream and convert it to glycogen; it is performed in a manner similar to that of a glucose tolerance test.

Galactosuria. Presence of galactose in the urine.

Galacturonic acid. A sugar acid resulting from the oxidation of the primary alcohol group of galactose to a carboxyl ($-COOH$) group. It occurs in various vegetable sources such as pectins and certain plant gums.

Gallstones. See *Cholelithiasis.*

Gamma-aminobutyric acid (GABA). An important neurotransmitter synthesized from glutamic acid; found in the brain, heart, lungs, and kidneys.

Gastrectomy. Surgical removal of all or part of the stomach. *Dietary management:* routine pre- and postoperative diets are followed after partial or minor gastrectomy. Special dietary modifications are needed after total gastrectomy because of the resulting nutritional problems like diarrhea, weight loss, malabsorption, and the dumping syndrome. The absence of intrinsic factor may eventually lead to macrocytic anemia, unless monthly injections of 100 μg vitamin B_{12} are given. The first 2 to 3 weeks after surgery, follow a progressive diet consisting of small, frequent feedings of easily digested, soft, low-fiber foods. As the patient's condition improves, give five to six small meals high in protein, moderate in fat, and relatively low in carbohydrate, especially simple sugars. It is best to take fluids between meals rather than with meals to retard the rapid emptying of hypertonic food into the duodenum and jejunum. Small amounts of milk and lactose-free nutritional products are better tolerated if there is milk intolerance due to a lactase deficiency. Maintain a healthy weight and watch for signs of general malabsorption. Use of medium-chain triglycerides (MCT oil) and supplemental vitamins and minerals, especially folate, iron, calcium, and vitamin D, may be indicated. Vitamin B_{12} should be given parenterally in total gastrectomy.

Gastric. Pertaining to the stomach or gastric glands.

Gastric acidity. Amount of hydrochloric acid in the stomach, which may be present in two forms—as *free acid* or as *combined acid* (in combination with protein from food, regurgitated duodenal secretion, saliva, and mucus). The sum of the free and combined acids is termed "total acidity." Protein foods stimulate more acid secretion than do carbohydrates and fats. Protein foods have an initial buffering effect, with less free acid to erode tissues.

Gastric bypass (stapling). A surgical procedure designed to restrict or divert normal intake of food as a method of controlling weight in morbid obesity. The stomach is divided by means of several rows of staples into a small proximal pouch of about 50–60 ml in capacity and a nonfunctioning distal pouch. The proximal pouch is then attached to the jejunum. This procedure results in rapid filling of the reduced stomach, giving a feeling of early satiety with small meals and consequent decrease in food intake. However, there are side effects, such as dehydration due to persistent vomiting, vitamin B_{12} and iron deficiency, and severe weight loss associated with malabsorption and hepatic dysfunction. *Dietary management:* postoperative progression from clear to full liquids, then blenderized and soft, semisolid foods in small quantities (30–60 ml). Frequent feedings are necessary to meet energy and protein needs. Gradually increase the volume to 120–150 ml and introduce soft foods, with gradual progression to reg-

ular foods. Monitor intake. Supplemental vitamins and minerals, especially the B-complex vitamins and iron, may be necessary.

Gastric enzymes. Pepsin, rennin, and gastric lipase. See Appendix 11.

Gastric juice. A colorless secretion of the gastric gland containing mucus, hydrochloric acid, enzymes, and intrinsic factor.

Gastric ulcer. See *Peptic ulcer disease.*

Gastrin. Hormone elaborated by the pyloric mucosa that stimulates hydrochloric acid secretion by the parietal cells.

Gastritis. Acute or chronic inflammation of the mucous lining of the stomach. It is due to a variety of causes, including allergy, ingestion of poison or irritants, and dietary indiscretion (i.e., rapid eating, overeating, or large intakes of fibrous or highly seasoned foods). Gastritis may also accompany cancer. *Dietary management:* correct faulty eating habits and provide nutritionally adequate meals. For chronic gastritis, depending on the patient's tolerance of solid foods, a soft diet is given in six small feedings, with vitamin and mineral supplements, particularly iron and vitamin B_{12}. In acute gastritis, withholding food for 24 hours to allow the stomach to rest may be indicated, followed by clear fluids the next day before a full liquid to soft diet is started.

Gastroenteritis. Inflammation of the stomach and intestine, usually due to viral infection. Characterized by diarrhea, vomiting, and abdominal pain with or without fever. *Dietary management:* see under *Gastritis.*

Gastroenterostomy. Surgical formation of a communication between the stomach and the small intestine, usually performed to short-circuit the food around a stomach ulcer.

Gastrointestinal tract (GIT). Also called the *"alimentary tract."* Refers to the entire digestive tract from the mouth through the stomach, intestines, and anus.

Gastroparesis. Partial paralysis of the stomach which may be related to local neuritis. It is a result of inadequate or absent contractions of the gastric muscles. There is delayed gastric emptying, as seen in diabetic autonomic neuropathy. Symptoms include anorexia, nausea, vomiting, constipation or diarrhea, and abdominal pain and distention. Symptoms are of varying degree and severity, and may lead to weight loss and *bezoar* formation. *Dietary management:* patients with mild to moderate gastroparesis may tolerate oral feedings of easy-to-digest foods given in small amounts. Patients with severe disease may need tube feedings. An elemental formula is usually the initial feeding. Tolerance to the feeding and adequacy of hydration should be monitored.

Gastroplasty. Surgical procedure reducing the volume of the stomach to only 50 ml, or about 2 liquid ounces. See *Gastric bypass (stapling).*

Gastrostomy. Opening into the stomach from the outside, usually for artificial feeding. The introduction of a nutrient formula through this gastrostomy tube is sometimes called "gastrogavage." Gastrostomy can be accomplished using either percutaneous endoscopic methods or an open surgical approach.

Gaucher's disease. A rare familial disease caused by an enzyme deficiency. Characterized by disturbance in lipid metabolism; accumulation of *kerasin* in the liver, spleen, lymph nodes, and bone marrow; and abnormal bone growth. Mortality is high in infancy and early childhood. *Dietary management:* milk formula low in fats but otherwise adequate in other nutrients and calories for infants. For children, provide the daily diet meeting the recommended dietary allowances according to age, controlling the fat level to 20–25% of total caloric intake.

GDM. Abbreviation for *gestational diabetes mellitus.*

Gemfibrozil. A lipid-lowering drug that decreases serum triglycerides, principally very-low-density lipoprotein triglycerides and to a less extent low-density-lipoprotein triglycerides; used in the management of type IV and mild type V hyperlipoproteinemia. The most frequent side effects involve the gastrointestinal tract and may cause dry mouth, anorexia, abdominal and epigastric pain, diarrhea, flatulence, nausea, and vomiting. The brand name is Lopid.

Gentamicin. An aminoglycoside antibiotic; active against many aerobic gram-negative bacteria and some gram-positive bacteria and used for treatment of skin and eye infections. Gentamicin increases the urinary excretion of potassium and magnesium, and may induce hypokalemia and hypomagnesemia. Brand names are Garamycin, Gentafair, Genoptic, Gentacidin, and Gentak.

Gerovital. A buffered solution of procaine hydrochloride; a compound that is being promoted as one that alleviates symptoms of aging and has been designated by some as "vitamin H_3" or "vitamin GH_3." These claims have not been supported, and gerovital is not recognized as a vitamin.

Gestational diabetes mellitus (GDM). High blood glucose level (hyperglycemia) developed during pregnancy which usually disappears after the baby is delivered. One cause is an overproduction of hormones by the placenta that antagonizes the action of insulin. Women who have a family history of diabetes or who are overweight have a greater chance of exhibiting GDM, which may recur with subsequent pregnancies. About 60% of the cases of GDM develop later in life as Type II or adult-onset diabetes. It is important to note that normal glucose levels in pregnancy are lower than in the nonpregnant state. Fasting blood glucose levels during pregnancy should be within 60–110 mg/dl, and 2 hours after a meal the acceptable range is 80–140 mg/dl. Self blood glucose monitoring (SBGM) and food records are very important, along with regular exercise and prescribed medications. The urine must be ketone-free. Total weight gain during pregnancy should be within 24 to 28 lb. *Dietary management:* give 30 kcal/kg/day, of which 50% should be provided by carbohydrates. Distribute the carbohydrates as follows: 10% for breakfast, 30% for lunch, 30% for dinner, and 10% each for in-between snacks. Breakfast is small and low in carbohydrate because of the tendency during pregnancy for peak postprandial glucose levels to occur early in the day. Avoid simple sugars and emphasize complex carbohydrates, which are more slowly absorbed and converted into glucose. Provide about 20-25% of the total calories from proteins, emphasizing proteins of high biologic value, supplied by a quart of milk a day, and the rest by lean meats, cheese, fish, and eggs. Encourage liberal intake of fluids. See also *blood sugar level* and *Diabetes mellitus.*

Gevral. Brand name for a high-protein, low-sodium supplement in powder form for use in high-protein, sodium-restricted diets. The protein source is from calcium caseinate; $^1/_3$ cup powder provides 95 kcal, 16 gm protein, 7 gm carbohydrate, and less than 1 gm fat. See Appendix 39.

GFR. Abbreviation for *glomerular filtration rate.*

Gingivitis. Inflammation of the gums (gingiva). Gingivitis is seen in association with vitamin C deficiency and is characterized by spongy, swollen gums that bleed readily. This may result in a high susceptibility to infection; teeth may become loose if the condition is not corrected.

GIT. Abbreviation for *gastrointestinal tract.*

Gland. Cell, tissue, or organ that produces a product used by the body (secretion) or eliminated from the body (excretion). Examples of glands that *secrete* are adrenal and thyroid glands; examples of glands that *excrete* are sweat and oil glands.

Gliadin. Glutamine-bound fraction of protein in wheat, oats, rye, and barley; a simple protein which lacks lysine and is classified as a partially complete protein. See also *Gluten.*

Glipizide. A sulfonylurea oral hypoglycemic agent for management of noninsulin-dependent diabetes mellitus (NIDDM). It has a metallic taste. Side effects are dose related and may cause nausea and vomiting. Alcohol may induce flushing and headache, and hypoglycemia may occur with prolonged exercise without caloric supplementation or with alcohol consumption. The brand name is Glucotrol.

Globin. A colorless basic protein often found in combination with other proteins; soluble in water, acid, or alkali and coagulable by heat. See Appendix 9.

Globulins. Group of plant and animal proteins slightly soluble in water but extremely soluble in salt solution; an important component of human blood. Fractionation of plasma globulins by electrophoresis gives alpha, beta, and gamma globulins. See Appendix 9.

Glomerular filtration rate (GFR). Number of milliliters of blood that is passed through the glomeruli in 1 minute. The normal GFR is approximately 130 ml/min. A polysaccharide such as inulin can be used to measure the GFR, since it is filtered but not reabsorbed by the kidney tubules. The amount of inulin in the urine corresponds to the amount that has been filtered from the plasma. This test is used to estimate the degree of function of the kidney. Aging and some disease conditions reduce the GFR. In chronic renal failure, the GFR helps determine the daily protein intake as follows: protein is restricted to 0.5 to 0.6 gm/kg/day (about 40 gm protein/day) if the GFR is 5-10 ml/min and to 0.7 gm/kg/day (about 50 gm protein/day) if the GFR is 15 ml/min. For every 50% reduction in GFR, the serum creatinine level will double. For example, with a GFR of 100 ml/min, the serum creatinine concentration is 1.0 mg/dl. As GFR decreases to 50 ml/min, the serum creatinine level increases to 2.0 mg/dl.

Glomerulonephritis. Inflammatory disease of the kidneys affecting chiefly the glomeruli. It may be acute or chronic and generally follows streptococcal infections of the respiratory tract such as tonsillitis, sinusitis, pneumonia, and influenza. Symptoms include nitrogen retention, presence of albumin and blood in the urine, and varying degrees of hypertension, edema, and uremia preceding convulsions and death. *Dietary management:* protein is restricted to 0.3 gm/kg/day when there is nitrogen retention. This may progress to 0.5 gm/kg/day and gradually increased as the patient's condition improves. Potassium is restricted to

2 gm/day if hyperkalemia is present. Sodium is restricted (1-2 gm/day) in edematous conditions. Replace fluids for normal diuresis, but if oliguria is present, restrict fluids to 600 ml/day. See *Nephritis.*

Glomerulus. Pl. "glomeruli." A coil or cluster of blood vessels projecting into the expanded end of each secreting tubule of the kidney.

Glossitis. Inflammation of the tongue (glossa); usually due to biting, burning, or injuring the tongue. It may also be a symptom of a gastrointestinal disorder or a nutritional deficiency. Deficiencies in niacin, riboflavin, vitamin B_{12}, folic acid, and iron may all give rise to glossitis. It is a feature of pellagra, sprue, and the various types of nutritional anemias. In acute glossitis, the tongue is swollen, the papillae are very prominent, and the color is characteristically red or purplish blue. Deep, irregular fissuring is common and shallow ulcers may occur, especially on the sides or tip. In chronic atrophic glossitis, the tongue is small and the surface appears smooth or has fine fissuring.

Glucagon. A hyperglycemic-glycogenolytic hormone of the pancreas that is protein in nature. Also found in gastric and duodenal mucosa, as well as in some commercial insulin preparations. It increases the blood sugar level by stimulating the breakdown of glycogen into glucose in the liver.

Glucerna. Brand name of a nutritional product, low in carbohydrate and with fiber, for patients with diabetes mellitus and stress-induced hyperglycemia. Made of sodium and calcium caseinates, hydrolyzed cornstarch, fructose, safflower and soy oils, and fiber from soy polysaccharide (14.3 gm fiber/liter). See Appendix 39.

Glucoascorbic acid. An analog of ascorbic acid; acts as an antivitamin C and can cause scurvy even in animals that do not normally require the vitamin in their diet.

Glucocorticoids. Steroid hormones secreted by the adrenal cortex or synthetic analogs of these hormones. These include corticosterone, cortisone, and cortisol. Glucocorticoids act primarily on carbohydrate, lipid, and protein metabolism, and also have anti-allergic and antiinflammatory effects. Prolonged use may cause protein wasting, decrease bone density, decreased glucose tolerance, increased appetite, weight gain, hypercholesterolemia, sodium and water retention, and peptic ulcer.

Glucogenesis. Formation of glucose; may arise from any of the intermediates in glycolysis or from glucogenic substances such as glycerol and some of the amino acids that can be converted into one of the intermediates in carbohydrate metabolism.

Glucola. Brand name of a drink that may be used in place of a 100-gm carbohydrate meal for a glucose tolerance test. A 7-oz bottle contains the equivalent of 75 gm of glucose; the rest of the carbohydrate is in the form of a partial hydrolysate of cornstarch dissolved in a cola-flavored solution that is also carbonated.

Glucolysis. Metabolic breakdown of glucose. See *Glycolysis.*

Gluconeogenesis. Formation of glucose or glycogen from noncarbohydrate sources such as glycerol and glucogenic amino acids.

Glucosamine. Amino sugar in which carbon atom 2 of glucose contains an amino group. Results from the hydrolysis of chitin and occurs in various mammalian polysaccharides, including heparin, hyaluronic acid, and several bacterial polysaccharides.

Glucose. Also called "dextrose," "grape sugar," or "blood sugar"; a 6-carbon monosaccharide occurring naturally in plant tissues and obtained from the complete hydrolysis of starch. It is the chief form in which carbohydrate is absorbed into the bloodstream. Physiologically, glucose is considered the most important sugar, and hence is referred to as the "physiologic sugar." It is the only source of energy for the brain which needs about 140 gm/day. It is the form in which carbohydrate is circulated in the blood and can be utilized by all cells. Glucose can be converted to glycogen or fat for future energy needs.

Glucose/nitrogen (G/N) ratio. The ratio between the amount of glucose and the amount of nitrogen excreted in the urine following induction of diabetes by phlorizin. It is an indication of the proportion of sugar that can be derived from protein. The ratio varies with the severity of the diabetes, reaching a maximum value of about 3.65.

Glucose tolerance factor (GTF). The biologically active form of chromium bound to an organic compound. It potentiates the action of insulin and increases the uptake of glucose by the cell. GTF is present in the liver, blood plasma, and other cells, and is also found in brewer's yeast, black pepper, and whole grains.

Glucose tolerance test (GTT). Also called the "oral glucose tolerance test (OGTT)." Test that measures the ability of the body to utilize a known amount of glucose. It is performed after a 12-hour fast. The subject is given orally 50 to 100 gm of glucose or an allowance of 1.75 gm/kg body weight. Blood samples for glucose analysis are taken after ½ hour and then at hourly intervals for the next 4 or 5 hours. A normal individual shows a rise in blood sugar about ½ hour after ingestion of glucose, but the blood sugar level returns to normal after 2 hours. A diabetic person shows a much higher rise in blood sugar after ½ hour, a rise that continues even after 2 hours and remains higher than normal after 4 hours. The plotted results of blood sugar values form the glucose tolerance curve.

Glucuronic acid. A sugar acid resulting from the oxidation of the primary hydroxyl group of glucose to COOH. It is present in various complex polysaccharides, and many toxic substances in the body are excreted in combination with glucuronic acid as *glucuronides.*

Glutamic acid. Alpha-aminoglutaric acid, a nonessential amino acid that is a constituent of *folic acid.* It is involved in transamination and deamination reactions and in the synthesis of glutathione, *GABA,* and glutamine. The monosodium salt of glutamic acid (MSG) is widely used as a flavoring agent.

Glutamine. Compound formed from glutamic acid and ammonia in the liver, brain, and kidneys. It plays an important role in transamination reactions and serves as a source of ammonia in the kidneys for base conservation. Glutamine can cross the blood-brain barrier, thus providing a source of glutamic acid for brain oxidation. The splitting of glutamine to glutamic acid and ammonia is catalyzed by the enzyme *glutaminase.* Long considered a nonessential amino acid, glutamine is now recognized for its role in wound healing.

Glutathione. A tripeptide composed of glutamic acid, cysteine, and glycine; widely distributed in nature and isolated from yeast, muscle, and liver. It is the prosthetic group of glyceraldehyde phosphate dehydrogenase and is believed to help maintain the sulfhydryl-containing enzymes in the reduced state that is essential for their activity.

Glutelin. A simple protein found in cereals; insoluble in water and neutral solutions but soluble in dilute acids and alkalis. Examples are *glutenin* in wheat, *oryzenin* in rice, and *hordein* in barley. See Appendix 9.

Gluten. Protein fraction of wheat and other cereals that gives flour the elastic property which is essential for bread making. It is composed of two fractions: gliadin and glutenin. It is believed that the gliadin portion is responsible for the malabsorption syndrome in susceptible individuals with gluten-sensitive enteropathy. This condition is corrected by eliminating wheat, oats, rye, and barley from the diet. See also *Diet, gluten-free.*

Gluten-sensitive enteropathy. Also called "gluten-induced enteropathy," "celiac disease," and "celiac sprue"; a form of malabsorption primarily affecting the proximal portion of the small intestines and characterized by damage to villus epithelial cells in response to ingestion of gluten. The cause of the intolerance is as yet unclear; a lack of brush-border enzyme and an immune reaction to alpha-gliadin have been proposed. It occurs in both children and adults. The principal abnormality is the failure of the jejunal mucosa to absorb digested substances adequately because of villus atrophy and a resultant reduction in the number of functioning absorptive cells. As a consequence, there is general malabsorption of fat, carbohydrate, protein, vitamins, and minerals. The condition is characterized by loss of weight, nausea and vomiting, abdominal pain, weakness, and diarrhea consisting of pale, bulky, frothy, foul-smelling stools. There is generalized wasting, and signs of multiple vitamin and mineral deficiencies develop, such as anemia, cheilosis, glossitis, peripheral edema, tetany, rickets, and hypoprothrombinemia with a tendency to bleed. The condition is completely relieved if *gluten,* derived chiefly from wheat, oat, and rye, is excluded from the diet. See *Diet, gluten-free.*

Glutethimide. A sedative and hypnotic used primarily in short-term treatment of insomnia. It probably induces inactivation of 25-hydroxyvitamin D_3, and thus may increase vitamin D turnover and bone resorption; it may also cause polyneuropathy, dry mouth, and gastric irritation. It is excreted in milk. The brand name is Doriden.

Glyburide. A sulfonylurea antidiabetic agent used in the management of noninsulin-dependent diabetes mellitus. Hypoglycemia may occur with inadequate food intake and prolonged exercise or with alcohol consumption. Simultaneous alcohol ingestion may cause flushing, headache, nausea, and vomiting. The drug has a metallic taste. Brand names are DiaBeta and Micronase.

Glycemic index. Measurement of the 2-hour glucose response to different foods given alone and compared with the value obtained after ingestion of bread as a standard. Glycemic index values are expressed as a percentage of that for bread. The results obtained thus allow foods to be compared on a rating scale where foods at the top of the scale raise blood glucose to a greater degree than foods at the bottom of the scale. This enables comparisons between different foods. In general, the lower glycemic index foods are kidney beans and legumes, while the higher ones are potatoes and refined cereals.

Glyceraldehyde. Glyceric aldehyde, the simplest form of carbohydrate, containing only 3 carbon atoms. In the form of phosphate ester, it acts as an intermediate product in the anaerobic breakdown of carbohydrate; it also serves as a precursor of glycerol.

Glycerol. Also called "glycerin"; trihydroxypropane, a trihydroxy alcohol. It is a clear, colorless, sweetish, and viscous liquid obtained from the hydrolysis of fats and oils. Esters of glycerol with fatty acids are called "glycerides." Glycerol possesses three hydroxy groups; it can combine with three molecules of fatty acid to form a *triglyceride* or simple fat.

Glycine (Gly). Formerly called "glycocoll"; aminoacetic acid, the simplest amino acid. It is sweet-tasting. It is an essential constituent of body tissues, a precursor of bile acid, and a participant in the detoxication mechanism and synthesis of purine, creatine, glutathione, and porphyrins. It is not considered a dietary essential except for growing chickens.

Glycinuria. Condition characterized by excessive excretion of glycine in the urine and elevated glycine blood levels accompanied by metabolic acidosis, respiratory distress, seizures, hematologic abnormalities, and mental retardation, leading to death. It is considered an inborn error of metabolism, although the specific enzyme defect has not been identified; it is probably due to a failure of conversion of glycine to glyoxalate. Symptoms are controlled by a low-protein diet with arginine and pyridoxine supplementation.

Glycocholic acid. One of the *bile acids,* yielding glycine and cholic acid on hydrolysis.

Glycogen. Animal starch; a branched-chain polysaccharide composed of glucose units. It is the chief carbohydrate storage material in animals, especially in the liver and muscles. In a well-nourished adult, glycogen is about 2-8% of the weight of the liver. Although muscle contains less glycogen (approximately 1%) than the liver, the greater mass of the muscle accounts for a considerable quantity of this storage form of carbohydrate. The amount of reserve glycogen stored in the liver and muscle depends largely on the nature of the diet and the amount of exercise. Fasting results in a rapid depletion of liver glycogen, and muscle glycogen is depleted during continuous or violent exercise.

Glycogenesis. Formation or synthesis of glycogen. Glycogenic substances are hexoses, as well as a wide variety of other compounds, e.g., glycogenic amino acids, glycerol derived from lipids, intermediates in glycolysis such as lactic acid and pyruvic acid, and products structurally related to hexoses.

Glycogenolysis. Breakdown or splitting up of glycogen, as opposed to glycogenesis. The conversion of glycogen to glucose occurs in several steps involving phosphorylation, rearrangement, dephosphorylation, and condensation or hydrolysis, with each step requiring a specific enzyme.

Glycogenosis. Type II glycogen storage disease characterized by extreme deposition of glycogen in the heart. The heart enlarges to as much as five times its normal weight. Infants affected by this condition usually die of heart failure before the age of 2 years. They resemble cretins or mongoloids, have poor appetites, and fail to grow. The specific enzyme defect is lysosomal α-1,4 glucosidase.

Glycogen storage disease. One of a group of genetically inherited metabolic disorders characterized by an abnormal accumulation of glycogen in the liver and other tissues. The condition is due to a deficiency in one of several enzymes involved in the interconversion of glycogen and glucose. The clinical manifestations vary with the enzyme deficiency and may include fasting hypoglycemia, hepatomegaly and liver cirrhosis, failure to thrive, convulsions, and muscular atrophy. Treatment requires frequent feedings, including a late-night snack of carbohydrate in the form of glucose or starch; a high protein intake is also beneficial. See *von Gierke's disease* and Appendix 44.

Glycolipid. Lipid that yields a carbohydrate, a fatty acid, and an alcohol on hydrolysis.

Glycolysis. Also called "Embden-Meyerhof pathway"; a series of reactions involving the anaerobic breakdown of glycogen (or glucose) in the tissues, with lactic or pyruvic acid as the end product. The net result is the synthesis of two molecules of adenosine triphosphate (ATP) per mole of glucose catabolized; oxygen is not consumed in the overall process. In the presence of oxygen, pyruvic acid is completely oxidized to carbon dioxide and water in the mitochondria by way of the Krebs tricarboxylic acid cycle and its associated oxidative phosphorylation. Although the yield of ATP from glycolysis is small compared to the net yield of 38 moles of ATP/mole of glucose with complete oxidation, glycolysis provides a means of rapidly obtaining ATP (hence, energy) in a relatively anaerobic organ such as muscle.

Glyconeogenesis. Former term for *gluconeogenesis.*

Glycoprotein. Conjugated product composed of a polysaccharide bound to protein such as ovomucin in egg white.

Glycosuria. Presence of sugar in the urine. It may be due to *diabetes mellitus,* a lowered renal threshold for glucose without any accompanying blood glucose elevation, a brain tumor or injury, or temporary emotional tension or worry.

Glycosylated hemoglobin (HbA$_{1c}$). A compound formed in the red blood cells by the irreversible reaction of hemoglobin A with glucose. The glycosylated hemoglobin concentration indicates the average blood glucose level over the previous 6 to 8 weeks. The rate of formation increases when the blood glucose level is elevated, as in uncontrolled diabetes mellitus. Normal values in nondiabetics are about 5% of the total hemoglobin, while uncontrolled diabetics have more than 10%. It is a reliable tool for evaluating long-term management of diabetes mellitus.

Glymidine. Sulfonylpyrimidine derivative that has a hypoglycemic action; used for the oral treatment of diabetes mellitus.

G/N ratio. Abbreviation for *glucose/nitrogen ratio.*

Goiter. Enlargement of the thyroid gland due to lack of iodine (simple goiter), overproduction of the thyroid hormone in hyperthyroid states (exophthalmic goiter or thyrotoxicosis), or decreased production of the thyroid hormone in hypothyroid states (cretinism and myxedema).

   Exophthalmic g. Also called "thyrotoxicosis," "Graves' disease," or "Basedow's disease"; results from hyperthyroidism and is characterized by a high basal metabolic rate leading to loss of weight, excessive nervousness, protruding eyeballs (exophthalmos), and enlarged thyroid gland. See also *Hyperthyroidism.*

Simple g. Enlargement of the thyroid gland, producing no symptoms either of hypothyroidism or of hyperthyroidism. It may be due to a deficiency in iodine, a constituent of the thyroid hormone *thyroxine,* or to antithyroid agents such as *goitrogens* in food, thiourea, thiouracil, or some of the sulfonamides that interfere with the synthesis of thyroxine by the thyroid gland. *Dietary management:* the most practical treatment is to supply iodine adequately, which is accomplished by iodization of salt. The fortification level used in the U.S. is 76 micrograms of iodide per gram of salt. Other rich sources of iodine include seafoods, especially seaweeds, although their iodine content depends on the level in the water. Drug therapy is still the primary treatment.

Goitrogens. Substances present in some foods that are capable of producing goiter by interfering with the production of the thyroid hormone. These have been identified as *arachidoside,* present in the red skin of peanuts, and *thiooxazolidone,* present in plants of the genus *Brassica* (e.g., cabbage, cauliflower, and turnip). Goitrogens are destroyed by heat.

Gooseflesh. Also called "goose pimples"; term given to rough skin characterized by erection of the hair follicles, as from cold or shock. Also seen in vitamin A deficiency. See *Keratosis.*

Gout. A disorder of purine metabolism characterized by abnormally high uric acid levels in the blood and deposits of sodium urate in soft and bony tissues like joints, cartilage, and tendons. The hyperuricemia of gout may be due to overproduction of uric acid or inadequate excretion by the kidney. *Dietary management:* some limitation in dietary purines may be advisable to prevent a needless increase in the uric acid pool. As an adjunct to drug therapy, a purine-restricted diet will reduce the excretion of uric acid by 200 to 400 mg/day and lower the mean serum uric acid level by 1 mg/100 ml. Other dietary considerations include weight control and maintenance of desirable body weight, high fluid intake to prevent urate precipitation in the kidneys, and moderate alcohol consumption since alcohol inhibits renal excretion of urates. See *Diet, purine-restricted.*

Grape sugar. Glucose or dextrose. See *Glucose.*

Griseofulvin. An antifungal antibiotic used for treatment of mycoses of the skin, hair, and nails. It may cause altered taste acuity, dry mouth, epigastric distress, nausea, and vomiting. Concurrent ingestion with alcohol may also cause tachycardia, headache, and flushing. High-fat meals increase drug absorption. Brand names include Fulvicin, Grifulvin, and Grisactin.

Growth factor. Any factor, such as a mineral, a vitamin, or a hormone, that promotes the growth of an organism.

Growth hormone. See *Somatotrophin (somatotropic hormone).*

GTT. Abbreviation for *glucose tolerance test.*

Guanethidine. A postganglionic adrenergic agent used in the treatment of hypertension. Long-term use may cause weight gain due to sodium and fluid retention; it may also cause dry mouth, taste disturbances, diarrhea, and possible anemia. Brand names are Ismelin and Esimil.

Guillain-Barré syndrome. A neurologic disorder characterized by an acute postinfectious polyneuritis, involving numbness, increasing fatigue, pain, and paralysis. This syndrome indicates respiratory failure and fluctuating blood pressure, coupled with weakening of the lower extremities, and even personality changes. *Dietary management:* total parenteral nutrition may be needed in certain cases. Increase calories and proteins as necessary. Monitor fat intake to prevent overproduction of carbon dioxide. As the patient improves, introduce a soft to regular diet with frequent snacks. Provide supplemental vitamins and minerals if the patient has problems with oral intake.

H

Haldane apparatus. Open-circuit type of respiration apparatus that applies the principle of *indirect calorimetry*. A small animal placed in the chamber is weighed before and after the experiment. The difference in weight represents carbon dioxide and water eliminated and oxygen consumed. The first two are directly measured by weighing the flasks containing soda lime and sulfuric acid that absorb them. Oxygen consumed is indirectly determined by subtracting the sum of carbon dioxide and water losses from the total weight loss of the animal.

Halibut liver oil. Expressed oil from fresh halibut liver standardized to contain approximately 100 times the amount of vitamin A and 10 to 30 times the amount of vitamin D.

Hamwi formula. A quick estimate for ideal body weight (IDW) that is easy to remember:

IBW for adult males (in lb)
= 106 lb for five feet plus 6 lb per inch over 5 feet.

IBW for adult females (in lb)
= 100 lb for five feet plus 5 lb per inch over 5 feet.

HANES. Abbreviation for Health and Nutrition Examination Survey. See *NHANES.*

Haptoglobin (Hp). Serum mucoprotein that binds hemoglobin. Its major role appears to be the conservation of body iron by binding hemoglobin and preventing its loss from the body. Increased levels of Hp are found in individuals with inflammatory or neoplastic disease. Plasma levels are decreased in acute hepatitis and hemolytic conditions.

Harelip. Congenital cleft or defect in the upper lip, usually due to failure of the median nasal and maxillary process to unite. *Dietary management:* individualize the diet for the infant or child according to age to meet the recommended dietary allowances. Modify the consistency of the diet from liquid to pureed or semisoft foods, depending on the seriousness of the defect. Special feeding tools may be needed in certain cases. See also *Cleft palate.*

Harris-Benedict formula. Formula for estimating basal energy expenditure (BEE) based on body weight and standing height. It is used to calculate the basal metabolic rate (BMR) (was originally termed BEE by Harris and Benedict, who in 1919 devised the formula):

BEE or BMR (men)
$$= 66.473 + 13.752 \, W + 5.003 \, H - 6.755 \, A$$

BEE or BMR (women)
$$= 66.096 + 9.563 \, W + 4.676 \, H - 4.676 \, A$$

where W is weight in kilograms, H is standing height in centimeters, and A is age in years.

Hartnup disease. Also called "H disease"; a genetic abnormality in the renal and intestinal transport of amino acids, especially alanine, threonine, phenylalanine, and tryptophan. The most striking feature is a pellagra-like skin rash sensitive to light, which is most likely due to nicotinamide deficiency secondary to the tryptophan malabsorption. There is also aminoaciduria and some growth retardation and psychological changes. The only treatment needed is nicotinamide supplementation (50 to 200 mg/day). A high-protein diet is recommended to counter amino acid loss in the urine.

Hb. Abbreviation for *hemoglobin.*

Head Start program. Provides children from low-income families with individualized and specialized services to "overcome the physical, social, and emotional deprivation of poverty in order that they may achieve social competence." It offers nutritional care services to develop positive food habits, provides well-balanced and nutritious meals and snacks, and educates families on the importance of food and nutrition in promoting good health, as well as physical, mental, emotional, and social well-being. See *Project Head Start.*

Health. State of physical, mental, and emotional well-being, and not merely freedom from disease or the absence of any ailment.

Healthy People 2000. A broad-based initiative to improve the health of all Americans over the next decade. Led by the U.S. Public Health Service, more than 300 national organizations form the Health Objectives Consortium. Priorities in the development of the objectives include health promotion, health protection, disease prevention, clinical preventive services, and age-related health problems. Some of the nutrition objectives are to reduce coronary heart disease to no more than 100 per 100,000 people; reverse the rise in cancer deaths to achieve a rate of no more than 130 per 100,000 people; reduce overweight to a prevalence of no more than 20% among people aged 20 and older and no more than 15% among adolescents aged 12 through 19; reduce growth retardation among low-income children aged 5 and younger to less than 10%; reduce iron deficiency to less than 3% among children aged 1 through 4 and among women of childbearing age; increase to at least 90% the proportion of school lunch and breakfast services and child care food services, with menus that are consistent with the nutrition principles in the Dietary Guidelines for Americans; and increase to at least 75% the proportion of primary care providers who provide nutrition assessment and counseling and/or referral to qualified nutritionists or dietitians.

Heart. A hollow, muscular, contractile organ; the center of the circulatory system. It is divided into four cavities: a left and a right atrium (or auricle) and a left and a right ventricle. The main function of the heart is to pump blood throughout the body. If this stops for even a short time, irreversible changes occur and death quickly ensues. See also *Nutrition, heart disease.*

Heartburn. Epigastric pain just below the sternum, often accompanied by regurgitation of acid and the presence of gas in the stomach. It may occur 10 to 15 minutes after eating a heavy meal, especially when the person is in a recumbent position. It is a common symptom of many disorders, such as hiatal hernia and esophageal dysfunction. During pregnancy, heartburn results from upward displacement of the esophageal sphincter because of increased intra-abdominal pressure. *Dietary management:* avoid spices, gas formers, alcohol, and large meals. Encourage the patient to eat slowly six to eight small meals a day.

Heat. Sensation of an increase in temperature; measured as a quantity of energy. See *Calorie.*

Heat of combustion. Amount of heat produced (usually expressed in calories) when a unit weight of a substance is oxidized.

Helium dilution. A gasometric procedure for determining body density. The animal or human is enclosed in a chamber of known volume, and a measured volume of helium gas is injected into the chamber. After a period of time long enough to allow mixing of the helium and air in the chamber, a sample is removed and analyzed. The degree to which helium gas is diluted is inversely proportional to the volume or space occupied by the animal or human. The smaller the subject, the more diluted the helium gas will be.

Hematin. Ferriprotoporphyrin hydroxide, a neutral compound in which iron is in the ferric state.

Hematocrit (HCT). The packed cell volume of erythrocytes, expressed as a percentage of the total blood volume. Originally, the term meant a flat-bottomed centrifuge tube used to separate red blood cells. When normal blood is centrifuged in this tube, approximately 45% of the volume is separated as cells and the remaining 55% as plasma. It is useful in clinical analysis of blood and can detect decreases (hemoconcentration) or increases (hemodilution) in plasma volume. See Appendix 30.

Hematopoiesis. See *Hemopoiesis.*

Heme. Ferroprotoporphyrin or ferroheme, a nonprotein, iron-containing portion of hemoglobin with no net charge. Contains divalent iron and combines with various nitrogenous bases, forming hemochromogens.

Hemeralopia. Glare blindness or day blindness; defective vision in bright light. A term used to describe the condition of reduced *dark adaptation* resulting from vitamin A deficiency, although there may be other causes such as diseases of the retina.

Hemicellulose. Indigestible polysaccharide found in plant cell walls, particularly in woody fibers and leaves. Hydrolysis by alkalis and acids yields xylose, a pentose sugar, other monosaccharides, and uronic acid. It may be digested to some extent by microbial enzymes. See also *Dietary fiber* under *Fiber.*

Hemin. Ferriprotoporphyrin or ferriheme, a nonprotein, iron-containing portion of hemoglobin with a net positive charge. Contains trivalent iron.

Hemochromatosis. Disorder of iron metabolism characterized by abnormal deposits of *hemosiderin* in the liver, spleen, and other tissues, causing cellular damage and degeneration. It is due to a genetic defect in the uptake of iron in the intestines and the reticuloendothelial system; more than the ordinary amount of iron is absorbed and stored. Features of the disorder include bronzing of the skin, jaundice, cirrhosis of the liver, abdominal pain, and sclerosis of the pancreas. *Dietary management:* reduce the intake of iron, maintaining adequate levels of the other nutrients for the patient. Control weight by maintaining a proper caloric level.

Hemodialysis. Blood is passed through a semipermeable membrane that is continually bathed in a hypotonic dialyzing fluid. The dialyzing machine acts as an artificial kidney. In this way, nitrogenous wastes can be removed from the blood. This method is used in acute and chronic kidney failure and in cases of poisoning where an overdose of a substance usually removed by the kidneys has been taken. *Dietary management:* the aims of the diet are to control edema, avoid nitrogen loss, replace amino acids, and prevent excessive interdialytic buildup of nitrogenous waste products. In hemodialysis, 6 to 8 gm of free amino acids and 3 to 4 gm of bound amino acids are lost per treatment. Thus, protein is usually calculated at 1.0 to 1.2 gm/kg body weight/day. Sodium is restricted to 2 gm/day if edema is present. The potassium level is monitored to avoid hyperkalemia, which may cause cardiac arrest. Caloric intake is calculated to prevent catabolism of lean body mass, with nonprotein calories provided by simple carbohydrates, fats, and oils. Additional restrictions may be prescribed, such as specific levels of fluid intake (e.g., 1200 or 1500 ml/day), calcium, and phosphorus (800 to 1200 mg/day or 15 mg/gm protein).

Hemoglobin (Hb). The oxygen-carrying pigment of red blood cells; a conjugated protein with the prosthetic group, *heme,* attached to the protein moiety, *globin.* A single red blood cell has about 280 million moles of Hb, each of which has a molecular weight of about 64,500. Of the 10,000 atoms in Hb, only 4 are iron atoms. The globin molecule accounts for the "species specificity" of Hb among animals. All types of human Hb have the same molecular weight and physical properties, but they differ in the globin portion because of a change in amino acid sequence. Normal Hb values for adults are about 14 to 16 gm/100 ml blood. The main function of Hb is to carry oxygen from the lungs to the tissues and transport carbon dioxide back to the lungs. A low Hb content of the blood is a useful indicator of nutritional anemia, which may be caused by a deficiency in iron, copper, folic acid, vitamin B_{12} and protein. See also *Anemia* and *Hemopoiesis.*

Hemolysis. Destruction of red blood cells with the liberation of hemoglobin. May be brought about by various hemolytic agents, such as bacterial toxins, bile salts, and the venoms of certain poisonous snakes, or by the production in the body of specific *hemolysins,* a class of immune substances or antibodies elicited as a result of injection of incompatible blood.

Hemopoiesis (hematopoiesis). More appropriately termed "erythropoiesis" or the formation of red blood cells (RBC). The average life span of an RBC is 4 months or about 127 days. RBC are continually destroyed and replaced. The process takes place mainly in the bone marrow, and to some extent in the liver and spleen. The primitive RBC matures by passing through several stages in the following order: *proerythroblast* (large cell with a granular nucleus); *basophilic normoblast* (the nucleus is more compact and less granular); *eosinophilic normoblast* (the cell acquires more hemoglobin and becomes acidophilic); *reticulocyte* (an immature or young RBC devoid of a nucleus but rich in ribosomes and nucleic acids); and finally, the mature RBC or erythrocyte. The hemoglobin (Hb) remains in the RBC throughout its life span until the worn-out cell is removed from the circulation by cells of the *reticuloendothelial system* (bone marrow, liver, and spleen). On destruction, the heme portion of Hb is split into *bilirubin* and other pigments that are carried to the liver and secreted in the bile. The released iron can be reutilized to form Hb. Factors needed for normal hemopoiesis include a hormonal factor (erythropoietin, a hematopoietic hormone found in the plasma); a maturation factor (folic acid); and other nutritional factors (good-quality protein, folic acid, ascorbic acid, iron, copper, etc.). In general, all nutrients, plus sufficient calories, are involved directly or indirectly in hemopoiesis.

Hemorrhage. Bleeding; profuse escape of blood from the vessels, which may be due to various causes. There may be *pulmonary hemorrhage* (from the lungs); *primary hemorrhage* (as an immediate result of injury); *renal hemorrhage* (as in glomerulonephritis); or *spontaneous hemorrhage* (in hemophilia), among others. Hemorrhaging is a common cause of *anemia.*

Hemosiderin. A dark yellow pigment of an iron-protein complex; a storage form of iron found in the liver, spleen, and bone marrow. Unlike *ferritin,* which is a water-soluble complex of iron and protein, hemosiderin is insoluble and granular.

Hemosiderosis. Condition of increased *hemosiderin* accumulation in the liver and other tissues; it occurs when excess iron can no longer be stored as *ferritin* and hemosiderin storage has reached its normal limits. It has been observed with excess iron intake (such as from prolonged iron therapy in non-iron-deficient individuals) and in chronic alcoholism, chronic liver disease, pernicious anemia, and certain types of refractory anemia. Hemosiderosis is increased iron storage without tissue damage, whereas *hemochromatosis* refers to increased storage with associated tissue damage.

HEP. Abbreviation for *high-energy phosphate.*

Heparin. A mucopolysaccharide with a molecular weight of about 18,000; it contains glucuronic acid, glucosamine, and sulfate ester groups. It acts as an anticoagulant by preventing the conversion of prothrombin to thrombin.

HepatAmine. Brand name of an 8% amino acid solution with high branched-chain amino acids (36% BCAA) for parenteral nutrition support in patients with liver disease and hepatic encephalopathy; it is high in arginine and low in methionine. See Appendix 39.

Hepatic. Pertaining to the liver (hepatic gland).

Hepatic Aid II. Brand name of a powdered nutritional supplement containing essential and nonessential amino acids, maltodextrins, sucrose, partially hydrogenated soy oil, and lecithin. It is high in branched-chain amino acids (46% BCAA) and arginine, and low in aromatic amino acid and methionine, for the dietary management of patients with chronic liver disease. See Appendix 39.

Hepatic coma. A neurologic disorder indicating extensive liver damage, characterized by varying degrees of consciousness, stupor, and lethargy. Other symptoms include personality change, trembling of the hands, loss of memory, hyperventilation, convulsions, and respiratory alkalosis. Endogenous or exogenous products toxic to the brain are not neutralized in the liver, and death may occur. *Dietary management:* the basic principle of the diet is to avoid tissue protein catabolism and to reduce ammonia production. It is not always necessary to reduce protein intake. When antibiotic therapy is not sufficient or effective, it may be necessary to restrict dietary protein. The level of protein restriction is very low—about 0.2 gm/kg body weight. Protein restriction should be used for as short a time as possible because protein is important in healing the liver tissue. As the patient's condition improves, increase the protein intake by 10 gm/day until a normal allowance is consumed. Provide sufficient calories from carbohydrate and fat (2000 kcal/day or more) to keep body tissue breakdown to a minimum. See *Diet, protein modified.*

Hepatic encephalopathy. Also called "liver failure." A disorder causing brain damage with ammonia intoxication. Clinical signs include disorientation for time and place, ascites, and general edema, bleeding, and hepatic coma. *Dietary management:* similar to that of *hepatic coma,* although some patients requiring tube feeding respond to solutions high in branched-chain amino acids (BCAA). Supplemental vitamins, particularly the B complex, C, and A, are recommended.

Hepatic insufficiency. Disorder that occurs in severe hepatic disease, characterized by a tendency to hemorrhage. Prothrombin and fibrinogen levels are decreased, and blood clotting is delayed. For dietary management, see *Hepatic encephalopathy.*

Hepatitis. Inflammation of the liver. May be caused by infectious agents such as viruses and bacteria, toxic drugs such as arsenicals, or toxic solvents such as carbon tetrachloride. Main symptoms are marked anorexia, fever, headache, rapid and marked weight loss, jaundice, and abdominal discomfort. Chronic hepatitis may lead to *cirrhosis* of the liver. *Dietary management:* a high-calorie, liberal-protein, high-carbohydrate, and moderate-fat intake is recommended. The objectives of the diet are to aid the regeneration of the liver tissue, to rest the liver, to assist in maintaining nitrogen balance, and to ensure glycogen storage. During the acute phase of the disease, a full liquid diet is given, which progresses to a soft diet and eventually to a regular diet as the patient's condition improves. Six to eight small feeding spaced throughout the day are beneficial.

Hepatoflavin. Name given to *riboflavin* isolated from the liver. See *Vitamin B2.*

Hepatomegaly. Enlargement of the liver. It is seen in certain infections; in diseases of the liver, blood, and heart; and in some nutritional deficiency states, such as kwashiorkor.

Herpes. Inflammatory skin disease characterized by the formation of small vesicles or blisters on the skin or mucous membranes. There are many types, but the most common is an acute viral type called *herpes simplex.* Type I is likely to cause oral infections and Type II affects the genitalia and anus. *Dietary management:* provide adequate calories and liberal amount of protein. Monitor the side effects of drugs used for reducing infection and fever.

Herpes zoster. A viral infection that is usually concentrated at a specific nerve tract, with neuralgic pain. Varicella virus may be an indication, and acuteness varies with age. Children may be detected with varicella or "chicken pox." *Dietary management:* replenish calorie and fluid losses. Avoid malnutrition by giving adequate protein, vitamins, and minerals. Administer frequent feedings with increased fiber and vitamin E.

Hexose monophosphate shunt (HMS). Also called the "pentose phosphate pathway," "Warburg-Dickens-Lipmann pathway," "phosphogluconate shunt," or "oxidative" shunt; one of two major pathways of glucose metabolism; the other is anaerobic *glycolysis* or the Embden-Meyerhof (EM) pathway. HMS is an aerobic process, whereas the EM pathway is anerobic; the latter occurs almost exclusively in muscles, whereas HMS is the major pathway in the mammary glands, testes, adipose tissues, leukocytes, and adrenal cortex. Both pathways occur in the liver simultaneously; about 50% of glucose is degraded by the EM pathway and the rest by the HMS. The HMS provides the pentoses, particularly ribose, needed for DNA and RNA synthesis. It yields NADPH (TPNH), which is needed for fat, steroid, and cholesterol synthesis and is important in photosynthesis. Many reactions and enzyme systems (e.g., transketolase, aldolase, dehydrogenase, and isomerase) involved in the HMS are identical to those observed in dark-reaction photosynthesis.

Hexuronic acid. 1. Acid derived from hexose sugar by the oxidation of the group on carbon atom 6. The hexuronic acid derived from glucose is glucuronic acid. 2. Name originally given to a substance isolated from lemon juice, later identified as vitamin C.

Hg. Chemical symbol for mercury.

5-HIAA. Abbreviation for 5-hydroxyindole acetic acid.

Hiatal hernia. The diaphragm opening called the "hiatus" is enlarged due to the protrusion of part of the stomach above the diaphragm. Usual symptoms include difficulty in swallowing, reflux, heartburn, and even vomiting of blood. *Dietary management:* see *Reflux esophagitis.*

High-density lipoprotein (HDL). A plasma lipoprotein that has a density of 1.063-1.210 g/dl; classified as the alpha fraction on the basis of electrophoresis. HDL contains about 33% protein, 29% phospholipid, 30% cholesterol, and 8% triglyceride. HDL is involved in the turnover of tissue cholesterol and in the transport of excess cholesterol to the liver, where it is metabolized to bile acids and eventually excreted. An increase in the concentration of HDL is believed to be linked to a decrease in the incidence of atherosclerosis.

High-energy phosphate (HEP). Compound that contains a labile phosphate bond that yields free energy, varying from 5 to 12 kcal/mole, when the bond is dissociated. Examples are adenoside triphosphate, creatine phosphate, and acetyl phosphate. See also *Phosphate bond energy.*

Hippuric acid. Conjugation product of benzoic acid and glycine; a normal constituent of the urine. Formed largely, if not solely, in the liver as a *detoxication* product of benzoic acid.

Histamine. Amine formed by the decarboxylation of histidine; occurs as a decomposition product of histidine and is prepared synthetically. It is a powerful vasodilator and can lower blood pressure. It can be useful in treating various allergies and as a stimulant for gastric pancreatic secretion and visceral muscles. It is used as a diagnostic agent in testing gastric secretion (histamine test). It promotes the contraction of smooth muscles, increases nasal secretions, and relaxes blood vessels and respiratory airways.

Histidine (His). Beta-imidazole alanine, an *essential amino acid.* Although its essentiality for infants and children was established years ago, it was only recently that studies confirmed that adults also need a dietary source of histidine. It is a component of carnosine, anserine, and hemoglobin and a precursor of histamine. See Appendix 9.

Histidinemia. Elevated blood level of histidine and its consequent excretion in the urine (histidinuria). It is a genetic disorder due to lack of the enzyme histidase. The condition is harmless for the majority of affected individuals, although some may develop speech and hearing defects and mental retardation. Avoidance of a high protein intake to restrict dietary histidine may be helpful, although this has not been proven effective.

Hodgkin's disease. Malignant, enlarged lymph nodes causing fatigue, weight loss, slight fever, cough, dyspnea, and chest pain. *Dietary management:* a diet high in calories, protein, and fluids is recommended. Monitor electrolyte balance and correct weight loss.

Homeostasis. Constancy of the internal environment. The ability of the body to maintain a balance among its physiochemical processes; these are dependent on *dynamic states* of metabolism. Homeostatic mechanisms in the body include fluid and pH balance; regulation of body temperature, blood sugar level, heart rate, and pulse rate; and hormonal control.

Homocysteine. A demethylated product of methionine; a homolog of cysteine. Present in cells as an intermediate metabolite; capable of conversion to methionine by direct transfer of a methyl group from compounds such as choline and betaine.

Homocystinuria. Inborn error of metabolism due to lack of the enzyme cystathionine synthetase, which is essential for the conversion of homocysteine to cystathionine, both of which are intermediate products formed in the metabolism of methionine. Plasma levels of methionine and homocysteine are elevated, and large amounts of homocystine are excreted in the urine. A similar condition can result from vitamin B_6 insufficiency, since cystathionine synthetase requires the vitamin as a cofactor. The characteristic symptoms of homocystinuria include mental retardation, dislocated lenses, glaucoma, osteoporosis, skeletal deformities, mild mental retardation, thromboembolism, and early atherosclerosis. A marked biochemical response to high doses of pyridoxine (vitamin B_6) is seen in about half of the individuals affected. Those who do not respond adequately to pyridoxine require a low-methionine, high-cystine diet and monitoring of plasma methionine and homocysteine levels. Supplementary betaine or choline may help promote remethylation of homocystine. See *Diet, methionine-restricted.*

Homogentisic acid. Intermediate product in the metabolism of phenylalanine and tyrosine. It is excreted in the urine in alkaptonuria and becomes oxidized to a blackish pigment on exposure of urine to air. See *Alkaptonuria.*

Hormone. Organic substance produced by groups of cells or an organ and discharged directly into the bloodstream for specific regulatory action on other organs or tissues remote from its original source. With a few exceptions, hormones are generally manufactured by the endocrine glands. Certain hormones are protein in nature (e.g., parathormone and insulin); some are amino acid derivatives (e.g., thyroxine and epinephrine); and others are steroids (e.g., estrogens and androgens).

Hp. Abbreviation for *haptoglobulin.*

Hunger. Craving for food more pronounced than appetite. A feeling of intermittent, brief cramping sensations of pressure and tension in the epigastric region, later accompanied by weakness and irritability. See *Nutrition, hunger.*

Huntington's chorea. An inherited disorder characterized by chronic, progressive chorea and mental deterioration terminating in dementia. It is usually evident in the fourth decade and becomes fatal after 15 years. *Dietary management:* give a high-protein, high-calorie diet modified in consistency from pureed to soft to prevent choking. Semisolid foods are easier to swallow than liquid foods. If necessary, the patient may be tube fed. Since there is loss of control of voluntary movements, most patients need assistance in feeding.

Hyaluronic acid. A viscous, high-molecular-weight mucopolysaccharide containing glucuronic acid and acetylglucosamine. It is found in connective tissue and acts as an intercellular cement that holds the cells together. It also binds water in the interstitial spaces and acts as a shock absorber in the joints.

Hydralazine. An antihypertensive agent used in the management of moderate to severe hypertension and congestive heart failure. Hydralazine is a pyridoxine antagonist and may cause pyridoxine depletion and peripheral neuropathy. Long-term use of the drug may also cause anorexia and retention of sodium and fluid. It is excreted in breast milk. Brand names include Apresazide, Apresoline, Serapes, Serpasil, and Unipres.

Hydrochloric acid (HCl). Also called "muriatic acid." A compound composed of hydrogen and chlorine. It is a normal constituent of the gastric juice in humans and other mammals. Its functions in digestion are to denature protein, activate pepsinogen to pepsin, provide an acid medium for absorption of iron, and stimulate the opening of the pylorus.

Hydrochlorothiazide. A thiazide diuretic used in the management of edema and hypertension. The drug enhances the urinary excretion of riboflavin, potassium, magnesium, zinc, and sodium, and thus cause deficiency states if the dietary intake is not adequate. It may also elevate blood glucose, lipid, and uric acid levels and cause dry mouth, increased thirst, loss of appetite, stomach cramping, and constipation or diarrhea. Hydrochlorothiazide is excreted in breast milk. Brand names include Aldoril, Aquazide, Esidrix, Hydrodiuril, Moduretic, and Oretic.

Hydrocortisone. See *Cortisol.*

Hydrogen (H). An inflammable, colorless, odorless, gaseous chemical element. It is the lightest of all known substances and has the smallest atomic weight. It is present in proteins, carbohydrates, fats, and water. It makes up approximately 10% of the body weight.

Hydrogenation. A process by which molecular hydrogen is added to the double bonds in the unsaturated fatty acids of triglycerides. Oils are changed to solid fats; the process reduces the biologic value of essential fatty acids when these polyunsaturated fatty acids become saturated.

Hydrolysis. Splitting a substance into smaller units by reaction with water.

Hydrostatic pressure. Pressure exerted by a liquid on the surfaces of the walls containing the liquid. In the body, it refers to the blood pressure, which maintains the fluid volume and circulation in the blood vessels.

Hydroxocobalamin. Form of vitamin B_{12} in which the cyanide group is replaced by a hydroxyl group.

Hydroxyapatite. A naturally occurring mineral crystal of the general formula $3Ca_3(PO_4)_2 \cdot Ca(OH)_2$. The minerals in the bone are deposited in the organic matrix in a crystal formation similar to that of hydroxyapatite, except that the hydroxyl groups are partially substituted by other elements and radicals such as fluoride and carbonate.

25-Hydroxycholecalciferol (25-HCC). Also called "25-hydroxyvitamin D_3"; now called "calcidiol." See *Vitamin D.*

5-Hydroxyindole acetic acid. Abbreviated as 5-HIAA; product formed from the breakdown of *serotonin.*

Hydroxylysine. Lysine to which a hydroxyl group has been added. One of the nonessential amino acids, it is found in the structural protein collagen.

Hydroxyproline. Proline to which a hydroxyl group has been added. One of the nonessential amino acids, it is found in the structural protein collagen.

Hydroxyprolinemia. Metabolic disorder due to lack of the enzyme hydroxyproline oxidase. Blood and urine accumulate large amounts of free hydroxyproline, and the condition may lead to mental retardation. At present, no therapy is available.

Hyperaldosteronism. A disorder characterized by increased production of aldosterone by the adrenal cortex. Among the signs and symptoms are muscle spasms of the extremities, hypertension, headache, cardiomegaly, retinopathy, hypokalemia, and paresthesia. *Dietary management:* a diet high in potassium may be required. Restrict sodium intake and hydrate adequately.

Hyperalimentation. Also called "total parenteral nutrition (TPN)" or "total parenteral alimentation (TPA)"; the parenteral administration of all nutrients for patients with gastrointestinal dysfunctions. Although the term "hyperalimentation" is commonly used to designate total or supplemental nutrition by intravenous feedings, it is not technically correct because the procedure does not always involve an abnormally increased or excessive amount of feeding. See *Parenteral feeding (nutrition).*

Hyperammonemia. An inherited metabolic disorder characterized by an elevated blood ammonia level. It is due to a deficiency of the enzyme ornithine transcarbamylase, which catalyzes the reaction between carbamyl phosphate and ornithine to form citrulline. The symptoms include ammonia intoxication, vomiting, lethargy, hypotonia or spasticity, and cerebral and cortical atrophy. Restriction of dietary protein intake (0.5 gm/kg body weight/day) is the mainstay of long-term treatment and results in a reduction of blood ammonia to near-normal levels. Life-threatening hyperammonemic crises are apt to recur unpredictably, especially during infectious illness; they may require a further reduction of protein to a minimum (0.2-0.3 gm/kg body weight/day). If protein intake from common food sources is to be kept very low, supplementary essential amino acids may be needed.

Hypercalcemia. Abnormally high level of calcium in the blood. It occurs in various clinical disorders, such as hyperparathyroidism; solid tumors of the breast, ovary, and lungs; hyperthyroidism; and toxicity in vitamins A and D. It may also be drug related, involving, for example, the use of thiazide diuretics, chlorthalidone, lithium, and large amounts of calcium-containing antacids. Hypercalcemia may result in vomiting, nausea, muscular weakness, high blood pressure, and renal calculi. A calcium-restricted diet is recommended.

Hypercarotenosis. Condition characterized by high levels of carotene in the blood and skin and manifested by a yellow jaundice-like coloration of the skin that is particularly evident in the nasolabial folds, forehead, palms, and soles. But unlike jaundice, in which bile pigments accumulate in the body, the eyes do not become yellow. The condition is benign and slowly disappears upon reduction of the intake of carotenoid-rich foods from the diet.

Hypercatabolism. Excessive breakdown of reserve tissue or cellular materials to the extent that nutrients are depleted at an abnormally fast rate. The end result of an untreated hypercatabolic state could be fatal. Hypercatabolism is seen in advanced cases of AIDS, burns, severe injuries, cancer, and malnutrition. Immediate nutrition intervention is needed.

Hyperchloremia. Elevated blood chloride level; may be caused by dehydration, excess solute loading, diabetes insipidus, brain stem injury, or excessive administration of solutions containing chloride.

Hyperchlorhydria. Excessive hydrochloric acid (HCl) in the stomach due primarily to increased secretion of the gastric juice.

Hypercholesterolemia. Condition in which blood cholesterol is above the normal limits (about 200 mg% or more). It is associated with atherosclerosis and other cardiovascular diseases, obstructive jaundice, hyperlipidemia, and excess adrenocorticotropic hormone. The etiologic factors implicated in high serum cholesterol levels are many and varied, but the exact mechanisms are not well understood. Hormonal, genetic, nutritional, and environmental factors have been implicated. *Dietary management:* weight reduction for the obese, reduction of cholesterol intake to 200 mg/day, moderate restriction in fat, and replacement of saturated fats with mono- and polyunsaturated fatty acids. See *Diet, cholesterol-restricted, fat-controlled,* and *Hyperlipoproteinemia.*

Hyperemesis. Severe vomiting which may lead to nutritional inadequacy. Hyperemesis *gravidarum* is abnormal, protracted vomiting seen in pregnancy, causing weight loss and dehydration. *Dietary management:* serve dry meals in frequent small feedings. Avoid forced feedings. Provide high-carbohydrate, dry foods like soda crackers and melba toast. Beverages should be drunk between meals, not with food. Vitamin and mineral supplements are recommended. Electrolyte imbalance should be corrected.

Hyperglycemia. Increased glucose concentration in the blood above normal limits. Glucose levels are above 140 mg/100 ml of blood. This may occur in the following conditions: *diabetes mellitus* due to lack of insulin; increased *epinephrine* secretion; following ingestion of a very high carbohydrate intake (called "alimentary" hyperglycemia); *hyperthyroidism* due to increased hepatic glycogenolysis; increased intracranial pressure (as a result of skull fracture, cerebral hemorrhage, or brain tumor); administration of anesthetics such as ether, chloroform, and morphine; and *hyperpituitarism*. For dietary management of hyperglycemia in diabetes mellitus, see *Diabetes mellitus, complications*. See also *Blood sugar level* and *Glucagon*.

Hyperglycemic-glycogenolytic factor (HGF). Another name for *glucagon*.

Hyperglycemic, hyperosmolar, nonketotic syndrome (HHNK). A metabolic disorder in which blood glucose is highly elevated (greater than 600 mg/dl) without ketosis. It leads to high serum osmolarity. Symptoms include polyuria, severe dehydration, polydipsia, and tachycardia. It commonly occurs with Type II diabetes mellitus and is considered one of its acute complications. *Dietary management:* restore electrolyte balance promptly. Rehydration is the mainstay of therapy. Monitor the levels of potassium and blood glucose and adjust the diet accordingly.

Hyperinsulinism. Condition of excessive insulin in the body. Caused either by an overdose of insulin (as in insulin shock) or by overproduction of insulin by the pancreas. The latter is commonly known as *reactive* or *stimulative hypoglycemia* or *functional hyperinsulinism*. See also *Hypoglycemia* and *Insulin*. *Dietary management:* dietary modifications vary, depending upon the cause. Give glucose solution or fruit juice containing natural sugars in case of insulin overdose. In functional hyperinsulinism, restrict carbohydrate intake to 100 gm/day to minimize insulin production. A high protein intake (120 gm/day or more) is recommended; fat furnishes the remaining calories. Provide six small meals, with equal distribution of carbohydrate, protein, and fat. Nonnutritive sweeteners may be used.

Hyperkalemia. Also called "hyperpotassemia"; abnormally high potassium level in the blood. A toxic elevation of serum potassium is observed in cases of renal failure, acute dehydration, Addison's disease, and excessive administration of potassium in the presence of renal insufficiency; it may also be due to massive release of potassium from cells, such as in crash injury, major surgical operations, and gastrointestinal hemorrhage. Symptoms, involving chiefly the cardiac and central nervous systems, include numbness, mental confusion, bradycardia, paralysis of the extremities, and cardiac arrest.

Hyperkeratosis. 1. Hypertrophy of the horny layer of the skin. 2. Hypertrophy of the cornea. See also *Follicular keratosis*.

Hyperkinesis. Also called "hyperactivity" or "attention deficit disorder (ADD)," in children. Condition observed with some children who are excessively restless, inattentive, and disruptive at home or in school due to their abnormally high level of energy. Believed to be due to eating foods with artificial colors and flavors. Studies done to recommend a dietary regimen are not conclusive. See *Diet, Feingold*.

Hyperlipidemia. Nonspecific term that refers to an elevation of one or more lipid constituents of the blood, including glycolipids, lipoproteins, and phospholipids. The preferred term is *hyperlipoproteinemia*.

Hyperlipoproteinemia. Elevation of blood lipoproteins, i.e., elevated plasma cholesterol and/or triglycerides. The five major types are:

Type I. Characterized by hyperchylomicronemia or an extremely high triglyceride level, with normal or elevated cholesterol levels. It is extremely rare. *Dietary management:* restrict fat intake to 20% or less of calories (30 gm/day for adults). The cholesterol intake is normal, and the caloric level is adjusted to attain a healthy weight. Alcohol is not allowed.

Types IIa and IIb. In both types, there are increased serum cholesterol levels because the low-density lipoproteins are elevated. In type IIa, very-low-density lipoproteins and triglycerides are normal; in type IIb, both are increased. *Dietary management:* type IIa requires a restricted cholesterol intake (150 to 200 mg/day) and adequate calories, of which 30% is supplied by fats high in unsaturated fatty acids.

The U/S ratio should be 1:1. Alcohol is permitted; it should be used in moderation.

Type III. Identified by the presence of elevated prebetalipoproteins, elevated plasma cholesterol, and elevated triglycerides.

It is relatively uncommon and is referred to as "broad beta disease." *Dietary management:* if weight reduction is indicated, reduce caloric intake; a maximum of 30% is provided by fats with low saturated fatty acids or a U/S ratio of 1:1. Cholesterol is restricted to about 200 mg/day. Alcohol is limited to 25 gm/day. Complex carbohydrates with dietary fiber are recommended. Nonnutritive sweeteners may be used for calorie-restricted diets.

Type IV. Characterized by elevated prebetalipoproteins, elevated triglycerides, and normal or slightly elevated cholesterol levels. It is also called "carbohydrate-induced hyperlipidemia" or "essential familial hyperlipoproteinemia." It occurs often and is associated with diabetes mellitus, obesity, and artherosclerosis. *Dietary management:* weight loss by caloric restriction usually lowers the triglyceride level of the blood and normalizes glucose tolerance. Limit cholesterol, saturated fats, and sugars.

Type V. A plasma lipoprotein pattern of hyperchylomicronemia and elevated prebetalipoproteins indicates intolerance to both endogenous and exogenous fat sources. Glucose tolerance and uric acid levels are also abnormal, as seen in cases of diabetic acidosis, obesity, nephrosis, and alcoholism. *Dietary management:* weight reduction is needed for the obese person. Restriction of calories, 25% of which are provided by fats and oils of any kind, is recommended. Cholesterol is limited to 300 mg/day. Alcohol and concentrated sweets are not permitted.

Hypermagnesemia. Presence of excessive amounts of magnesium in the blood; almost always the result of renal insufficiency and the inability to excrete excess magnesium in foods and drugs, especially antacids. Symptoms include muscle weakness, confusion, and a fall in blood pressure.

Hypernatremia. Abnormally high blood sodium level; may be caused by dehydration due to inadequate fluid intake, respiratory loss with fever, hyperventilation of dyspnea, skin losses with burns, or metabolic acidosis; may also be due to excessive solute loading, as with concentrated feedings high in protein and salts without adequate supplemental water intake. Symptoms include thirst, flushed loose skin, tachycardia, hypotension, and hyperosmolarity.

Hyperoxaluria. A rare metabolic disease characterized by increased excretion of oxalate in the urine. The basic difficulty is the inability to metabolize glyoxylic acid. As a result, excess oxalic acid is produced and is precipitated as calcium oxalate in the kidney. The individual usually dies of renal failure in infancy. Calcium oxalate deposits may be found in other tissues.

Hyperparathyroidism. Abnormally increased secretion of parathyroid hormone leading to withdrawal of calcium from the bones. Features of this endocrine disorder include tenderness of the bones, muscular weakness and pain, abdominal cramps, and spontaneous fractures.

Hyperphosphatemia. High blood phosphate level; may be due to acute renal failure, chronic renal insufficiency, hypoparathyroidism, and hypervitaminosis D.

Hyperpituitarism. Pathologic condition due to increased activity of the *hypophysis* (pituitary gland). Symptoms vary, depending on the pituitary cells affected and the type of hormone secreted in excessive amounts. *True hyperpituitarism* is overactivity of the eosinophilic cells (excess growth hormone) resulting in gigantism in children and *acromegaly* in adults.

Hyperprolinemia. Disorder in the metabolism of proline probably resulting from a lack of the enzyme proline dehydrogenase. Symptoms include fever, vomiting, diarrhea, drowsiness, frequent convulsions, and hearing loss. Fasting levels of blood plasma proline are three to five times normal; urinary levels of proline, hydroxyproline, and glycine are also elevated.

Hypersensitivity skin test. Intradermal injection of three to five antigens to which most individuals have received prior sensitization (*Candida albicans,* mumps, tuberculin, streptokinase-streptodornase, *Trichophyton*). The diameter of the induration, measured after 24–48 hours, is graded 0 if nonreactive, 1 if 5 mm reactive, and 2 if more than 5 mm reactive. A normal positive response in a healthy individual is demonstrated by an area of inflammatory induration more than 5 mm in diameter; relative anergy is a response between 1 and 4 mm, and anergy is a negative response to all antigens. See *Anergy.*

Hypertension (HPN). Also called "high blood pressure"; persistent elevation of *blood pressure* above normal. Blood pressure varies considerably among individuals, depending on many factors, such as age, physical constitution, occupation, and health. For adults the average systolic/diastolic pressure is about 120/80 mm mercury (Hg). Hypertension may occur at any age, but more frequently in persons over 40 years old, with overweight or obesity as a predisposing factor. About 85 to 90% of the cases are *essential hypertension* (hypertension of unknown cause), which may be genetic or familial. Hypertension accompanies many renal and cardiovascular disorders, tumors of the adrenals, and emotional disturbances. Hypertensive persons usually suffer from dizziness, frequent headaches, impaired vision, shortness of breath, chest pain, failing memory, and sometimes gastrointestinal disturbance. *Dietary management:* restrict sodium to 250–500 mg/day in severe hypertension. When diuretics are used, 1000–2000 mg sodium is recommended. Weight reduction is indicated for obese patients. Restrict alcohol and caffeine use. Low dietary levels of calcium, potassium, and magnesium have been suggested to be part of the etiology of hypertension, but the dietary implications are still debatable.

Hyperthyroidism. Endocrine disorder caused by excessive secretion of the thyroid hormone as a result of overmedication with potent thyroid drugs, hyperactivity of the thyroid gland, or tumor (toxic adenoma of the thyroid). The clinical syndrome is generally called *exophthalmic goiter* because

two-thirds of the patients show exophthalmos (i.e., protruding eyes with wide-open lids). Other symptoms include thyroid enlargement, increased basal metabolic rate and pulse rate, nervousness and muscle tremors, and loss of weight. *Dietary management:* a high-calorie, liberal-protein, liberal-carbohydrate diet with calcium, phosphorus, and vitamins D and B complex supplementation is recommended. The basic aim of the diet is to compensate for the increase in basal metabolic rate (3500 to 4000 calories) and nitrogen metabolism (90 to 120 gm protein). A high carbohydrate intake will replenish depleted liver glycogen stores. Vitamin D is essential for the utilization of calcium and phosphorus, and the B complex vitamins are needed because of the increased caloric intake and high basal metabolic rate.

Hypertriglyceridemia. Increased blood levels of triglycerides. See *Hyperlipoproteinemia.*

Hypervitaminosis. Vitamin toxicity; a condition in which the level of a vitamin in the blood or tissue is high enough to cause undesirable symptoms. Hypervitaminosis has long been associated with excessive intake of the fat-soluble vitamins, especially vitamins A and D, which are not generally excreted from the body. Toxic effects have also been observed with some of the water-soluble vitamins when these are taken in excessively high therapeutic doses. Some of the toxic effects of vitamins are violent headache, swelling and pain of long bones, and rough skin (vitamin A); renal calcinosis, soft tissue calcification, and bone demineralization (vitamin D); hemolytic anemia, jaundice, and albuminuria (vitamin K); and flushing, tingling, and epigastric pain (nicotinic acid).

Hypoalbuminemia. Abnormally low serum albumin concentration. Depressed serum albumin concentrations have been associated with both decreased albumin synthesis and increased albumin degradation. Conditions associated with decreased albumin synthesis include malnutrition, cirrhosis, carcinoma, hypothyroidism, and acute stress due to surgery, trauma, burns, and infection.

Hypoalbuminemia may also follow exposure to various hepatic toxins, including alcohol and carbon tetrachloride. Conditions associated with albumin degradation are those leading to marked catabolism. Hypoalbuminemia results in impaired healing of soft and bony tissues, decreased resistance to infection, depressed gastric and intestinal motility, impaired intestinal absorption of water and electrolytes, and dependent edema and ascites.

Hypocalcemia. Abnormally low blood calcium level; may be due to hypoparathyroidism, chronic renal failure, chronic use of anticonvulsants, vitamin D-deficient rickets, and malabsorption syndromes. Hypocalcemia may result in cardiac cramps, seizures, choreiform movements, increased neuromuscular irritability, and paresthesias of the extremities. *Dietary management:* if intravenous feeding is initially required, give Ca^{++} gluconate. Provide adequate vitamin D_3. Select foods enriched with calcium.

Hypochloremia. Abnormally low plasma chloride level; may be dilutional with hyponatremia, as in expanded extracellular fluid following trauma and water retention, or due to chloride loss from the gastrointestinal tract, as in vomiting and gastric suctioning, adrenal steroid administration with sodium retention and potassium and chloride loss in urine, and diuretic use with loss of chloride in excess of sodium.

Hypochlorhydria. Abnormally low amount of hydrochloric acid in the stomach; observed in pernicious anemia, sprue, chronic gastritis, and pellagra. Some cases occur in nephritis, diabetes, cholecystitis, and cancer.

Hypoglycemia. Condition characterized by abnormally low blood glucose level. *Spontaneous hypoglycemia,* which occurs without the administration of exogenous insulin, is brought about by any of the following etiologic factors: *hyperinsulinism* (e.g., tumor or hypertrophy of the pancreas), *hepatic disease* (toxic hepatitis and von Gierke's disease), *adrenal hypofunction* (e.g., Addison's disease), *pituitary hypofunction* (e.g., Simmonds' disease), and certain *inborn errors of metabolism* (e.g., sugar malab-

sorption and leucine-induced hypoglycemia). The symptoms are characteristic of those seen in insulin reaction and include extreme hunger, nervousness, flushing of the skin with profuse sweating, dizziness, palpitations, and apathy. On the basis of *dietary management,* hypoglycemias are grouped into fasting and stimulative types:

Fasting h. Blood sugar level is below 60 mg% before breakfast or after fasting. This may also occur in adrenal or pituitary hypofunction, liver diseases, and other conditions. In contrast to the stimulative type, fasting hypoglycemia becomes more severe if carbohydrate intake is restricted. Thus the dietary treatment consists of readily available glucose (high-carbohydrate, high-protein diet), which should be constantly and regularly supplied (frequent meals with snacks).

Reactive (stimulative) h. Also called "spontaneous hypoglycemia" or "functional hyperinsulinism"; hypoglycemia in the absence of an organic lesion. Carbohydrate intake stimulates the pancreas to secrete higher than normal levels of insulin. As a consequence, hypoglycemia occurs 2 to 4 hours after meals; there is no hypoglycemia following fasting and omission of meals. *Dietary management:* provide adequate calories based on individual needs. Carbohydrate restriction is not necessary but refined carbohydrates should be avoided, especially sugars and concentrated sweets. Protein and fat should be taken whenever carbohydrate is consumed to delay gastric emptying and to blunt the postprandial insulin response to carbohydrate. Rather than three large meals, it is better to divide the daily food allowance into six small protein-containing meals. A high-fiber diet is beneficial in controlling blood glucose levels.

Hypoglycemia, diabetes mellitus. The most common acute complication among diabetics which may be a result of too much medication, too little food, too much exercise without adequate caloric supply, or alcohol consumption in the absence of food. When blood glucose falls within 50 to 60 mg/dl, the early signs of hypoglycemia are dizziness, pallor, sweating, nervousness, hunger, weakness and tachycardia. When blood glucose falls below 40 mg/dl, impaired central nervous system functions are manifested, such as confusion, lethargy, slurred speech, lack of motor coordination, and mood changes. Eventually seizures and unconsciousness develop, unless treatment is given immediately. Insulin-dependent diabetics are more prone to hypoglycemia, although it may also occur in noninsulin-dependent persons. *Dietary management:* the initial treatment for the alert person is to give 10 to 20 gm of simple carbohydrate, like oral glucose, orange juice or apple juice, to raise the blood glucose level quickly. A blood glucose test is performed after 20 to 30 minutes and if necessary, give another 20 gm of simple carbohydrate. Recheck blood glucose after 30 minutes and if it has improved, give eight ounces of nonfat milk and half a sandwich. In severe hypoglycemia when the patient is comatose or unable to swallow, the administration of glucagon or intravenous glucose is necessary.

Hypoglycemic agents. Substances that lower blood glucose levels, such as *insulin* and *oral hypoglycemic agents.* See also *Blood sugar level.*

Hypokalemia. Abnormally low plasma potassium level; may be due to decreased potassium intake, gastrointestinal tract losses (diarrhea, prolonged vomiting or gastric suction, small bowel fistulas), renal losses with potassium-depleting diuretics, and metabolic alterations with secondary potassium loss (surgical trauma, sepsis, burns). The undesirable effects of hypokalemia include impaired glucose tolerance with impaired insulin secretion, muscle weakness, metabolic alkalosis, and heart failure. *Dietary management:* parenteral administration of potassium fluids is required. The diet should include potassium-rich foods such as orange juice, bananas, milk, and potatoes.

Hypokinesis. "Deconditioning" of the body due to lack of exercise or physical activity. Prolonged physical inactivity results in stiffness, fatigue, weakness, sensitivity, incoordination, instability, muscular atrophy, ataxia, myocardial ischemia, urolithiasis,

and osteoporosis. See also *Nutrition, motor performance.*

Hypomagnesemia. Abnormally low blood magnesium level; may be due to malabsorption (inflammatory bowel disease, gluten enteropathy, radiation enteritis), increased loss (renal magnesium wasting, chronic diarrhea, laxative abuse), inadequate intake, or endocrine disorders. Primary hypomagnesemia is a rare genetic defect due to the inability of the intestinal mucosa to absorb magnesium. Symptoms include muscle cramps, athetoid movements, jerking, tetany with facial twitching, and disorientation.

Hyponatremia. Abnormally low blood sodium level; may be due to chronic wasting illnesses (cancer, liver disease, ulcerative colitis), abnormal loss of sodium without adequate replacement (excessive sweating, adrenal insufficiency, diarrhea), or prolonged, strict sodium restriction with drugs (chlorothiazide, mercurial diuretics, ethacrynic acid, or furosemide). Symptoms include loss of appetite, nausea, vomiting, weakness, irritability, confusion, and muscle weakness.

Hypophosphatasia. A genetic metabolic disorder resulting from serum and bone alkaline phosphatase deficiency leading to hypercalcemia. Clinical manifestations include severe skeletal defects resembling vitamin D-resistant rickets, dyspnea, cyanosis, failure to thrive, beading of the costochondral junction, and rachitic bone changes.

Hypophosphatemia. Abnormally low blood phosphate level; may be due to diminished intake and absorption (starvation, malabsorption syndrome, small bowel bypass) and increased loss (hyperparathyroidism, renal tubular defects, uncontrolled diabetes mellitus). Complications ascribed to hypophosphatemia include osteomalacia, congestive heart failure, respiratory failure, and kidney stones.

Hypophysis. Preferred name for *pituitary gland.* An endocrine gland about the size of a lima bean located beneath the brain and protected by a saddlelike depression called the *sella turcica.* It is composed of three portions: the anterior, intermediate (*pars* *intermedia*), and posterior lobes. Each lobe secretes important hormones that regulate vital processes in the body. The anterior lobe secretes somatotropin, thyrotropin, gonadotropins (luteinizing hormone, follicle-stimulating hormone, luteotropic hormone), and adrenocorticotropic hormone. The intermediate lobe elaborates the melanocyte-stimulating hormone, and the posterior lobe secretes oxytocin and vasopressin. The hypophysis is called the "master gland" or the "king of all glands" because it regulates the action of many of the other endocrine glands through the different hormones elaborated by its three lobes.

Hypopituitarism. Decreased activity of the *hypophysis* (pituitary gland) caused by a tumor, infarct, hemorrhage, or atrophy. Forms include pituitary myxedema, which is due to lack of the thyroid-stimulating hormone and is similar to myxedema of hypothyroidism; panhypopituitarism, which involves all the hormonal functions of the hypophysis (as in Simmonds' disease); and pituitary dwarfism, which is characterized by cessation of growth and diminished metabolic activities. *Dietary management:* a high-calorie, high-protein diet is recommended, supplemented with vitamins and minerals. Provide frequent, small feedings and avoid dehydration.

Hypotension. Reduced arterial systolic blood pressure below normal. May result from injection of drugs that lower blood pressure, hemorrhage or shock, and suppression of renal blood flow. Primary hypotension is not a disease but is common among young asthenic women. Secondary hypotension is associated with diseases such as myocardial infarction, vascular accidents, cachexia, and fever. Postural hypotension may occur in some debilitated or elderly persons when they assume the upright position and there is exaggerated venous pooling.

Hypothalamus. Area lying at the base of the brain just below the thalamus. It is responsible for the maintenance of body temperature, blood pressure, water regulation, control of satiety and appetite, and other basic functions necessary to life. Because of its close anatomic connection to the pituitary gland, it has been implicated in the control of endocrine gland function.

Hypothyroidism. Endocrine disorder resulting from the decreased activity of the *thyroid gland.* The effects of a decreased thyroid hormone supply in the body are *myxedema* in adults, particularly in women, and *cretinism* in children. Clinical signs are reduced basal metabolic rate as low as 40% below normal; puffy face, hands, and eyelids; easy fatigability; apathy and dullness; and reduced gastrointestinal motility. Blood lipids are often increased. Children have retarded growth and development. Drug therapy is the treatment of choice. *Dietary management:* restrict calories for obese persons. Limit intake of fats and cholesterol-rich foods. Liberal fluid and fiber intake prevents constipation.

I

I. Chemical symbol for iodine.

Iatrogenic. Term meaning "caused by medical treatment or diagnostic procedures." *Iatrogenic malnutrition* is an induced nutritional deficiency due to drug therapy or certain medical procedures, unless carefully monitored, to prevent any nutritional complication. The condition is observed with prolonged use of oral contraceptives, antibiotics, and anticonvulsive drugs; total parenteral nutrition lacking certain elements, particularly trace minerals; complications from ostomies; and gastric stapling in morbid obese patients.

IBC. Abbreviation for *iron-binding capacity.*

Ibuprofen. A nonsteroidal anti-inflammatory agent; also an antipyretic and analgesic. Used for treatment of rheumatoid arthritis and osteoarthritis and for relief of aches and pains. Its most frequent adverse effects involve the gastrointestinal tract and may cause anemia due to gastrointestinal bleeding and peptic ulceration; it may also cause stomatitis, epigastric pain, cramping, decreased appetite, and weight gain due to fluid retention. It should be taken with milk or food. Alcohol should be avoided. Brand names include Advil, Medipren, Midol, Motrin, Nuprin, and Pamprin.

IBW. Abbreviation for *ideal body weight.* See *Weight.*

Icteric. Pertaining to icterus or jaundice. See *Jaundice.*

Icteric index. Measure of the yellow color in blood plasma; expressed by comparing the color of the serum with the color of a 1:10,000 potassium dichromate solution. The normal range is from 4 to 6. Values higher than 6 are indicative of jaundice or icterus.

IDDM. Abbreviation for insulin-dependent diabetes mellitus. See under *Diabetes mellitus.*

Idiopathic. 1. Without any known origin; self-originated. 2. Pertaining to disease of unknown cause (e.g., idiopathic celiac disease).

Idiopathic thrombocytopenic purpura (ITP). Bleeding into the skin, gums, nose, and other organs caused by platelet destruction. Acute ITP in children may be due to a viral infection which lasts for periods ranging from several weeks to a few months. Chronic ITP is more common in adults and adolescents and lasts for a longer period. *Dietary management:* since treatment is usually by drugs (corticosteroids) and splenectomy, nutritional guidelines are directed to the side effects of corticosteroids and to surgical care.

IDL. Abbreviation for *intermediate-density lipoprotein.*

IEM. Abbreviation for *inborn errors of metabolism.*

Ileitis. Acute or chronic inflammation of the lower ileum, although other parts of the intestine may also be affected by edema, fibrosis, and ulceration. Clinical symptoms include abdominal cramps, loss of weight, bloody diarrhea, and progressive anemia. *Dietary management:* correct the diarrhea and lessen the abdominal pain and irritation with an elemental diet for acute cases. Correct anemia and weight loss with a high-calorie, high-protein diet, with vitamin-mineral supplementation. For chronic cases, maintain a normal diet but monitor any fat and lactose intolerance. Supplementary iron and B complex vitamins may be needed.

Ileostomy. A surgical opening is created from the ileum to empty fecal matter outside the abdomen via an intestinal tube. May be needed in patients suffering from cancer of the intestines, Crohn's disease, or ulcerative colitis. *Dietary management:* a low-residue diet is given several days before the operation, with fluid restriction 24 hours before surgery. After surgery, a colostomy bag is connected to the stoma for fecal matter disposal. An average ileostomate drains about 0.5 to 1 liter of fluid per day from the intestinal contents, carrying with it sodium and potassium salts. Electrolyte and fluid losses must be replaced immediately. A low-fiber diet in small, frequent feedings will lessen watery stools during the first month after surgery, after which fiber intake is gradually increased. Bile salt deficiency in ostomies requires fat restriction. The use of medium-chain triglycerides and fat-soluble vitamin supplementation aids recovery. In many cases, a vitamin B_{12} injection is indicated. Ostomates vary greatly in their food tolerances, which need careful nutritional assessment and individualized meal plans.

Ileum. Third and last portion of the small intestine, extending from the jejunum to the large intestine. It is the site for absorption of bile salts, vitamin B_{12} and intrinsic factor, disaccharides, and mineral salts. See also *Absorption, nutrients.*

IM. Abbreviation for "intramuscular."

Imipramine. A tricyclic antidepressant. Has a peculiar taste and may cause anorexia, stomatitis, weight loss, and riboflavin depletion. It is excreted in milk in small quantities. Alcohol should be avoided completely. The drug can increase the intoxicating effects of alcohol. Brand names include Imavate, Presamine, and Tofranil.

Immobilization. Patients who need prolonged bed rest, and those who have paralysis, fractures and multiple trauma, and the like, excrete large amounts of calcium and go into negative nitrogen balance. Because of the demineralization during immobilization, the serum calcium level is elevated. This does not require increased dietary intake, but can be reversed by quiet standing for a few hours or by changes in weight-bearing activities.

Immunity. Security against any particular disease; power of an organism to resist or overcome infection. Immunity may be natural (inborn), or may be acquired by having the disease or by injection, inoculation, or vaccination with an antigen. See *Nutrition, immune system.*

Impact. Brand name of a tube-feeding formula for critically ill patients with depressed immune function. Has added arginine, omega-3 fatty acids, RNA nucleotides, and all the known immunologically relevant essential nutrients. See also Appendix 39.

Inanition. Wasting of the body due to complete lack of food; a state of starvation.

Inborn error of metabolism (IEM). A large group of inherited disorders due to a deficiency or absence of a protein involved in the metabolic pathway either as an enzyme, carrier, receptor, or other functional role. Examples are galactosemia, phenylketonuria, and tyrosinemia. Treatment for many of these disorders may require dietary intervention. The benefits obtained from dietary modification vary from marginal relief of symptoms to effective palliation and control. See *Nutrition, genetics* and Appendix 44.

Incomplete protein. See *Protein classification* and *Protein quality.*

Index of nutrient quality (INQ). A ratio indicating the *nutrient density* of a food, calculated as follows:

$$INQ = \frac{\%RDA \text{ of a nutrient for an individual}}{\% \text{ energy requirement for an individual}}$$

Thus, INQ varies among different individuals. In general, if a food has an INQ of 1 and if a serving portion provides at least 2% of the recommended dietary allowance (RDA) for a nutrient, that food is said to be a good source for the nutrient. Food with an INQ of 1.5 and a serving portion furnishes 10% of the U.S. RDA is considered an excellent source for the nutrient.

Indigestion. Also called *dyspepsia.* Faulty or incomplete digestion of food; often accompanied by heartburn, abdominal pain, and flatulence. Usually a functional disorder which may be due to nervous or emotional upsets, poor eating habits, or poor cooking methods. If indigestion is associated with an organic disease, treatment is directed to the causative factor.

Indomethacin. A nonsteroidal anti-inflammatory agent for the relief of joint pains and inflammation associated with arthritis. Adverse nutritional effects include decreased serum ascorbic acid level, decreased absorption of amino acids and xylose, iron deficiency anemia secondary to gastrointestinal blood loss, and anorexia. The drug may also cause sodium and fluid retention, abdominal distress, and bloating. Excreted in breast milk. Brand names are Indocin and Indocin-SR.

Infant feeding. Breast feeding is generally accepted as the most desirable method of feeding an infant. Human milk is considered ideal. Except for iron and vitamins C and D, it contains adequate amounts of all nutritional factors needed by the newborn infant. The other advantages of breast feeding are as follows: babies are less likely to be overfed; breast milk is always fresh, bacteriologically safe, and nonallergenic; dental development is promoted; and breast milk contains immune bodies that make the infant more resistant to infection. Other maternal benefits are convenience, less cost, and suppression of ovulation. Contraindications to breast feeding include a history of tuberculosis, severe chronic illness, mastitis, insufficient milk production, certain medications, drug abuse, poor maternal health, acute infections, emotional and mental stress, alcoholism, and another pregnancy. In such cases, artificial feeding or bottle feeding with cow's milk or a commercially prepared infant milk formula is satisfactory for infants. Sometimes mixed feeding or a combination of breast feeding and artificial feeding is used, especially when breast milk is not sufficient or when the mother works outside the home. For the composition of milk and selected formulas for infant feeding, see Appendix 37. See also *Nutrition, infancy.*

Infantile colic. A disorder among infants characterized by unexplained paroxysms of crying and even agonized screaming, irritability, and distended stomach. About 25% of infants who develop colic in the first weeks of life may outgrow it after 4 months of age. The exact etiology is not known, although hypersensitivity to cow's milk and excessive intestinal gas are possible causes. It has been observed that the mother's smoking habit and exposure to maternal drugs may cause infantile colic. *Dietary management:* if there are no symptoms of food intolerance, dietary changes are not necessary. The baby should be fed in the upright position and trained for slow sucking to minimize the amount of swallowed air by limiting the periods of sucking to 10 minutes.

Infantile eczema. Also called "atopic dermatitis." A disorder of unknown etiology seen in infants. Associated with physical, emotional, and hypersensitivity factors. Some symptoms are fragility of the skin with lesions, accompanied by severe itchiness, dryness, and crusting; capillary dilatation; and edema and erythema. *Dietary management:* if hypersensitivity to milk is involved, give a hypoallergenic formula. If the infant is ready for solid foods, determine which items are allergens and follow the approach used for food allergy. See *Food allergen.*

Infection. Transfer of disease; entrance and development of pathogenic microorganisms and parasites in the body. Any disease caused by growth of pathogenic microorganisms in the body is called an "infectious disease." It may or may not be contagious. See also *Nutrition, infection* and *Sepsis.*

Infectious mononucleosis. Also called "glandular fever." May be caused by the Epstein-Barr herpes virus. Characterized by chills, headache, sore throat, fever, stomach aches, chest pains, breathing difficulty, and visible swelling of the neck and other glands. *Dietary management:* maintain fluid, protein, and electrolyte balance. Provide liberal calories with an N:C ratio of 1:150 (N = nitrogen in gm/day and C = kcal/day).

Inflammatory bowel disease (IBD). Term for chronic ulcerative colitis and Crohn's disease, which are two distinct disorders, although both involve mucosal inflammation of the intestines. For further details, see *Crohn's disease* and *Ulcerative colitis.*

Ingestion. 1. Eating; taking in foods or beverages. 2. Process by which a cell takes up foreign matter, such as bacilli or smaller cells.

INH. Abbreviation for isonicotyl hydrazide. See *Isonicotinic acid hydrazide.*

Inositol. Water-soluble, cyclic, 6-carbon compound closely related to glucose. It exists in nine forms, but only myoinositol demonstrates any biologic activity. Myoinositol is present in relatively large amounts in the cells of practically all animals and plants. In animal cells, it occurs as a component of phospholipids; in plant cells, it is found as *phytic acid,* an organic acid that binds calcium, iron, and zinc in an insoluble complex and interferes with their absorption. In addition to occurring in foods, inositol is synthesized in the cells. It is stored largely in the brain, muscles, liver, and kidneys. Like choline, inositol has a lipotropic effect and exists in cells as a phosphatide (phosphatidylinositol). It is not classified as a vitamin, since it is present in practically all plants and animal tissues in concentrations higher than those normally associated with vitamins. There is no demonstrable requirement for inositol in humans, although there is growing evidence of altered inositol metabolism in certain clinical situations likely to induce deficiency, such as diabetes mellitus and multiple sclerosis. Experimental animals fed semipurified diets lacking in inositol develop alopecia, dermatitis, retarded growth, and fatty liver.

Insensible fluid losses. Fluid excreted from the body not readily seen or felt, such as losses from *insensible perspiration,* vaporization from the lungs, and losses from fecal matter.

Insensible perspiration. Water lost through the skin which is not noticeable because evaporation takes place immediately. It is important for the maintenance of body temperature. About 400 ml of water is lost by diffusion in insensible perspiration, in contrast to about 300 ml in sweating. This loss of body weight through vaporization of water can be measured within a short period of time, using a sensitive balance, and may be used as an indirect method for estimating the basal heat production of a person.

Insulin. Hormone secreted by the beta cells of the islets of Langerhans of the pancreas. It is a protein with a molecular weight of 6000 and is composed of two polypeptide chains, A and B, with 21 and 30 amino acids, respectively. Insulin secretion is stimulated by carbohydrates, amino acids, and pancreozymin. Before active insulin is released, it exists as proinsulin. The latter has a connecting peptide called "C-peptide" which is cleaved off, leaving the active insulin molecule. The C-peptide has no hormonal function but is useful as a diagnostic test for *diabetes mellitus.*

Insulin-dependent diabetes mellitus (IDDM). A form of diabetes mellitus that requires insulin administration to maintain normoglycemia. Persons with IDDM are prone to ketosis. See under *Diabetes mellitus.*

Insulin, functions. The only hormone that lowers blood sugar, insulin inhibits the breakdown of glycogen into glucose; promotes glycogenesis, or the conversion of glucose to glycogen in the liver; fosters lipogenesis, or the formation of fat from glucose; and increases cell permeability to glucose. In the muscles, insulin stimulates protein synthesis by inhibiting protein breakdown to glucose. Lack of insulin leads to *diabetes mellitus.* See also *Hyperglycemia, Hypoglycemia,* and *Hyperinsulinism.*

Insulin preparations. Insulin is commercially prepared in amorphous or crystalline form from beef, pork, and sheep pancreas or bacteria. It is sold either unmodified (regular insulin), in combination with basic proteins (globin and protamine), or with crystalline zinc salts (PZI) to make the compound less soluble and less absorbable, thus effecting a longer duration of action.

Globin i. Insulin preparation modified by the addition of globin to make it more insoluble for prolonged action. This permits less frequent injections than when regular insulin is used. The duration of action is about 16 to 20 hours.

Human i. A preparation that has been biosynthetically produced from two strains of *Escherichia coli* using recombinant DNA technology. Human insulin is useful for individuals who are allergic to animal insulin.

Isophane i. Preparation of insulin combined with protamine in an isophane ratio of approximately 0.5 mg protamine for each 100 units of insulin. NPH insulin is an isophane insulin.

Lente i. Insulin preparation crystallized from an acetate buffer in the presence of zinc. By varying the conditions of preparation, it is possible to obtain insulin preparations of varying particle size and duration of action. *Semilente* is a suspension of amorphous insulin particles with a duration of action of 12 to 18 hours; *Lente* is a suspension of insulin crystals of small particle size with a duration of action of 24 hours; and *Ultralente* is a suspension of insulin crystals of large particle size with a duration of action of over 30 hours.

Neutral protamine Hagedorn (NPH) i. An isophane insulin developed by Hagedorn; consists of crystals of insulin, protamine, and zinc suspended in a buffered medium. The duration of globin insulin is less than that of *protamine zinc insulin (PZI).*

Protamine zinc i (PZI). Preparation of insulin combined with zinc and a protamine present in the sperm of fish. This combination makes insulin more stable and produces a prolonged action (20 to 30 hours) because of its relative insolubility.

Regular i. Also called "amorphous," "ordinary," or "soluble insulin"; it is an unmodified preparation now seldom used alone because of its very short duration of action (6 hours), requiring many injections each day. However, it becomes the insulin of choice in emergencies such as ketosis, infection, and surgery; it is also used in combination with the slow-acting insulins.

Another classification of insulin products is based on its onset (O), peak (P) of action, and duration (D) of action as follows:

Intermediate-acting i. (O = 1 to 2 hours; P = 6 to 15 hours; D = 16 to 24 hours; examples of products are Humulin N, Insulated NPH, Lente, Lente Iletin, Novolin L, Novolin NPH, NPH, NPH Iletin.

Long-acting i. (0 = 4 to 6 hours; P = 8 to 30 hours; D = 24 to 36 hours; examples of products are Humulin U, Protamine Zinc and Iletin I, Ultralente, and Ultralente Iletin.

Rapid-acting i. (O = ½ hour; P = 2 to 5 hours; D = 6 to 8 hours; examples of products are Humulin R, Novolin R, Regular, Semilente, and Vesolin R.

For ease of injection, mixtures are also available, such as Novolin 70/30 and Mixtard (70% NPH and 30% Regular). In choosing the type of insulin product to use, one has to consider the species source, purity, antigenicity, duration of action, kinds of binding agents, concentration, need for mixed insulins, and suitability for the patient's condition and lifestyle.

Insulin pump. A means of providing insulin by inserting a syringe subcutaneously; this is a portable unit that can be operated manually or attached to a microcomputer that regulates insulin flow. The main purpose of this infusion device is to maintain euglycemia for 24 hours without interfering with the person's daily activities. There are several kinds one can choose from, depending on factors like an alarm feature, cost, size, simplicity of operation, dependability, multiple basal doses, and supplemental and accumulative dose features. It is more expensive than injection and a more difficult method to master, but with professional and peer support, highly motivated persons find it effective for their lifestyles. There are "pump clubs" for assisting those who encounter difficulties. Only regular or rapid-acting insulin is used for pump therapy, which can be given as a continuous infusion, called the "basal rate," or as an intermittent bolus given prior to eating to control the postprandial rise in blood glucose.

Insulin shock. The preferred term is "insulin reaction" or "hypoglycemic episode"; a reaction of the body due to a very low blood sugar level because of overdosage of insulin. It is characterized by a feeling of hunger, weakness, nervousness, double vision, shallow breathing, sweating, pallor, headache, and dizziness. If the blood glucose level falls below 40 mg/dl, the patient develops mental confusion, slurred speech, muscular twitching, convulsions, loss of consciousness, and eventually coma. *Dietary management:* see under *Hypoglycemia.*

Insulin unit. The physiologic activity of insulin is expressed in *international units (IU).* One IU is equivalent to 0.125 mg of the international standard preparation or $1/23$ mg of a standard preparation of crystalline zinc insulin.

Interferon. A family of glycoproteins that interferes with the replication of various viruses (hence the name) and also affects cell growth and immunologic processes by activating or suppressing selected components of the immune system. Interferons are released by cells in response to a variety of agents, including viruses, microorganisms, and endotoxins.

Intermediary metabolism. Synthesis (anabolism) and degradation (catabolism) of the cell constituents of living organisms. In the intact cell, both processes go on simultaneously, and energy released from the degradation of some compounds may be utilized in the synthesis of other cellular components. In a broad sense, intermediary metabolism refers to all the chemical reactions taking place inside the body, ranging from the ingestion of foodstuffs to the discharge of ultimate chemical products and excretion of metabolic end products. See Appendices 9, 10, and 11.

Intermediate-density lipoprotein (IDL). A subclass of lipoprotein with a density between that of very-low-density lipoprotein and low-density lipoprotein; classified as the broad beta fraction on the basis of electrophoresis. It is formed in plasma from the action of lipoprotein lipase on chylomicrons and very-low-density lipoprotein. Cholesterol and phospholipids are the lipids present in greatest amount.

International Dietetic Association. Organization whose aim is to raise the level of the dietetics profession in member countries. Every 4 years, an annual convention is held in a host country for the International Congress of Dietetics.

International Life Sciences Institute (ILSI). A nonprofit, worldwide foundation established in 1978 to advance the understanding of scientific issues relating to nutrition, food safety, toxicology, and environmental safety. It is affiliated with the World Health Organization and with the Food and Agriculture Organization for specialized consultation services. See also *Nutrition Foundation, Inc.*

International unit (IU). Figure that represents the biologic activity of a nutrient or substance. It is a specific reference standard of known potency that produces specific effects over a specified period of time in a laboratory animal.

Interstitial. Situated in the interspaces of tissue or between parts. See interstitial fluid under *Water compartment, body.*

Intestinal juice. *Succus entericus.* A straw-colored alkaline fluid secreted by the intestinal mucosa; contains enzymes that complete the hydrolysis of carbohydrate, protein, and fat. Mixed with it are the pancreatic secretions containing enzymes and the hormone enterokinase. See Appendix 11.

Intestinal lipodystrophy. Also called "Whipple's disease." A rare disease with insidious onset, more common in males than in females; characterized by infiltration of the small intestines with macrophages containing glycoprotein and bacilli. Clinical signs include malabsorption, anemia, endocarditis, hypoproteinemia, lymphadenopathy, edema, and abnormal skin pigmentation. Central nervous system involvement may be serious. This systemic disease is usually fatal. *Dietary management:* correct weight loss, anemia, malabsorption, and hypoproteinemia with a high-calorie (about 1.2 to 1.5 times the basal energy expenditure), high-protein (1.5 gm/kg/day), and moderately low-fat diet supplying 25% of caloric needs. Supplemental vitamins and minerals, especially iron, calcium, and fat-soluble vitamins, promote recovery. Edema, dehydration, and electrolyte losses should be corrected.

Intestinal lymphangiectasia. Disorder characterized by increased intestinal pressure dilating the lymphatics and discharging fluids into the bowel. Protein loss is lessened when the fluid is digested and reabsorbed. In addition, the absorption of fats and fat-soluble vitamins is reduced. *Dietary management:* provide adequate calories and protein and monitor fat absorption. A diet using medium-chain triglycerides is beneficial. Supplemental fat-soluble vitamins prevent deficiencies.

Intestine. Part of the digestive tract that extends from the stomach (pylorus) to the anus; divided into the small and large intestines.

Large i. The last portion of the gastrointestinal tract, extending from the ileum to the anus. It is about 5 feet long and is divided into three parts: the *cecum, colon,* and *rectum.* Although no digestion takes place in the large intestine, it serves as the site for absorption of water and unabsorbed products of digestion and for temporary storage of feces until they are eliminated. The microflora inhabiting the large intestine can synthesize some vitamins (especially vitamin K) and can hydrolyze crude fiber to some extent. See also *Fiber.*

Small i. The portion that extends from the pylorus to the large intestine at the cecum. It is about 20 feet long and divided into three parts: the *duodenum, jejunum,* and *ileum.* The small intestine is the main site for the digestion and absorption of food. See also *Absorption, nutrients.*

Intralipid. Brand name of a 10% or 20% fat emulsion for intravenous administration; made of soybean oil, egg yolk, phospholipid, and glycerin. Provides 1.1 kcal (at 10%) and 2 kcal (at 20%) per milliliter. See also Appendix 41.

Intrinsic factor. A glycoprotein in the gastric juice that combines with vitamin B_{12} and aids in its absorption from the small intestine. A deficiency in this factor results in *pernicious anemia.*

Introlite. Brand name of half-strength tube feeding formula for the transitional or intolerant feeder; provides 0.5 kcal/ml. See also Appendix 39.

Inulin. Polysaccharide composed of *fructose* units; found in Jerusalem artichoke and dahlia tuber. It is used as a test for kidney function, since it is completely filtered by the glomerulus and is not reabsorbed or excreted by the kidney tubules. See also *Kidney.*

Inversion. Conversion of sucrose in solution into equal amounts of glucose and fructose by the action of acid or enzyme (invertase). The mixture is called *invert sugar.*

Iodine (I). A trace mineral that is a dietary essential; an important constituent of the thyroid hormones *thyroxine* and *triiodothyronine,* which are necessary for several metabolic functions, including lipid, carbohydrate, and nitrogen metabolism; growth development and reproduction; oxygen consumption; and regulation of basal metabolic rate. Iodine also plays an important role in fetal brain development independent of its action via the thyroid hormones. A deficiency in iodine leads to a wide range of diseases that vary in severity with the degree of iodine deficiency, from *simple goiter* with a barely visible to grossly enlarged thyroid gland to *cretinism* with mental retardation. Endemic goiter and the more severe forms of iodine deficiency continue to be a worldwide problem. The introduction of iodized salt in the United States sharply reduced the incidence of endemic goiter, although isolated cases are still seen in certain areas. Various *goitrogens,* such as those found in the cabbage family and cassava, can also prevent the thyroid from accumulating iodine and converting it into active thyroid hormones. The iodine level in foods varies greatly, depending upon the environment in which they are grown and produced. Seafoods are the richest natural source; iodized salt is another reliable source, providing 76 μg iodine per gram of salt. Iodine is rapidly and almost completely absorbed and transported to the thyroid gland, where it is found in greatest concentration, although all body tissues and secretions contain trace amounts; excretion is mainly in the urine. Excess iodine ingestion is regulated, within limits, by decreased iodine uptake by the thyroid and increased excretion in the urine. Chronic toxicity with grossly excessive intake can cause *thyrotoxicosis,* an enlarged, hyperactive thyroid, seen among some inhabitants of Japan, who consume as much as 25,000 μg iodine from seaweed, and in Tasmania, among the elderly population accustomed to low iodine intakes, when iodine was substantially increased by iodization of bread.

Iodine 131. Radioactive isotope of iodine; it has a half-life of 8 days. Useful in the diagnosis and treatment of thyroid gland disorders, determination of blood plasma volume and cardiac output, and as a diagnostic aid prior to surgery for the location of brain tumors.

Iodine number. Also called "iodine value"; the number of grams of iodine taken up by 100 gm of fat. It is a quantitative value that reflects the amount of fatty acids and the degree of unsaturation of a fat or an oil. The value ranges from 10 for coconut oil to 200 for safflower oil.

Iodized salt. Table salt that contains 1 part sodium or potassium iodide per 5000 to 10,000 parts (or 0.01%) of sodium chloride.

Iodopsin. Visual violet; a light-sensitive violet pigment of the cones in the retina that is important for vision. It contains vitamin A.

Iodothyroglobulin. Globulin-iodine complex found in the thyroid gland; serves as the prosthetic group of *thyroxine.*

Ion. Atom or chemical radical carrying an electric charge that is positive (cation) or negative (anion) or both (zwitterion). *Ionization* is the dissociation of a substance in solution into its constituent ions.

Iron (Fe). A trace mineral essential to the body; a constituent of hemoglobin, myoglobin, and various oxidative enzymes. Iron is necessary for the prevention of nutritional anemia and plays an important role in respiration and tissue oxidations. The hemoglobin of the red blood cells and the myoglobin of the tissue cells is vital for oxygen transport to the cells and storage within the cells, whereas the iron-containing enzymes within the cells are associated with metabolic oxidation. Good food sources are liver and other glandular organs, meats, eggs, seafoods, whole-grain or enriched cereals, and dried fruits. There are two forms of food iron: heme (organic) and nonheme (inorganic). Heme iron is absorbed more efficiently than nonheme iron and is independent of vitamin C and iron-binding chelating agents. The absorption of nonheme iron can be enhanced by ascorbic acid when the two nutrients are ingested together. It can be inhibited by several factors, such as calcium phosphate, bran, phytates, polyphenols in tea, and antacids. Only about 10% of dietary iron is absorbed in the upper part of the small intestine; absorbed iron is transported by blood as *transferrin* to the bone marrow for hemoglobin synthesis, or is removed from blood by cells for use by respiratory enzymes and as cell constituents. Iron is stored in the liver and other tissues as *ferritin* and *hemosiderin.* Absorbed iron is lost only by desquamation from the alimentary, urinary, and respiratory tracts and by skin and hair losses; iron released from the breakdown of hemoglobin is reutilized. In adult men, the total iron loss that needs replacement is about 1 mg/day; in adult women, there is an additional 5-32 mg/month menstrual loss. A deficiency of iron results in *anemia* of the hypochromic, microcytic type. Some people are genetically at risk from iron overload, or *hemochromatosis.* About 2000 cases of iron poisoning occur each year in the United States, mainly in young children who ingest the medicinal iron supplements formulated for adults. Other than long-term ingestion of home brews made in iron vessels, there are no reports of iron toxicity from foods in people without genetic defects that increase iron absorption.

Iron-binding capacity (IBC). The relative saturation of the iron-binding protein transferrin. This protein is usually 25-30% saturated, representing the serum iron content. In iron deficiency there is decreased saturation to less than 18%. The amount of transferrin bound to iron in relation to the amount remaining free to combine with iron determines the iron-binding capacity (IBC), and the amount of additional iron that can be bound to transferrin is called the "unsaturated iron-binding capacity (UIBC)." Both values together represent the *total iron binding capacity (TIBC)*.

Isoalloxazine. A heterocyclic yellow flavin that is a constituent of riboflavin together with ribose.

Isoascorbic acid. A geometric isomer of ascorbic acid with only slight vitamin C activity. It is a strong reducing agent, and is used in food as an antioxidant and in cured meats to speed up color fixing.

Isocal. Brand name of a lactose-free, isotonic, low-residue nutritional product for oral or tube feeding; contains calcium and sodium caseinates, soy protein isolate, maltodextrin, soy oil (80%), MCT oil (20%), and lecithin. Also available with a higher nitrogen content (Isocal HN) for mildly stressed patients; as a high-calorie, high-protein formula (Isocal HCN) for hypermetabolic patients; and in a flexible pouch (Isocal II Entri-Pak) for closed enteral feeding systems. See Appendix 39.

Isoleucine (Ile). Alpha-amino-beta methylvaleric acid. An essential branched-chain amino acid rarely limiting in foods. See also *Amino acid* and *Maple syrup urine disease*.

Isolife. Brand name of a liquid nutritional product made of whey protein concentrate, soy protein, hydrolyzed cornstarch, corn oil (70%), MCT oil (30%), and lecithin. It is low in residue, lactose free, and isotonic. See Appendix 39.

Isomil. Brand name of a milk-free formula for infants with milk protein hypersensitivity and intolerance to lactose or galactose; made of soy protein isolate, corn syrup, sucrose, coconut oil, and soy oil. Also made without added sucrose (Isomil SF) for infants and children with sucrose intolerance. See Appendix 37.

Isoniazid. Generic name for *isonicotinic acid hydrazide*.

Isonicotinic acid hydrazide (INH). An antituberculosis drug chemically related to pyridoxine that acts as an antagonist to vitamin B_6. Its prolonged administration induces pyridoxine deficiency; it may also interfere with vitamin D metabolism and cause niacin and folate depletion. It has a mild monoamine oxidase inhibitor effect and can cause a tyramine-type reaction with certain foods. Other adverse effects include nausea and vomiting, loss of appetite, epigastric distress, dry mouth, and cheilosis. Vitamin B_6 supplementation may be indicated with longterm use. Brand names are Hydrazid, INH, Laniazid, Rifamate, and Rimactane.

Isoriboflavin. An isomer of riboflavin; acts as a metabolic antagonist and competes with the vitamin.

Isosource HN. Brand name of a high-nitrogen, lactose-free nutritional liquid supplement; made of sodium and calcium caseinates, maltodextrin, MCT oil, and corn oil. See also Appendix 39.

Isotein HN. Brand name of a powdered, lactose-free, high-protein product for oral and tube feeding; also gluten-free and low in sodium and residue. Made of delactosed lactalbumin, maltodextrin, monosaccharides, partially hydrogenated soybean oil, and MCT oil. See also Appendix 39.

Isotretinoin. Synthetic analog of vitamin A used in the treatment of severe acne when other treatments are ineffective. Adverse effects resemble those associated with vitamin A toxicity and may cause liver damage, increased risk of coronary heart disease, and peripheral vascular disease. It is contraindicated during pregnancy and may damage a developing fetus. The brand name is Accutane.

Isovaleric acidemia. A genetic disorder of leucine metabolism due to a deficiency of the enzyme isovaleryl CoA dehydrogenase. This leads to increased levels of isovaleric acid in the blood and urine. Affected infants have vomiting, metabolic acidosis, mental retardation, and a characteristic odor similar to that of sweaty feet. The condition may be treated by restricting the intake of leucine. This is done by lowering the intake of protein until the amount of leucine ingested equals that required for growth. Supplemental glycine and carnitine may be beneficial.

ITP. See *Idiopathic thrombocytopenic purpura*.

IU. Abbreviation for *international unit*.

IV. Abbreviation for *intravenous*.

J

J. Symbol for *joule.*

Jaundice. Also called "icterus." The yellowish discoloration of the skin, mucous membranes, and certain body fluids due to the accumulation of bile pigments in the blood. It may be due to increased production of bile pigments from hemoglobin or may result from the failure of the liver to excrete bilirubin because of an injury to the liver cells or obstruction to the flow of bile. Jaundice is generally classified into three types—hemolytic, obstructive, and toxic.

Hemolytic j. Due to abnormally large destruction of red blood cells, as in pernicious anemia, malaria, yellow fever, and other infections. There is increased production of bile pigments from hemoglobin in excess of the amount that can be excreted by the normal, healthy liver.

Obstructive j. Due to complete or partial interference with the flow of bile anywhere along its course from the hepatic lobules to the duodenum. The obstruction may be due to the presence of gallstones, parasites, tumors, or inflammation or thickening of the mucosa of the common bile duct.

Toxic j. Due to damage or injury of the liver cells by toxic substances such as various poisons, drugs, and viral infections. The agent prevents the damaged liver from manufacturing bile and therefore causes dumping of the pigments into the bloodstream.

In all types of jaundice, treatment should be directed to the cause and not to the symptoms. *Dietary management:* the anorexia, nausea, and vomiting that accompany jaundice require small feedings of foods that are tolerated. In chronic obstructive jaundice, steatorrhea can be controlled by restricting the intake of long-chain fatty acids. The use of medium-chain triglycerides (2 tablespoons/1000 kcal) should be considered in severe cases of steatorrhea, especially when a high caloric intake is needed. Supplementation with fat-soluble vitamins is recommended. See also *Hepatitis.*

JCAHO. Abbreviation for *Joint Commission on the Accreditation of Healthcare Organizations.*

Jejunal hyperosmotic syndrome. Preferred term for dumping syndrome.

Jejunostomy. Creation of an artificial opening through the abdominal wall into the jejunum for feeding. *Dietary management:* small, frequent feedings, with extra care to avoid diarrhea and gas formation, should be used. Since jejunostomy bypasses the stomach, there is likelihood of the dumping syndrome. See also *Ostomy.*

Jejunum. The second portion of the small intestine between the duodenum and the ileum; it is about 8 feet long. For its role in digestion and absorption of nutrients, see Appendix 11 and *Absorption, nutrients. Jejunitis* is the inflammation of the jejunum. *Jejunectomy* is the excision of all or part of the jejunum. See also *Jejunostomy.*

Jevity. Brand name of a lactose-free, isotonic tube feeding formula containing 14 gm fiber per liter; made of calcium and sodium caseinates, hydrolyzed cornstarch, soy polysaccharide, MCT oil, and corn oil. See Appendix 39.

JODM. Abbreviation for *juvenile-onset diabetes mellitus.*

Joint Commission on the Accreditation of Healthcare Organizations (JCAHO). A private, nonprofit agency that sets guidelines for the operations of hospitals and other health care facilities to ensure high standards of patient care. A staff of medical inspectors is drawn from members of the American College of Physicans, American College of Surgeons, American Hospital Association, and American Medical Association. The team of inspectors (who examine the operation of the hospital by invitation) submits a written report and recognizes compliance with standards by granting a certificate of accreditation for 1-3 years.

Joule. In the metric system, energy is measured in joules. One joule (kJ) equals 4.184 kcal.

Junk food. Layman's term for food with low nutrient value except calories. Usually rich in fats, simple sugars, and/or starches. Similar to foods with "empty" calories.

Juvenile-onset diabetes mellitus (JODM). Diabetes mellitus among the young, in some cases starting in childhood. Classified as insulin-dependent *diabetes mellitus.* See under *Diabetes mellitus.*

Juvenile-onset obesity (JOO). Obesity that develops during childhood; characterized by large amounts of fat stored. The child also has an excessive number of adipose cells.

K

K. 1. Chemical symbol for potassium. 2. Symbol for "kilo," as in kilogram (kg).

K 40. Potassium 40, a radioactive isotope naturally present in the body. Potassium 40 measurement is used to determine body composition. It is based on the assumption that body potassium is found in constant concentration in the muscles and lean portions of the body but is not present in fat. Body potassium therefore becomes an index of lean body mass.

Kaposi's sarcoma. A cancer of the reticuloendothelial cells usually associated with AIDS and lymphomas. Characterized by brownish or purplish papules on the skin that progressively spread to the viscera and lymph nodes. *Dietary management:* if the patient is receiving chemotherapy and radiotherapy, management is similar to that of cancer. See also *Nutrition, cancer.*

Kerasin. A cerebroside occurring in the brain. On hydrolysis, it yields a fatty acid, galactose, and sphingosine.

Keratin. Insoluble protein of hair, hooves, nails, and feathers. Contains a large amount of sulfur and is a commercial source of the amino acid cystine. Not hydrolyzed by digestive enzymes of humans.

Keratinization. Process of becoming horny due to the development of *keratin.* In vitamin A deficiency, keratinization of epithelial tissue occurs throughout the body, first in the salivary glands and then in the respiratory tract, eyes, and skin. Secondary infections from cracks in this dry layer in the respiratory tract lead to pneumonia and, in the eyes, to *xerophthalmia.*

Keratitis. Inflammation of the cornea of the eye. May be due to infection, vitamin A deficiency, allergy, or injury to the eye.

Keratomalacia. Softening and death of cells of the cornea of the eye. The earliest sign is dryness of the conjunctiva, which may lead to ulceration and infection. Effective treatment at this stage is followed by corneal scarring and opacity. If the process is not stopped by treatment, it leads to perforation of the cornea, prolapse of the iris, and infection of the whole eyeball. Healing results in scarring of the whole eye and frequently in total blindness. Keratomalacia is seen in severe vitamin A deficiency, although it may also be due to other diseases causing corneal lesions, such as trauma, bacterial infection, measles, and repeated exposure to excessive dust.

Keratosis. Any skin disease characterized by horny growth. In *follicular keratosis,* the skin becomes rough, dry, and scaly, and the hair follicles are blocked with plugs of keratin, which appear as prominent projections along the upper forearm and thighs, as well as along the shoulders, back, abdomen, and buttocks. Because of its appearance, the condition is commonly called "gooseflesh" or "toad skin." It is seen in vitamin A deficiency.

Keshan disease. Syndrome named after the region in China where it is endemic. It is considered to be due primarily to a deficiency in *selenium.* Symptoms include low blood and hair selenium levels and cardiomyopathy with high mortality in children and women of childbearing age.

Keto-. Prefix denoting the presence of the ketone or carbonyl group (C=O). A *keto acid* is a compound that contains both the carbonyl group (C=O) and the carboxyl group (−COOH).

Ketoacidosis. Accumulation of ketones in the body resulting in an abnormal increase in hydrogen ion concentration (acidosis). Occurs in faulty carbohydrate metabolism and is a complication of *diabetes mellitus;* characterized by nausea, vomiting, dyspnea, fruity odor of the breath, and mental confusion. It leads to coma if untreated.

Ketogenesis. Formation of ketone or acetone bodies in the liver. Ketone bodies formed in the liver are oxidized in other tissues, especially in the muscles. When ketone formation exceeds ketone oxidation, ketone bodies accumulate and cause *ketosis*.

Ketogenic. Capable of being converted into ketone bodies. The ketogenic substances in metabolism are the fatty acids and certain amino acids. See also *Diet, ketogenic,* and *Ketogenic amino acid* under *Amino acid.*

Ketogenic-antiketogenic ratio. Ratio between substances in the diet that give rise to ketone bodies (ketogenic factors) and those that favor ketone oxidation (antiketogenic factors). The *ketogenic factors* are precursors of ketone bodies such as fatty acids and the ketogenic amino acids. The *antiketogenic factors* are precursors of glucose; these include carbohydrates, glucogenic amino acids, and the glycerol portion of fat. For clinical purposes, the following simplified ratio may be used:

$$\frac{\text{Ketogenic factors}}{\text{Antiketogenic factors}} = \frac{0.5\,P + 0.9\,F}{0.5\,P + 0.1\,F + 1.0\,C}$$

where P, F, and C represent, respectively, the number of grams of protein, fat, and carbohydrate in the diet. A ketogenic diet with a ketogenic/antiketogenic ratio of 3:1 will produce a state of ketosis.

Ketone. Compound containing the carbonyl group (C=O); derived from oxidation of a secondary alcohol. The ketone test in the urine is done with a dipstick reagent or a test tablet. See also *Ketonuria.*

Ketone bodies. Also called "acetone bodies"; collective term given to the intermediate products of fatty acid degradation. These include acetoacetic acid, beta-hydroxybutyric acid, and acetone and are present in the blood in very small amounts under ordinary conditions. Ketone bodies formed in the liver are normally oxidized in other tissues. However, ketone bodies tend to accumulate when the rate of production becomes so great that the organism cannot burn them at a sufficiently rapid rate. See *Ketosis.*

Ketonemia. Presence of ketone (acetone) bodies in the blood above normal levels; characterized by a fruity breath odor.

Ketonuria. Presence of ketone (acetone) bodies in the urine. Abnormal amounts in the urine indicate rapid catabolism of fats, as in uncontrolled diabetes mellitus, starvation, or other disorders associated with increased fat metabolism.

Ketose. Carbohydrate containing the ketone group. Fructose is a ketose.

Ketosis. Clinical condition in which *ketone bodies* accumulate in the blood and appear in the urine; characterized by a sweetish acetone odor of the breath. Ketosis may be caused by a disturbance in carbohydrate metabolism (as in uncontrolled diabetes mellitus), by a dietary intake quite low in carbohydrate but very high in fat (as in a ketogenic diet), or by a diminution in carbohydrate catabolism with consequent high mobilization of body fats (as in starvation). Uncontrolled ketosis leads to *acidosis*. It causes a decrease in the alkali reserve in plasma, hyperventilation, low CO_2 tension in alveolar air, and an increase in urinary ammonia; in advanced states, it causes low blood pH.

Ketoxylose. Also called "xylulose." One of the few L-sugars found in nature. It is excreted in the urine of humans with a hereditary abnormality in pentose metabolism.

Kidney. One of a pair of bean-shaped organs located in back of the abdominal cavity on either side of the spine just below the spleen on the left and the liver on the right. The functioning unit is the *nephron,* which consists of a *glomerulus,* or tuft of capillaries, that is surrounded by *Bowman's capsule.* This capsule is attached to a long, winding *tubule* through which passes the fluid from the blood contained in the glomerulus. Urine is produced in the nephron and emptied into the *pelvis* of the kidney. From here, urine flows into the *ureter,* which is a muscular tube extending from the kidney to the *urinary bladder.* The chief functions of the kidney are to maintain constant blood composition and volume by its unique filtering system; to maintain normal pH of body fluids by excreting an acid urine and by synthesizing ammonia whenever necessary; and to excrete body wastes or metabolic by-products. There are at least 2 million nephrons, which filter more than 2500 pints of blood daily. The pituitary hormone (antidiuretic hormone) helps the kidneys to regulate *water balance*. See also *Urine*.

Kidney (renal) clearance test. Test of *kidney function* by measuring the ability to excrete waste products such as creatinine, urea, inulin, or dye in the urine. The quantity excreted per minute divided by the amount present in 1 ml of plasma is the urinary clearance.

Kidney transplantation. When a patient receives a normal kidney from a donor, he or she is usually given high doses of immunosuppressive drugs (such as prednisone azathioprine and cyclosporine A) to prevent immune rejections. Mineral balance, particularly for calcium and phosphorus, may be affected by these drugs; thus, their intake should be increased 1.5 times the normal recommended dietary allowance. Hyperglycemia and edema are other side effects which require carbohydrate and sodium restriction. Following successful kidney transplantation, protein restriction is no longer needed, as nitrogen retention is not a problem. Maintain desirable body weight and monitor any hyperlipidemia, hypercholesterolemia, and hypertension. With prednisone therapy, however, increase protein intake to 1.5 to 2 gm/kg/day for adults. In cases of transplant rejection, resume monitoring of protein, fluid, and electrolytes, especially sodium and potassium. Dialysis may be resumed, depending on the severity of rejection.

Kilocalorie (kcal). See *Calorie*.

Kinky hair disease. See *Menke's disease*.

Kjeldahl method. Method of determining the amount of nitrogen in an organic compound by digestion with sulfuric acid and conversion of the amine group in the amino acid to ammonia. Nitrogen is calculated by measuring the amount of ammonia formed. In foods, most of the nitrogen comes from protein (about 16% nitrogen). Thus the *crude protein* content in foods may be determined by multiplying the total "Kjeldahl nitrogen" by the factor 6.25.

Knee height. An anthropometric measurement used to estimate the stature of a person who is bedfast or chairbound or who has spinal curvature. The formulas are given below:

Stature for men (in cm)
$$= (2.02 \times \text{knee height}) - (0.04 \times \text{age}) + 64.19$$

Stature for women (in cm)
$$= (1.83 \times \text{knee height}) - (0.24 \times \text{age}) + 84.88$$

Knee height is measured in cm (or in. $\times$ 2.54) and age is rounded to the nearest whole year. To measure knee height accurately, use a sliding broad-blade caliper that is commercially available. It is best to measure knee height when the person is in a recumbent position. See also *Weight, computed*.

Koagulation vitamin. See *Vitamin K*.

Kofranyi-Michaelis respirometer. Lightweight portable *respirometer* that makes possible the systematic measurement of energy expenditure during work. The instrument weighs only about 5 lb and can be worn on the back.

Koilonychia. Spoon-shaped nails; a nail deformity in which the outer surface becomes concave. Occurs in severe iron deficiency anemia.

Koladex. Brand name of a cola-flavored beverage containing 100 gm dextrose per 10-oz bottle. It is used for the standard glucose tolerance test.

Korsakoff's syndrome. Set of symptoms characterized by confusion, loss of memory, and irresponsibility. Often, degenerative changes occur in the thalamus as a result of thiamin and vitamin B_{12} deficiencies. Seen in chronic alcoholism, usually together with *Wernicke's encephalopathy*.

Krebs cycle. Tricarboxylic acid cycle or citric acid cycle. It is a cycle of reactions in which acetylcoenzyme A combines with oxalacetate, forming seven intermediary products —*citrate, cis-aconitate, isocitrate, alpha-ketoglutarate, succinate, fumarate,* and *malate*—and eventually re-forming *oxalacetate,* which is set free to unite with another molecule of acetylcoenzyme A, thus repeating the cycle. The Krebs cycle is considered the final common pathway in the oxidation of carbohydrate, protein, and fat to carbon dioxide and water, with the release of energy. The acetylcoenzyme A that unites with oxalacetate may come from the anaerobic phase of carbohydrate metabolism, from fatty acid breakdown, and indirectly from ketogenic amino acids. Some of the intermediate products in the cycle may also be formed from glucogenic amino acids and during fatty acid breakdown. For details, see Appendix 15.

Krebs-Henseleit cycle. Also called "ornithine cycle" in urea formation. See *Urea.*

Kwashiorkor. Nutritional deficiency disease due to inadequate intake of protein; seen principally in children shortly after weaning to a diet high in starch and low in protein. Unlike *marasmus,* kwashiorkor occurs even with adequate caloric intake. It is characterized by retarded growth, anemia, edema, fatty infiltration of the liver, pigmentary changes of the skin and hair, gastrointestinal disorders (especially diarrhea), muscle wasting, delayed wound healing, and psychomotor changes. Water and electrolyte imbalance is brought about by hypoalbuminemia, diarrhea, and decreased cell enzyme and endocrine functions. Severe dehydration may cause heart failure. Kwashiorkor is a public health problem in many countries where the quality and/or quantity of protein intake are below minimal requirements. Although this severe protein deficiency syndrome is especially prevalent in malnourished children, it may also occur in hospitalized patients suffering from long-term illness who are in hypercatabolic states with insufficient nutritional support. *Dietary management:* immediate measures should be taken to correct dehydration and electrolyte imbalance. As the patient improves, a high-protein diet (3 to 4 gm/kg ideal body weight/day for young children) is initially provided by nonfat milk solids or skimmed milk powder added to a mixed diet. Refeeding should be gradual. Provide sufficient calories from carbohydrate to spare protein. If necessary, use tube feeding. Currently, many commercial nutrient formulas of high protein-calorie density are available. Mineral and vitamin supplementation is recommended, since magnesium and potassium depletion and vitamin A deficiency may be serious. Compare kwashiorkor with *Marasmus.*

Kynurenine. An intermediate product in tryptophan metabolism. Kynurenine in mammalian liver may be hydrolyzed to anthranilic acid and alanine, requiring pyridoxal phosphate as a cofactor. Large amounts of kynurenine are excreted in the urine in pyridoxine deficiency. It is found in normal urine in trace amounts but may be temporarily increased after tryptophan administration.

Kyphosis. Also called "humpback." Abnormal curvature of the spine. Often the result of bad posture, vitamin D deficiency, certain types of arthritis, osteoporosis, or tuberculosis of the spine.

L

L. Symbol for liter or lung.

Labeling. Accompanying printed information about the product (food, drug, cosmetics, tool, etc.), usually following established regulations. See *Food labeling* and *Nutritional labeling.* See also Appendix 3.

Lactaid. Commercial preparation of liquid *lactase* enzyme, which can hydrolyze up to 99% of the *lactose* in milk when added 24 hours before use; also available in caplet form for oral ingestion with foods containing lactose.

Lactalbumin. One of the milk proteins; the others are casein and lactoglobulin. It is identical to serum albumin and is not easily precipitated by acids. The soft, flocculent curds are easy to digest, in contrast to the large, hard curds of casein. Thus the higher ratio of lactalbumin to casein in human milk (one-half of human milk protein is lactalbumin) is an advantage for infant feeding. Although the total amount of protein in cow's milk is about two times that of human milk protein, the ratio of lactalbumin to casein is only 1:5. Also, the higher lactose/protein ratio in human milk is favorable. See *Infant feeding* and *Lactose.*

Lactase. Enzyme that splits *lactose* into glucose and galactose. It is present in the intestines of all young mammals but may become deficient with age and in certain conditions affecting the small intestine. Lactase deficiency causes intolerance to lactose, which is characterized by bloating, cramping, flatulence, and diarrhea. See *Lactose intolerance.*

Lactase deficiency. See *Lactose intolerance.*

Lactation. The period of milk secretion; the secretion of milk by the mammary gland. The amount of milk produced is affected by several factors, including the nutritional status of the mother, frequency of sucking by the young, ingestion of medicinal or food galactogens, and hormonal control. See Appendix 1 for the recommended dietary allowances for lactation.

Lacteals. Tiny vessels in the villi of the wall of the small intestine through which chylomicrons are absorbed. These ducts empty into the lymphatic system.

Lactic acid. An acid produced by fermenting lactose (milk sugar); also formed from sucrose, glucose, or maltose by the action of lactic acid bacteria. In mammalian tissues, lactic acid is formed by the reduction of pyruvate when oxygen is lacking and pyruvate cannot be oxidized and is channeled into the *Krebs cycle.*

Lactic dehydrogenase (LDH). Enzyme that reversibly catalyzes the reduction of pyruvic acid to lactic acid or the oxidation of lactic acid to pyruvic acid. It is present in the tissues and released into the blood when there is tissue necrosis, as in liver damage, myocardial infarction, and renal tubular necrosis.

***Lactobacillus bifidus* factor.** A protective factor in human milk that encourages growth of beneficial bacteria in the infant's intestines; one of the reasons for encouraging breast feeding.

***Lactobacillus bulgaricus* factor.** A growth factor for certain microorganisms identical to *pantothenic acid,* a water-soluble vitamin.

***Lactobacillus casei* factor.** Former name for *folic acid,* a water-soluble vitamin.

Lactoflavin. Riboflavin of milk; the name given to the greenish-yellow fluorescent flavin pigment of whey. A former name is "lactochrome." See *Vitamin B$_2$.*

Lactose. Also called "milk sugar"; a disaccharide that occurs naturally only in the milk of mammals. It is hydrolyzed by acid or the enzyme lactase into the monosaccharides glucose and galactose. Lactose is less readily digested than other disaccharides. The undigested lactose passes into the large intestine, where it is fermented by normal colonic bacteria to form lactic acid and hydrogen. These fermentation products can osmotically draw water into the lumen, causing cramping and diarrhea.

Lactose intolerance. Condition characterized by intestinal symptoms like bloating, cramping, flatulence, and diarrhea that follow the ingestion of lactose. Lactose intolerance varies in degree among individuals and may be primary or secondary. *Primary* lactose intolerance is due to lack of the enzyme lactase. Congenital lactase deficiency is rare, but the condition may develop after weaning and with maturity. Adult lactase deficiency is quite common in many nonwhite and ethnic populations, including blacks, Orientals, Jews, Mexicans, and American Indians. *Secondary* or acquired lactose intolerance is due to diseases affecting the intestinal mucosa (as in acute enteritis, celiac sprue, inflammatory bowel disease), and can occur after small bowel or gastric surgery and after periods of disuse of the intestinal tract (as in starvation and prolonged parenteral nutrition), causing lactase deficiency with atrophy of the small intestine. Secondary lactose intolerance is transient and disappears when the disease resolves. Primary lactose intolerance seems to be permanent, although the extent of intolerance varies and the severity of symptoms is related to the amount of lactose ingested. Most lactose-intolerant individuals usually have no difficulty handling small amounts of lactose. See *Diet, lactose-restricted.*

Lactose tolerance test. Measurement of the blood glucose level following the ingestion of a lactose dose. In the adult, an increase less than 20 mg/dl after a 50-gm lactose load is strongly suggestive of lactase deficiency.

Lactulose. A synthetic derivative of lactose used as a laxative and as an adjunct to protein restriction in the treatment of fulminant hepatic failure. Because lactulose cannot be digested, colonic bacteria metabolize it to lactic acid, which removes ammonia from the blood and reduces the degree of hepatic encephalopathy. Lactulose also increases the water content of the stools. Brand names include Cephulac, Cholac, Chronulac, Constilac, and Constulose.

Laënnec's cirrhosis. Also called "portal" or "alcoholic cirrhosis"; the end result of prolonged dietary inadequacy, particularly of protein, coupled with the toxic effects of alcohol on the liver. See *Cirrhosis.*

Laetrile. The compound 1-mandelonitrile-*B*-glucuronic acid, found in the seeds of certain fruits and nuts. It has been claimed, but not supported experimentally, that laetrile has therapeutic value in the treatment of cancer due to the cyanide it contains, which acts specifically to destroy the cancer cells. Normal animal cells, however, lack the enzymes required to release cyanide from mandelonitrile. Laetrile has also been erroneously promoted as vitamin B_{17}; there is no evidence of physiologic or biochemical abnormality when it is not included in the diet.

Large-for-gestational-age infant (LGAI). An infant with accelerated fetal growth and birth weight well above normal, usually beyond the 90th percentile of appropriate weight for gestational-age infants. Often influenced by maternal diabetes mellitus and Beckwith's syndrome. Signs include hypoglycemia and respiratory distress.

Lauric acid. A saturated fatty acid containing 12 carbon atoms; found in coconut oil, laurel oil and spermaceti.

Lavage. The washing out of an organ such as the stomach or bowel.

LBM. Abbreviation for *lean body mass.*

LBWI. Abbreviation for *low-birth-weight infant.*

LCT. Abbreviation for *long-chain triglycerides.*

LDH. Abbreviation for *lactic dehydrogenase.* See also *Serum enzymes.*

LDL. Abbreviation for *low-density lipoprotein.*

Lead (Pb). Trace element required in very small amounts for normal growth and health. Experimentally induced lead deficiency is associated with growth retardation; hypochromic anemia with decreased iron stores in the blood, liver, and spleen; and decreased hepatic concentrations of glucose, triglycerides, and phospholipids. The average intake of lead is about 300 μg/day, although this is highly variable. The lead content of foods varies with soil and environmental conditions; in addition, smaller amounts of lead are ingested with drinking water and with foods from lead-soldered cans, and are inhaled from the atmosphere and from cigarette smoke. Absorption is age dependent; infants and children absorb nearly 40%, whereas adults absorb only 5-10%. In the body, most of the lead is deposited in the bone (about 90%) and the rest in soft tissues, notably the liver and kidney. The observation that humans accumulate lead slowly and gradually with age implies that the capacity for excretion is not adequate to maintain overall homeostasis. Lead intake is of concern not for its beneficial properties but rather for its toxic effects, which can be especially damaging to children. The most common consequences of lead intoxication are anemia, stunted intellectual development, hypertension, and renal damage.

Lean body mass (LBM). Active tissue mass; the part of the body weight concerned with energy metabolism. It is a measure of body composition, taken as the difference between body weight and the total mass of the adipose tissue, the extracellular fluid, and the skeleton. The minimum essential fat content is only about 2%.

Lecithin. Phosphatidyl choline, a phosphatide consisting of glycerol, two molecules of fatty acids, phosphoric acid, and choline. It is widely distributed in animal cells, especially nerves. Lecithin exists in the cell as a dipolar ion; choline is a strong base, and phosphoric acid is a moderately strong acid. This is significant in fat transport. See *Lipotropic agent (factor)* and *Phospholipid.*

Leucine (Leu). Alpha-aminoisocaproic acid; an *essential amino acid* that is strongly ketogenic; acetoacetic acid is its chief catabolic product in the liver.

Leucine-induced hypoglycemia. A rare inborn error of metabolism due to a deficiency of a lyase enzyme needed in the degradation of leucine. Infants with this disorder fail to thrive and may have convulsions, delayed mental development, severe acidemia, and life-threatening, profound hypoglycemic attacks. Acute management is directed at correcting the profound hypoglycemia. Longer-term management is directed at reduction of leucine intake by moderate protein restriction in small, frequent meals and with nocturnal feedings if required to avoid hypoglycemia. See *Diet, leucine-restricted.*

Leucovorin. Generic drug name for the calcium salts of folinic acid, an active metabolite of folic acid. Folinic acid circumvents the metabolic block produced by folic acid antagonists (such as methotrexate) and is used as an antidote to these drugs. It is also used to treat megaloblastic anemia due to folate deficiency.

Leukemia. Type of blood cancer due to proliferation of leukocytes and decreased production of red blood cells. The etiology is unknown, although ionizing radiation, the effects of certain chemicals, heredity, and hormonal abnormalities may be causative factors. There are two kinds: acute and chronic. Generally, leukemia is characterized by diffuse replacement of bone marrow with proliferating leukocyte precursors, abnormal numbers and forms of immature white blood cells in the circulation, and infiltration of lymph nodes, spleen, liver, and other organs. Usually occurs with sudden onset; visible signs are fatigue and extreme weakness. Patients have frequent hemorrhaging and mouth ulcers. Some patients have been successfully treated with aminopterin and other folic acid antagonists and with bone marrow transplantation. *Dietary management:* for acute leukemia, serve meals at proper temperatures. Stabilize the patient's nutritional status prior to bone marrow transplantation. A diet high in protein, calories, vitamins, and minerals is recommended. In febrile conditions, ample fluids are needed. Encourage small, frequent feedings.

Leukocyte (leucocyte). Also called "white blood cell (WBC)"; the nonpigmented, nucleated cell of the blood. WBC play an important role in the body's defense mechanisms. They can destroy disease-causing organisms. The normal WBC count is about 5000 to 10,000/mm^3. This is increased in acute infections and leukemia and decreased in *leukopenia.*

Leukopenia. An abnormal reduction in the number of white blood cells as a result of decreased production by the bone marrow or increased destruction of the cells, usually in the spleen. The condition may be congenital or brought about by malignancy, folic acid deficiency, or some unknown causative factor (pernicious type).

Levan. Also called "fructosan"; a *homopolysaccharide* composed of fructose units. It is derived chiefly from Jerusalem artichokes and certain grasses. *Inulin* is a levan.

Levodopa. The levorotatory isomer of dihydroxyphenylalanine and the metabolic precursor of dopamine. It is used in the treatment of parkinsonian syndrome. The drug's effectiveness is decreased by high intakes of protein and pyridoxine; vitamin supplements containing pyridoxine should be avoided. Levodopa increases the need for ascorbic acid and vitamin B$_6$; decreases the absorption of tryptophan, phenylalanine, and tyrosine; and increases the urinary excretion of sodium and potassium. It may also cause anorexia, nausea, vomiting, and abdominal distress. It may be present in breast milk. Long-term use and high doses may cause vitamin B$_6$ deficiency and hypokalemia, especially if laxatives and potassium-losing diuretics are taken concurrently. Brand names are Bendopa, Dopar, Laradopa, and Sinemet.

Levulose. Another name for *fructose* or fruit sugar to indicate that it is levorotatory.

LGAI. Abbreviation for *large-for-gestational-age infant.*

Light adaptation. Changes occurring in the eye opposite in nature to those observed in *dark adaptation,* i.e., constriction of the pupil, diminished sensitivity of the retina, bleaching of the visual purple, and a change in pH from an alkaline to an acid reaction.

Lignin. An indigestible compound occurring in the cell walls of plants. It is a noncarbohydrate, insoluble *dietary fiber* and consists of a multiringed alcohol network. It is resistant to hydrolysis by digestive enzymes, strong acids and alkalis, and is not attacked to any extent by intestinal microorganisms.

Linoleic acid. An *essential fatty acid;* a polyunsaturated fatty acid with 18 carbon atoms in its chain and two double bonds, one of which is in the omega-6 position. It is the major omega-6 fatty acid in foods; it is found in linseed, safflower, cottonseed, and soybean oils, fish oils, and animal tissues. Human milk contains about four times more linoleic acid than cow's milk. Linoleic acid is a dietary essential (i.e., the body cannot synthesize it). It is essential for growth and prevention of dermatitis, and helps form hormone-like compounds called *eicosanoids.* The omission of linoleic acid together with two other polyunsaturated fatty acids, *linolenic* and *arachidonic acids,* from the diet results in failure of growth, scaly skin, hair loss, and delayed wound healing. Linoleic acid deficiency was reported in the early 1970s among hospitalized patients fed exclusively with intravenous fluids without fat. Patients with malabsorption, as in cystic fibrosis, may also be deficient in linoleic acid. Infants receiving milk formula lacking in polyunsaturated fatty acids develop an infantile eczema characterized by leathery skin with desquamation and oozing. Addition of trilinolein to the diet (5 to 7% of total calories) results in the disappearance of symptoms. The need for *essential fatty acids* will be met if linoleic acid is present in the diet at a level of at least 1% of total caloric requirements. See also *Fat intake, recommended.*

Linolenic acid. The alpha form is an essential fatty acid. It is a polyunsaturated fatty acid with 18 carbons and three double bonds, one of which is in the omega-3 position. It is found chiefly in linseed oil and fish oils. Alpha linoleic acid is the major omega-3 fatty acid in foods. It is considered a nutrient because of its growth-promoting effect; it plays a vital role in the immune system of the body. It produces hormone-like compounds called *eicosanoids.*

Lipemia. An increased level of blood lipids. *Temporary absorptive lipemia* occurs after a fatty meal as chylomicrons discharged into the blood plasma cause a rapid rise in lipid, chiefly as triglycerides, along with a small amount of protein. *Idiopathic lipemia* (unknown etiology) is frequently observed in diabetic acidosis and glycogen storage disease.

Lipid. Member of a large group of organic compounds insoluble in water and soluble in fat solvents, e.g., chloroform, ether, benzene, petroleum, and carbon disulfide. Lipids are divided into two groups: nonpolar lipids, which occur mainly as esters of fatty acids, which are water-insoluble and have to be hydrolyzed before entering the body; and polar or amphipathic lipids, which have fatty acids plus a polar radical such as a carbohydrate, lecithin, sphingomyelin, or phosphate-containing amino alcohol. Lipids of nutritional importance are *fatty acids,* particularly essential fatty acids; triglycerides or neutral *fats;* phosphatides, especially *lecithins;* terpenes, especially *carotene;* and steroids such as *cholesterol* and the *adrenocortical steroids.* Lipids are essential components of the cell and for energy storage. See Appendix 10.

Lipid malabsorption. Interference with lipid absorption brought about by bile deficiency, lack of the pancreatic enzyme *lipase,* defective intramucosal metabolism (as in nontropical sprue and adrenal hormone insufficiency), lymphatic obstruction, and impaired lipoprotein synthesis.

Lipochromes. Plant pigments that are soluble in fats and organic solvents. Examples are chlorophyll and carotenoids.

Lipofuscin. Ceroid pigments which occur as brown spots on the skin when lipid breakdown products accumulate.

Lipogenesis. 1. Synthesis of lipids or formation of body fat. 2. Specifically, the formation of fatty acids in the liver. Any dietary constituent that supplies acetate (e.g., carbohydrate and protein metabolites) may contribute to lipogenesis. In obese persons, the rate of lipogenesis may be five times greater than normal.

Lipoic acid. 6,8-Dithio-*n*-octanoic acid, a cyclic disulfide. It is also called "thioctic acid," "protogen," "pyruvate oxidation factor (POF)," and "*L. casei* acetate factor." It is needed for oxidative decarboxylation of alpha keto acids such as pyruvic acid and alpha-ketoglutaric acid. Lipoic acid functions as a hydrogen and an acyl acceptor. It is an essential growth factor for various organisms. Although its function is closely associated with that of thiamin, lipoic acid is not considered a vitamin since it appears to be synthesized in adequate amounts in the mammalian cell. See also *Lipothiamide pyrophosphate.*

Lipoid. A substance resembling fat in appearance and solubility but containing groups other than glycerol and fatty acids, which make up the true fats.

Lipolysis. 1. Breakdown or degradation of lipids. 2. Specifically, the splitting of fat into glycerol and fatty acids in the liver. Glycerol enters the pathway of carbohydrate metabolism as glycerol-3-phosphate. The fatty acids are degraded by a series of reactions leading to the ultimate product, *acetyl CoA.*

Lipomul-Oral. Brand name of a corn oil emulsion providing 3 kcal/ml; used as a concentrated source of calories in protein-restricted diets. It can be mixed with many foods. See Appendix 39.

Lipoprotein. Compound protein formed when a simple protein unites with a lipid. It has the solubility characteristics of protein; hence it is involved in lipid transport from the intestinal tract and liver to a variety of tissue sites. Five types circulate in the blood: *chylomicrons;* alpha lipoprotein or *high-density lipoprotein (HDL);* prebeta lipoprotein or *very-low-density lipoprotein (VLDL);* beta lipoprotein or *low-density lipoprotein (LDL);* and broad beta or *intermediate-density lipoprotein (IDL).* Levels of lipoproteins in the blood are influenced by diet, age, weight change, emotions and stress, drugs, illness, and a number of hormones (insulin, thyroxine, adrenal hormones, and anterior pituitary hormones). See *Blood lipids* and *Hyperlipoproteinemia.*

Lipoprotein lipase. Also called *clearing factor;* this lipase catalyzes the hydrolysis of fats present in chylomicrons and lipoproteins. It is found in various tissues and is important in the mobilization of fatty acids from depot fats.

Liposyn. Brand name of a 10% and a 20% fat emulsion for intravenous administration; made with safflower oil, soybean oil, egg phosphatides, and glycerin. Each milliliter provides 1.1 kcal (10% emulsion) and 2.0 kcal (20% emulsion). See also Appendix 41.

Lipothiamide pyrophosphate (LTPP). A conjugate of thiamin pyrophosphate and *lipoic acid* believed to be the active catalyst in the oxidative decarboxylation of alpha keto acids such as pyruvic acid.

Lipotropic agent (factor). Any substance capable of transporting or mobilizing fat and preventing or correcting the fatty liver of choline deficiency. The lipotropic agents are choline, betaine, methionine, inositol, serine, and lecithin. The exact mechanism by which these substances prevent fatty liver is not known. However, it has been suggested that neutral fats are converted to choline-containing *phospholipids* to mobilize the fat and thus prevent deposition in the liver.

Lithiasis. Formation of stones, or calculi, as in cholelithiasis and pancreatic lithiasis.

Liver. Also called "hepatic gland"; largest gland of the body, comprising about 3% of body weight, and located in the upper right quadrant of the abdomen. It is said that no other organ is concerned with so many varied functions as the liver, so that it is fittingly called the "warehouse and chemical manufacturer" of the body. Its physiologic roles include manufacture of vital substances (bile, prothrombin, fibrinogen, heparin, and urea); regulation of bodily processes (detoxification, reticuloendothelial activity, blood volume, and blood sugar level); metabolism of carbohydrate, protein, lipid, vitamins, and minerals; and storage of nutrients and other substances (protein reserves, glycogen, iron, copper, and vitamins A, D, K, and some B complex vitamins).

Liver disorder. A disease in which liver cells are damaged with some degree of severity, scarring the tissues. Causes include infections, biliary obstruction, heart disease; in some cases, the causes are congenital or unknown. *Dietary management:* a diet high in protein, carbohydrate, and calories with vitamin supplementation, particularly fat-soluble vitamins, is necessary. Alcohol is not allowed. Sodium intake should be restricted in ascites, and protein should be curtailed in hepatic coma. Foods should be soft and low in fiber in the presence of bleeding esophageal varices. See the recommended diets for ascites, cirrhosis, hepatitis, and hepatic coma. See *Ascites, Cirrhosis, Hepatitis,* and *Hepatic coma.*

Liver transplant. It is recommended in hepatic failure, usually caused by chronic liver disease, hepatitis, cirrhosis, and primary biliary cirrhosis. *Dietary management:* correct malnutrition and increase branched chain amino acid (BCAA) intake. Lessen aromatic amino acids (tyrosine and tryptophan). Provide protein at 1.3-1.5 gm/kg/day and calories at 35-45 kcal/kg/day or 1.5-1.75 × basal energy expenditure. Increase medium-chain triglyceride intake and monitor sodium and potassium profiles.

Load test. Also called "saturation test"; a method of assessing the nutritional status of a particular nutrient by measuring its urinary excretion after administration of a test dose to a person on a controlled intake. It is assumed that an individual whose tissues are saturated with the nutrient will retain little and excrete most of the dose, whereas one with low nutrient reserves will retain a large amount in order to saturate tissue levels.

Lofenalac. Brand name of an infant formula that is low in phenylalanine; used in the dietary treatment of *phenylketonuria.* It is prepared by enzymatic digestion of casein followed by chemical treatment to remove 95% of the phenylalanine. See also Appendix 37.

Lonalac. Brand name of a low-sodium, high-protein product in powder form prepared from casein, lactose, and coconut oil; used as a dietary source of protein when sodium restriction is severe, as in congestive heart failure, nephrosis, and hepatic cirrhosis with ascites. See also Appendix 39.

Long-chain triclycerides (LCT). Fats containing fatty acids longer than lauric acid (C12). Naturally occurring fats are composed predominantly of LCT containing palmitic (C16), stearic (C18), oleic (C18 with one double bond), and linoleic (C18 with two double bonds) acids. LCT should be restricted in the dietary treatment of *malabsorption syndromes* and replaced with *medium-chain triglycerides (MCT)*.

Lo-Sal. Brand name for an antacid low in sodium.

Lovastatin. A lipid-lowering drug used for the treatment of type IIa and type IIb hyperlipoproteinemia; it reduces serum low-density lipoprotein (LDL) cholesterol and increases high-density lipoprotein (HDL) cholesterol. The brand name is Mevacor.

Low-birth-weight infant (LBWI). The infant is considered LBW if the birth weight is less than 2500 gm (5½ lb), regardless of gestational age. Infants born before 25 weeks rarely survive. If the weight is less than 1500 gm (3½ lb), the infant is considered very low-birth-weight. Tiny premature infants encounter problems such as feeding intolerances, respiratory distress, fluid and electrolyte imbalances, intracranial hemorrhaging, anemia, immunulogic abnormalities, cardiovascular difficulties, and hypoglycemia. *Dietary management:* LBW infants usually need intensive care. Intravenous glucose solution and electrolytes are immediately given. Later, parenteral nutrition is introduced gradually, especially for infants with gastrointestinal problems. Care is taken to prevent protein-energy malnutrition with a proper choice of commercial formulas. As the infant improves, he or she can be gradually weaned from hyperalimentation to enteral feeding. The energy needs of LBW infants who receive parenteral nutrition are usually less (about 70–90 kcal/kg/day) than those who receive enteral feeding (120–130 kcal/kg/day) because the latter allows for nutrient losses due to poor digestion and absorption capacity. Protein needs range from 2 to 3 gm/kg/day. The initial protein source is in the form of crystalline amino acid solutions. Fluid requirements are variable because of environmental and physiologic factors. Initially, 40 to 80 ml/kg/day of fluids may be given. After the second week of life, most LBW infants receive 120 to 180 ml/kg/day. Glucose is the typical carbohydrate source, calculated at 3.4 kcal/gm. However, it is important to monitor glucose intolerance (hyperglycemia), which is especially common among VLBW infants.

Low-density lipoprotein (LDL). A plasma lipoprotein that has a density of 1.019–1.063 g/ml; classified as the beta fraction on the basis of electrophoresis. LDL contains 20-25% protein, 15-22% phospholipid, 45-50% cholesterol, and 10-13% triglycerides. LDL cholesterol is the most atherogenic lipoprotein. Individuals with elevated LDL have type II hyperlipidemia. Since LDL is difficult to measure, the level is calculated by the following formula (all values in mg/dl):

$$LDL = \text{Total cholesterol} - \left(\frac{\text{triglycerides}}{5} + HDL\right)$$

Low-sodium milk (LSM). Milk from which about 90% of its natural sodium is removed by an ion-exchange process. One quart of low-sodium milk may contain as little as 50 mg sodium compared to 500 mg in 1 quart of regular milk.

Low-sodium syndrome. Disturbance characterized by the following set of symptoms: weakness, lethargy, loss of appetite, nausea and vomiting, confusion, acid-base disturbance, and abdominal pain with general muscular cramps, renal damage, oliguria and later uremia, and possibly convulsions and shock. It is caused by prolonged periods of very low sodium intake, adrenal cortical insufficiency, and marked losses of body fluids and electrolytes, as in very hot weather or excessive perspiration, severe burns, marked diarrhea, and vomiting. Prompt provision of salt will correct the condition.

Luteotropic hormone (LTH). Also called "luteotropin," "prolactin," and "lactogenic hormone"; a hormone secreted by the anterior lobe of the hypophysis (pituitary gland). It is helpful in the development of the mammary glands and also initiates milk secretion. It stimulates the corpus luteum to synthesize progesterone and estrogens.

Lycopene. The principal red pigment present in tomatoes, watermelon, and pink grapefruit. It is an isomer of carotene but has no vitamin A activity.

Lymph. Fluid obtained from lymphatic ducts; one of the circulating fluids of the body. It is yellowish and alkaline in reaction. Occasionally, it is pinkish due to the presence of some red blood cells. When fat globules are present, it turns milky. It resembles blood plasma in appearance and composition, except that lymph contains colorless cells (lymphocytes) and has a lower protein content than plasma. Its main function is to nourish and bathe cells by circulating substances from the blood into the tissues. It is important in fat absorption.

Lymph node. Small bean-shaped body occurring at intervals along the lymphatic vessels. It removes foreign particles from the lymph by filtration and by *phagocytosis.*

Lymphocyte. Type of white blood cell that arises in the reticular tissue of the lymph glands. The nucleus is single and surrounded by a nongranular protoplasm. Lymphocytes are important for antibody formation. See *Total lymphocyte count.*

Lymphoma. Malignant, enlarged lymph nodes, spleen, and general lymphoid tissues causing fatigue, weight loss, slight fever, cough, dyspnea, and chest pain. *Dietary management:* give foods as tolerated; increased protein, calorie, and fluid intake is recommended.

Lysin. An *antibody* with destructive action on cells and tissues, causing dissolution or breakdown.

Lysine (Lys). An *essential amino acid;* the limiting amino acid in many cereal proteins, especially gliadin. Deficiency in humans may cause nausea, vomiting, dizziness, and anemia, in addition to growth failure in the young. In the tissues, this basic amino acid readily converts its epsilon carbon to carbon dioxide and helps to form glutamic acid. However, it does not exchange its nitrogen with other circulating amino acids, a property unique to lysine. See also *Amino acid.*

Lysine intolerance. Also called "hyperlysinemia." A congenital metabolic disorder caused by the inability to hydrolyze the amino acid lysine due to insufficient levels of the enzyme lysine ketoglutarate reductase. Symptoms include nausea, vomiting, mental retardation, episodes of coma, and high blood levels of lysine, arginine, and sometimes ammonia. Whether or not dietary treatment is effective in hyperlysinemia is controversial. It may be prudent to restrict protein intake to 1 gm/kg body weight.

Lysolecithin. A substance obtained by partial hydrolysis of lecithin, with only one fatty acid liberated. It aids in the emulsification of dietary lipids.

Lysophosphatides. Substances that are destructive to red blood cells. They are produced from lecithin by the action of the enzyme lecithinase, which is present in the venom of poisonous snakes.

Lysozyme. Enzyme that digests certain high-molecular-weight carbohydrates and some gram-positive bacteria. It is present in tears, saliva, mucus and nasal secretions, and other body fluids. Its activity is reduced by generalized malnutrition, particularly by vitamin A deficiency.

Lytren. Brand name of an oral electrolyte solution used in replacing water and electrolyte losses; it also contains dextrose. See Appendix 38.

M

M. 1. Symbol for mega- or molar concentration. 2. Abbreviation for metastasis, as in the malignant stage of cancer.

MAC. Abbreviation for *mid-arm circumference.*

Macrocyte. A giant red blood cell. *Macrocythemia* is an abnormal number of macrocytes in the blood. *Macrocytic anemia* is a type of anemia in which the red blood cells are unusually large, as in folic acid or vitamin B_{12} deficiency.

Macronutrients. Nutrients that are present in relatively high amounts in the body, constituting about 0.005% of body weight (50 ppm) or above. Protein, fat, water, and major minerals are macronutrients. See also *Nutrient classification.*

Macrophages. Cells of the reticuloendothelial system; they ingest foreign particles such as bacteria and cellular debris by *phagocytosis.*

Magnacal. Brand name of a high-calorie liquid formula that is low in residue and lactose-free; provides a concentrated source of calories (2 kcal/ml) for patients with restricted fluid allowance or increased energy needs. Suitable as an oral supplement or for tube feeding. Contains sodium and calcium caseinates, sucrose, maltodextrin, and soy oil. See also Appendix 39.

Magnesium (Mg). A major mineral essential to plants and animals; a component of chlorophyll in green plants. In humans, it is needed in relatively large amounts. In adults, it comprises about 0.05% of body weight, 60% of which is in bones and teeth, about 40% in the muscle and soft tissues, and the remainder in extracellular fluids. As a cofactor in reactions involving adenosine triphosphate, magnesium is important in carbohydrate, protein, and fat metabolism. More than 300 enzymes are known to be activated by magnesium. It also plays an important role in neuromuscular transmission and activity. Dietary magnesium deficiency is uncommon since it is widely distributed in nature, particularly in legumes, nuts, and unrefined grains; other good sources are cocoa, soybeans, and green leafy vegetables. Magnesium deficiency, or hypomagnesemia, occurs when the dietary intake is poor and associated with disease states involving intestinal malabsorption and/or decreased renal function, as in protein-calorie malnutrition, chronic alcoholism with malnutrition, and renal disease involving tubular dysfunction. Magnesium deficiency also occurs in long-term use of magnesium-free parenteral feeding; when there is excessive loss from the body, as in burns; and in increased urinary magnesium excretion with drugs like the cardiac glycosides and the loop diuretics, furosemide and ethacrynic acid. Deficiency states affect the neuromuscular, cardiovascular, and renal systems; characteristic symptoms are muscular twitching and muscle weakness, convulsions, tachycardia, nausea, and vomiting. Magnesium toxicity and hypermagnesemia occur primarily when there is severe renal insufficiency and when magnesium salts or magnesium-containing antacids and cathartics are administered in large doses. Signs of toxicity include nausea and vomiting, hypotension, paralysis of voluntary muscles, and somnolence. See Appendix 1 for the recommended dietary allowances.

Malabsorption syndrome. Set of symptoms indicating defective absorption of nutrients, which may include carbohydrates, protein, fat, vitamins, and minerals, as well as total calories. It may occur as a result of structural changes in the alimentary tract or its adjacent organs, failure of food to reach the absorptive surfaces, maldigestion, diver-

147

sion of foodstuffs to intestinal organisms, failure of the absorptive mechanism, or intestinal resection. Symptoms include abdominal distention and pain, steatorrhea and diarrhea, anorexia and muscle wasting with loss of weight, and anemia. Examples of disorders that show the malabsorption syndrome are *celiac disease, cystic fibrosis, carbohydrate intolerance,* and *pancreatic insufficiency.*

Malacia. Morbid softening or softness of a tissue or part, as in *osteomalacia,* or softening of bones.

Malaria. An infectious disease caused by one of four species of *Plamodium,* a protozoan transmitted by *Anopheles* mosquito bites. It may also be spread by blood transfusion or by the use of an infected hypodermic needle. *Dietary management:* see *Fever.* Frequently, the liver is enlarged and liver functions are impaired; in this case, dietary modifications for liver disease are followed.

Malnutrition. 1. Simply stated, any disorder of nutrition; bad or undesirable health status due to either *lack* or *excess* of a nutrient supply. 2. State of impaired biologic activity or development due to a discrepancy between the nutrient supply and the nutrient demand of cells. Malnutrition may be classified into three categories: malnutrition associated with poverty or an inadequate food supply; malnutrition associated with ignorance and indifference; and malnutrition secondary to such factors as diseases, alcoholism, drug abuse, and mental illness. See also *Deficiency disease* and *Nutritional deficiency (inadequacy).*

Maltase. Also called "alpha-glucosidase"; an enzyme found in yeast and intestinal juice. It hydrolyzes *maltose* to two glucose units.

Maltose. Also called "malt sugar"; a disaccharide made up of two molecules of glucose. It is formed as an intermediate product of starch hydrolysis. During digestion, maltose is hydrolyzed by the enzyme maltase to two glucose units.

MAMC. Abbreviation for *mid-arm muscle circumference.*

Manganese (Mn). An essential trace mineral widely distributed in plant and animal cells. The human body contains 12–20 mg manganese, which is concentrated in the liver, pancreas, kidney, skin, muscles, and bones. Manganese is a component of two metalloenzymes and is a catalyst for a number of enzymes involved in glucose and fatty acid metabolism and urea formation. It is also needed for bone development, skin integrity, and utilization of thiamin. Main food sources are nuts, legumes, and unrefined grains; tea, leafy vegetables, and fruits contain moderate amounts. Dietary manganese deficiency in humans has not been observed. Experimentally induced deficiency results in weight loss, transient dermatitis, retarded growth of hair and nails, changes in hair color, and decreased serum cholesterol and triglycerides. Cases of suboptimal manganese status have been found in selected populations, such as in children with inborn errors of metabolism (phenylketonuria, maple syrup urine disease, and galactosemia), in children and adults with epilepsy, and in persons with exocrine pancreatic insufficiency and active rheumatoid arthritis. Individuals with these conditions may have a special need for manganese. Toxicity from dietary sources appears to be highly unlikely. The few cases of manganese toxicity have resulted from ingesting large doses of the mineral supplement for 4 to 5 years, drinking well water contaminated with manganese from buried batteries, and prolonged exposure and inhalation of ore dust. Toxicity results in dementia and a psychiatric disorder resembling schizophrenia, followed by a crippling neurologic disorder that is similar to Parkinson's disease. See Appendix 2 for the estimated safe and adequate dietary intake.

Mannitol. A sugar alcohol obtained from the hydrogenation of *mannose.* Commercially it is extracted from certain seaweeds. It has a sweetening power, as does glucose, but yields only half as many calories because it is only partially absorbed.

Mannose. A monosaccharide containing 6 carbon atoms (a hexose); does not occur free in nature. It is found in legumes in the form of *mannosan,* a partially digestible polysaccharide.

MAO. Abbreviation for *monoamine oxidase.*

Maple syrup urine disease (MSUD). Also called "branched-chain ketoaciduria." An inborn error of metabolism due to a defect in the oxidative decarboxylation of the branched-chain amino acids leucine, isoleucine, and valine. This leads to the accumulation of these keto acids in the blood and cerebrospinal fluid and consequent excretion in the urine, to which they impart an odor of maple syrup or burnt sugar. Symptoms usually appear within the first week of life; these include difficulty in feeding with jerky aspirations, vomiting, periods of rigidity and flaccidity, seizures of the grand mal type, hypoglycemia, and possibly death. Survivors generally have severe brain damage. Treatment consists of restricting the dietary intake of leucine, isoleucine, and valine. See *MSUD Diet Powder.*

Marasmus. 1. Form of extreme undernutrition primarily due to a lack of calories and protein. It was formerly called "protein-calorie malnutrition" (PCM). The preferred designation now is "energy-protein malnutrition (EPM)" or "protein-energy malnutrition (PEM)." 2. Infantile atrophy that occurs almost wholly as a sequel to acute disease, especially diarrheal diseases. Marasmus is characterized by loss of weight, retarded growth and development, loss of subcutaneous fat, and wasting of muscle tissue. The word "marasmus" comes from a Greek word meaning "wasting." Other clinical symptoms due to protein deficiency are edema, skin changes, anemia, enlarged liver, and increased susceptibility to infections, accompanied by high fever. Marasmus is a major public health problem affecting as many as 50% of children in the developing countries. *Dietary management* depends on the presence of complications such as dehydration, electrolyte imbalance, vitamin deficiencies, and infections. Fluid and electrolyte imbalances should be corrected promptly. Oral or parenteral feeding high in protein and calories is needed.

Maxamaid XP. An orange-flavored powder free of phenylalanine and formulated for the 2- to 8-year-old child with phenylketonuria. Contains L-amino acids, carbohydrate, minerals, trace elements, and vitamins.

Maxamum XP. A phenylalanine-free powdered product designed for children 8 years of age and older and for pregnant women with phenylketonuria.

MBF. Abbreviation for *meat-based formula.*

MCT. Abbreviation for *medium-chain triglycerides.*

MCT oil. Commercially available for use as a substitute for or as a supplemental source of fat calories for patients in whom conventional food fats are poorly digested, absorbed, or utilized. It is made from fractionated coconut oil and contains 67% octanoic (C-8) and 23% decanoic (C-10) fatty acids; provides 115 kcal/tablespoon. See *Medium-chain triglycerides.*

MCV. Abbreviation for *mean corpuscular volume.*

ME. Abbreviation for *metabolizable energy.*

Meal. Portion of food eaten at a particular time to satisfy the appetite. *Meal patterns* are plans or guides for the inclusion of certain foods at stated intervals during the day, usually for the main meals—breakfast, lunch, and dinner.

Meals-on-Wheels. Community meals, especially for senior citizens; volunteers and paid employees prepare meals and deliver them to the recipient's home 5 days a week. Generally, a hot noon meal and a packaged evening meal are provided. The charge is based on the ability of the individual to pay for this service.

Mean corpuscular volume (MCV). Determined from the following formula:

$$MCV = \frac{HCT}{RBC} \times 10$$

where HCT and RBC represent values for hematocrit and red blood cell count, respectively. Elevated levels may indicate macrocytosis due to a deficiency of folate or vitamin B_{12} or excess alcohol consumption. Depressed levels indicate microcytosis due to iron deficiency or malabsorption, increased iron requirement, and blood loss.

Meat-based formula (MBF). Brand name of a milk-free formula for infants with galactosemia, lactose intolerance, and allergy to cow's milk protein. Contains sucrose, tapioca starch, beef heart, and sesame oil. See also Appendix 37.

Medical history. Record of pertinent information about an individual or patient that includes past illnesses, familial tendencies toward certain diseases, general health status since birth, and present complaints. Routinely taken when a patient is admitted to a hospital or seeks a medical consultation. It is a diagnostic aid in the management of a patient and a technique used in *nutrition surveys* and *nutritional assessment* to detect conditioning factors in nutritional inadequacy.

Medium-chain triglycerides (MCT). Fats composed of fatty acids shorter than lauric acid, predominantly saturated fatty acids with 6 to 10 carbon atoms. Compared with long-chain triglycerides, MCT have the following advantages: lower melting point, faster rate of hydrolysis, less need for bile acids, easier dispersion in water, smaller quantity incorporated into lipid esters, and less tendency to storage in the liver. MCT preparations are useful in the dietary management of *malabsorption syndromes* such as pancreatitis, postgastrectomy, sprue, cystic fibrosis, and chyluria.

Megacolon. An enlarged bowel due to an abnormality in the dilatation of the colon. Usually affects elderly persons who have constipation problems or use excessive amounts of laxatives. Tumors and strictures may also cause obstruction of the elimination process. Signs are distention, flatulence or incontinence, nausea, fatigue, and headache. *Dietary management:* provide adequate fluids and fiber, particularly prune juice, fresh fruits, leafy vegetables, legumes with skin, and whole-grain cereals.

Megaloblastic anemia. Type of anemia characterized by an increased level of *megaloblasts,* which are primitive nucleated red blood cells much larger than the mature normal erythrocytes. The megaloblastic anemias of pregnancy and infancy respond readily to folic acid therapy and an adequate balanced diet. See also *Anemia.*

Megavitamin therapy. Use of massive doses of vitamins to cure hyperactivity and other behavioral abnormalities. Advocates of megavitamin therapy or orthomolecular psychiatry propose that optimum molecular concentrations of vitamins are essential for proper mental functioning. However, this theory was based on studies which failed to meet the requirements of a proper scientific protocol. Currently, the American Academy of Pediatrics and the American Psychiatric Association feel that megavitamin therapy is unproved in terms of safety and efficacy.

Menadione. Synthetic compound with vitamin K activity; used in the prevention and treatment of hypoprothrombinemia secondary to factors that limit absorption or synthesis of vitamin K. It is two to three times more potent than the naturally occurring vitamin K. The brand name is Synkavite.

Menaphthone. Vitamin K_3 or *menadione.*

Menaquinone. Vitamin K_2; a homolog of vitamin K synthesized in animals. It is found in meats, especially liver, and in eggs and cheese, but the major source is bacterial synthesis in the intestines. Formerly called "farnoquinone."

Meniere's syndrome. A chronic disorder of the ear with signs of vertigo, nausea and vomiting, blurred vision, and nerve deafness. In some cases, allergy, trauma, or infection accompanies the disorder or may be the cause. *Dietary management:* restrict fluid and salt intake to reduce the pressure on the labyrinth. Eliminate any allergenic food.

Menetrier's disease (hypertrophic gastritis). A pathologic disorder characterized by enlargement of the gastric mucosa with hyperplastic cells. *Dietary management:* see under *Gastritis.*

Meningitis. Inflammation of the *meninges,* the membranes covering the brain and spinal cord. Symptoms include fever, severe headaches, nausea and vomiting, stiff neck, and tachycardia. *Dietary management:* intravenous fluids and nasogastric tube feeding may be required until dehydration is corrected. Monitor caloric intake to avoid weight loss and to offset the catabolic effects of fever.

Menke's disease. Also called "kinky hair disease." An inborn error of *copper* metabolism characterized by brittle, kinky hair texture resembling steel wool, accompanied by all the overt symptoms of gross copper deficiency except anemia. It is due to the intestinal failure to absorb copper, which accumulates in the intestinal mucosa. The liver becomes refractory to copper intake. Some improvement is achieved with parenteral copper administration (not by the oral route), which restores the *ceruloplasmin* level to normal, although the neurologic abnormalities do not improve. The disease is usually fatal.

Menstruation. Also called "menses"; the periodic cycle, usually 28 to 30 days, characterized by uterine bleeding or menstrual flow. It is peculiar to women from puberty to menopause. It normally lasts for 3 to 7 days, with a bloody discharge of about 125 ml; it contains materials sloughed off from the uterine wall plus blood that is devoid of fibrinogen and prothrombin and hence does not clot. Iron lost during menstruation can be as much as 1.5 mg/day, with an average of 0.7 mg/day, which is taken into consideration in establishing the recommended dietary allowance for women who are still menstruating. See also *Premenstrual syndrome.*

Mental illness. Also called "psychiatric disorder." Any disturbance in the adaptive and emotional balance of an individual. *Dietary management:* nutritional care must be individualized. Among the feeding problems that may be encountered are the following: a depressed patient loses interest or appetite; an overactive patient may not sit long enough to eat; a delusional patient may develop fears and suspicions about food; an emotionally insecure patient may indulge in overeating for personal satisfaction; a patient with anorexia nervosa is difficult to feed; and a patient undergoing shock therapy may need a high caloric intake.

Mercaptopurine. A chemical analog of the physiologic purines adenine and hypoxanthine; a component of various chemotherapeutic drugs used in the treatment of acute leukemia. It may antagonize pantothenic acid and produce a sprue-like syndrome. It may also cause weight loss, anemia, nausea, vomiting, and diarrhea. The brand name is Purinethol.

Mercapturic acid. A complex of cysteine with naphthalene or various halogenated aromatic hydrocarbons in which the latter compounds are detoxified and excreted in the urine.

Mercury (Hg). Heavy liquid metal used in thermometers and other scientific instruments; also used as a dental amalgam. Its salts are used as antiseptics, diuretics, fungicides, and parasiticides. The environmental concern for mercury in the food supply focuses on its toxic effects on the tissues, particularly the brain. Toxicity is due to the binding of tissue proteins and interference with cellular metabolism. The dangerous forms of mercury are the alkyl derivatives methylmercury and ethylmercury. Population outbreaks of poisoning have been reported from the ingestion of fish and seafood exposed to methylmercury contamination and of seed grains previously treated with mercurial fungicides. Characteristic symptoms of mercury poisoning are visual abnormalities, tremors, proteinuria, apathy, and mental deterioration. The U.S. Department of Agriculture has set a safe level guideline of 0.5 ppm mercury in fish.

Meritene. Brand name of a milk-based nutritional product, in liquid or powder form, for oral supplementation or tube feeding. Made with milk, corn syrup solids, corn oil, sucrose, and mono- and diglycerides; contains 55 gm lactose/1000 ml. See Appendix 39.

Metabolic body size. Also called "physiologic size"; the active tissue mass of an individual. It is determined by raising the body weight in kilograms to the three-fourths power.

Metabolic cart (MC). A portable cart used for indirect *calorimetry.* It measures the amount of oxygen and carbon dioxide in a respiratory gas sample. Data are used to calculate the resting energy expenditure

(REE) and respiratory quotient (RQ) as follows:

$$REE = 3.9 \, VO_2 + 1.1 \, VCO_2 \times 1.44$$

where VO_2 is oxygen consumed (ml/min) and VCO_2 is carbon dioxide produced (ml/min).

$$RQ = VCO_2 \div VO_2.$$

Metabolic chamber. A room-sized chamber that permits continuous and long-term analysis of exhaled gases; used in indirect *calorimetry.*

Metabolic pool. 1. Phrase descriptive of the manner in which a nutrient can change, combine with, or participate in metabolic reactions. 2. Components, indistinguishable as to origin, that may be employed for either synthetic or degradative processes. When the end products of digestion (e.g., amino acids, fatty acids, glycerol, and glucose) are absorbed, they enter the metabolic pool and intermingle with other substances, or they are metabolized for various bodily functions.

Metabolic water. See under *Water.*

Metabolism. The sum of all the chemical changes in the body. There are two phases: *anabolism,* or constructive metabolism, which is concerned with the building up of materials and tissues; and *catabolism,* or destructive metabolism, which is the breaking down of materials and tissues. See also *Intermediary metabolism.*

Metabolizable energy (ME). The portion of gross food energy capable of transformation in the body for useful work (or net energy) and for basal metabolism. It does not include heat losses from urinary and fecal excretions.

Metalloprotein. A compound protein; a protein combined with a metal-containing prosthetic group. Examples are ferritin (iron-containing protein), carbonic anhydrase (zinc-containing protein), and ceruloplasmin (copper-containing protein). See also Appendix 9.

Metaprotein. Denatured protein formed by the action of dilute acid or alkali on native proteins, usually albumin and globulin.

Methemoglobin. Also called "ferrihemoglobin." A hemoglobin molecule in which the iron component is oxidized to the ferric state and can no longer carry oxygen. It is present in the blood as a product of normal metabolic activity in trace amounts only. See *Hemoglobin.*

Methionine (Met). An *essential amino acid;* contains sulfur and the labile methyl group. It is one of the *lipotropic agents* and participates in methylation reactions; hence it is important in protein and fat metabolism.

Methotrexate. A folic acid antagonist; a potent anticancer drug. It inhibits dihydrofolate reductase and thus decreases the formation of tetrahydrofolic acid. It also causes malabsorption of folate, vitamin B_{12}, fat, and carotene. Other adverse effects include anorexia, weight loss, stomatitis, gingivitis, megaloblastic anemia, nausea, vomiting, and diarrhea. It is excreted in breast milk. Brand names are Folex and Mexate.

Methylcellulose. Preparation of indigestible polysaccharide that provides bulk and satiety value. It is prescribed for constipation and in the dietary management of obesity.

Methyldopa. An antihypertensive agent which is structurally related to *catecholamines* and their precursors. It increases the need for folic acid and vitamin B_{12}, and may also cause glossitis, dry mouth, constipation, and weight gain due to salt and fluid retention. It is excreted in breast milk. Brand names are Aldocor, Aldomet, and Aldoril.

3-Methylhistidine. Compound released during the breakdown of actin and myosin. The 24-hour urinary excretion of 3-methylhistidine is an indicator of change in skeletal muscle mass and in the rate of muscle protein breakdown.

Metoprolol. A beta-adrenergic blocking agent used in the management of hypertension, myocardial infarction, and angina. It may cause dry mouth, nausea, vomiting, abdominal cramping, and constipation or diarrhea; it may also increase blood urea nitrogen and serum triglycerides. The brand name is Lopressor.

Metronidazole. An antibacterial and antiprotozoal agent used for the treatment of trichomonal infections and intestinal amebiasis. It has a sharp, unpleasant, metallic taste. May cause loss of appetite, altered taste, dry mouth, glossitis, nausea, vomiting, epigastric distress, and abdominal cramping. It is excreted in breast milk. It should not be taken with alcohol due to the risk of a disulfiram-like reaction. Brand names are Femazole, Flagyl, Metronid, Metryl, Protostat, and Satric.

Mg. Chemical symbol for magnesium.

MI. Abbreviation for *myocardial infarction.*

Micelle. 1. Dispersed particles in a colloidal system that are held in a particulate form because of their special physicochemical properties. 2. One of the submicroscopic structural units of protoplasm. 3. It is an essential step in the digestion and absorption of fats; an emulsified compound formed by positioning the hydrophobic radicals of the molecule toward the center and the hydrophilic part toward the outside. Thus, the compound becomes more water-miscible.

Microbiologic assay. Means of analyzing nutrients, especially vitamins and amino acids, by the use of microorganisms. A suitable microorganism is inoculated into a medium containing all the needed growth factors except the one nutrient under examination. The rate of growth is proportional to the amount of the particular nutritional factor added to the medium. The commonly used test microorganisms and the vitamins determined are as follows: *Lactobacillus fermentum 36* (thiamin), *Lactobacillus casei* (riboflavin and folic acid), *Saccharomyces carlsbergensis* (vitamin B_6 and inositol), and *Lactobacillus leichmannii 313* (vitamin B_{12}).

Microcyte. Red blood cell that is smaller than normal. *Microcytic anemia* is a type of anemia in which the red blood cells are smaller than normal. This is seen in iron-deficiency anemia.

Microlipid. Brand name of a safflower oil supplement to oral or tube feeding formulas; used as a concentrated source of calories when protein and carbohydrate need to be restricted, as in renal failure and chronic obstructive pulmonary disease. Provides 4.5 kcal/ml.

Micron (μ). Unit of length measurement equal to one-millionth of a meter. A millimicron (μm) is one-thousandth of a micron.

Micronutrients. Nutrients present in the body in amounts less than 0.005% of body weight (50 ppm). Examples are trace minerals, vitamin B_{12}, and pantothenic acid.

Mid-arm circumference (MAC). Also called "upper-arm circumference." Measurement (in centimeters) at the midpoint between the tip of the acromial process of the scapula and the olecranon process of the ulna. MAC is an indicator of fat stores. Measurements greater than the 50th percentile are acceptable; the 40th to 50th percentile indicates mild fat depletion; the 25th to 39th percentile indicates moderate fat depletion; and measurements below the 25th percentile indicate severe fat depletion.

Mid-arm muscle circumference (MAMC). Measurement of mid-arm muscle circumference provides an indirect assessment of skeletal muscle protein reserves. This is obtained by measuring the mid-arm circumference (MAC) and the triceps skinfold (TSF). The mid-arm muscle circumference (in centimeters) is then determined from the following formula:

$$MAMC = MAC - (0.314 \times TSF)$$

where MAC and TSF, respectively, represent values for mid-arm circumference (in centimeters) and triceps skinfold (in millimeters) measurements. Values greater than 85% are considered acceptable; 76-85% indicates mild depletion; 65-75%, moderate depletion; and less than 65%, severe depletion. See Appendix 23.

Milk-alkali syndrome. Occurs in persons with peptic ulcer who consume large amounts of milk and alkalis for a long period of time. The symptoms are hypercalcemia, calcium deposition in soft tissues, vomiting, gastrointestinal bleeding, and high blood pressure.

Mineral. An inorganic element that remains as ash when food is burned. Analysis of mineral ash may show as many as 40 kinds, but only 19 are essential to human nutrition. The criteria that determine the essentiality of a mineral are as follows: a deficiency state occurs with a diet considered adequate in all respects except for the mineral under study; there is a significant response (growth or alleviation of signs of deficiency) when a supplement of the mineral is given; the response is repeatedly demonstrable; and the deficiency state correlates with a low level of the mineral in the blood or tissues. The major minerals (macrominerals) are *calcium, phosphorus, potassium, sodium, magnesium, sulfur,* and *chlorine.* The trace minerals (microminerals) needed by humans are *iron, zinc, selenium, molybdenum, iodine, copper, manganese, fluorine, chromium, arsenic, nickel,* and *silicon.* Probably also essential are *boron, tin,* and *vanadium.*

Mineral functions. Minerals make up about 4% of body weight. In general, the role of minerals in the body is classified as *structural* or *regulatory.* The function of a mineral is structural when it is an integral part of a cell, tissue, or substance, e.g. calcium, phosphorus, and magnesium in bones and teeth; sulfur in hair, insulin, and thiamin; iron in hemoglobin; and chloride in hydrochloric acid of gastric juice. Regulatory functions include maintenance of water and acid-base balance, muscle contractility, nerve irritability, and actions as cofactors of enzyme systems.

Mineral oil. Liquid petrolatum preparation used as a lubricant laxative. It has no caloric value, but it interferes with the absorption of carotene and the fat-soluble vitamins A, D, E, and K; it also decreases the absorption of calcium and phosphorus. Brand names are Agoral, Kondremul, Petrogalar, and Zymenol.

Mn. Chemical symbol for *manganese.*

Mo. Chemical symbol for *molybdenum.*

Moducal. Brand name of a refined, readily digestible carbohydrate source for use in patients with increased caloric requirements or limited intake. It is bland and nearly tasteless, and can be mixed with foods and beverages without appreciably altering their taste. Consists of glucose polymers and small amounts of glucose, maltose, and isomaltose. Provides 3.8 kcal/gm powder.

Molality. Number of moles of solute per 1000 gm of solvent; usually designated by a small "m." A *1-molal solution* contains 1 mole (gram molecular weight) of solute in 1000 gm of solvent. See *Osmolality.*

Molarity. Number of moles of solute per liter of solution; usually designated by a capital "M." A *1-molar solution* contains 1 mole (gram molecular weight) of solute in 1 liter of solution. See *Osmolarity.*

Molybdenum (Mo). An essential trace mineral; it functions as a constituent of enzymes involved in the metabolism of sulfur and purines and the transfer of electrons for the oxidation/reduction process. Molybdenum deficiency in goats fed purified rations results in decreased food intake, retarded weight gain, impaired reproduction, and shortened life expectancy. Molybdenum deficiency has been reported in one individual on long-term total parenteral nutrition who developed a variety of symptoms, including headache, night blindness, lethargy, disorientation, hypermethioninemia, and increased urinary excretion of xanthine and sulfite. Treatment with molybdenum resulted in clinical improvement and normalization of sulfur metabolism. The congenital deficiency of molybdenum-pterin cofactor leads to a lack of sulfite oxidase and xanthine dehydrogenase, causing mental retardation, bilateral dislocation of the lens, and severe neurologic dysfunction. Little is known about the chemical form or bioavailability of molybdenum in foods. The estimated average intake from food and water is about 0.2 mg/day. Good food sources are milk and milk products, whole grains, legumes, and cereals. Molybdenum is rapidly absorbed from the gastrointestinal tract and is excreted mainly in the kidneys. Since molybdenum is antagonistic to copper, the adverse effects of molybdenum toxicity are similar to those of copper deficiency. Toxicity in animals results in severe diarrhea, anemia, retarded growth, weakness, stiffness, and loss of hair color. See Appendix 2 for the estimated safe and adequate daily dietary intake.

Mongolism. See *Down's syndrome.*

Monoamine oxidase (MAO). An enzyme, found mainly in nerve tissue and in the liver and lungs, that catalyzes the oxidative deamination of various amines, including epinephrine, norepinephrine, dopamine, and serotonin. Inhibition of MAO results in an increase in the concentration of these amines throughout the body. The increase in free serotonin and norepinephrine and/or alterations in the concentration of other amine neurotransmitters in the central nervous system are believed to have an antidepressant effect. Thus the *MAO inhibitor* drug is used in patients with neurotic or atypical depression. The drug may cause a hypertensive reaction, severe headache, tachycardia, and intracranial hemorrhage when taken with foods high in *tyramine* and caffeine. Brand names are Eutonyl, Marplan, Nardil, and Parnate. See also *Diet, tyramine-restricted.*

Monosaccharides. Group of carbohydrates that are simple sugars; composed of one sugar unit that cannot be hydrolyzed into smaller units. They are classified according to the number of carbon atoms they contain as triose, tetrose, pentose, and hexose (3, 4, 5, and 6 carbon atoms, respectively). Monosaccharides of nutritional importance are glucose, ribose, fructose, and galactose. See also Appendix 8.

Monosodium glutamate (MSG). Chemical used to enhance flavor in foods. It is used extensively in Asian cookery and is thought to cause the *Chinese restaurant syndrome.* This food additive is avoided in restricted sodium diet below 2 gm/day.

Morbidity. 1. Diseased or unhealthy condition. 2. Prevalence of a disease. *Morbidity rate* is expressed as the number of reported cases of a given disease present at a given time per 100,000 population.

MOSF. Abbreviation for *multiple organ systems failure.*

Motor neuron disease (Lou Gehrig's disease). A disorder indicating a malfunction in the transmission of nerve impulses by the nerve cells. It may be the result of injury to peripheral or upper neurons resulting in malfunctions in the nerve system, depending on the location of damage. *Dietary management:* assist the patient with self-feeding problems. Maintain weight and provide a nutritionally adequate diet in small, frequent feedings. Modify the consistency of foods as tolerated.

Mottled teeth. Also called "dental fluorosis"; condition of the teeth in which the enamel appears dull, rough, and chalky, with white patches separated by yellow or brown staining, giving the characteristic mottled appearance. In severe cases, pits and depressions may be present on the surface. All the teeth may be affected, but mottling is usually seen on the incisors of the upper jaw. The condition does not impair health. It is common in many parts of the world where the fluoride content of the water is high (3-5 ppm). However, it occurs only when high fluoride ingestion takes place during tooth development and ceases afterward. Other conditions (genetic and other nonnutritional factors) may also cause mottling.

Moxalactam. An antibiotic used in the treatment of infections of the abdominal, lower respiratory, and urinary tracts caused by susceptible organisms. It can cause bleeding due to vitamin K deficiency, especially in patients with liver disease. It may also cause a disulfiram-like reaction when taken with alcohol. The brand name is Moxam.

MPF. Abbreviation for *multipurpose food.*

MSUD. Abbreviation for *maple syrup urine disease.*

MSUD Diet Powder. A product formulated with an amino acid mixture free of branched-chain amino acids (BCAA) leucine, isoleucine, and valine, and containing corn syrup solids, modified tapioca starch, and corn oil. It is designed for the dietary management of maple syrup urine disease in infants and children, and may be helpful in other disorders of BCAA metabolism like hypervalinemia, leucine-induced hypoglycemia, and isovaleric acidemia.

Multiple organ systems failure (MOSF). A disorder of two or more organs, such as a combination of failures in the cardiac, respiratory, renal, or hepatic systems. *Dietary management:* provide close monitoring of blood levels of nutrients to ensure appropriate nutrition, particularly amino acids, glucose, and vitamins. Energy and protein needs generally parallel increases in metabolism and skeletal muscle breakdown. Evaluate the necessity for parenteral or tube feeding if oral intake is inadequate.

Multiple peripheral neuritis. See *Guillain-Barré syndrome.*

Multiple sclerosis. Central nervous system disorder of unknown etiology. It develops as an acute disease and runs intermittently, with exacerbations at weekly, monthly, or yearly intervals. There is destruction of the myelin sheaths of the brain and spinal cord. The symptoms are weakness, incoordination, strong jerky movements of the limbs, and slurred speech. *Dietary management:* dietary modification is highly individualized, depending on the severity of the neural damage. Tube feeding is given if the person cannot chew or swallow. Use oral feeding as long as the gastrointestinal tract is functional. Otherwise, parenteral nutrition may be needed.

Muscular dystrophy. Disorder of striated or skeletal muscles characterized by progressive atrophy, increased urinary creatinine excretion, increased oxygen consumption, and necrosis of muscle fibers leading to paralysis. It is rare in humans, and if it does occur, its onset is during childhood. Usually the child cannot close the lips, chew, or swallow easily. Lack of physical activity may lead to overweight. *Dietary management:* modify the consistency of foods if there is difficulty in chewing and swallowing. Encourage self-feeding with special devices. In serious cases of dysphagia, tube feeding of a prepared formula is recommended. Monitor body weight to avoid obesity. See also *Diet, dysphagia.*

Myasthenia gravis. Syndrome of fatigue and exhaustion of the muscular system without sensory disturbance or atrophy. It may affect any muscle of the body, but especially those of the face, lips, tongue, throat, and neck. It may be due to lack of acetylcholine. Other symptoms are fatigue, dysphagia, faint voice, and pneumonia. *Dietary management:* encourage feeding by mouth unless the dysphagia is severe. Allow plenty of time for feeding, with rest periods during the meal. Modify the consistency of the diet and use foods high in nutrient density. Lecithin and choline have been proven successful in certain patients, although more research is needed.

Myelin sheath. Whitish cylindrical covering of nerve fibers rich in lipids.

Myeloma. Cancer of the plasma cells which have invaded the bone marrow, resulting in abnormal immunoglobulin. The bones usually affected are the vertebrae, ribs, pelvic bone, and flat bones of the skull. Symptoms include nausea and vomiting, anorexia, weight loss, severe pain of the bones, susceptibility to infections, easy fatigability, fragility of bones, and a tendency to bleed. *Dietary management:* adjust the calorie level to correct weight loss. The main feeding challenge is to increase the patient's appetite, which is further decreased if the patient receives radiotherapy and steroid therapy. For further dietary guidelines, see *Cancer.*

Myelomeningocele. A congenital condition due to the failure of the neural tube to close during the development of the embryo. Symptoms usually include varying degrees of paralysis of the lower extremities, musculoskeletal defects, joint deformities, and hip dysplasia, which are all detectable at birth. *Dietary management:* maintain adequate nutrition and monitor fluid and electrolyte balance according to individual needs. Folate supplements during pregnancy may reduce the incidence of myelomeningocele in subsequent pregnancies.

Myocardial infarction (MI). Also called "coronary thrombosis" and commonly called "heart attack." It results in the death of part of the heart muscles. Acute MI causes permanent damage of a heart muscle, as in a thrombotic occlusion of a branch of an atherosclerotic coronary artery. It is accompanied by severe pain, shock, and cardiac dysfunction and may result in sudden death. *Dietary management:* on the first day, give caffeine-free and clear liquids; during the next few days, provide full liquid to semisolid foods in small, frequent feedings to avoid heart strain. Avoid gas formers. Depending on the patient's progress, introduce regular foods, following the *prudent* diet.

Myogen. Muscle protein present in the sarcoplasm and not within the muscle fibrils. It comprises about 20% of the total muscle protein.

Myoglobin. Hemoglobin of muscle. It is an iron-protein complex responsible for the color of muscle meat. Oxygen is stored temporarily as oxymyoglobin; that is, oxygen is loosely bound to the ferrous iron, giving a bright red color. *Metmyoglobin* is a brown pigment formed when ferrous iron is oxidized to the ferric state.

Myoinositol. The biologically active form of *inositol*. It is present in relatively large amounts in the cells of practically all animals and plants. See *Inositol.*

Myosin. A muscle protein found in the fibrils that constitutes about 65% of the total muscle proteins. It combines with actin to form *actomyosin,* which is responsible for the contractile and elastic properties of muscle.

Myristic acid. Saturated fatty acid containing 14 carbon atoms. It is found in nutmeg, butter, coconut oil, and spermaceti.

Myxedema. *Hypothyroidism* in adults. It is more prevalent in women than in men; usually insidious, with gradual retardation of physical and mental functions. The disorder is characterized by decreased basal metabolic rate, dry, thick skin, puffy face and eyelids, enlargement of the tongue, sparse dry hair, husky voice, and slurred speech. There is general mental deterioration and decreased reproductive activity. The symptoms may be completely reversed by suitable therapy with thyroid preparations.

N

Na. Chemical symbol for *sodium*.

NAD. Abbreviation for *nicotinamide adenine dinucleotide*.

NADP. Abbreviation for *nicotinamide adenine dinucleotide phosphate*.

Nasogastric (NG) tube. Tube that is inserted into the nose and passed through the esophagus and then the stomach. See *Tube feeding*.

National Academy of Sciences (NAS). A private, nonprofit organization of distinguished scholars engaged in scientific and engineering research for the furtherance of science and technology. It advises the federal government of the United States on scientific and technical matters. In 1916, NAS organized the *National Research Council (NRC)*.

National Center for Nutrition and Dietetics (NCND). The public education initiative of the American Dietetic Association (ADA) and its foundation. The purposes of the center include identifying and providing food and nutrition information to meet the needs of dietitians and consumers; working closely with librarians and at least 300 data bases to locate and obtain the needed information; and providing a hotline staffed by dietitians to answer consumers' calls about food and nutrition.

National Child Nutrition Project. Nonprofit, voluntary agency that works with individuals, state, and local groups to improve delivery of nutrition services. Initiates *Hunger Task Forces* to extend food assistance benefits to those in need, and supports food stamp outreach campaigns. It publishes *Food Action*.

National Cholesterol Education Program (NCEP). A nationwide program launched in 1985 by the National Heart, Lung and Blood Institute (NHLBI) to educate the American people about the relationship between cholesterol and health. The main goal for adults is to keep total serum cholesterol under 200 mg/dl and low-density-lipoprotein (LDL) cholesterol under 160 mg/dl, or below 130 mg/dl in persons with two or more risk factors such as obesity, hypertension, a family history of coronary heart disease, and diabetes.

National Dairy Council (NDC). Nonprofit research and educational organization supported by the dairy industry. Serves as a national resource agency in nutrition education, maintaining cooperative relations with government, professional, educational, and consumer group. Publishes the *Dairy Council Digest* bimonthly.

National Food Consumption Surveys (NFCS). The U.S. Department of Agriculture conducts nationwide food consumption surveys to evaluate the kinds and amounts of foods people are eating and to gather other related information on food consumption to guide in the development of food plans and policies. To cite one survey, the sixth NFCS, conducted in 1977-1978, included 8661 individuals from a statistical sample of households from 48 states. Dietary data from 24-hour recall and 2-day food records were analyzed for nutrient density for 14 nutrients, and these were related to factors such as income level, race, employment status, educational level of the head of the household, and geographic region. Alcohol consumption was also studied.

National Health and Nutrition Examination Survey (NHANES). A continuing national program to obtain information on the health and nutritional status of the American people. NHANES I, conducted from 1971 to 1974, included 28,043 persons sampled statistically from 48 states ranging in age from 1 to 74 years. Dietary data, biochemical tests, clinical examinations, and anthropometric measurements were evaluated. NHANES II was conducted from 1976 to 1980 in 50 states with a total of 27,801 persons surveyed, including 6-month-old infants. The methods used were the same as those for NHANES I, except that a special study was made on iron, zinc, and copper, and more information was collected about vitamin and mineral supplements. The Hispanic Health and Nutrition Examination Survey (HHANES), conducted from 1982 to 1984, included about 16,000 Hispanics in the United States, using the same methods of study as NHANES II. To date, NHANES III is in progress. Results from NHANES surveys are reported in several journals.

National Institutes of Health (NIH). Research unit of the Public Health Service in the U.S. Department of Health and Human Services engaged in clinical research on diseases of public health importance. The NIH supports research and training programs in nutrition related to health maintenance, disease prevention and treatment, and human development throughout the life cycle.

National Nutrition Consortium, Inc. An organization composed of professional societies in the fields of nutrition, food, and dietetics. Provides leadership in the development and coordination of food and nutrition policies at national and local levels. Publications include materials on nutrition labeling and interpretation of complicated nutrition information for public understanding.

National Nutrition Monitoring System (NNMS). Set of activities to provide the scientific foundation for the maintenance and improvement of the nutritional status of the population and the nutritional quality and healthfulness of the national food supply in the United States. The objectives of the NNMS are to ensure the adequacy of nutrients for all Americans, ensure the safety and quality of the food supply, develop a better data base for decisions on national nutrition policies, and guide appropriations

for nutrition and health. The NNMS coordinates the data of the *National Health and Nutrition Examination Survey (NHANES)* and the *National Food Consumption Surveys (NFCS),* especially on the following components: nutritional surveillance, food production and marketing, food consumption and nutritional status surveys, dissemination of nutrition information, and development of methods for these components or activities.

National Research Council (NRC). Organized in 1916 by the National Academy of Sciences (NAS), it engages in research and advises the federal government on scientific and technical matters. The NRC functions in accordance with general policies determined by the NAS and is currently the main operating agency for the NAS in providing services to the government, the public, and the professional communities. The 10th edition of the Recommended Dietary Allowances (RDA: see Appendix 1) was a project approved by the NRC's governing board, whose members were drawn from the councils of the National Academy of Sciences, the National Academy of Engineering, and the Institute of Medicine. The 10th edition of RDA was mainly the work of the *Food and Nutrition Board (FNB).*

National School Lunch Program (NSLP). See *School Lunch Program.*

National Science Foundation (NSF). This foundation was established in 1950 to improve scientific research and education in the United States. Grants are awarded to universities and other nonprofit institutions to support research. The foundation also maintains a register of scientific personnel.

NE. Abbreviation for *niacin equivalent.*

Necrotizing enterocolitis (NEC). Infection of the intestinal tract mucosa by enteric pathogens, characterized by respiratory distress syndrome, vomiting, distended abdomen, diarrhea and sepsis. *Dietary management:* initially, give nothing by mouth; use parenteral feeding only. As the patient's condition improves, a progressive liquid diet is given, later advancing to semisolid foods that are easy to digest and given in small, frequent feedings. Protein intake should be about 1.5 times the recommended dietary allowance. Commercial protein hydrolysates supplemented by vitamins and minerals, especially iron and zinc, speed recovery.

NEFA. Abbreviation for *nonesterified fatty acid.* See under *Fatty acid.*

Neonate. A newborn infant. See *Nutrition, neonatology.*

Neopham. Brand name of a 6.4% solution of essential and nonessential amino acids for intravenous infusion in total parenteral nutrition.

NephrAmine. Brand name of a 5.4% solution of essential amino acids plus histidine for parenteral nutrition of patients with renal failure. It is designed to be infused with a concentrated source of calories. See also Appendix 39.

Nephritis. Also called "Bright's disease"; inflammation of the kidney; a diffuse, progressive, degenerative or proliferative lesion affecting the renal parenchyma, the interstitial tissue, and the renal vascular system. The disease is called *glomerulonephritis* if the inflammation is primarily of the glomeruli. It is called *pyelonephritis* if it is caused by bacterial invasion from the urinary tract. Nephritis may follow such diseases as scarlet fever, tonsillitis, and influenza. *Dietary management:* the basic dietary objective is to reduce the work of the kidneys by minimizing the rate of excretion of waste products, especially urea and salts. The diet also aims to prevent edema, uremia, and electrolyte imbalance, especially of sodium, potassium, and chloride. For further details of dietary modifications, see *Glomerulonephritis.*

Nephrolithiasis. Formation of stones in the kidney or the disease condition that leads to their formation. Kidney stones are of various types, shapes, and sizes. Causes include chronic infection of the kidney, stagnation of the urine, prolonged confinement in bed, dietary factors (e.g., excessive oxalates, urates, calcium or magnesium trisilicate), and certain congenital biochem-

ical abnormalities. A hot climate may contribute to the formation of kidney stones. See also *Diet, ash.*

Nephrosclerosis. Also called "arteriosclerotic Bright's disease"; hardening of the renal arteries seen in renal hypertension and often associated with arteriosclerosis. As a rule, it occurs in adults after 35 years of age and may be benign for many years. Characterized by albuminuria and nitrogen retention, retinal changes, fibrosis of the glomeruli, degeneration of the renal tubules, and, ultimately, renal insufficiency. Death usually results from circulatory failure. *Dietary management:* protein intake of 1 gm/kg/day should consist of good-quality proteins to replace losses, especially albumin. Sodium is restricted to 2 gm/day to reduce edema and help control hypertension. Fluid restriction is recommended in renal failure. Cholesterol and fat should be monitored as necessary. Weight reduction is recommended for the obese to lessen the work of the circulatory system. Vitamin and mineral losses should be replaced.

Nephrosis. Also called "nephrotic syndrome" or "degenerative Bright's disease"; degeneration or disintegration of the kidney without signs of inflammation. The primary lesion occurs in the capillary basement membrane of the glomerulus, causing the loss of proteins into the urine. The main symptoms are massive edema, marked proteinuria, decreased serum albumin, and oliguria. *Lipoid nephrosis* is a rare chronic condition frequently seen in children and characterized clinically by proteinuria, edema, and hypercholesterolemia. *Dietary management:* modifications of the diet aim to correct proteinuria, edema, and hypercholesterolemia. Therefore, a moderately high protein intake characterizes the diet. As much as 30 gm protein may be lost in the urine daily, which can be replaced by allowing a protein intake of at least 1.2 gm/kg/day, emphasizing protein foods of high biologic value. Caloric intake should be high to ensure efficient utilization of protein, allowing 50 kcal/kg/day. Sodium is restricted to 1 gm/day in the presence of edema. A more severe sodium restriction would present problems in planning a diet high in animal protein foods, especially if the patient does not like low-sodium milk. Supplemental iron and vitamins are beneficial.

Net protein utilization (NPU). Proportion of the nitrogen intake that is retained in the body. It is calculated by multiplying the biologic value of a protein by its digestibility factor.

Neuritis. Inflammation of a nerve or nerves; usually associated with pain, anesthesia or paresthesia, paralysis, muscle degeneration, and loss of reflexes. Symptoms vary according to the cause, the location, and the nerves involved. See also *Polyneuritis.*

Newtrition. Brand name of a line of lactose-free formulas for tube feeding; available as Newtrition Half Strength, One and a Half, Isotonic, High Nitrogen, and Isofiber (with 14 gm/liter soy fiber). See also Appendix 39.

NHANES. Abbreviation for *National Health and Nutrition Examination Survey.*

Ni. Chemical symbol for nickel.

Niacin. Generic name for pyridine-3-carboxylic acid (nicotinic acid) and its corresponding amide (nicotinamide or niacinamide); a member of the B complex water-soluble vitamins. The term "niacin" was originally proposed to avoid association of the vitamin with nicotine of tobacco. Nicotinamide is a constituent of two coenzymes, nicotinamide adenine dinucleotide (NAD) and nicotinamide adenine dinucleotide phosphate (NADP), which act as hydrogen and electron acceptors and donors, respectively, and which function in the metabolism of carbohydrate, fat, and protein, rhodopsin synthesis, and cellular respiration. Niacin also has two pharmacologic actions at high dosage: peripheral vasodilation (mainly nicotinic acid) and serum cholesterol reduction. Niacin deficiency may be one of the features of a general nutritional deficiency. A multiple deficiency syndrome, called *pellagra,* is seen in maize-eating areas in association with diets providing low levels of niacin equivalents. The characteristic symptoms are dermatitis, diarrhea, inflammation of the mucous membranes, and dementia in severe cases. Niacin is found in most animal and plant foods, but often in a form that is unavailable. Good food sources are meats, fish, poultry, liver, and enriched cereals. Another source of niacin is by biosynthesis from the amino acid tryptophan; 1 mg niacin is formed from 60 mg tryptophan. This conversion requires *pyridoxal phosphate*-dependent enzymes and hence adequate dietary intake of pyridoxine, or *vitamin B₆*. Ingestion of large doses of nicotinic acid, but not of the amide, may produce a transient sensation of burning, flushing, and tingling or stinging of the skin; long-term use may cause xerostomia, activation of peptic ulcer, blurred vision, hyperglycemia, jaundice, and liver damage. See Appendix 1 for the recommended dietary allowances.

Niacinamide. Also called "nicotinamide"; the amide form of nicotinic acid. See *Niacin.*

Niacin equivalent (NE). Sum of the two forms in which niacin is made available to the body, as the preformed niacin and that derived from tryptophan (60 mg tryptophan = 1 mg niacin).

Nickel (Ni). A trace element essential to several animals which is probably also required by humans. Its precise biologic role has not been clearly defined, although recent findings indicate that nickel functions as a cofactor or structural component in specific enzymes involved in intermediary metabolism. Nickel deficiency in animals results in depressed growth and hematopoiesis, and in changes in the levels of iron, copper, and zinc in the liver. Nickel interacts directly or indirectly with at least 13 essential minerals. Of the dietary interactions, the one with iron is perhaps the most significant; nickel affects the absorption and metabolism of iron. In humans, about 10 mg of nickel is present in the body, with the largest proportions in the skin and bone marrow. Liver and muscle concentrations appear to be most responsive to the level of dietary intake, which is about 0.3 to 0.6 mg/day, mainly from plant foods. Rich food sources are nuts, dried beans and peas, chocolate, and grains. Average absorption is about 3% and is enhanced during pregnancy and with high intake. Nickel is a cause of allergic contact dermatitis. Toxicity through oral intake is unlikely, although chronic exposure and inhalation of substantial quantities in animal studies resulted in degeneration of heart muscle, brain, lung, liver, and kidney.

Nicotinic acid. Pyridine-3-carboxylic acid, a member of the B complex vitamins. See *Niacin.*

Night blindness. Also called "nyctalopia"; a condition of defective or reduced vision in the dark, especially after coming from bright light. When temporary, it may be due to vitamin A deficiency, and it responds to suitable vitamin supplementation. Night blindness occurs when there is insufficient vitamin A to bring about prompt and complete regeneration of the *visual purple.* Night blindness not responsive to vitamin A supplements may be due to diseases of the retina and other factors not related to vitamin A. See also *Dark adaptation.*

NIH. Abbreviation for *National Institutes of Health.*

Nitrofurantoin. An antimicrobial used for prevention and treatment of infections in the urinary tract. It may decrease serum folate and cause megaloblastic anemia; it may also cause peripheral neuritis, anorexia, and abdominal cramps. It may be present in breast milk. Brand names include Furadantoin, Furantoin, Furalan, Macrodantin, and Nitrex.

Nitrogen (N). A chemical element essential to life; found free in the air and in combinations of proteins and other organic compounds. Plants can use nitrogen from the soil, and nitrogen-fixing bacteria can use free nitrogen from the air. Animals and humans, however, can utilize nitrogen only when it is supplied from foods. It is an important constituent of all animal and plant tissues and a unique element in *proteins.* See also *Amino acid.*

Nitrogen balance. Measurement of the state of nitrogen equilibrium in the body. An organism is said to be in nitrogen balance or equilibrium when the nitrogen intake (from food eaten) equals the nitrogen output (in urine, feces, and perspiration). A *positive nitrogen balance* exists when nitrogen intake is above output. This can be brought about by growth, pregnancy, lactation when the mother is storing protein as milk, or recovery from illness or trauma. A *negative nitrogen balance* exists when intake is below output, as in fasting, fever, surgery, burns, or shock following an accident. A negative nitrogen balance is undesirable because body protein is being broken down more rapidly than it is being built up. A method of determining nitrogen balance is as follows:

Nitrogen balance

$$= \left(\frac{\text{protein intake}}{6.25}\right) - (\text{UUN}+4)$$

where protein intake (gm) is calculated from a 24-hour food record and urinary urea nitrogen (UUN), also in grams, is analyzed from a 24-hour urine specimen of the same period. The factor 4 is additional nitrogen lost from the feces and skin. To be assured of a positive nitrogen balance, a three-day average value of more than 0.04 gm of nitrogen/kg body weight/day is desirable.

Nonesterified fatty acid (NEFA). Also called "free fatty acid." See under *Fatty acid.*

Nonprotein nitrogen (NPN). The total nitrogen of the blood, excluding that from protein. This may come from urea, uric acid, creatine, creatinine, etc.

Norepinephrine. Also called "noradrenaline." A catecholamine hormone secreted by the *adrenal medulla.* It is a demethylated epinephrine synthesized from tyrosine and liberated at the ends of sympathetic nerve fibers after stimulation. It causes an increase in blood pressure by increasing peripheral resistance, with little effect on cardiac output. Unlike epinephrine, it has little effect on carbohydrate metabolism and oxygen consumption. See also *Epinephrine.*

Norleucine. An amino acid, alpha-amino-*n*-caproic acid.

Nortriptyline. A tricyclic antidepressant used for the relief of emotional depression. It has a peculiar taste and may cause dry mouth, irritation of the tongue and mouth, fluctuation of blood sugar levels, and constipation. It may be present in breast milk. Brand names are Aventyl and Pamelor.

Novamine. Brand name of an amino acid solution for intravenous administration in total parenteral nutrition by peripheral vein or central infusion. Contains both essential and nonessential amino acids and is available in 8.5%, 11.4%, and 15% concentrations. See also Appendix 40.

NPN. Abbreviation for *nonprotein nitrogen.*

NPU. Abbreviation for *net protein utilization.*

NRC. Abbreviation for *National Research Council.*

NSF. Abbreviation for *National Science Foundation.*

NSLP. Abbreviation for National School Lunch Program.

Nucleic acid. A highly complex portion of nucleoproteins that yields a mixture of purines and pyrimidines, a ribose or deoxyribose component, and phosphoric acid on complete hydrolysis. The two general types of nucleic acid are *ribonucleic acid (RNA)* and *deoxyribonucleic acid (DNA).*

Nucleotide. Phosphate ester of the nucleoside. Examples are adenylic acid, guanylic acid, and cytidylic acid. Nucleotides of importance in metabolism are the adenosine phosphates adenosine diphosphate and adenosine triphosphate. See *Adenosine phosphates.*

Nursoy. Brand name of a hypoallergenic formula for infants sensitive to milk and lactose; contains soy protein isolate, sucrose, tapioca, dextrose, oleo, coconut oil, and soy oil. See also Appendix 37.

Nutramigen. Brand name of a hypoallergenic formula for infants sensitive to intact protein, cow's milk, and/or lactose; contains a high percentage of free amino acids. The remainder of the protein is in the peptide form.

Made with casein hydrolysate, sucrose, modified cornstarch, and corn oil. See also Appendix 37.

Nutren. Brand name of a lactose-free nutritional supplement; made with casein, maltodextrin, corn syrup, sucrose, MCT oil, and corn. Available in concentrations providing 1.0, 1.5, and 2.0 kcal/ml. See Appendix 39.

Nutri-1000. Brand name of a high-fat nutritional supplement for oral or tube feeding; made with skim milk, sucrose, corn oil, and coconut oil. See also Appendix 39.

Nutrient. Any chemical substance needed by the body for one or more of the following functions: to provide heat or energy, to build and repair tissues, and to regulate life processes. Although nutrients are found chiefly in foods, some can be synthesized in the laboratory (e.g., vitamins) or in the body (biosynthesis). See also *Nutrition.*

Nutrient classifications. Nutrients are classified according to the amount present in the body, chemical composition, essentiality, and function:

   Amount present in the body. See *Macronutrients* and *Micronutrients.*

   Chemical composition. The two categories are *inorganic* (water and minerals) and *organic* (carbohydrate, protein, fat, and vitamins). These six major groups of nutrients are composed of individual nutrients as listed on page 164.

   Essentiality. All nutrients, by definition, are *physiologically essential;* a nutrient that performs one function is as *important* as another nutrient that performs three functions. The term "nonessential nutrient" is misleading and should be revised to "nondietary essential." For further details and examples, see *Amino acid, Dietary requirement, Fatty acid, Recommended dietary allowances,* and Appendix 1.

   Function. Nutrients are grouped according to three general functions: *source of energy* (carbohydrate, protein, and fat); *growth and repair of tissues* (protein, minerals, vitamins, and water); and *regulation of life processes* (protein, minerals, vitamins, and water).

CARBOHYDRATE	MINERALS	VITAMINS
Glucose	*Major Minerals*	*Fat-soluble Vitamins*
	Calcium	A
FAT	Chloride	D
Linoleic acid	Magnesium	E
α-Linolenic acid	Phosphorus	K
	Potassium	
PROTEIN	Sodium	*Water-soluble Vitamins*
Essential Amino Acids	Sulfur	Ascorbic acid
Histidine		Biotin
Isoleucine	*Trace Minerals*	Cobalamin
Leucine	Arsenic	Folacin
Lysine	Boron	Niacin
Methionine	Chromium	Panthothenic acid
Phenylalanine	Cobalt	Riboflavin
Threonine	Copper	Thiamin
Tryptophan	Fluoride	Vitamin B_6
Valine	Iodine	Vitamin B_{12}
	Iron	
Nonessential Amino Acids	Manganese	**WATER**
Alanine	Molybdenum	
Asparagine	Nickel	
Aspartic acid	Selenium	
Cysteine	Silicon	
Cystine	Tin	
Glutamic acid	Vanadium	
Glycine	Zinc	
Hydroxylysine		
Hydroxyproline		
Proline		
Serine		
Tyrosine		

Nutrient interrelationships. Cellular metabolism is an integrated, coordinated chain of reactions, and interference with any reaction affects the whole system, which includes all nutrients. The close interrelationship of the six major groups of nutrients is best summarized as follows: Protein, fat, and carbohydrate metabolites enter a common pathway to yield energy with the help of enzyme systems containing vitamins and minerals as cofactors. Water is the circulating medium for all reactions. Specific interrelationships can exist between two nutrients, such as iron-copper, calcium-phosphorus, cobalamin-cobalt, water-sodium, and folic acid-vitamin C. Specific interrelationships also exist among several nutrients, such as calcium-phosphorus-magnesium-vitamin D, cobalt-iron-zinc, and niacin-tryptophan-pyridoxine. One recent example is the involvement of manganese, zinc, and copper in preventing peroxidation or breaking up of polyunsaturated fatty acids. See also Appendix 15.

Nutrient stores. Nutrient stores or reserves in the body affect the pathogenesis of deficiency diseases. The capacity to store and the duration before nutrient stores are depleted vary with each nutrient. The body cannot store amino acids for more than a few hours, but it can store minerals in the bones for a few years. Calcium reserves last as long as 7 years. Water loss after 4 days is critical. Iron stores for menstruating women are depleted in 3 months, compared to 2 years for men. Thiamin reserves are depleted faster than those of the other B vitamins, i.e., 2 months and 5 months, respectively. More studies are needed to confirm the length of time needed to deplete nutrient stores in the body.

Nutrisource. Brand name of a line of modular products, in liquid or powder form, for oral and enteral use. Intended as an additional source of carbohydrate, amino acids, medium-chain triglycerides, or long-chain triglycerides. See Appendix 39.

Nutrition. Simply stated, the study of food in relation to health. As defined by the Food and Nutrition Council (of the American Medical Association), nutrition is the "science of food, the nutrients and other substances therein, their action, interaction and balance in relation to health and disease, and the processes by which the organism ingests, digests, absorbs, transports, utilizes and excretes food substances." Nutrition deals with the physiologic needs of the body in terms of specific nutrients, the means of supplying these nutrients through adequate diets, and the effects of failure to meet nutrient needs. In addition, nutrition is concerned with the social, economic, cultural, and psychological implications of food and eating. The basic concepts in nutrition may be summarized as follows: (1) Adequate nutrition is essential for health. (2) A number of compounds and elements broadly classed as protein, fat, carbohydrate, minerals, vitamins, and water are needed daily in the food of humans. (3) An adequate diet is the foundation of good nutrition, and it should consist of a wide variety of natural foods. (4) Many nutrients should be provided preformed in food, while a few may be synthesized within the body. (5) Nutrients are interrelated, and there must be metabolic balance in the body. (6) Body constituents are in a dynamic state of equilibrium. (7) Human requirements for certain nutrients are known quantitatively within certain limits. The search for quantitative determination for the others has been going on for over a century. (8) The effects of nutritional inadequacy are more than physical; behavioral patterns and mental performance are also affected. (9) The nutritional status of populations and individuals can be measured for certain nutrients. However, for other nutrients, techniques of assessment (dietary, clinical, and biochemical) have yet to be refined. (10) Proper education, technical expertise, and the use of all resources in applied nutrition and food technology will help upgrade the nutritional status of people. (11) The biologic meaning of food is attributable to the three functions of nutrients. To an individual or family, food is eaten for more than its physiologic, social, and aesthetic values. (12) The study of nutrition as a subject or course has a broad scope and is interrelated with many allied fields, such as physiology, biochemistry, food technology, dietetics, public health, behavioral sciences (sociology, anthropology, and psychology), and many branches of medicine (anatomy, preventive medicine, pediatrics, etc.). For nutrition objectives for the next decade, see *Healthy People 2000.*

Nutrition, adolescence. The adolescent period is characterized by an accelerated growth rate and intense activity with physical, social, emotional, and mental changes. It is a transition period between childhood and adulthood; girls mature earlier than boys. The nutritional needs of adolescents are unique, conditioned primarily by the building of new body tissues, the demands of increased physical activity, and to some extent the emotional changes attending maturation. In general, the growing adolescent requires a high caloric intake, an abundance of good-quality protein, and a liberal intake of minerals and vitamins. Because of the onset of menstruation, adolescent girls have specific nutrient needs, especially for iron, protein, and other nutrients essential for blood formation. Nutrition education is focused on the eating habits of adolescents because of the following problems that affect nutrient intake: (1) irregularity of meals and skipping breakfast; (2) poor choice of snack items, with a tendency to eat foods with empty calories or junk foods such as cakes, cookies, and soft drinks; and (3) anxiety about figure development, which causes some girls not to eat enough. Anorexia nervosa and bulimia may occur in this group. For recommended dietary allowances, see Appendix 1.

Nutrition, adulthood. Adulthood is the period of life when one has attained full growth and maturation. The onset of this stage varies among individuals, and there are no clear-cut age boundaries. However, in relation to dietary needs, adulthood pertains to the years between ages 25 and 50 without stresses such as pregnancy, lactation, and convalescence. Proper nutrition needs emphasis in adulthood, since it is the longest period of the life cycle and possibly the years of peak productivity. Ideally, one should reach adulthood with broad familiarity with and acceptance of different foods, as well as sound food habits. Adults tend to resist changes in their food habits, hence the importance of proper training both in food selection and in regularity of eating as early in life as possible. Another aim of good nutrition throughout adulthood is the maintenance of a healthy body weight. It is recommended that the daily caloric allowances be reduced with increasing age. See *Nutrition, aging process,* and *Nutrition, geriatric.* See also Appendix 1.

Nutrition, aging process. Theoretically, aging is a continuous process from conception until death. However, in the young growing organism, the building-up processes exceed the breaking-down processes, so that the net result is a picture of growth and development. Once the body reaches adulthood, the process is reversed. Although the rate of degenerative changes is slow during middle adulthood, it increases as the individual approaches the geriatric age. See *Nutrition, geriatric.*

Nutrition, alcoholism. Chronic alcoholism is a complex condition involving psychological, social, and physiologic factors. Excessive intake of alcohol is a prominent contributor to and causative factor in cirrhosis of the liver, one of the 10 leading causes of death in the United States. An alcoholic usually has faulty eating habits and an inadequate diet, consuming as much as 50 to 60% of the total caloric intake from ethanol. *Cirrhosis of the liver* in chronic alcoholism is caused mainly by dietary deficiencies, particularly thiamin and other B complex vitamins and protein. The metabolic explanation for vitamin B-induced deficiencies is based in part on the involvement of the B complex vitamins in enzyme systems needed to oxidize alcohol (1 gm alcohol yields 7 kcal), which takes place in the liver. Excess alcohol has toxic effects on the central nervous system (e.g., alcoholic dementia and Korsakoff's psychosis), heart, kidneys, and other organs of metabolism. Nutritional inadequacy is sometimes aggravated by chronic gastritis resulting from habitual drinking. See also *alcohol, Fetal alcohol syndrome,* and *Wernicke-Korsakoff syndrome.*

Nutrition, anemias. Nutritional anemias probably constitute the most common nutritional diseases in humans. This statement is not difficult to believe because of the many etiologic factors that lead to anemia. Nearly all nutrients are involved directly or indirectly. *Protein* is needed for the globin portion of hemoglobin (Hb); *iron* is an integral part of heme; *copper* catalyzes the utilization of iron both in the intestinal tract and at the tissue level; *pyridoxine* helps in the formation of the pyrrole ring of Hb; *riboflavin* is important in protein synthesis; *ascorbic acid* increases the absorption of iron by keeping it in its ferrous state and catalyzes the conversion of folic acid to folinic acid; and *cobalamin* and *folinic acid* are needed for normal maturation of red blood cells and in the synthesis of methyl groups needed for heme structure. Because of their interrelationships, other nutrients are indirectly involved. See also *Anemia* and *Hemopoiesis.*

Nutrition, antibiotics. The increasing use of antibiotics necessitates a review of how nutrition is affected by this special group of drugs. There are several mechanisms or modes of action to explain their nutritional influence. Many antibiotics have direct effects on the gastrointestinal tract (e.g., nausea, anorexia, glossitis, stomatitis, and diarrhea). Certain antibiotics bind some nutrients (e.g., tetracycline binds protein, and penicillin and sulfonamides bind serum albumin). Other antibiotics increase the volume and/or frequency of stools. In general, antibiotics alter microflora and inhibit bacterial synthesis of certain vitamins. See also *Nutrition, drug-nutrient interactions.*

Nutrition, bone. Bone is a metabolically active tissue, constantly turning over through resorption or breakdown of bone cells and formation of osteoblasts or bone mineralization. These processes are necessary for the reshaping and repositioning of bones to bear the changing weight shifts of the body. Bone formation starts with fetal development. Rapid bone growth and calcification occur up to adolescence. Peak bone mass is attained in the early twenties, at age 23 on the average. Bone is made up of an organic matrix that contains the protein collagen, which acts as the supporting material for mineral crystals. The process of depositing calcium and phosphorus in the form of hydroxyapatite is called "calcification" or "ossification." The bone shaft, which is the rigid part, also contains sodium, zinc, fluoride, and carbonates. The nutritional implications of bone formation are focused not only on protein and mineral needs, but also on other nutrients, like vitamins C and D, and on the proper ratio of calcium to phosphorus (about 1:1) for the growing years. See *Nutrition, dental health* and *Nutrition, growth and development.* See also *Osteoporosis.*

Nutrition, cancer. To date, cancer is the second leading cause of death in the United States. Present knowledge about the relationship of nutrition and cancer is not conclusive for two main reasons: (1) the causative factors of malignant tumors are numerous and often undetermined, and (2) the carcinogenic stimulus affects the organism in varying degrees, depending on factors such as the amount or dose of the stimulus, the period of exposure, and the susceptibility of the individual. The observation that cancers of the stomach and liver are the most prevalent types is of interest, since these organs are directly involved in nutrient utilization. In addition, certain substances found in foods are carcinogenic. Among these are the aflatoxin of moldy peanuts, cycasin in cycad meal, polyphenols in tea, excess selenium in the diet, and a toxic substance developed in overheated fats. The question of limiting or increasing a certain nutrient or specific nutrients in the diet of patients with cancer is not yet resolved. However, some trends in humans need further study; for example, a diet excessively high in phosphates may stimulate nucleic acid synthesis, as well as malignant growth of tumors; restriction of essential amino acids (e.g., phenylalanine) may inhibit the cancerous growth of cells; a diet low in pyridoxine may be beneficial, since pyridoxine tends to stimulate malignant growth; antioxidants like vitamins C and E can protect DNA, which is the genetic "coder" of a cell; cruciferous vegetables have a role as cancer inhibitors; and the excessive intake of certain food additives and nonnutritive sweeteners may promote or cause cancer. Dietary fiber bind carcinogens in the feces. Dietary fat should be limited to 20–30% of total caloric intake per day to reduce the risk of breast cancer. Maintenance of desirable body weight is emphasized because some forms of cancer are linked to obesity and lack of physical activity.

Nutrition, chemical dependency. Chemical dependency is a disorder resulting in biologic, psychological, and social problems due to addiction to alcohol and drugs like cocaine, heroin, marijuana, morphine, and nicotine. The effects of alcoholism have been well studied; although little research has been done on the other addictive drugs, there is no doubt about the need for nutritional intervention because most drug users have impaired food habits. Besides the primary factor of malnutrition (i.e., inadequate food ingestion), the conditioning factors of malnutrition observed with chemical dependency include digestive malfunctions, malabsorption, increased nutrient requirements to metabolize the drug, poor utilization due to inactivated enzymes, and impaired nutrient storage. The nutritional care of drug addicts undergoing treatment include: an evaluation of the addict's nutritional status; supervision of nutritional rehabilitation through delivery of palatable, nourishing meals and supplements; monitoring of body weight; monitoring of gastrointestinal problems (e.g., anorexia, nausea, vomiting, diarrhea), especially during the initial phase of detoxification; and provision of nutrition counseling. Dietary guidelines for a recovery diet are as follows: eat balanced meals at regular times with nourishing snacks between meals; avoid all drugs including caffeine in coffee, tea, colas, and chocolate; avoid alcoholic beverages; eat more complex carbohydrates and reduce intake of concentrated sweets; and ensure a liberal supply of good quality protein foods. Improved nutritional status certainly speeds up treatment and rehabilitation. Nutrition counseling does not stop at the discharge of patients, but should be continued by providing an aftercare plan which involves not only the dietitian, but also the other members of the rehabilitation team, with a physician or psychiatrist as the leader of the team. The ultimate goals are to prevent relapse and to rehabilitate the patient to a long-range stable, healthy lifestyle.

Nutrition, childhood. Childhood is the period of life between infancy and puberty, generally from ages 1 to 12 years. Nutritional needs during this period cannot be generalized because of the following factors: spurts of growth occur, and growth patterns among children vary; the kind and size of food servings should be adjusted with age, development, and appetite; and outside influences such as school activities and play affect eating habits; and so on. Thus nutritional needs for specific ages from 1 to 12 years are considered separately. See *Nutrition, preschool age; Nutrition, schoolchildren;* and *Nutrition, toddler.*

Nutrition, dental health. The time intervals involved in the development of *teeth* are important considerations in any discussion of the relationship of nutrition to tooth development. The life history of a tooth may be divided into three main eras: the period during which the crown of the tooth is forming and calcifying in the jaw; the period of maturation when the tooth is erupting into the oral cavity and its root or roots are forming; and the maintenance period when it is in full function in the oral

cavity. Prenatal factors affect *deciduous teeth* (baby teeth) far more than factors after birth. At the early stage of the 6th fetal week, the tooth buds start to form; calcification begins on the 16th week. Eruption of baby teeth starts at around the age of 7 months; the last baby molar comes out at the age of 2 years. Calcification of the permanent teeth starts soon after birth, and eruption of the first permanent tooth occurs at about 6 years of age, when the child is starting to lose baby teeth. Hence, an adequate diet is imperative as early as the first trimester of pregnancy. All nutrients, directly or indirectly, play an important role in dental development, as does the maintenance of dental health. The nutrients directly involved are *protein,* for organic matrix formation; *calcium, phosphorus, magnesium,* and *vitamin D* for deposition of the mineral compound *apatite* into the matrix structure; *ascorbic acid,* involved in mineral utilization and for cementum formation to connect the tooth to the bone structure and to the gum tissues; *vitamin A* for the proper functioning of enamel-forming cells to achieve a smooth, even enamel as well as a deposit of sound dentin; and *fluorine* to harden the enamel and prevent dental caries. Although nutrition influences dental health profoundly, nonnutritional factors are also important, such as oral hygiene, regular visits to the dentists, and fluoridation of the community water supply.

Nutrition, dermatology. The *skin* is a tough but resilient covering of the body with protective, regulatory, excretory, and sensory functions. The first layer (epidermis) is the site of keratin and vitamin D synthesis; the second layer (dermis), which is rich in blood vessels, nerves, and sweat and sebaceous glands, is a storehouse for water, blood, and electrolytes. The innermost layer (subcutaneous tissue) is a storehouse for body fats and helps to support the body. Protein deficiency results in dryness, scaliness, pallid appearance, and inelasticity of the skin, often with brownish pigmentation on the face. In kwashiorkor there is extensive hypopigmentation and dryness of the skin and hair, with the characteristic "flag sign" of the hair. Lack of *essential fatty acids* results in eczematous skin lesions that are probably related to the seborrheic dermatitis of *pyridoxine* deficiency. The skin changes caused by lack of *vitamin A* include desquamation of epithelial cells, keratinization, and dry, rough gooseflesh with follicular hyperkeratosis. On the other hand, excessive carotene (provitamin A) results in jaundice-like yellow discoloration of the skin. In *riboflavin* deficiency, dermatitis is of the seborrheic type, with fine oily scales, especially around the nose and lips. Symmetric dermatitis, (i.e., dark red eruptions and desquamation appearing bilaterally) is characteristic of pellagra (*nicotinic acid* deficiency). Dry, "crackled," and scaly dermatitis is observed in *biotin* deficiency. *Ascorbic acid* deficiency results in inelastic skin with a tendency to petechial hemorrhages.

Nutrition, diet therapy. Also called "therapeutic nutrition" or "nutritional therapy." In the dietary management of diseases (diet therapy), the prescribed diet has certain nutritional effects, depending on the type of therapeutic diet and the length of time it is used. For example, the clear liquid diet is nutritionally inadequate; sodium-restricted diets reduce the palatability of food; fat-restricted diets decrease absorption of fat-soluble vitamins; a high polyunsaturated fatty acid diet tends to lower serum cholesterol; a high protein intake increases the requirement for riboflavin and pyridoxine; a high-carbohydrate diet tends to elevate serum triglycerides and to increase the thiamin requirement; and prolonged sodium restriction, especially at the 200-mg level, leads to the *low-sodium syndrome*. For further details, see *Diet* and *Diet therapy*.

Nutrition, diseases. The nutritional effects of diseases are collectively considered as secondary factors or "conditioning factors" of nutritional inadequacy. In general, a diseased condition leads to anorexia. Bed rest increases calcium and nitrogen excretion; diarrheal diseases increase motility of the intestines, and the frequent bowel movements obviously cause reduced nutrient intake, maldigestion, and malabsorption. Many diseases, particularly gastrointestinal disorders, are characterized by nausea and vomiting, affecting electrolyte and water balance. Renal diseases increase the loss of nitrogen. For other examples of the nutritional effects of diseases, see the discussion under each disease. Medical treatment of diseases usually involves the use of drugs, which affect nutrition in many ways. See *Nutrition, drug-nutrient interactions.*

Nutrition, drug-nutrient interactions. The trends in modern chemotherapy are of interest because of the effects of certain drugs on nutrient availability or utilization. To cite the most common examples, antacids destroy thiamin; appetite depressants such as amphetamines may irritate the gastric mucosa and cause nausea and vomiting; mineral oil decreases absorption of fat-soluble vitamins; chelating agents bind many minerals and reduce their availability; cation-exchange resins also reduce available sodium, potassium, and calcium; antimetabolites for cancer therapy antagonize the physiologic role of some vitamins; barbiturates have antivitamin action against folic acid; and corticosteroids alter electrolyte, carbohydrate, and fat metabolism. This dictionary contains the names of 120 drugs, entered alphabetically, and discusses the nutritional implications of each drug. See also *Nutritional deficiency* and *Nutrition, antibiotics.*

Nutrition, emergency feeding. Refers to the provision of meals to persons suddenly deprived of food as a result of either artificial or natural catastrophes such as famines, floods, industrial accidents, fires, and wars. In emergency feeding, the long-range objective is to sustain adequate nourishment until the victims return to their normal pattern of life. The immediate aim, however, is to provide water and warm food to maintain body temperature and to give nourishment as soon as possible. Less emphasis is placed on dietary adequacy, especially when the emergency is brief. Distribution of food should be orderly, and the feeding program should include the rescue workers. Special attention should be given to vulnerable groups such as infants, children, pregnant women, and those under pathologic stress. The food relief personnel or volunteers should help allay fears and anxiety, avoid panic, and maintain morale. See *Emergency feeding.*

Nutrition, emotional stability. Well-nourished individuals generally have a cheerful disposition and a positive attitude toward changes and can adjust easily to various situations. By contrast, undernourished individuals tend to be nervous, tense, apathetic, dull-looking, and irritable. Examples of the relationship between nutrition and emotion include the following: (1) women who are emotionally distressed require a higher intake of calcium (and possibly other nutrients) than happy, relaxed women; (2) the well-known depression of pellagra starts with irritability, headache, and sleeplessness in the early stages, followed by loss of memory, hallucinations, and severe depression in the advanced stages; (3) persons starved for a long time are prone to excitement and hysteria; (4) fear, anger, and worry stimulate adrenaline secretion, which in turn increases the loss of nitrogen from the body; and (5) thiamin-deficient individuals show moodiness, uneasiness, and disorderly thinking. The allusion to thiamin as the "morale vitamin" originated from its ability to alleviate certain mental and emotional depressions. See also *Nutrition, mental health* and *Nutrition, stress.*

Nutrition, exercise. It is now common knowledge that regular exercise is important to one's physical, mental, and emotional health. Exercising conditions the body for greater stamina, increases energy output for weight reduction, maintains normal serum cholesterol and blood glucose levels, and relieves stress. During exercise, more endorphins, which are natural tranquilizers, are secreted. Regular exercise maintains a healthy cardiovascular system. Persons confined to bed lose muscle tone and show mineral imbalance (see *Immobilization*). Normally, it is not necessary to consult a physician for an exercise regimen. Some individuals will need medical clearance before starting an exercise program (e.g., cardiac disease, hypertension, breathing problems, some types of chronic illness). See also *Nutrition, physical health* and *Nutrition, sports.*

Nutrition, eye changes. See *Nutrition, opthalmology.*

Nutrition Foundation, Inc. A public nonprofit institution established in 1941 for "the advancement of nutrition knowledge and its effective application in improving the health and welfare of mankind." It is supported by food and allied industries. The foundation publishes *Nutrition Reviews,* monographs, and pamphlets for the layman. It also sponsors conferences on nutrition. In 1985, the Nutrition Foundation, Inc. merged with the International Life Sciences Institute (ILSI) becoming the North American branch for ILSI. In 1990, ILSI-NFI published the sixth edition of the nutrition classic, *Present Knowledge in Nutrition.*

Nutrition, gastronautic. See *Nutrition, space feeding.*

Nutrition, genetics. Every person is genetically unique because of various hereditary factors. The multifactorial inheritance pattern results from the interaction of genes, such as from parents to offspring, or with environmental variables. The relationship between genetics and nutrition is best observed in disorders known as *inborn errors of metabolism (IEM).* These inherited enzyme malfunctions of absorption, reception action, or utilization may lead to malnutrition and specific damage to a given organ system. See Appendix 44.

Nutrition, geriatric. Nutrition in the aged or persons over 65 years of age. The changes peculiar to the aging process present problems that contribute to *nutritional inadequacy.* These include poor dentition or loss of teeth, loss of appetite and acuity of taste and smell, reduced secretions of digestive enzymes, lack of neuromuscular coordination, reduced cellular metabolism, reduced circulatory and excretory functions, hormonal changes, and a tendency to develop osteoporosis, pernicious anemia, and many metabolic disorders. Aside from these physiologic changes are socioeconomic and psychological factors that affect nutriture. Most common among the aged are depression, boredom, inactivity, lack of interest in the environment, anxiety, faulty eating habits that resist change, and economic insecurity. Considering these changes, dietary principles that govern feeding the aged are as follows: reduced caloric intake; liberal intakes of protein, vitamins, and minerals; liberal water intake to prevent constipation, which is common among elderly people; and small, frequent feedings of palatable meals that are easy to manage and digest. See Recommended Dietary Allowances, Appendix 1.

From the public health standpoint, people over 65 years of age represent 11% of the U.S. population. About 85% of them have nutrition-related medical problems, such as osteoporosis, obesity, hypertension, cardiovascular diseases, and diabetes mellitus. Approximately one-third of the elderly use dietary supplements, mostly as vitamins and minerals. One-half of the federal budget for health is spent for the senior citizens. The creation of the National Institute on Aging is a positive approach by the government to meet the needs of the elderly. Nutrition programs like Meals-on-Wheels and Congregate Meals provide one-third of their RDA.

Nutrition, growth and development. In a broad sense, growth and development refers to the increase in the size and number of cells, as well as cell maturation for functional processes of the body. Thus, the study of nutrition as related to growth and development covers the whole life cycle of an individual. For nutrition principles for each period of life, see *Nutrition, adolescence; Nutrition, adulthood; Nutrition, geriatric; Nutrition, infancy; Nutrition, pregnancy; Nutrition, preschool age; Nutrition, schoolchildren;* and *Nutrition, toddler.*

Nutrition, heart disease. Heart disease is the leading cause of death in the United States (1988 report of the National Health Center for Statistics). Coronary heart disease (CHD) comprises about two-thirds of the heart diseases and is responsible for about 500,000 deaths each year. Most cases of CHD result from *atherosclerosis.* The major risk factors identified in CHD are a family history of heart disease, hypercholesterolemia (especially elevated low-density-lipoprotein cholesterol), hypertension and other vascular disorders, obesity, hyperlipidemia, diabetes mellitus, reduced physical activity, cigarette smoking, and a stressful lifestyle. The incidence of CHD is higher among males than among females. The National Institutes of Health urges people over 20 years of age to have their total serum cholesterol, serum high-density-lipoprotein and low-density-lipoprotein cholesterol, and triglyceride levels checked for preventive measures against early heart diseases. Many national programs (like the National Cholesterol Program, HeartGuide, National High Blood Pressure Education Program, and NHLBI Smoking Education Program) aim to reduce the incidence of heart diseases. See also *Healthy People 2000* and Appendix 7.

Nutrition, hunger. Hunger is discomfort, weakness, or pain caused by lack of food. It is the consequence of being unable to obtain food from nonemergency channels due to poverty, environmental isolation, food inaccessibility, and other factors. Food shortages occur predominantly in Asia, Africa, and Latin America. All together, these areas account for 50% of the world's population, but they have only 25% of the world's food supply. World food production has not increased at a rate faster than or equal to the rate of population growth. World population is expected to double by the year 2026. Unfortunately, at present, many depressed areas of the world are already experiencing famine and hunger. The United Nations reported that over 500 million people in the world are malnourished. Over 20 million people die each year due to hunger-related causes and lowered resistance to infections because of malnutrition. At least one-third of these deaths involve children below 5 years of age. In the United States, 20 million Americans are said to suffer from hunger and inadequate nutrition for several weeks due to domestic interruption, poverty, family dislocation, and other situational problems. A national program to fight domestic hunger should include: strengthening key government food programs such as the Food Stamp Program, the School Breakfast Program the School Lunch Program, the Summer Food Program, and the Home Delivered Meal Program for senior citizens; coordinating private and government services to create both short-term and permanent programs to alleviate hunger, such as the Self-Help and Resource Exchange (SHARE), the Food Policy Councils, and Farmers' Market Coupon Program; increasing funding for nutrition education programs, such as the Expanded Food and Nutrition Education Program (EFNEP) and the Nutrition Education and Training Program (NETP); implementing a comprehensive and responsive national nutrition monitoring system to track trends and evaluate intervention efforts; and providing job training, child care and housing assistance, adequate minimum wages, extended unemployment benefits, equitable public assistance benefits, and charitable tax incentives. The ultimate objective of a national program to prevent hunger is to provide food security, which means that nutritionally adequate and affordable meals are available at all times through conventional food sources.

Nutrition, immune system. The immune system of the body is a biochemical complex of *structures* (lymphocytes, T cells, and B cells; the Kupffer's cells of the liver and leukocytes) and *processes* (formation of antigens and antibodies, phagocytosis, etc.) to protect against disease-producing organisms and foreign bodies like tumor cells and toxins. Malnutrition is the most common cause of acquired immunodeficiency or reduced resistance to infections. To cite a few cases, a breakdown of the first barrier against infection (skin) may be due to deficiencies in protein, zinc, and the A, C and B complex vitamins. Lack of protein reduces biosynthesis of lymphocytes and immunoglobulins or antibodies. Iron is

needed for optimal immune function of neutrophils and lymphocytes. Selenium promotes antibody production and protects the phagocytic function of the neutrophils. *Anergy* occurs in protein-energy malnutrition (PEM), which is observed in cancer, bacterial and viral infections, multiple trauma, burns, uremia, liver disorders, and other debilitating diseases. Immunologic reactions to food, commonly called "food allergies," are examples of diet-immune system relationships. See also *Food allergen, Nutrition, infection,* and *Nutrition, resistance to disease.*

Nutrition, infancy. The first 12 months of life are characterized by the most rapid rate of growth and development of the entire lifetime; thus, an infant's nutritional needs merit special attention. Recommended caloric intake is about 110 to 117 kcal/kg/day, using the higher level for the first months of age. About two-thirds of the caloric needs should come from milk and the rest from added carbohydrates and, later, from supplementary foods. *Protein* needs should be within 2 to 2.2 gm/kg/day, which is easily supplied by adequate milk intake. *Fat* is important primarily to provide essential fatty acids comprising at least 1 to 2% of total caloric needs. This is adequately supplied by human milk or whole cow's milk. *Fluid* requirement is about 4.5 to 5 oz/kg/ day; it is the most variable nutrient need because of fluctuations in the infant's activities and the environmental temperature. *Mineral* needs are generally met during the first 3 months of age by human milk or by the prescribed milk formula. However, after 3 months, the infant's iron stores are depleted, and there is need for other foods and supplementation. *Vitamins* needed by the infant are ample in the milk supply except for vitamins A, D, and C, which must be supplemented (see Appendix 1). See also Appendix 37 for the composition of milk and selected formulas for infant feeding. The following are the main criteria of normal growth and development during infancy: *steady weight gain* of 5 to 8 oz/week, which slows down toward the end of the first year to about 4 oz/week (this means that an average infant should have doubled and tripled his or her birth weight at the end of 5 and 12 months, respectively); *normal increase in body length* is about 10 inches (50% more) at the end of the first year; firm, well-formed muscles with moderate subcutaneous fat; normal sleeping habits and happy disposition; and normal dental and motor development. See *Nutrition, dental health; Nutrition, mental health;* and *Nutrition, motor performance.*

Nutrition, infection. Blood levels of vitamin A are sufficiently reduced in acute infections that xerophthalmia and keratomalacia frequently develop in children receiving diets deficient in this vitamin. Any intestinal infection producing malabsorption interferes with the absorption of fats and fat-soluble vitamins. Clinical manifestations of thiamin, folic acid, vitamin B_{12}, and ascorbic acid deficiencies are all related to a preceding infection of a vulnerable host. Increased losses of calcium and phosphorus are seen in tuberculosis. Losses of sodium, chloride, potassium, and phosphorous are seen in diarrheal diseases of infectious origin. Hookworm infections can be responsible for enough loss of blood to induce anemia. See also *Nutrition, immune system* and *Nutrition, resistance to disease.*

Nutrition, lactation. Nutrient requirements of the mother during *lactation* are increased to provide for normal secretion of milk and for recovery from pregnancy and delivery. Thus, the *caloric requirement* is increased by 500 to 750 calories over that of the non-pregnant woman. This is approximately 90 kcal/100 ml of milk secreted to provide for energy expenditure of the secretory function and for the caloric content of milk. Similarly, intakes for *protein, minerals* (particularly *calcium*), and *vitamins* are increased (see Appendix 1). See also *Infant feeding* and *Lactation.*

Nutrition, mental health. The relationship of nutrition and mental health is well established; proper nourishment is conducive to mental efficiency, the ability to concentrate, and the ease of adjustment to environmental changes. By contrast, nutrient inadequacy may result in permanent changes in the size or chemical composition of the brain, thus affecting mental capacity; inborn errors of metabolism retard mental development (e.g., phenylketonuria and galactosemia); and specific nervous lesions occur as a result of nutrient deficiencies, as in *pellagra, kwashiorkor, marasmus,* and *beriberi.* For further details, see also *Nutrition, emotional stability; Nutrition, nervous system;* and *Nutrition, psychiatry.*

Nutrition, motor performance. The ability of the body to coordinate its movements and to perform other physical activities has its roots in the motor development during infancy and childhood. Evidence of the importance of adequate nutrition for motor development comes from studies of kwashiorkor, beriberi, and other deficiency diseases; phenylketonuria and other inborn errors of metabolism; and *hypokinesis.* Lack of exercise and prolonged immobilization, as in bedridden patients, lead to negative nitrogen and mineral balances. The physiologic effects of moderate exercise on nutriture and good health in general are as follows: it promotes pulmonary ventilation, circulation, and oxidation processes; it stimulates appetite, flow of digestive juices, and peristalsis; it improves muscle tonus and sleep habits; and it increases strength, mental acuity, and resistance to infection. See also *Nutrition, exercise,* and *Nutrition, sports.*

Nutrition, neonatology. The study of specialized care of newborn infants. The first 4 weeks after birth is called the "neonatal period." Newborn care is categorized into Level I: full-term neonates; Level II: normal (full term) neonates, but considered high-risk for various medical reasons; and Level III: critically ill neonates requiring intensive care. The last group is classified as either low-birth-weight (LBW) infants weighing less than 2500 gm (5½ lb) at birth or very-low-birth-weight (VLBW) infants weighing less than 1500 gm (3½ lb). Level III neonates have a smaller metabolic reserve than those in Levels I and II and are unable to store fat and glycogen during the last period of gestation. Their glycogen reserve may be only 110 kcal/kg, and their fat reserve may be only 1% of their total body weight (compared to 16% in the full-term baby). Since the basal metabolic need of LBW infants is 50 kcal/kg, careful monitoring and adequate provision of energy intake are very important. High-risk neonates can be given parenteral feedings of dextrose, amino acids, electrolytes, vitamins, minerals, and trace elements. See also *Nutrition, prematurity.*

Nutrition, nervous system. Proper nutrition is important for the integrity of nerve cells and the normal functioning of the nervous system. An obvious example is the feeling of restlessness or irritability when one is hungry. All nutrients are involved in maintaining a healthy nervous system, notably the following: *carbohydrate* (specifically, glucose) is the chief energy source utilized by the brain; *protein* is needed to synthesize the enzyme systems to oxidize glucose; and *B complex vitamins* are involved as cofactors for these enzymes. Certain vitamin deficiencies lead to neurologic changes varying from mild symptoms to gross anatomic nerve lesions; for example, lack of *thiamin* results in neuromuscular incoordination (nystagmus, hyperesthesia, ataxia, cramps, and loss of tendon reflexes), brain lesions and degeneration of nerve fibers and myelin sheaths, with death of the parent nerve cells; *riboflavin* deficiency is characterized in the early stages by photophobia and affects nicotinic acid metabolism, in which riboflavin is indirectly involved; lack of *nicotinic acid* is associated with the psychosis of pellagra; and *pyridoxine* deficiency leads to sensory neuritis, convulsions, hyperesthesia, and loss of positional sense. See also *Nutrition, alcoholism; Nutrition, emotional stability; Nutrition, mental health;* and *Nutrition, psychiatry.*

Nutrition, ophthalmology. It has long been established that the muscles, nerves, and mucous membranes of the eyes, as well as the visual process, are affected by nutrition. The ability to see or adapt in dim light depends in part on adequate *vitamin A* intake.

Ocular changes associated with a lack of vitamin A are xerosis, keratomalacia, Bitot's spots, night blindness, and xerophthalmia. *Riboflavin* deficiency leads to corneal vascularization, conjunctivitis, photophobia, and burning and itching of eyes. Lack of *pyridoxine* results in angular blepharitis and conjunctivitis. The *essential amino acids, vitamin C,* and *nicotinic acid* maintain the integrity of the eye lens and prevent cataracts.

Nutrition, parasitism. Infestation of the human host with *parasites,* particularly in the digestive tract, is a conditioning factor of nutritional inadequacy. The common intestinal parasites are tapeworms, hookworms, pinworms, whipworms, ascarides, flukes, *Trichinella,* and *Trichuris.* The extent of their harmful effects depends on the tissues invaded, the types of secretion they produce, their rate of growth and multiplication, and the ability of the body to protect itself from these effects. The principal ways in which parasites harm the host are as follows: mechanical injury (tissue lesions and hemorrhage), inflammation, and pain; obstruction (e.g., blocking ducts); toxicity of their secretions; and robbing the host of its nutrient supply, especially proteins and vitamins. The nutritional implications of these parasitic effects do not need further elaboration. Preventive measures against parasitism include *nutrition education* (a well-nourished body can build antibodies that neutralize the toxic effects of parasites); *environmental sanitation* (e.g., proper sewage disposal, safe water and food supplies, educated food handlers and consumers); and *parasitic control* (medical attention and use of chemicals or other means of interfering with the life cycle of the parasite). See also *Nutrition, resistance to disease.*

Nutrition, physical health. The state of nutrition is easily reflected in a person's appearance. The physical signs of good nutrition are normal weight for height, body frame, and age; firm, moderately padded muscles; clear and slightly moist skin with good color; well-formed jaw and teeth; soft, glossy hair and clear, bright eyes; a well-formed trunk; good appetite and abundant energy; endurance of physical work and resistance to disease; and, in general, a happy personality. See also *Nutrition, sports.*

Nutrition, preadolescence. See *Nutrition, puberty.*

Nutrition, pregnancy. Good nourishment during pregnancy is important for meeting not only the mother's needs but also those of the growing fetus (prenatal nutrition). Good maternal nutrition results in a lower incidence of abortion and miscarriage; fewer stillborn and premature infants and infants with congenital malformations; fewer complications during pregnancy (e.g., toxemias and anemias) and delivery (e.g., prolonged labor, premature separation of the placenta, and hemorrhaging); healthier full-term babies; and reduced infant mortality and morbidity rates. Pregnancy imposes a physiologic stress on the mother, and the most important changes with nutritional implications are an increase in basal metabolic rate (about 25% in the latter half of pregnancy); a tendency to retain water; decreased gastric acidity and intestinal motility, with frequent impairment of digestion and absorption in the early stage and constipation in the last trimester; simple glycosuria; hormonal changes (increased activities of progesterone, gonadotropin, estrogen, and adrenal steroid hormones); and a positive nitrogen balance and an increase in plasma volume, with corresponding decrease in hemoglobin concentration. With these significant changes in mind, dietary intakes try to provide for the increased maternal metabolic activities; the nutrient needs of the growing fetus; the development of reproductive tissues (uterus, placenta, etc.) and the mammary glands; and the nutrient reserves to allow for losses during delivery. In general, all nutrient requirements are increased from the nonpregnant to the pregnant state. For further details, see Appendix 1. Noteworthy is the need to regulate weight gain during pregnancy. The desirable weight gain is about 20 to 25 lb throughout the gestation period, distributed as follows: normal weight of the infant at birth = 7 to 7½ lb; weight of the uterus, placenta, and membrane = 3 to 3½ lb; weight of amniotic fluids = 2 lb; weight of the mammary glands and tissues = 1 to 1½ lb; and the remaining weight is in the form of maternal body water and increased blood volume. The total weight gain of 23 lb (average) should be about 5, 8, and 10 lb for the first, second, and third trimesters, respectively. In view of the rapid fetal growth and development that occur as early as the second month of pregnancy, it is recommended that *protein, mineral,* and *vitamin* intakes be increased as early as possible. See also *Nutrition, teenage pregnancy.*

Nutrition, prematurity. Premature infants have special nutritional needs because their nutrient requirements are high relative to their body size and weight. Their digestive capacity is usually small; the sucking and swallowing reflexes are not well developed; respiration is irregular, with a tendency to regurgitate and aspirate foods; achlorhydria is common; and fat absorption is poor, resulting in a loss of fat-soluble vitamins and calcium along with fecal fat. The dietary management of a premature infant has to be individualized, depending on the anatomic facilities and physiologic condition. Daily nourishment should provide at least 125 kcal/kg and 4.5 gm protein/kg body weight with vitamin and mineral supplementations. A recommended feeding regimen for a premature infant is as follows: for the *first 12 hours,* nothing is given orally; for the *next 24 hours,* a 5% glucose solution is given at 2- to 3-hour intervals, starting first with a half teaspoonful and gradually increasing by half teaspoonfuls; for the *fourth 12 hours,* the mixed formula is given at 2- to 3-hour intervals, gradually increasing the amount; for the *third day* and thereafter, a full concentration of the prescribed formula is given, starting with small amounts and gradually increasing as tolerated by the infant. Vitamin and mineral supplements are given by the second week. See also *Nutrition, infancy* and *Nutrition, neonatology.*

Nutrition, preschool age. The group composed of 1- to 5-year-old children constitutes a far more nutritionally vulnerable group than infants. Recognizing that ages 1 to 5 years are the most formative years of child development in all aspects of personality (physical, mental, and social), the importance of nutrition cannot be overemphasized. For a quantitative evaluation of dietary adequacy for ages 1 to 3 and 4 to 6 years, see Appendix 1.

Nutrition, psychiatry. Humans associate varying emotional experiences with food, such as social acceptance or rejection, feelings of security or anxiety, pleasure or pain, satisfaction or frustration, and many other feelings. In the mentally ill, these associations are often exaggerated, and feeding problems are more difficult to manage. Well-known conditions with underlying psychological disorders are obesity with uncontrollable overeating, anorexia nervosa, chronic alcoholism, and drug addiction. For successful dietary management, the dietitian must know the background of the patient (social, economic, educational, etc.), especially the underlying psychiatric defect. The feeding regimen is part of the patient's total rehabilitation program, which requires the teamwork approach including the physician or psychiatrist, dietitian, nurse, social worker, and psychotherapist and others. See also *Diet therapy* and *Nutrition, emotional stability.*

Nutrition, puberty. Puberty is the period during which the reproductive organs become functionally operative and secondary sex characteristics start to develop, with accompanying increased rates of growth and metabolism. Its onset varies from 10 to 15 years of age, with 12 to 13 years of age being the average for boys and 2 years earlier for girls. For nutritional considerations, see also *Nutrition, adolescence.*

Nutrition, public health. The theory and practice of nutrition as a science through organized community efforts, with the family as the smallest unit under study. The overall aim of public health nutrition is to improve or maintain good health through proper nutrition. Various agencies, governmental and nongovernmental, are concerned with nutrition work at local, national, or international levels. See Appendix 47.

Nutrition, resistance to disease. There are two ways in which nutrition can affect host resistance to disease: antibody synthesis and cellular immune response. Protein malnutrition impairs the production of circulating antibodies in response to certain viral and bacterial antigens. Malnutrition and the depletion of protein reserves result in atrophy of the liver, spleen, bone marrow, and lymphoid tissues, from which phagocytes and lymphocytes originate. Lysozyme activity is also reduced by generalized malnutrition. Nutritional deficiencies cause tissue changes that lower body resistance and affect wound healing and collagen formation. Deficiencies in protein, vitamin A, ascorbic acid, and niacin are especially likely to cause tissue changes that lower resistance to disease. See also *Nutrition, immune system.*

Nutrition, schoolchildren. Dietary principles in feeding schoolchildren are the same as those for preschoolers, but food intake differs in quantity and variety. Due to school activities, children from 6 to 12 years of age are more independent, and this includes their choice of food outside the home. Unless supervised by nutrition educators, as in the case of *school lunch programs,* feeding time and food selection may be erratic. Hurried meals, skipping breakfast, poorly selected snacks, and lack of appetite due to social and school interests are the common feeding problems faced by parents and teachers.

Nutrition, skin condition. See *Nutrition, dermatology.*

Nutrition, space feeding. Also called "gastronautics"; the preferred name is "astrophysiologic dietetics," signifying that feeding an organism beyond the earth's environment is both an art and a science. Space begins about 120 miles above the earth and is devoid of air, friction, gravity, and oxygen. Thus, the very nature of a trip into space causes nutritional problems. Although the water requirement remains the same, caloric needs are reduced because of weightlessness and confinement, resulting in sedentary activity. About 50% of the total caloric intake should come from fat (this is an advantage, since fat catabolism requires less oxygen); 15% of calories is provided by protein; and the rest is carbohydrates. Fecal losses are minimized by the use of low-residue diets. Mineral levels for calcium, sodium, potassium, and magnesium are increased by 10% above normal needs. Foods used should be specially prepared to tolerate weightlessness; sudden fluctuations of pressure, temperature, light, radiation, and humidity; and other conditions during the flight. The overall aim of the feeding system is to promote maximum efficiency of the crew, whose movements are restricted even in mastication. Evidently, there are changes in ingestion and digestion, taste acuity, nitrogen and calcium needs, and metabolism of food. Besides providing nutrient adequacy, foods should be palatable, easy to manage, and not subject to deterioration. Thus, the types of foods chosen are bite-sized finger foods, precooked foods, and freeze-dried foods, each packaged to serve three purposes—storage container, food utensil, and eating device.

Nutrition, sports. Recommended intakes of calories and the major nutrients for an athlete vary according to age, sex, body size, type of sports activity, and duration and intensity of the athletic event or training. For example, a large-framed teenage male athlete on endurance training needs more than an adult female tennis player. The caloric needs of an athlete should, therefore, be individualized and calculated accordingly. Half (50%) of total calories should come from complex carbohydrates, 5% from simple carbohydrates, 15% from protein, and 30% from fats. Contrary to popular myth, a very-high-protein diet is not recommended. With an intake of at least 3000 kcal/day, vitamin and mineral requirements should be adequately met, using the dietary guidelines and recommended food groups. Athletes should avoid alcohol and caffeine. Five to six meals and snacks, properly spaced throughout the day, are better than three big meals. A pre-game meal is best eaten 3 hours before the event to allow for digestion. Avoid gas-forming foods and replace fluid losses. An athlete may lose more than 2 liters of sweat per hour in a hot environment while performing or during prolonged exercise. Electrolytes lost by sweating can be replaced easily from foods eaten. There is no need for special tablets when natural foods rich in sodium, potassium, and magnesium will supply these minerals. See also *Carbohydrate loading.*

Nutrition, starvation. A state of malnutrition arises from prolonged starvation caused by any of the following circumstances: lack of food, as in famine, war, or poverty; the presence of a conditioning factor, especially disorders of the digestive tract and malabsorption syndrome; and the effect of certain toxemias that may be metabolic or infectious in origin. The outstanding changes in starved individuals are generalized atrophy, or wasting of tissues, with loss of body fat and increased extracellular fluids; shrinkage of lean tissues, with muscular weakness and loss of skin elasticity; disturbance of water balance as a result of loss of plasma proteins and electrolyte changes, with consequent nutritional edema; digestive and renal disorders, especially nocturia and "starvation diarrhea"; lack of hormone and enzyme production, leading to decreased metabolic activities; loss of sexual function; amenorrhea in women; lowered blood pressure; mental restlessness and physical apathy; cancrum oris; and many other clinical and anatomic lesions, depending on the severity of starvation (partial or complete deprivation of food) and the length of time an individual is starved. The rehabilitation of the starved person should be gradual. Immediately correct any existing electrolyte imbalances. Thereafter, dietary needs are met by calories in the form of warm, easily digested, bland foods given in small, frequent feedings and then gradually increased as tolerated. Recommended first foods are skim milk and simple carbohydrates. Medical supervision and parenteral feedings are needed for severely starved persons. See also *Nutrition, hunger* and *Starvation.*

Nutrition, stress. Stress is any stimulus that interferes with the normal equilibrium of the body with varying rate of wear and tear on vital activities. Stress factors may be internal or "built-in" ones such as genetic disposition, age or sex, or they may be external or manageable ones such as poor diet, alcoholism, and drug abuse. Therefore, stress management has become a necessary consideration in nutrition assessment, care, and planning based on human needs and an essential component in current promotional programs. Factors that disturb the normal equilibrium of the body are called "physiologic stresses." They include physical; mental; emotional stimuli, such as pain, anxiety, fear, time pressure, and worry; and metabolic factors. Physiologic stresses stimulate the sympathetic nervous system. The initial responses include: increased catecholamines and hormones leading to hyperglycemia, glucogenesis, gluconeogenesis, and increased secretions of glucagon, glucocorticoid and antidiuretic hormones. Respiratory rate and heart rate are elevated. Peristalsis is decreased and nutrient absorption is reduced. A person under stress may experience nausea, vomiting, anorexia and oliguria. Energy requirement may increase as much as 100%, depending on the severity of stress factors (see Appendix 24). The body's basal protein needs may increase as much as 300% in severe trauma. Undoubtedly, other dietary factors (e.g., fats, vitamins and minerals) play important roles in the overall process of nutrition and stress interactions.

Another group of stress factors are environmental in nature and are called "psychosocial" factors. They include poverty, feelings of isolation, insecurity, or powerlessness, and others. These are perpetuated by society's values and attitudes. Emotional tension from multiple causes is the most common agent of human stress. It can contribute to cardiac and gastrointestinal diseases, especially if the body is conditioned by malnutrition, faulty diet, or poor housing, as in the case of high-risk families in the grip of poverty. Both physiologic and psychosocial stresses can depress the immune function of the body and decrease its resistance to disease.

Nutrition, teenage pregnancy. Adolescent or teenage pregnancy is still a major public health problem in the U.S. Pregnant adolescents are nutritionally at risk and require nutritional care throughout the gestation period. Because of the accompanying complex effects of socio-economic, emotional, and physical factors, teenage pregnancy presents the the greatest challenge for nutrition counseling. Assessment and management of nutrition services for pregnant adolescents should be done by a dietitian of an established adolescent program, with prenatal health clinic visits and parent sessions. The latter involve educating parents to continue supportive counseling at home. Significant nutrient-related risk factors for pregnant teenagers include: low pregnancy weight gain; low pregnancy weight for height and other evidence of malnutrition; excessive prepregnancy weight for height; low gynecological age, i.e., age of onset of pregnancy minus age of menarche; unhealthy lifestyle such as the use of drugs, alcohol, or cigarettes; a history of eating disorders; and the presence of anemia, toxemia, and other chronic diseases. To ensure optimal fetal development and growth, at the same time provide for her own needs as a growing adolescent, a pregnant teenager requires increased intakes of calories and nutrients that exceed the dietary allowances for a mature pregnant woman. See Appendix 1.

Nutrition, therapeutic. See *Nutrition, diet therapy.*

Nutrition, toddler. The nutritional problem of the child from 1 to 3 years of age is only an extension of his or her needs from infancy. The primary concern is to increase gradually the kind and amount of food and to lessen the number of feedings to three meals with in-between snacks. Significant in this period is the establishment of proper food habits at home, hence the need for nutrition education for mothers. For quantitative consideration of nutrient needs for children ages 1 to 3 years, see Appendix 1.

Nutrition, tongue and mouth conditions. Certain oral changes are associated with specific nutrient deficiencies. Two striking examples are the tongue and mouth lesions caused by a lack of riboflavin and nicotinic acid. In *ariboflavinosis,* angular stomatitis, cheilosis, and a purplish or magenta tongue are the characteristic lesions. In *pellagra,* the tongue is swollen and has a beefy red color; its papillae are smooth or denuded, and the tongue assumes a mushroom appearance. Mucous membranes and lips are also red and often fissured. The tongue and mouth lesions associated with lack of other B complex vitamins are as follows: a clean, pale, and smooth tongue (chronic atrophic glossitis) in pernicious anemia due to *vitamin B*$_{12}$ deficiency; seborrheic angular dematitis in *vitamin B*$_6$ deficiency; and endematous glossitis resulting from a lack of *folic acid.*

Nutrition, vegetarism. Most vegetarian diets can be nutritionally adequate with careful planning. In general, the more variety of food products used, especially the addition of some animal protein foods, the easier it is to provide all nutrient needs. Hence, persons who add milk, cheese and/or eggs to their vegetarian diet, are less likely to encounter nutritional deficiencies than the pure vegetarians. The vegans, fruitarians, and persons who observe the Zen macrobiotic diet, may have difficulties in providing good quality protein, riboflavin, vitamin B$_{12}$, vitamin D, iron, calcium, and zinc, unless carefully planned by using a wide variety of plant foods and by adding supplements. See *Protein, supplementary value* and *Vegetarian.*

Nutrition, weight control. Weight control is concerned with bringing a person's body weight to its healthy level. An increase of body weight of 20% or more than the so-called ideal weight in the form of adipose tissues is an established health hazard (see *Obesity*). Body weight as a parameter is the sum of fat, water, protein, and minerals in the skeletal system. The first two components are particularly variable. The currently used height-weight tables according to body frame should be considered guidelines only, because there are other varying factors among individuals that affect body weight, such as age, body composition, nutritional status, and state of health. Other methods to estimate body lean mass or subcutaneous fat should be used, such as

skinfold and circumference measurements, body density, and bioelectric impedance analysis (BIA). Of the weight control problems, obesity is the most studied, because of its prevalence and its physiological and psychological consequences. It is estimated that 25% of the American population weighs more than 20% over the ideal body weight. Over 20 million adult Americans who are obese need a weight control program that is effective for long-range maintenance of healthy body weight. There is a high dropout rate among weight reducers which is not surprising, given the complexity of obesity from the standpoint of etiology or origin; genetic make-up; physiological factors; dietary regimen used; physical activities; and psychological, emotional, and social factors. Metabolic variabilities that exist are due in part to the many hormones involved in the regulation of hunger, appetite, satiety and energy utilization. At least 20,000 weight-loss methods have been surveyed by the Health, Weight and Stress Program at Johns Hopkins University; less than 6% have been found effective or safe. The recommended weight control programs use a multidisciplinary approach including dietary means, behavioral changes, regular exercise, and monitoring of gradual weight loss with the help of a support group and professionals. Professional supervision is especially needed in treating morbid obesity using a very-low-calorie diet (500 to 800 kcal/day). Other weight-loss methods that require medical supervision are the use of surgical procedures and drug therapy; these have side effects which should be carefully considered. Two main problems of treating morbid obesity are recidivism or the tendency to regain lost weight, and the high cost of some weight loss programs. In addition to obesity, extreme underweight conditions also need medical attention. See *Anorexia nervosa* and *Bulimia.*

Nutritional adaptation. Maintenance of a fairly constant blood or tissue composition despite deficiencies or excesses of nutrients in the food supply. Any change in the diet that would create a condition of nutritional stress is checked by the body's ability to adapt itself to maintain constancy in nutrient composition. An increased supply of a nutrient leads to the accentuation of systems associated with excretion of this excess nutrient, increased metabolism, or the preferential use of the nutrient as a source of energy. A reduced supply of a nutrient leads to decreased activity of systems associated with its metabolism, e.g., the unusual thrift in the use of a scant supply seen in fasting. Eventually, an adaptive increase or decrease in the utilization of a nutrient takes place.

Nutritional anthropometry. Measurement of the physical dimensions and gross composition of the body at different age levels and degrees of nutrition. These measurements include height; weight; circumference of the arm, chest, and hip (ACH index); skinfold thickness, waist-hip ratio, elbow breadth, growth charts, and many others. Nutritional anthropometry is a useful aid in the assessment of the nutritional status of an individual or a population group. See Appendices 18 to 23.

Nutritional assessment. This is a comprehensive process of identifying and evaluating the nutritional needs of a person using appropriate, measurable methods. Nutritional assessment consists of gathering information and evaluating the data using four techniques: history taking, nutritional anthropometry, physical examination, and biochemical tests. *History taking* includes medical, social, dietary and related background information about the client or patient. Risk factors associated with nutrition from history-taking include drastic weight loss or gain; anorexia, chronic illnesses, and recent major surgery; chewing and swallowing difficulties; drug addiction; habitual intake of oral contraceptives, catabolic steroids, antibiotics, and other drugs with significant nutrient-drug interaction; and socio-economic factors like poverty, lack of education, and inadequate or poor food habits. The latter may be assessed by a 24-hour food recall and/or by keeping a food record from 3 to 7 days. *Anthropometric measurements* include data on height and weight, frame size, body mass index (BMI), skinfold thickness, mid-

arm muscle circumference (MAMC), upper arm muscle area (UAMA), and knee height. See Appendices 18 to 23 for details. *Physical examination* can reveal possible deficiency signs of malnutrition based on clinical signs and symptoms associated with lack of a nutrient as summarized in Appendix 26. *Biochemical tests* include data from laboratory analysis for various nutrients and related substances from the blood and urine. Common biochemical indices include: serum albumin, serum albumin/globulin ratio, serum transferrin, total iron binding capacity, total lymphocyte count, complete blood cell profile, lipid profile, somatomedin-C, nitrogen balance, creatinine-height index, serum enzyme levels, urinary ketones, urinary nitrogen, and others. For details, see Appendices 27 to 31. A meaningful nutritional evaluation consists of interpreting the results from these four techniques of measuring nutritional assessment. This should be followed by a nutritional intervention/plan of action to correct any deficiency and to aid in therapy.

Nutritional care. A set of activities to provide a diet adequate in nutrients needed by an individual and to help with proper eating habits. The nutritional care process starts with *nutritional screening*. This is followed by *nutritional assessment* and *nutritional counseling*. In healthcare facilities, the patient's medical record is the basic means of communication among health professionals. An organized system of charting that is commonly used is the problem-oriented medical record (POMR) system. It starts with the collection of a data base and identifying any problem concerned with providing quality healthcare to the patient. The problem could be medical, nursing, nutritional, behavioral, economic, psychosocial, environmental, and others. Examples of nutritional problems include anorexia, food allergies, dysphagia, missing teeth, inability to self-feed, and drug-nutrient interactions. Each problem is clearly defined, followed by specific treatment plans, implementation, patient education and follow-up. A suggested format in charting is to use the acronym SOAP as an outline which stands for subjective (S), objective (O), assessment or analysis (A) and plan (P). The nutritional plan includes intervention, monitoring, and follow-up, written as progress notes.

Nutritional counseling. Providing expert advice to help a person with current or potential nutrition problems. The process involves a great deal of knowledge and skill in interviewing and educating people. Trying to make dietary changes is difficult because of a person's lifetime habits, personal tastes, ethnic or cultural background, educational level, attitudes toward food, economic obstacles, social lifestyle, and other factors. Effective nutritional counseling should start with establishing rapport, stating the objectives of the session and the benefits derived from dietary adherence, and identifying possible problems which the client may encounter with the dietary regimen or meal plan. After the initial counseling session, an aftercare plan or follow-up is essential. Long-term adherence and positive results leading to the client's recovery or maintenance of good nutritional status are the most challenging aspects of nutritional counseling.

Nutritional deficiency (inadequacy). Condition of the body that may arise as a result of a lack of one or more nutrients in the diet (primary factor of nutritional inadequacy) and/or a breakdown of one or more of the bodily processes concerned with nutrient utilization (secondary factor of nutritional inadequacy). The underlying reasons for a dietary lack, either in quantity or in quality, may in turn be due to poverty, ignorance of proper nutrition practices, faulty selection of food, lack of facilities for preservation and storage, and overpopulation. The secondary factors are sometimes referred to as "conditioning factors of nutritional inadequacy" (i.e., nutrient deficiencies occur even if the diet is adequate) because they interfere with bodily processes, as listed below:

1. *Factors that interfere with ingestion:* loss of teeth, anorexia, self-feeding problems, neuropsychiatric disorders, and therapy that reduce taste acuity and appetite.

2. *Factors that interfere with digestion and absorption:* diarrhea, achlorhydria, biliary disease, gastrointestinal surgery, and therapy with mineral oil.

3. *Factors that interfere with utilization:* liver disease, diabetes mellitus, hypothyroidism, malignancy, alcoholism, and antimetabolite and sulfa drug therapy.

4. *Factors that increase nutritive requirements:* strenuous physical activity, fever, delirium, hyperthyroidism, growth, pregnancy, and lactation.

5. *Factors that increase excretion:* polyuria, lactation, excessive perspiration, and therapy that causes diuresis.

6. *Factors that increase nutrient destruction:* achlorhydria, lead poisoning, and alkali and sulfonamide therapy.

See also *Deficiency disease, Nutrition,* and *Nutritional status.*

Nutritional labeling. A format or system of identifying the nutritional qualities of foods to help consumers. In the United States, the Food and Drug Administration (FDA) has the task of establishing nutrient labeling regulations. Currently, the FDA's proposal requires nutrition labeling of most foods "that are meaningful sources of calories and nutrients," e.g., foods that provide 2% or more of the Reference Daily Intake (RDI) per serving for protein, vitamin A, vitamin C, iron, or calcium; more than 40 kcal per serving or more than 0.4 kcal per gram of the food; or more than 35 mg of sodium per serving. The label must include a listing of caloric content, serving size, number of servings per container, grams of protein, carbohydrate and fat, milligrams of sodium; and percentage of the US recommended dietary allowance for protein, vitamin A, vitamin C, thiamin, riboflavin, niacin, calcium, and iron. Total fat should include triglycerides and saturated fat content. Total carbohydrate should include total starch, sugars, polyols, and dietary fiber. Other information on optional nutrients and nutritionally related components can be added voluntarily. However, if claims are specified on the label about any of these components, amounts must be declared. For example, other vitamins and minerals should be declared quantitatively if added. If claims are made on dietary fibers, total fiber, soluble and insoluble fiber contents must be declared. Descriptive terms have to follow legal definitions. For example, "sodium-free" and "very low sodium" mean that the products contain less than 5 mg and 35 mg sodium per serving, respectively. Sugar-free products cannot contain sucrose, honey, fruit juice, molasses or other simple sugars. "Cholesterol-free" products must contain less than 2 mg cholesterol per serving, and "low cholesterol" foods must contain less than 20 mg per serving. See Appendix 3 for the US reference daily intakes (USRDI) for labeling purposes. The ingredient list should be introduced by the words "From Most to Least." Virtually all foods at the retail level should be nutritionally labeled.

Nutritional monitoring. Process of providing information on a regular basis about the role and status of nutritional factors that relate to health. Nutrition monitoring, therefore, extends over a period of time, with repeated nutritional assessment to measure changes. See also *National Nutrition Monitoring System.*

Nutritional screening. The preliminary step to nutritional assessment in order to prioritize patients who need extensive nutritional care. Examples of first priority-patients (those at highest nutritional risk, who should be given attention as soon as possible) are those admitted for multiple trauma, sepsis, severely underweight, renal dialysis, major surgery, carcinoma, insulin-dependent diabetes, and major burns.

Nutritional status. Also called "nutriture." State of the body resulting from the consumption and utilization of nutrients. Clinical observations, biochemical analyses, anthropometric measurements, and dietary studies are used to determine this state. See *Nutritional assessment.*

Nutritional survey. Study of the nutritional status of a population group in a given area of operation. The population may be homogeneous (e.g., teenage girls or diabetics) or heterogeneous (e.g., hospital patients). The survey may be focused on various factors, such as age, sex, race, or socioeconomic, geographic, physiologic, or pathologic condition, depending on the aims of the study. In general, the main objectives of the nutrition survey are to determine the extent of malnutrition and ascertain feeding problems, to provide ways and means of correcting or preventing nutritional problems, and to help in nutrition education, economic planning, and other programs for the improvement of the health status of the population or group. The main techniques used in nutrition surveys are: *dietary surveys,* which are food consumption data to detect inadequate diets and faulty food habits (e.g., food accounts, food frequency questionnaires, food recall, and food records); *medical history* to know the past and present illnesses and identify secondary factors of nutritional deficiencies; *clinical tests* or *physical examinations* to detect signs and symptoms of malnutrition; *biophysical tests* that reveal anatomical or tissue changes related to malnutrition; and *biochemical analyses* (e.g., analysis of blood and urine constituents) to detect abnormal nutrient levels. Examples of nutritional surveys conducted in the United States include the Ten-State Nutrition Survey, the National Health and Nutrition Examination Survey (NHANES) I, II, and III, and the United States Department of Agriculture Nationwide Food Consumption Surveys (NFCS).

Nutritional tool. Any material, device, instrument or technique used to carry out the nutritional activities and services of a nutritionist; includes a wide array or variety of resources, such as the basic food guides, the recommended dietary allowances (RDA), medical and food records, anthropometric measurements, growth charts, food exchange lists, food and nutrient labels, food composition tables, meal plans and recipes, food models, printed materials, software and other audiovisual aids, and many others. See Appendices.

Nutritionist. A professional who teaches and/or applies the science of nutrition for the improvement of health and control of disease. He or she may organize and conduct training programs for paraprofessionals and members of allied professions on food and nutrition, coordinate the nutritional activities of public and private health and related agencies, plan and conduct meetings on nutrition, and participate in nutritional surveys.

Nutrition Today Society. A nonprofit professional organization that aims to increase public awareness of new developments in nutrition. It publishes *Nutrition Today* and produces audiovisual learning materials and other nutrition resources.

Nyctalopia. See *Night blindness.*

Nystagmus. Also called "nystaxis." Involuntary rapid and rhythmic eye movements. Seen in thiamin deficiency, certain eye diseases, and a number of neuromuscular disorders.

O

O. Chemical symbol for oxygen. O_2 is molecular oxygen.

OA. Abbreviation for *Overeaters Anonymous.*

Obesity. Also called "adiposity"; state of malnutrition in which the accumulation of depot fat is so excessive that functions of the body are disturbed. An individual is considered *obese* when the body weight is 20% or more above the desirable weight because of adiposity. Obesity is classified as mild (20 to 40% overweight), moderate (41 to 100%), and morbid (over 100% overweight). There are several causative factors (genetic, traumatic, environmental, etc.), but ultimately, the overall picture is the result of caloric intake in excess of caloric output. *Simple obesity* is due to overeating (sometimes called *exogenous obesity*), reduced physical activity, decreased basal metabolism, or a combination of these factors. Many cases of overeating are psychological in nature (to relieve tension, worry, depression, and frustration, or to provide security and pleasure). Some cases of obesity are due to a metabolic disturbance that favors adiposity, as in hypothyroidism, lesions of the hypothalamus, hypofunction of the gonads, hyperfunction of the adrenal cortex, and pituitary obesities. Obesity is now considered a disease for the following reasons: it shortens life expectancy, it may complicate pregnancy and surgery, it is a social and physical handicap, and it predisposes the person to disease (e.g., renal, cardiovascular, and gallbladder diseases, gout, diabetes, and arthritis). Managing obesity is not only dietary but needs behavioral modifications, with emphasis on motivation, goal setting, support group intervention, increased physical activity, and exercise. For further details, see *Nutrition, weight control.* See also *Low-calorie diet* under *Diet, calorie-modified; Energy balance;* and *Overweight.*

Occult. Obscure or hidden, such as *occult blood,* which is not recognizable with the naked eye and can only be detected by chemical tests or the use of a microscope.

OGTT. Abbreviation for oral glucose tolerance test. See *Glucose tolerance test.*

OHA. Abbreviation for *oral hypoglycemic agent.*

Oils. Simple lipids chemically similar to *fats* but differing in that they are generally liquid at room temperature. There are several kinds, e.g., *animal* and *vegetable* oils used in cooking, medicine, and food processing; *volatile* or *essential* oils distilled from flowers, leaves, and other parts of plants; and *mineral* oils used for fuel.

Oleic acid. Monounsaturated fatty acid containing 18 carbon atoms. The double bond is in the *cis* configuration. It is one of the most abundant fatty acids in nature, occurring widely in animal and vegetable fats and oils.

Oligosaccharides. Group of *carbohydrates* that yield 2 to 10 simple sugars or monosaccharide units on hydrolysis. See Appendix 8.

Omega fatty acid. A fatty acid with several double bonds, indicated by the position of one double bond closest to the methyl end of the carbon chain. For example, omega-3 fatty acid has one double bond from the methyl ($CH3-$) end between the third and fourth carbons. See *Fatty acid.*

Oncotic pressure. Pressure exerted by proteins that helps to regulate the distribution of fluids on both sides of a semipermeable membrane. In this manner, plasma proteins regulate water balance in the body. The oncotic pressure gradient is the pressure difference between the osmotic pressure of the blood and that of the lymph or tissue fluids. It maintains the water balance of these two compartments. If it is disrupted, as in hypoalbuminemia, fluid accumulates in the interstitial tissues, resulting in edema. See also *Osmotic pressure.*

Opsin. Protein occurring in both the rods and the cones of the retina. It reacts with retinaldehyde in the dark to form the visual pigment rhodopsin.

Opsonin. Form of antibody that can render bacteria and cells more susceptible to *phagocytosis.*

Oral contraceptive. Commercial preparation of an estrogen-progestin combination for prevention of conception. Oral contraceptives may produce a wide variety of metabolic changes and may cause alterations in carbohydrate and lipid metabolism, decreased blood levels of vitamin B_6, vitamin B_{12}, ascorbic acid, folate, riboflavin, magnesium, and zinc, and increased urinary excretion of xanthurenic acid and kynurenine, indicating interference with the normal pathway of tryptophan metabolism. It may also cause nausea, vomiting, fluid retention, and weight gain. Brand names include Brevicon, Demulen, Loestrin, Nordette, Norlestrin, Ortho-Novum, Ovcon, and Ovral.

Oral glucose tolerance test (OGTT). See *Glucose tolerance test.*

Oral hypoglycemic agent (OHA). Medication taken by mouth which lowers the blood glucose level. The most commonly used OHAs are the sulfonylureas. At least six compounds are available, classified as first generation (*tolbutamide, acetohexamide, tolazamide, chlorpropamide*) and second generation (*glyburide* and *glipizide*). Their duration of action ranges from 6 to 72 hours. They stimulate pancreatic insulin release, increase the number of insulin receptor sites or decrease insulin resistance, and decrease glucose production in the liver. OHAs are indicated for Type II diabetics who are either obese or of normal weight but in whom hyperglycemia still persist, despite compliance with the prescribed meal plan and exercise regimen. They should not have complications such as acidosis,

infections, severe trauma, hepatic or renal dysfunction, or diarrhea. OHAs are *contraindicated* for patients with juvenile diabetes, gestational diabetes, and for those who will undergo surgery. Side effects of OHAs include hypoglycemia, skin rash itchiness, headache, nausea, diarrhea, and rarely, anemia. The side effects occur less often with second-generation sulfonylureas. Other OHAs include phenformin, biguanides, and metformin. However, these are not currently approved by the Food and Drug Administration. See also *Diabetes mellitus* and *Insulin.*

Oral rehydration therapy. Solution developed by the World Health Organization to rehydrate children suffering from diarrhea, especially in countries where intravenous therapy may not be readily available. It can be made at home using potable water and given as a drink by a family member; it costs much less than intravenous therapy. The formula (per liter of water) consists of 75 to 100 mEq sodium, 20 to 30 mEq potassium, 20 to 30 mEq bicarbonate, and 75 to 100 mmol glucose. The osmolarity of the solution is 270 to 360 mOsm/liter. This oral solution has been used successfully in most cases of diarrhea, but not in severe cases when there is fluid loss of more than 10 ml/kg body weight per hour. It is not used in cases of shock and malabsorption. See also Appendix 38.

Ornithine. Diaminovaleric acid, an amino acid obtained from arginine by the hydrolytic removal of urea. Together with citrulline, arginine, and aspartic acid, it is an intermediate product in the cyclic process of urea formation.

Osmolality. The number of osmols or milliosmols of solutes per kilogram of water. Osmolality refers to the number of particles (solutes) in 1 liter of solvent, whereas *osmolarity* refers to the number of particles per liter of the solution (solute plus solvent). The normal osmolality of extracellular fluid is 280 to 300 mOsm/kg. Above this range is a condition of hyperosmolality which is associated with certain clinical signs and symptoms, such as electrolyte depletion and dehydration. Hyperosmolality may be brought about by feeding formulas of high osmolality or osmolarity. Smaller particles like glucose, free amino acids, and electrolytes contribute more to osmolality than do bigger particles like proteins and carbohydrates. Fats do not increase osmolality because of their insolubility in water. Serum osmolality is one of the most reliable parameters of fluid balance. It can be calculated indirectly using the following formula:

Serum osmolality

$$= 2 \times Na \ (mEq/liter) + \frac{BUN}{3} + \frac{glucose}{18}$$

where BUN = blood urea nitrogen in mg/dl and glucose is in mg/dl.

A measured osmolality as reported in a chemistry profile is usually slightly higher than a calculated osmolality. See also *Osmolarity* and *Osmotic pressure.*

Osmolarity. The number of osmols or milliosmols per liter of solution. Osmolarity therefore considers both solute and solvent, and is affected by the temperature of the solution and the number of particles present in it. Thus, osmolarity is more appropriate in describing the characteristics of an enteral or parenteral nutritional solution. The terms *hypotonic, isotonic,* and *hypertonic* are used to compare the mOsm/liter of a particular solution with that of plasma. For example, a hypertonic enteral formula given by jejunostomy feeding may result in diarrhea. Serum osmolarity can be estimated by the following formula:

Serum osmolarity (mOsm/L)

$$= 2(Na + K) + \frac{Glucose}{18} + \frac{BUN}{3}$$

where Na + K are in mEq/liter and glucose and BUN (blood urea nitrogen) are in mg/dl. Normal range is 275 to 295 mOsm/liter.

Osmolite. Brand name of an isotonic, lactose-free liquid formula for tube feeding or oral supplementation; contains sodium and calcium caseinates, soy protein isolates, hydro-lyzed cornstarch, MCT oil, and corn oil. Also available as Osmolite HN. See Appendix 39.

Osmosis. Passage of solvent through a membrane from a dilute solution to a more concentrated one to equalize the osmolality of the fluids on both sides of the membrane.

Osmotic pressure. "Attractive" or drawing force that many substances in solution exert on water molecules (or solvents). It is the force exerted by a solute that causes the solvent to pass through the semipermeable membrane until the concentration on both sides is approximately equal. The osmotic pressure of body fluids is due to the presence of various electrolytes and crystalloids. It is the number of particles, and not their size, that influences osmotic pressure. This pressure is the fundamental force underlying physiologic processes such as the interchange of materials between the blood and tissue cells, the excretion of urine, and the regulation of blood volume. However, osmotic pressure in the body is not constant. It varies as a result of metabolic processes and the concentrations of various constituents of the intra- and extracellular fluids. See also *Oncotic pressure.*

Osseous tissue. Bony tissue; *os* is Latin word meaning bone. See *Bone.*

Ossification. Process of bone formation. The *organic matrix* becomes strong and rigid as a result of calcification or deposition of minerals, chiefly calcium and phosphorus salts plus magnesium, carbonate, citrate, fluoride, and others in trace amounts. The structure resembles that of *hydroxyapatite* crystals, and the process is catalyzed by *vitamin D.*

Osteoarthritis. Also called "degenerative" or "hypertrophic arthritis"; a joint disorder characterized by degeneration of the articular cartilage and bony outgrowths around the joints. It is a painful disease associated with advancing age and is often seen in overweight or obese persons. Extra body weight puts a strain on the weight-bearing joints such as the ankles and knees. *Dietary management:* a weight reduction program is recommended for the obese.

Osteomalacia. Also called "adult rickets"; softening of the bones resulting from a lack of vitamin D, calcium, and/or phosphorus. There is inadequate mineralization of the organic matrix of bones, resulting in skeletal deformities, pain of the rheumatic type in bones of the legs and lower part of the back, and spontaneous multiple fractures. It is common among women who have become depleted of calcium because of repeated pregnancies and those who have little exposure to sunlight. Osteomalacia may occur when there is interference with fat absorption or defective metabolism of vitamin D, such as seen in severe liver disease, end-stage renal failure, and prolonged use of anticonvulsant drugs.

Osteomyelitis. An infection of the long bones and bone marrow due to certain bacteria, like *Escherichia coli, Staphylococcus aureus,* and *Streptococcus pyogenes.* Fever, chills, nausea and vomiting, acute joint pain, regional muscle spasm, and pressure sores are the usual symptoms. The patient may be on parenteral antibiotics and bed rest for several weeks. *Dietary management:* maintain fluid balance and ensure a liberal calorie and protein intake.

Osteopenia. A condition of subnormal bone density; the rate of bone matrix synthesis is not great enough to equal the rate of bone lysis. May be caused by cancer or hyperthyroidism. Associated with deficiencies of copper, manganese, and zinc, with overall reduction of bone calcification. Osteopenia has been observed to increase the incidence of fractures among the elderly. Treatment is similar to that of osteoporosis, with emphasis on intake of trace minerals.

Osteopetrosis. Condition in which bones become hard, brittle, and marble-like, referred to as "marble bones" or "ivory bones." There is generalized increase in bone density, associated with excessive fluoride intake. Considered an inborn error of metabolism, this inherited disorder in its advanced state causes severe anemia and deformities of the skull, with compression of cranial nerves which may lead to blindness and early death.

Osteoporosis. Bone disorder characterized by a reduction in total bone mass without a change in chemical composition. It occurs when the rate of bone resorption exceeds the rate of formation, resulting in bone loss and increased porosity. Bone formation remains the same with age, whereas bone resorption increases with age. The result is a gradual loss of bone. Osteoporosis is seen in persons after age 50, especially in women after monopause. Practically all people begin to lose bone at age 55. Clinical manifestations are low back pain that is sometimes severe, kyphosis of the dorsal spine, and skeletal fractures. The etiology of osteoporosis is multifactorial and includes the following age-related changes: decreased estrogen production associated with menopause, long-time low intake of calcium and decreased absorption of calcium, reduced circulating level of calcitriol, increased urinary loss of calcium, and reduced physical activity and immobilization. Calcium absorption from the intestine decreases with age, as does the usual dietary intake of calcium. Although the role of dietary factors is not clear, calcium deficiency must be considered a possible risk. The severity of bone loss can be ameliorated if there is a liberal intake of calcium throughout life, especially among women. Those who chronically have low intakes of calcium and are inactive appear to have a higher risk of osteoporosis than those who are physically active and have developed maximum bone mass. However, not all persons with low calcium intake develop osteoporosis. Treatment of osteoporosis is aimed at reducing bone resorption and includes a variety of measures, such as exercise, estrogen replacement therapy, calcium and vitamin D (alone or in combination), calcitonin, and fluoride.

Osteosarcoma. A malignant bone tumor of unknown etiology. It occurs primarily in adolescents and elderly people. Clinical signs and symptoms include weight loss, fatigue, fever, and pain in the affected area. *Dietary management:* guidelines are directed to the use of anticancer drugs, weight loss, and fever. Maintain a well-balanced diet consisting of foods tolerated by the patient, given in six feedings per day.

Ostomy. The surgical procedure of creating an opening, or stoma, in the wall of the abdomen. A feeding ostomy allows a feeding tube to be passed, as in esophagostomy, gastrostomy, and jejunostomy. Disorders which usually need ostomy procedures include colon and rectal cancers, Crohn's disease, severe diverticulitis, ulcerative colitis, and familial polyposis. Nutritional intervention is important for ostomates to maintain good nutriture and to avoid foods that cause flatulence, unpleasant odors, and obstructions. If steatorrhea occurs, fat restriction to about 30 gm/day is recommended. The use of an MCT diet is beneficial. As the patient's condition improves, introduce fiber to the diet gradually. See also *Colostomy* and *Ileostomy.*

OTC. 1. Abbreviation for *oxytetracycline.* 2. Abbreviation for over-the-counter drugs or nonprescription medications.

Ouch-Ouch disease. Disease reported only in Fuchu, Japan. It resembles *osteomalacia* combined with proteinuria and glycosuria. The locally grown rice and soybeans contain large amounts of cadmium, lead, and zinc. It has been suggested that cadmium plays a role in this disease.

Ovalbumin. The albumin of egg white. Although it is considered a simple *protein* because of its solubility and other physical properties, some authorities classify it with glycoproteins, since it contains small amounts of carbohydrate (less than 4% hexose).

Overeaters Anonymous. A self-help support group of volunteer members who meet regularly to discuss problems and help each other in coping with compulsive eating, binging, purging, and other concerns about weight control.

Overweight. Term applied to a person whose weight is about 10 to 20% above the desirable weight. An athlete with well-developed muscles may be overweight but not obese. See also *Obesity* and *Weight control.*

Ovoflavin. Name give to *riboflavin* in egg. See also *Vitamin B₂.*

Oxalate. Salt of oxalic acid; the end product of both glyoxylic and ascorbic acid metabolism. It occurs primarily in foods of plant origin; rich food sources are spinach, beets, rhubarb, berries, plums, and tea. Oxalates form insoluble calcium salts, rendering calcium unavailable for absorption. Urinary excretion of oxalate (oxaluria) is normally less than 60 mg/24 hours; small increases in urinary oxalate concentration enhance the potential for crystal formation.

Oxidation. Any chemical reaction that involves the addition of oxygen, the removal of hydrogen, or, in general, a loss of electrons and an increase in valence. In biologic systems, oxidation requires energy.

Oxidation-reduction (oxido-reduction). Oxidation involves a loss of electrons, and reduction involves a gain of electrons. Thus the electron donor or acceptor is itself oxidized or reduced during the process. Oxidation and reduction reactions occur simultaneously in cellular respiration.

Oxycalorimeter. Apparatus that determines the caloric value of food by measuring the amount of oxygen consumed. It is used in *indirect calorimetry.*

Oxygen (O). Nonmetallic element occurring free in the atmosphere as a colorless, tasteless gas. It is present in many substances combined with other elements. It constitutes 20% of the atmosphere and makes up 65% of body weight as part of water. Oxygen is essential to life for *respiration* and *physiologic oxidation.*

Oxygen debt. Deficit of oxygen that arises during continuous or intense exercise when energy cannot be adequately supplied by oxidative means and lactic acid accumulates faster than it can be oxidized. When exercise is finished, the depth of respiration is increased to provide more oxygen to oxidize the excess lactic acid that has accumulated. See *Lactic acid.*

Oxythiamin. Analog of thiamin in which a hydroxyl group is substituted for the free amino group on the pyrimidine ring. It is an antimetabolite and displaces thiamin from the tissues.

P

P. Chemical symbol for *phosphorus.*

PAA. Abbreviation for *plasma amino acids.*

PABA. Abbreviation for *para-aminobenzoic acid.*

Paget's disease. Also known as "osteitis deformans." A nonmetabolic bone disease of unknown etiology; a strong familial origin is indicated. Bone destruction can be excessive, accompanied by pains, headaches, enlarged skull, a tendency to fractures and anemia, and heart failure. *Dietary management:* maintain a normal diet but monitor anemia, especially due to serum iron and vitamin B_{12} deficiency.

Pancreas. Glandular organ extending across the upper abdomen close to the liver. It secretes into the intestinal tract the *pancreatic juice,* which contains enzymes that act on protein, fat, and carbohydrate. It also produces the hormones *insulin, glucagon,* and *somatostatin* elaborated by its islets of Langerhans. For more information on pancreatic enzymes, see Appendix 11.

Pancreatic insufficiency. Deficiency of pancreatic secretion, especially of the digestive enzymes (see Appendix 11). It may be congenital, as in cystic fibrosis, or caused by a number of diseases, such as carcinoma of the pancreas and pancreatitis. It may also result from pancreatectomy or from the destruction of exocrine function by ligation of the pancreatic duct. Symptoms include recurrent attacks of abdominal pain, alteration of bowel habits, and steatorrhea. Weight loss and malnutrition are due to malabsorption of proteins, fats, and fat-soluble vitamins. *Dietary management:* weight loss is corrected with a high caloric intake, usually between 2500 and 3500 kcal/day. Protein intake is 1.5 to 2.0 gm/kg/day, and carbohydrate is the main source of energy (at least 60% of total calories) in the form of simple sugars and easy-to-digest starches. Fat, which is poorly tolerated, is provided as medium-chain triglycerides, about 4 tablespoons/day. Generally, pancreatic enzymes given with meals relieve the condition.

Pancreatic juice. Digestive juice produced by the pancreas and secreted into the duodenum. It is alkaline (pH 7.5 to 8.0) and contains some protein and electrolytes, mainly sodium, potassium, bicarbonate, and chloride ions. It contains a number of enzymes involved in the digestion of protein, fat, and carbohydrate. For further details, see Appendix 11.

Pancreatin. Commercial preparation made from the pancreas of animals, usually the ox or hog. It contains the enzymes of pancreatic juice and is used to correct pancreatic insufficiency.

Pancreatitis. Inflammation of the pancreas. *Acute pancreatitis* is characterize by severe epigastric pain, nausea, vomiting, fever, and decreased peristalsis. The serum amylase level is elevated. However, the serum calcium level is decreased in some patients. If chylomicronemia occurs, withdrawal of long-chain fatty acids from the diet effectively relieves the clinical sign. *Chronic pancreatitis* is characterized by a disturbance in the functioning of the pancreas, leading to inadequate production of digestive enzymes. About 25% of patients develop pancreatic insufficiency. As a result, stools become bulky and foul-smelling, with increased excretion of protein, carbohydrate, and fat. Pancreatitis is associated with alcoholism, biliary tract disease, abdominal trauma, and hyperlipidemia. *Dietary management:* the basic aim is to rest the pancreas by restricting foods that stimulate its action. In the acute stage, nothing is given by mouth, and liquids are gradually introduced from clear to full and semisoft, restricting the fat intake to 20% of total calories (about 35 to 40 gm/day). Eventually, a soft, low-fat diet (about 35 to 40 gm/day) is given in six small feedings. Fat as medium-chain triglycerides is well tolerated. For chronic pancreatitis, pancreatic enzymes with meals and a low-fat diet are effective therapeutic measures. In some cases, supplemental vitamin B_{12} may be needed. Avoid alcoholic beverages.

Pancrelipase. A substance containing the enzymes lipase, amylase, and protease. It is used in the treatment of malabsorption syndrome caused by pancreatic insufficiency, as in cystic fibrosis and chronic pancreatitis. The dosage is determined by the fat content of the diet. About 2000 USP units of lipase activity are given before or with each meal for each 5 gm of dietary fat. Pancrelipase may decrease folate absorption. Brand names are Cotazym, Ilozyme, Pancrease, and Viokase.

Pangamic acid. D-Gluconodimethylaminoacetic acid, a natural substance present in foods that was first prepared from apricot pits and later from rice, liver, blood, and yeast. Little is known about the role of pangamate at the molecular level, although scientists in Europe and the Soviet Union have recorded enhanced oxygen uptake and better adaptation to hypoxia and strenuous exercise. Some effects on cardiovascular function and lowering of cholesterol have also been reported. Because of these physiologic effects, pangamic acid has been designated "vitamin B_{15}." However, there is no evidence that its lack in the diet results in a deficiency disease.

Pantothenic acid. A B complex vitamin named from the Greek word meaning "from everywhere." It is present in all living cells and was formerly called "chick antidermatitis factor" and "filtrate factor." As a component of coenzyme A and of the acyl carrier protein, pantothenic acid plays an important role in acetylation and acylation reactions; oxidation of keto acids and fatty acids; synthesis of triglycerides, steroids, phospholipids, and fatty acids; formation of acetylcholine; and synthesis of porphyrin for hemoglobin formation. As *acetyl CoA,* the vitamin functions in the metabolism of carbohydrate, protein, and fat. It is also necessary for the maintenance of normal skin and for the development of the central nervous system. Pantothenic acid is widely distributed among foods; good sources are liver, egg, meat, whole grain cereals, and legumes. It is readily absorbed from the small intestine and stored to some extent in the liver and kidneys. Dietary deficiency in humans has not been observed, although pantothenic acid has been implicated in the *burning feet syndrome* observed among prisoners in World War II, which responded to pantothenic acid administration but not to other members of the vitamin B complex. Experimental deficiency states in humans fed a semisynthetic diet virtually free of the vitamin or given a metabolic antagonist (omega-methylpantothenic acid, pantoyl taurine, or phenyl pantothenate) produced a syndrome characterized by fatigue, dermatitis, muscle cramps, paresthesia in extremities, susceptibility to infection, and loss of antibody production. Large amounts of pantothenic acid appear to help humans withstand stress, perhaps due to its effect on the adrenal gland. Deficiency in animals results in a wide range of defects such as growth retardation, abortion, infertility, graying of hair, severe dermatitis, myelin degeneration, convulsions, gastrointestinal disorders, adrenal cortical failure, and sudden death. Pantothenic acid is relatively nontoxic; however, ingestion of large amounts may cause diarrhea and water retention. See Appendix 2 for the estimated safe and adequate daily dietary intake.

Para-aminobenzoic acid (PABA). Formerly classified with the B complex vitamins. However, present knowledge maintains that it is not a vitamin for humans, although it plays an indirect role as a component of *folic acid.*

Para-aminosalicylic acid (PAS). A synthetic antituberculosis agent, commercially available as the acid and the sodium salt. The most frequent adverse effects are gastrointestinal disturbances including nausea, vomiting, anorexia, abdominal pain, and diarrhea. Malabsorption of vitamin B_{12}, folic acid, iron, and lipids may also occur, possibly as the result of increased peristalsis. Brand names are P.A.S., Parasal, and Pasna.

Parasympathetic nervous system. Part of the autonomic nervous system comprising preganglionic fibers that arise from the midbrain, the medulla, or the sacral region of the spinal cord. It controls the activity below the level of consciousness, e.g., gland secretion, intestinal action, and heart function.

Parathormone (PTH). Parathyroid hormone or parathyrin, a protein consisting of a single polypeptide chain with alanine as its N-terminal amino acid. Secreted by the parathyroid glands, it exerts a profound effect on the metabolism of calcium and phosphorus. Administration of the hormone raises the blood calcium level and lowers the blood phosphorus level, increases the elimination of phosphorus in the urine, causes migration of calcium from the bones if there is an insufficient supply of this element in the food, and increases the *phosphatase* activity of the serum.

Parathyroid glands. Two pairs of small endocrine glands located in the posterior part of the thyroid gland, a pair in each lobe, one below the other. They are reddish or yellowish brown, egg-shaped bodies weighing a total of 0.1 to 0.2 gm in humans. Their secretion is concerned chiefly with calcium and phosphorus metabolism. Insufficient secretion results in a decrease of calcium and phosphorus ions in the blood, causing *tetany.* Oversecretion results in increased calcium in the blood and increased excretion of phosphate through the kidneys. As a result, there is muscular weakness, and calcium phosphate stones are formed.

Parenteral feeding (nutrition). A means of providing nutrients by routes other than through the mouth and digestive tract, such as subcutaneous, intramuscular, or intravenous feeding. A common example is the standard intravenous (IV) dextrose (D_5W) with added electrolytes through the peripheral veins. This provides an immediate source of energy (about 170 kcal/liter/day) until the patient can eat normally. Parenteral feedings can be used in addition to enteral feedings, or used alone. If parenteral feed-

ing is the main source of nutrition, other nutrients have to be given via the small veins, usually in the arm (called peripheral parenteral nutrition or PPN), or centrally into the superior or inferior vena cava or the jugular vein (called central parenteral nutrition or CPN). Central parenteral nutrition is also called total parenteral nutrition (TPN) or intravenous hyperalimentation (IVH) which is a misnomer since parenteral nutrition does not contain an excessive or "hyper" amount of any nutrient. The decision to use PPN or CPN is based on the number of calories needed and the osmolarity of the solution. Hypertonic solutions can not be given in peripheral veins which have low blood flow; the area can become infiltrated and inflamed, or a thrombosis can occur. If administered via CPN, a hypertonic solution can be quickly diluted by the rapid flow of blood. PPN is usually used for brief periods, but central vein parenteral nutrition (CPN) may be used for a longer time. See also *Total parenteral nutrition.*

Parenteral nutrients. Dextrose solutions and fat emulsions are the energy substrates commonly used. Synthetic crystalline L-amino acid solutions are used to provide nitrogen for protein synthesis. Vitamins, minerals, and fluid (water) are added to meet the patient's needs. See Appendices 40, 41, and 42.

Carbohydrate (dextrose). Carbohydrate is given as a dextrose monohydrate which provides 3.4 kcal/gm. Dextrose solutions are available in 5%, 10%, 20%, 30%, 50% and 70% solutions. The osmolarity of a dextrose solution increases with its concentration. See Appendix 43. The 5% solution is the only product within the range of normal serum osmolarity (275 to 296 mmol/kg); all the other solutions are hypertonic. The 5% and 10% solutions can be given by PPN; all the other solutions are given by CPN. The most widely used in parenteral nutrition is the 50% solution.

Fat emulsion. To prevent essential fatty acid deficiency, fat emulsion is given several times a week, if it is not used daily as a calorie source. Fat emulsions are derived from soybean oil and safflower oil; these are available in concentrations of 10% (provides 1.1 kcal/cc) and 20% (provides 2.0 kcal/cc). The emulsions are made isotonic by the addition of glycerol, giving an osmolarity of 270 to 340 mmol/liter. Fat infusion should be introduced slowly, and gradually increased in kind and amount.

Fluid (water). Provide a minimum of 1 ml/ kcal or 100 ml free water per gram nitrogen. Fluid is restricted immediately after myocardial infarction or in kidney failure, but is increased when fluid losses have to be replenished, as in wound drainage, diarrhea, fever, and other hypercatabolic states. Fluid monitoring is very important, especially with the elderly, infants, and young children.

Minerals. Mineral requirements should be adequately met. Electrolytes are added to some of the commercially prepared amino acid solutions (See Appendix 40). Specific electrolytes may be reduced, depending upon the disorder (e.g., sodium in cardiovascular and renal conditions, and potassium in scanty urinary output). Serum levels of the trace elements, in addition to those of the macro-minerals, must be monitored. Trace elements like copper, iodine, selenium, and zinc, have been found to be deficient in prolonged use of total parenteral nutrition. Supplementation that meets established guidelines for parenteral trace elements are also commercially available.

Protein (amino acids). Several amino acid formulations are available in 3.0%, 3.5%, 5.0%, 7.0%, 8.5%, 10.0%, and 15% solutions, with or without added electrolytes. Introduce protein solutions with care to avoid ammonia intoxication. For patients with renal or hepatic failure, the infusion rate is slower. Special formulations are available commercially for such conditions; those containing branched-chain amino acids have been effective.

Vitamins. The U.S. recommended dietary allowances for vitamins do not apply to parenteral nutrition, because the absorptive process is by-passed. Parenteral vitamin supplementation is based on recommendations by the American Medical Association Nutrition Advisory Group (AMA/NAG). Several commercial products are available that encompass these guidelines. See Appendix 42.

Paresthesia. An abnormal sensation characterized as burning, pricking, or tingling. It is seen in *beriberi* and other disorders involving the nerves and spinal cord.

Parietal. 1. Of or pertaining to the walls of a cavity. Parietal cells found on the margin of the peptic glands of the stomach that secrete hydrochloric acid. 2. The parietal bone that forms part of the sides and top of the skull.

Parkinson's disease. A neurologic condition marked by muscular rigidity and tremors, abnormal gait and balance, slurred speech, poor mastication, and dysphagia. It is a progressive disabling disease characterized by a low concentration of the neurotransmitter *dopamine* at the basal ganglia of the brain. Of unknown etiology, it responds to therapy with the drug *levodopa* or its combination with carbidopa (Sinemet). *Dietary management:* modifications focus on the dysphagia and difficulty in self-feeding, plus the nutrient-drug interactions. If the patient is taking levodopa, a high level of protein interferes with this drug. Restrict protein to 0.8 gm/kg/day. Patients responding poorly to levodopa may benefit from the intake of low protein meals for breakfast and lunch, followed by an evening meal that provides the balance of 0.8 gm/kg/day allowance for protein. Give proteins of high biologic value, modifying the consistency according to the chewing and swallowing abilities of the patient. Serve the protein-rich foods mainly in the evening meal. Tyrosine (a precursor of dopamine) may be beneficial. Limit the intake of pyridoxine to less than 5 mg/day to make levodopa more effective. Avoid constipation and encourage the intake of fluids. See also *Dysphagia*.

Parorexia. Abnormal craving for special foods, as opposed to *anorexia*.

Patch test. Skin test for allergy administered by applying the suspected antigen to a filter paper and placing it on a certain patch of skin. The area is uncovered after 2 to 4 days and compared with an unpatched skin area.

Pb. Chemical symbol for lead.

PBI. Abbreviation for *protein-bound iodine*.

PCM. Abbreviation for *protein-calorie malnutrition.*

Peak bone mass. Bone growth is characterized by an increase in longitudinal growth and in bone mass. Peak bone mass is attained about 5 to 10 years after adolescence or in early adulthood. Adequate dietary calcium (about 1200 mg/day for adults in their mid-twenties) is important for achieving peak bone mass. This is a preventive measure against *osteoporosis* in later life.

Pectic substances. Also called "pectins." Group designation for complex colloidal carbohydrate derivatives that occur in or are prepared from plants. They contain a large proportion of anhydrogalacturonic acids and are considered soluble fibers. See *Dietary fibers* under *Fiber.*

Pedialyte. Brand name of a ready-to-use oral electrolyte solution for maintenance of water and electrolytes during mild to moderate diarrhea in infants and children. Also available as Pedialyte RS for replacement of water and electrolytes during moderate to severe diarrhea. See Appendix 38.

Pediasure. Brand name of a lactose-free, isotonic, enteral formula for children aged 1 to 6 years old who are undernourished because of illness, poor appetite, or inability to eat.

Pellagra. From *pelle,* meaning "skin," and *agra,* meaning "rough." A deficiency disease due to lack of niacin (nicotinic acid); characterized by dermatitis, diarrhea, dementia, and eventually death if unremedied. These pellagrous symptoms are commonly referred to as the classic "four Ds." The skin changes occur in several stages: there is thickening and pigmentation with temporary redness similar to that of sunburn, then atrophic thinning with dark red eruption, and finally desquamation. In the severe stage the involved parts erupt and swell, with ulceration and infection. Typical pellagrous dermatosis is symmetric, clearly demarcated, and hyerpigmented. Parts of the body exposed to sunlight are commonly affected, e.g., the cheeks, neck, hands, and forearms. The digestive disturbances include sore mouth with angular stomatitis, bright red or scarlet tongue with glossitis, achlorhydria, and nausea and vomiting, followed by severe diarrhea. The neurologic disturbances include insomnia, irritability, poor memory, confusion, delusions of persecution, hallucinations, and dementia. See also *Casal's necklace.*

Pelvic inflammatory disease (PID). Inflammation of the pelvic cavity that affects the fallopian tubes and ovaries. Symptoms include abdominal, pelvic, and low back pains accompanied by fever and vaginal discharge. *Dietary management:* maintain a well-balanced diet and control body weight. Restore fluid and electrolyte balance. Increase caloric intake if fever is a serious problem. Frequent feedings are suggested, with supplementary vitamins and minerals.

PEM. Abbreviation for *protein-energy malnutrition.*

Penicillamine. A degradation product of all penicillins; used in the treatment of Wilson's disease, cystinuria, and lead intoxication. Penicillamine can chelate copper, cystine, mercury, lead, and other heavy metals by forming soluble complexes which are excreted by the kidneys. However, the drug can also chelate iron, zinc, and pyridoxine and may cause depletion of these nutrients. It may also cause partial or total loss of taste perception, particularly for saltiness and sweetness, as well as anorexia and weight loss. Adverse gastrointestinal effects include diarrhea, nausea, vomiting, dyspepsia, epigastric pain, colitis, and reactivation of peptic ulcer. Brand names are Cuprimine and Depen.

Penicillin. Natural or semisynthetic antibiotic produced by or derived from certain species of the fungus *Penicillium.* It is bacteriostatic for many microorganisms and useful in the treatment of infections caused by most of the gram-positive bacteria. Frequent adverse gastrointestinal effects are epigastric distress, nausea, vomiting, sore mouth or tongue, diarrhea, and colitis. It may also cause electrolyte imbalances, especially in patients with impaired renal function. Brand names include Bicillin, Pentids, Tegopen, and Wycillin.

Pentosan. Also called "pentan"; a homopolysaccharide or a complex carbohydrate of pentose units that is widely distributed in wood, straw, gums, hulls, and corncobs. It is not digested by humans, but it is hydrolyzed by acid to yield pentoses. Examples are arabans and xylans.

Pentose. A 5-carbon monosaccharide. Pentoses important to nutrition are arabinose, xylose, ribose, 2-deoxyribose, xylulose, and ribulose. The first four are aldoses and do not occur free in nature; the last two are ketoses. Arabinose is obtained by hydrolyzing various gummy substances; xylose is derived from wood and straw; ribose and deoxyribose are constituents of *nucleic acids;* xylulose is often the sugar found in the urine in *pentosuria;* and ribulose is found only as an intermediate metabolite in the *hexose monophosphate shunt.* See also *Pentosan* and *Riboflavin.*

Pentosuria. Excretion of pentose in the urine. *Alimentary pentosuria* occurs temporarily in normal individuals after ingestion of large amounts of prunes, cherries, grapes, and other foods rich in pentoses (mainly arabinose and xylose). *Congenital pentosuria* is due to an inborn error of metabolism; the body cannot metabolize L-xylulose.

Pepsin. Digestive enzyme in gastric juice that converts protein to peptones and proteoses. It occurs in the stomach as an inactive precursor, *pepsinogen,* which is converted to the active pepsin by hydrochloric acid.

Peptamen. Brand name of an isotonic, elemental formula containing enzymatically hydrolyzed whey protein, maltodextrin, starch, MCT oil, and sunflower oil. See also Appendix 39.

Pepti 2000. Brand name of an elemental enteral formula of short-chain peptides as the primary protein source. Contains hydrolyzed lactalbumin, maltodextrin, MCT oil, and corn oil. See also Appendix 39.

Peptic ulcer disease (PUD). Ulceration on the mucous membranes of the esophagus, stomach, or duodenum caused by hyperacidity, lowered cellular resistance, insufficient mucus secretion, local trauma, and predisposing factors. The exact etiology is not known, although individuals prone to peptic ulcer include those with a family history of recurrent episodes; emotional, highly stressed persons; chronic users of alcohol and of certain drugs, like aspirin; and possibly those with susceptibility to the bacterium *Campylobacter pyloridis.* The main symptom of peptic ulcer is epigastric pain 1 to 3 hours after meals, characterized as a burning, gnawing, or sharp pain. This is relieved by eating or by using alkalis or antacids. Clinical signs include weight loss, low plasma protein, anemia, and hemorrhaging. *Dietary management:* with modern drug therapy, which is now the treatment of choice, dietary restrictions are minimal. The traditional bland diet is no longer used because of the wide variations among individuals as to which foods are irritating to them. The emphasis now is on the frequency and volume of feeding per meal or snack. Except for alcohol, caffeine, strong spices, and gas formers, the only foods avoided are those not tolerated. Soft and soluble fibers are encouraged to prevent constipation, which is a side effect of antacid use. See also *Diet, bland.*

Peptide. Compound formed when two or more amino acids are linked together by the

$$-\overset{\overset{\textstyle O}{\|}}{C}-\overset{\overset{\textstyle H}{|}}{N}-$$

linkage, called the *peptide linkage,* which is the main bond in protein structure. See also *Protein.*

Peptone. A secondary protein derivative. When protein is hydrolyzed, it is changed to proteoses, then to peptones, peptides, and finally amino acids. Peptones as distinguished from proteoses, are not precipitated by ammonium sulfate or tannic acid. *Peptonization* is the conversion of protein to peptones, using suitable proteolytic enzymes such as those found in *pancreatin* or pancreatic juice.

PER. Abbreviation for *protein efficiency ratio.*

Pericarditis. Inflammation of the pericardium; may be caused by trauma, infection, uremia, myocardial infarction, rheumatic fever, tuberculosis, or collagen disease. Symptoms are chest pains radiating to the shoulder and neck, dyspnea, dry cough, anxiety, mild fever, difficulty in breathing, and rapid pulse rate. *Dietary management:* initially, parenteral fluids may be required. As the patient recovers, oral feeding is given, following the dietary modifications for *myocardial infarction.*

Periodontal disease. Any pathologic condition of the supporting tissues surrounding the teeth. The main characteristic is the inflammation of the gums due to plaque and microbial flora buildup, caused by poor dental hygiene and *pyorrhea alveolaris.* Periodontal diseases are classified as inflammatory (gingivitis and periodontitis), dystrophic (trauma and periodontosis), and other abnormalities of the areas surrounding the teeth. *Dietary management:* ensure adequate intake of protein, calcium, and phosphorus. Maintain a normal calcium/phosphorus ratio. Supplement with fortified milk (for vitamins A and D), fluoride, and zinc. Raw vegetables and fruits are recommended.

Peristalsis. Normal wavy movement of the gastrointestinal tract characterized by alternate contraction and relaxation along the walls from the esophagus to the intestine, forcing the contents toward the anus. *Reverse peristalsis* is an abnormal backward movement of the intestine, as seen in pyloric obstruction and *diverticulitis.*

Peritoneal cavity. Region bordered by the parietal layer of the peritoneum. It contains all the abdominal organs except the kidneys.

Peritoneal dialysis. Process of removing excess fluid and metabolic waste products from the body by filtering the blood artificially using a hyperosmolar solution. The peritoneal membrane acts as the semipermeable membrane for the exchange of fluids. One method, known as "continuous ambulatory peritoneal dialysis (CAPD)," introduces the dialysate directly into the peritoneal cavity and is successfully used at home. A disposable container for the dialysate is permanently inserted by means of a catheter and is left in the peritoneum and exchanged manually 3 to 5 times a day. The

other type of peritoneal dialysis for home use is called "continuous cycling peritoneal dialysis (CCPD)." This technique uses an automated device for night therapy. Compared with CAPD, there is a minimal risk of peritonitis with CCPD. The most common dialysates are 1.5, 2.5, or 4.25% dextrose in 1.5 to 2 liters of solution. Protein is lost with each exchange of dialysis. As much as 30 gm protein may be lost per 24 hour treatment; protein loss increases with peritonitis. An estimation of protein loss is about 0.5 gm/l dialysate with a normal peritoneum and 1.0 gm/l with peritonitis. *Dietary management:* protein intake is increased to 1.2 gm/kg/day in CAPD or CCPD; as much as 1.5 gm/kg/day is needed in cases of peritonitis. Adjust the caloric intake depending on glucose absorption from the solution. On the average, 30 to 35 kcal/kg/day is allowed. If weight loss is desired, calorie intake is limited to 25 kcal/kg/day. Because this type of dialysis is continuous, sodium and potassium need not be restricted. However, monitor the serum levels of sodium potassium, and phosphorus and adjust intakes accordingly. Usually, 3 gm sodium, 2 gm potassium, and 1 gm phosphorus may be ordered. For hypotensive patients, a high-sodium diet is beneficial. Fluid intake is not restricted but should be limited when the weight gain between dialysis treatments exceeds 1 lb. Since water-soluble vitamins are lost during dialysis, supplementation is recommended.

Peritonitis. Inflammation of the peritoneum due to the introduction of bacteria or irritating substances into the abdominal cavity by a wound or perforation of an organ in the gastrointestinal or reproductive tract. It is accompanied by fever, abdominal pain, vomiting, and constipation. *Dietary management:* initially, the patient is given intravenous feedings and nothing by mouth. When gastrointestinal tract or bowel sounds are present, resume feeding by mouth, starting with clear liquids and progressing to a nutritional formula to supplement a full liquid diet. Monitor fluid and electrolyte balances. Provide soft to regular diets as the patient's condition improves, considering his or her food tolerances.

Permeability. Property or state of being penetrated. *Capillary permeability* is the property of the capillary walls that allows filtration and diffusion. This is important in the exchange of substances between the blood and tissue fluids. See also *Osmosis.*

Pernicious. Causing injury or death; destructive or incurable. *Pernicious anemia* is a misnomer since the advent of liver extract and vitamin B_{12} therapy. However, the term is retained traditionally to designate a clinical entity.

Pernicious anemia. A chronic macrocytic anemia found mostly in middle-aged and elderly persons. The red blood cells cannot be supplied by the bone marrow as rapidly as needed because of vitamin B_{12} deficiency conditioned by the lack of intrinsic factor. This factor is a glycoprotein found normally in gastric juice and is essential for the absorption of vitamin B_{12}. Pernicious anemia is characterized by disturbances in the gastrointestinal, nervous, and blood-forming systems. The symptoms are achlorhydria, atrophy of the gastric mucosa, diarrhea, glossitis, paresthesia, ataxia, degeneration of the lateral and posterior tracts of the spinal cord, macrocytosis that is often hyperchromic, and hyperplastic bone marrow. Treatment consists of intramuscular or subcutaneous injection of vitamin B_{12}. See also *Vitamin B_{12}.*

Peroxidation. Formation of peroxides as a result of the action of oxygen on polyunsaturated fatty acids. Vitamin E prevents lipid peroxidation in cells.

Perspiration. Also called "sweat"; secretion and exudation of fluid by the sweat glands of the skin, averaging about 700 ml/day. See also *Insensible perspiration.*

Petechiae. Small pinpoint-sized, nonraised, purplish-red spots on the skin formed by a subcutaneous effusion of blood. It is seen in vitamin C deficiency.

PGA. Abbreviation for *pteroylglutamic acid.*

pH. Symbol commonly used in expressing hydrogen ion concentration; a measure of alkalinity and acidity. It is the logarithm of the reciprocal of the hydrogen ion concentration. Examples of pH values of body fluids are as follows: blood serum, 7.35 to 7.45; cerebrospinal fluid, 7.35 to 7.45; gallbladder bile, 5.4 to 6.9; pure gastric juice, 0.9; pancreatic juice, 7.5 to 8.0; saliva, 6.35 to 6.85; and urine, 4.5 to 7.5.

Phagocyte. Cell that can engulf particles or cells that are foreign or harmful to the body. Phagocytes are present in the blood, lymph, lungs, liver, and spleen.

Phagocytosis. Also called "pinocytosis." Process of ingesting a moving or foreign particle through the cell membrane. It is one of the body's defense mechanisms against bacteria and other harmful substances. In this process, a portion of the cellular membrane envelops the foreign body by forming a small pocket outside the cell and then pinches it off from the surface to create an intracellular vacuole. Phagocytosis is also an important process in the absorption of certain nutrients. See *Absorption, nutrients.*

Phaseolin. A simple protein of the globulin type occurring in kidney beans.

Phenelzine. A monoamine oxidase inhibitor antidepressant agent. See *Monamine oxidase.*

Phenobarbital. A barbiturate used as a sedative, hypnotic, and anticonvulsant. It may cause vitamin D deficiency, especially in children, by inactivation of 25-hydroxyvitamin D. It may also decrease thiamin absorption, increase vitamin C excretion in urine, and lower serum levels of folacin, vitamin B_{12}, pyridoxine, magnesium, and calcium. It is excreted in breast milk. Brand names are Barbita, Luminal, and Solfoton.

Phenolphthalein. A stimulant laxative: a diphenylmethane derivative. Abuse of this drug can cause potassium depletion and decreased absorption of vitamin D, glucose, calcium, and other minerals. Brand names include Agoral, Alophen, Correctol, and Ex-Lax.

Phenylalanine (Phe). Alpha-amino-beta-phenylpropionic acid, an *essential amino acid* rarely limiting in protein foods. It is easily converted to *tyrosine,* but the reaction is not reversible. As a precursor of tyrosine, phenylalanine is also involved in reactions in which tyrosine plays a direct role, as in melanin formation. Phenylalanine participates in *transamination* and can be ketogenic as well as glycogenic. See also *Phenylketonuria.*

Phenylbutazone. A pyrazole derivative which is a nonsteroidal anti-inflammatory agent used in the treatment of gout and rheumatoid arthritis. It may decrease serum folate, increase urinary protein and uric acid, and cause weight gain due to sodium and fluid retention. Adverse gastrointestinal effects include abdominal and epigastric distress, stomatitis, dry mouth or throat, anorexia, gastritis, peptic ulcer, and gastrointestinal bleeding. Brand names are Azolid and Butazolidin.

Phenyl-free. Brand name of a phenylalanine-free supplement for older children with *phenylketonuria;* contains all the essential amino acids except phenylalanine, sucrose, corn syrup solids, modified tapioca, and corn oil. Its use allows a greater variety of natural foods containing phenylalanine. See Appendix 37.

Phenylketonuria (PKU). An inborn defect in phenylalanine metabolism due to a lack of the liver enzyme phenylalanine hydroxylase, which is needed in the conversion of phenylalanine to tyrosine. As a result, phenylalanine and its metabolite, phenylpyruvic acid, accumulate in the blood and tissues and are eventually excreted in the urine. Abnormal amounts of unmetabolized phenylalanine interfere with normal brain development and may cause severe mental retardation. There is also poor growth, nonspecific neurologic abnormalities, minor seizures, an eczema-like skin eruption, and reduced pigment production resulting in fair skin and blond hair. The treatment requires dietary restriction of phenylalanine. See *Diet, phenylalanine-restricted.*

Phenytoin. A hydantoin-derivative anticonvulsant used in the management of seizures. A high intake of folic acid (greater than 5 mg/day) can interfere with seizure control. However, long-term drug administration can induce folate deficiency, with the develop-

ment of megaloblastic anemia; vitamin D deficiency and a decrease in bone density, which may result in rickets in children and osteomalacia in adults; and vitamin K deficiency with bleeding, especially in the infants of mothers who have been taking the drug. The drug is excreted in breast milk. Brand names are Dilantin, Diphenylan, and Ditan.

Pheochromocytoma. A rare disease caused by a vascular tumor of the adrenal medulla that causes the production of abnormal amounts of *catecholamines.* Various cardiovascular and metabolic disturbances are associated with this disorder, such as hypertension, palpitations, hyperglycemia, and heart failure. *Dietary management:* modifications focus on the clinical signs and symptoms. Encourage intake of fluids without caffeine and give small, frequent feedings. If the patient has to undergo surgery, the standard surgical care procedures are observed. See also *Vanillylmandelic acid* and *Diet, VMA test.*

Phlorizin. Also spelled "phlorhizin"; a bitter-tasting glycoside from the root bark of apple, cherry, plum, and pear trees. It causes glycosuria by blocking the tubular reabsorption of glucose. It is used as a test for kidney function and to examine the formation of glucose from other ingredients of the diet.

Phosphatase. Enzyme that hydrolyzes monophosphoric esters, with the liberation of inorganic phosphate. It is found in practically all cells, body fluids, and tissues. Phosphatases constitute a large and complex group of enzymes, some of which appear to be highly specific.

Phosphate bond energy. Energy trapped in the phosphate bond of "phosphate carriers," which are of two categories: the relatively inert types, or those that release 3000 calories on hydrolysis, such as triose phosphates, and the active phosphate carriers that yield 5000 to 12,000 calories for each energy-rich bond hydrolyzed. To the latter group belongs creatine phosphate and adenosine di- and triphosphate. The energy released by the energy-rich bonds is used mainly for biologic oxidation in muscular work and maintenance of cell potential.

Phosphocreatine. Also called "creatine phosphate"; a constituent of the muscles that acts as a phosphate donor when hydrolyzed into creatine and phosphate. For its biologic role, see *Creatine.*

Phosphoinositide. Inositol-containing phosphatides. The synthesis and degradation of these compounds occur mainly in the brain. On hydrolysis, phosphoinositide yields glycerol, L-myoinositol, fatty acids, and phosphoric acid. These compounds are important in the transport processes of the cells and in hormone action.

Phospholipid. Also called "phosphatide"; substituted fat containing a phosphoric acid residue, nitrogenous compounds, and other constituents in addition to fatty acids and glycerol. Phospholipids include *lecithins, sphingomyelins, cephalins,* and *plasmalogens.* Sphingomyelins contain 4-sphingenine in place of glycerol. Phospholipids are essential components of the cell membrane. They play a role in electron transport, stimulate protein synthesis in special systems, affect cell permeability in ion transport, affect fat absorption and transport, and induce blood coagulation with the formation of thromboplastin.

Phosphoprotein. Conjugated protein compounds with a phosphorus radical other than nucleic acid (nucleoproteins) or lecithin. To this group belong the ovovitellin of egg yolk and the casein of milk.

Phosphorus. An essential mineral that comprises 22% of the total minerals in the body. Of this, 85% is in bones and teeth as insoluble calcium phosphate (apatite) crystals, and the rest occurs in soft tissues, cells, and in combination with enzymes, proteins, carbohydrates, and lipids and other compounds. Practically all biologic reactions need phosphorus to form adenosine triphosphate and in enzyme systems for energy metabolism. Phosphorus, together with calcium, gives rigidity to bones and teeth; is a constituent of a buffer system and helps to regulate the pH of blood; transports fatty acids as phospholipids; is a component of nucleic acids; and regulates osmotic pressure. Phosphorus is present in nearly all foods; hence, dietary lack is unlikely. Foods rich in protein and calcium are also good sources of phosphorus, such as milk, cheese, meats, whole grain cereals, and legumes. Phosphorus deficiency may occur with intravenous administration of glucose or total parenteral nutrition without sufficient phosphorus and with excessive use of a aluminum hydroxide antacid, which binds phosphorus and makes it unavailable for absorption. Characteristic symptoms of deficiency are similar to those of calcium deficiency and include weakness, malaise, pain, anorexia, and bone loss. Phosphorus deficiency may also be seen in small premature infants fed human milk exclusively. Such infants need more phosphorus than is contained in human milk for the rate of bone mineralization required; without additional phosphorus, hypophosphatemic rickets may develop. There is no evidence of phosphorus toxicity. See Appendix 1 for the recommended dietary allowances.

Photophobia. Abnormal sensitivity to light as seen in riboflavin deficiency.

Phylloquinone. Vitamin K_1; homolog of *vitamin K* synthesized by plants. It is especially abundant in alfalfa and green leafy vegetables, and probably accounts for most of the vitamin obtained from the diet.

Phytanic acid. An oxidation product of *phytol* which is found in a large variety of foods. An enzymatic defect in the metabolism of phytanic acid results in *Refsum's* disease, a rare autosomal recessive disorder.

Pica. An abnormal craving for unusual articles such as hair, clay, chalk, laundry starch, and dirt. Although this is rarely seen in humans, it presents a nutritional problem when it occurs. It has been associated with iron and zinc deficiencies. The cause is not well understood. It has been observed in hysteria, mentally defective children, and some pregnant women.

PID. Abbreviation for *pelvic inflammatory disease.*

PIH. Abbreviation for *pregnancy-induced hypertension.*

Pinocytosis. 1. Process whereby a cell absorbs liquids. The membrane invaginates and then closes to form a liquid-filled vacuole. It is similar to *phagocytosis,* whereby a cell engulfs solid particles.

Pituitary gland. See *Hypophysis.*

PKU. Abbreviation for *phenylketonuria.*

Placebo. An inactive substance or preparation that has no effect but is similar in appearance to a substance being tested. It is used in metabolic and controlled studies to determine the efficacy of substances.

Placenta. A highly vascular organ within the uterus that is the means of communication between the fetus and mother through the umbilical cord. The maternal and fetal blood supplies are separated by two thin membranes that eventually fuse. All fetal nourishment must pass through this barrier. The placenta also elaborates hormones needed for normal pregnancy.

Plasma. 1. The liquid portion of the blood in which corpuscles are suspended. (When fibrinogen is separated from the plasma by blood clotting, the remaining fluid is called *serum.*) 2. The lymph without its cells. 3. The cytoplasm or protoplasm.

Plasma amino acids (PAA). The amino acid levels in the plasma which can be used as a measure of protein quality. It is expressed as follows:

$$PAA = \frac{B - A}{Amino\ acid\ needs} \times 100$$

where A and B are plasma amino acid concentrations measured immediately before and after the meal. See also *Protein quality.*

Plasma protein. Any of the proteins in the blood plasma (e.g., albumin, globulin, fibrinogen, prothrombin). Plasma proteins constitute about 7% of the blood plasma in the body. They help maintain water balance, blood pressure, and blood viscosity. Fibrinogen and prothrombin are important in blood coagulation.

Plasma volume. The total volume of plasma in the body. The normal plasma volume in males is about 39 ml/kg of body weight; for females, it is about 40 ml/kg of body weight. Plasma volume is decreased in dehydration, Addison's disease and shock. It is increased in vitamin C deficiency and in liver disorders.

Plumbism. Chronic *lead* poisoning characterized by poor appetite, vomiting, headache, pain in the joints, pallor, colic, and increased restlessness. In severe cases, lead poisoning affects the bone marrow, kidneys, and nervous system, which may result in convulsions and coma. Lead interferes with the activity of several enzymes involved in hematopoiesis; the anemia resulting from lead toxicity can be severe. Damage to the kidneys leads to increased excretion of phosphates and amino acids and interferes with the formation of the active metabolite of vitamin D. Lead and lead compounds are found in lead-based paints in many old homes and homemade toys and furniture, and in ceramic glazes, leaded gasoline, and industrial processing. The absorption of lead is 5 to 10 times higher in children than in adults.

PNI. Abbreviation for *prognostic nutritional index.*

Poliomyelitis. An infectious disease caused by one of three polioviruses. The nonparalytic form lasts for periods ranging from a few days to a week and is characterized by fever, malaise, nausea and vomiting, and back stiffness. The paralytic form has all the clinical signs and symptoms of the nonparalytic type plus paralysis. The large proximal muscles of the limbs are often affected, and in the bulbar type of poliomyelitis, the brain stem and spinal cord are affected. *Dietary management:* nutrition intervention is very important due to the high fever, nausea, and vomiting. Tube feeding may be needed in some cases. Foods that tend to produce mucus, usually milk and cream, are generally not tolerated and should be avoided. The paralytic patient needs assistance in feeding. See *Dysphagia* and *Fever.*

Polycose. Brand name of a carbohydrate supplement consisting of glucose polymers in liquid or powder form. It is tasteless, mixes readily with foods and beverages, and requires little or no amylase for digestion. See also Appendix 39.

Polycythemia vera. Also called "Osler's disease." An acute, progressive disorder marked by increased erythrocyte or red blood cell levels. Other clinical signs are flatulence and fullness, headaches, vertigo, chest pain, gout, seizures, speech impairment, and flushed face and hands. Dietary management is similar to that of *congestive heart failure.*

Polydipsia. Excessive thirst due to loss of body fluids, especially from the urine, as seen in diabetes mellitus.

Polyneuritis. A condition that involves the inflammation of many nerves. It occurs in thiamin deficiency.

Polyneuropathy. Multiple noninflammatory degeneration of nerves. Nutritional polyneuropathy is caused by a lack of nutrients, particularly the B complex vitamins. It is characterized by bilateral lesions of the legs, with cramps, ataxia, foot drop, loss of vibratory and positional sense, and paresthesia. It is seen in beriberi, chronic alcoholism, and starvation.

Polypeptide. A long chain of amino acids (usually about 100 units) linked by the peptide bond. Polypeptides are smaller than proteins, but larger than proteoses.

Polyphagia. 1. Swallowing abnormally large amounts of food at a meal. 2. Excessive appetite as in diabetes mellitus.

Polysaccharide. A carbohydrate containing ten or more monosaccharide units. Those of nutritional significance are glycogen, starch, and dietary fiber. See Appendix 8.

Polyunsaturated fatty acid (PUFA). A fatty acid that has more than one unsaturated linkage in its carbon chain. See *Fatty acid.*

Polyuria. Excessive secretion and discharge of urine as seen in diabetes mellitus.

POMR. Abbreviation for *problem-oriented-medical record.*

Portagen. Brand name of a nutritionally complete product that contains 85% of the fat as *medium-chain triglycerides,* which are more readily hydrolyzed and absorbed than conventional long-chain fatty acids. It is used in infants and children with cystic fibrosis, pancreatic insufficiency, biliary atresia, and other disorders of fat malabsorption. See also Appendix 37.

Potassium. An essential mineral that is the chief cation in intracellular fluids. It is important in the maintenance of acid-base and water balances, osmotic equilibrium, muscle and nerve irritability, and normal blood pressure. Potassium is widely distributed in many foods but is especially abundant in nuts, whole grains, meats, and fruits. Dietary potassium deficiency does not occur under normal circumstances. However, secondary deficiency (hypokalemia) may occur when there is excessive loss of potassium with prolonged vomiting, chronic diarrhea, laxative abuse, and use of certain diuretics; some forms of renal disease, diabetic acidosis, and other metabolic disturbances may also lead to severe potassium loss. Symptoms of deficiency are lack of appetite, nausea, muscle weakness, mental disorientation, nervous irritability, and cardiac irregularities. Elevated blood potassium (hyperkalemia) is seen when there is tissue damage, as in myocardial infarction or renal failure.

PPN. Abbreviation for peripheral parenteral nutrition. See *Parenteral nutrition.*

Prazosin. A derivative of quinazoline, an adrenergic blocking agent used in the treatment of hypertension. It may cause weight gain due to fluid retention; it may also cause nausea, vomiting, diarrhea, constipation, and abdominal discomfort. Brand names are Minipress and Minizide.

Prealbumin. A plasma albumin that moves ahead of albumin on paper electophoresis. It is synthesized by the liver and serves as a carrier of retinol and thyroxine in the blood. Prealbumin is an early indicator of protein nutritional status; it has a short half-life (2-3 days). Prealbumin responds rapidly to refeeding, with a significant increase noted within 4 days. Normal plasma concentration is 15-30 mg/dl. Values of 10-15 mg/dl indicate mild depletion; 5-10 mg/dl, moderate depletion; and <5 mg/dl, severe depletion. The serum level is reduced in acute catabolic states, after surgery, and with infection, stress, trauma, liver disease, and hyperthyroidism; it is increased in patients with chronic renal failure on dialysis.

Pre-Attain. Brand name of a half-strength starter formula for tube feeding. It is lactose-free and contains sodium caseinate, malto-dextrin, and corn oil. See also Appendix 39.

Precision. Brand name of a line of polymeric and lactose-free products (Precision HN, Precision Isotonic, and Precision LR) made with egg albumin as the protein source for oral or tube feeding; also contains maltodex-trin, sucrose, and soy oil. See Appendix 39.

Precursor. A forerunner; something that can be used to synthesize another factor; for example, carotene is a precursor of vita-min A. See also *Provitamin.*

Prednisone. A synthetic corticosteroid used for its anti-inflammatory and immunosup-pressant effects. It is excreted in breast milk. See *Corticosteroid* for its adverse effects. Brand names are Deltasone, Meti-corten, Orasone, and Panasol-S.

Preeclampsia. A *toxemia* of pregnancy char-acterized by hypertension, albuminuria, and edema of the lower extremities. See *Pregnancy-induced hypertension.*

Preemie SMA. Brand name of a formula for premature and low-birth-weight infants. Con-tains whey, casein, glucose polymers, lactose, MCT oil, and coconut and soy oils. It has a whey/casein ratio of 60:40 (compared to 18:82 in standard infant formulas) and gives a better distribution of amino acids. See also Appendix 37.

Preformed. Ready for use by the body, in contrast to *precursor.*

Pregestimil. Brand name of a lactose-free for-mula for infants sensitive to intact protein and recovering from prolonged diarrhea. Contains casein hydrolysate, free amino acids, glucose polymers, modified tapioca starch, MCT oil, and corn oil. See also Appendix 37.

Pregnancy. Also called "gestation"; the con-dition of having a developing embryo or fetus in the body after the union of an ovum and a spermatozoon. In the mother's womb, the period of pregnancy is about 266 to 280 days. It is divided into three main phases: *implantation,* the first 2 weeks of gestation, during which the fertilized ovum becomes embedded in the wall of the uterus and the placenta develops; *organogenesis,* the next 6 weeks, during which the developing fetal tissue undergoes differentiation and is the most sensitive period for nutrition-induced birth defects; and *growth,* the remaining 7 months of pregnancy, characterized by rapid cell divi-sion and development. See also *Nutrition, pregnancy.*

Pregnancy-induced hypertension (PIH). High blood pressure developed by some preg-nant women with serious complications like edema, convulsions, and kidney failure. It may even be fatal to the mother and fetus. The exact etiology is not known, but nutri-tional intervention reduces the seriousness of this disorder. Formerly called "preeclamp-sia" (presence of hypertension and protein-uria) and "eclampsia" (with convulsive seizures). *Dietary management:* sodium intake is mildly restricted to 3 gm/day. Pro-tein intake is controlled to provide the opti-mal needs for pregnancy, avoiding excesses. Supplemental vitamins and minerals are recommended. Monitor the weight gain desirable for the gestational period.

Premature infant. A liveborn infant, regard-less of birthweight, born before the 37th week of the gestational period. There are many causes of premature birth, some of which are unknown. Undoubtedly, mater-nal malnutrition is a significant cause. See *Nutrition, prematurity.*

Premenstrual syndrome (PMS). A disorder seen in some women a few days just before the menstrual period; characterized by headache, bloating, depression and "moodi-ness," breast pain, back pain, and changes in metabolism. The appetite increases par-ticularly for carbohydrate foods. Research-ers have studied the relationship between nutrition and PMS, but the results are not conclusive. Some of the nutrients impli-cated are vitamin B_6, vitamin E, and magnesium. Treatment consists of alleviat-ing the symptoms, which disappear once the menstrual period has begun. *Dietary management:* small meals with moderate salt restriction, high protein, limited sugars and concentrated sweets, and avoidance of caffeine may help alleviate some symptoms of PMS.

Primidone. A structural analog of phenobarbital used in the management of seizures. Its adverse effects are the same as those of *phenobarbital.* It is also excreted in breast milk; infants should be watched for drowsiness. The brand name is Mysoline.

Probenecid. A sulfonamide-derivative uricosuric agent used in the treatment of gout. It increases the urinary excretion of riboflavin, calcium, magnesium, sodium, phosphorus, and chloride. It may also cause anorexia, sore gums, anemia, nausea, vomiting, and abdominal discomfort. Probenecid increases the concentration of uric acid in the renal tubules, which may crystallize and form stones if the urine is acidic, or in diets producing an acid-ash residue. Brand names are Benacen, Benemid, ColBenemid, and Probalan.

Problem-oriented medical record (POMR). See *Nutritional care.*

Probucol. An antilipemic agent used as an adjunct to diet therapy to decrease elevated serum cholesterol in type IIa hyperlipoproteinemia. The drug is structurally unrelated to other currently available antilipemic agents. Its adverse effects are generally mild to moderate in severity and of short duration. There may be diarrhea, nausea, vomiting, flatulence, and abdominal pain. The brand name is Lorelco.

Procalamine. Brand name of a 3% amino acid and a 3% glycerin solution with electrolytes for intravenous injection. It supplies 29 gm protein equivalent (4.6 gm nitrogen) and 130 nonprotein calories per 1000 ml. See Appendix 40.

Procarbazine. An antineoplastic hydrazine derivative; used in the treatment of advanced Hodgkin's disease and other lymphomas. Severe nausea and vomiting occur frequently following its administration, and there may be anorexia, stomatitis, dry mouth, and dysphagia. The drug is a pyridoxine antagonist and may cause depletion of the vitamin. Since it has some monoamine oxidase inhibitory activity, the drug should not be taken with alcohol and tyramine-containing foods to avoid a disulfiram-like reaction. The brand name is Matulane.

Prochlorperazine. A derivative of phenothiazine used for the control of severe nausea and vomiting of various etiologies. It is excreted in breast milk; avoid the use of the drug, if possible, when breast-feeding. It may also cause dry mouth, constipation, and difficulty in swallowing. Brand names are Combid and Compazine.

Product 3200AB. A special dietary product that is low in phenylalanine (11 mg/dl) and tyrosine (6 mg/dl) for use in infants with hereditary tyrosinemia. Contains enzymatically hydrolyzed and specially treated casein to reduce phenylalanine and tyrosine, corn syrup solids, modified tapioca starch, and corn oil.

Product 3200K. A low-methionine diet powder for use in infants with homocystinuria. Made of soy protein isolate, corn syrup solids, corn oil, and coconut oil.

Product 3232A. A mono- and disaccharide-free diet powder used in infant formulas for the nutritional management of disacchari-dase deficiencies (lactase, sucrase, and maltase) and for impaired glucose transport and fructose utilization. The desired carbohydrate is added to the formula base, which contains casein hydrolysate, modified tapioca starch, MCT oil, and corn oil.

Product 80056. A protein-free diet powder for use in the dietary management of amino acid disorders, such as hyperalanemia, propionic aciduria, hyperlysinemia, malonic aciduria, isovaleric acidemia, arginosuccinic aciduria, and maple syrup urine disease. Contains corn syrup solids, modified tapioca starch, and corn oil, plus vitamins and minerals.

Professional Standards Review Organizations (PSRO). Established in 1972, the aim of this agency is to evaluate the quality of patient care, including dietary services. Nutritional screening, assessment, monitoring, and education are examples of professional standards of practice needing review to ensure that they meet professional standards.

Profiber. Brand name of a high-fiber, isotonic, lactose-free tube feeding formula. Contains sodium caseinate, hydrolyzed cornstarch, corn oil, and 13 gm soy fiber per liter. See also Appendix 39.

Prognostic nutritional index (PNI). Predictive model relating morbid complications to four variables of nutritional status. Calculated from the following formula: PNI% = 158 − 16.6 (albumin, gm/dl) − 0.78 (triceps skinfold thickness, mm) − 0.2 (transferrin, mg/dl) − 5.8 (hypersensitivity skin test). The risk of morbidity and mortality, using the PNI, is divided into three categories: low risk, PNI <30%; intermediate risk, PNI 30-50%; and high risk, PNI ≥50%.

Project Head Start. Program started in 1965 by the Office of Economic Opportunity to help disadvantaged preschool children from poverty-stricken areas attain their potential in growth and physical and mental development before entering school. Nutrition is an important part of this project. Meals and snacks are provided at the Head Start centers. In addition, meal planning and preparation classes are held for the parents of these children.

Prolamine. Simple protein insoluble in water, neutral solvents, and absolute alcohol but soluble in 70 to 80% alcohol. Examples are *zein* (corn) and *gliadin* (wheat).

Proline. A heterocyclic nonessential amino acid. See *Amino acid.*

Promix RDP. Brand name of a powdered dietary supplement containing rapidly dispersing protein (whey) that is easily suspended in liquids. See Appendix 39.

ProMod. Brand name of a powdered protein supplement made of whey; provides 75 gm protein/100 gm powder. Can be mixed with food or liquids. See Appendix 39.

Propac. Brand name of a powdered protein supplement for enteral feeding; made of whey protein. Provides 75 gm protein/100 gm powder. See Appendix 39.

Propranolol. A beta-adrenergic blocking agent used in the management of hypertension or angina pectoris in patients with chronic obstructive pulmonary disease (COPD) or Type I diabetes mellitus. Uptake is enhanced when the drug is given with food. It may increase blood urea nitrogen and decrease carbohydrate intolerance; adverse gastro-intestinal effects include nausea, vomiting, diarrhea, epigastric distress, abdominal cramping, flatulence, and constipation. Excreted in breast milk. Brand names are Inderal and Inderide.

Prosobee. Brand name of a milk-free formula made with soy protein isolate, corn syrup solids, soy oil, and coconut oil. It is used for infants with protein hypersensitivity, lactose or sucrose intolerance, and galactosemia. See also Appendix 37.

Prostaglandins. New family of hormone-like compounds which are long-chain PUFA, with a 5-carbon ring. Several forms exist, varying slightly in structural formula; designated as PGD, PGE, PGF, PGG, PGH, and PGI, with numerical subscripts to indicate the number of double bonds. The polyunsaturated fatty acids serve as precursors for these compounds. Prostaglandins perform a variety of functions in the body, acting, for example, as blood pressure depressants, smooth muscle stimulants, and antagonists to several hormones.

Prosthetic group. Nonprotein molecule that confers characteristic properties on the complex protein. The binding to protein is very firm, as in the heme of hemoglobin. See also *Coenzyme* and *Cofactor.*

Protamine. A simple protein soluble in water or in ammonium hydroxide but not coagulated by heat. This basic polypeptide contains a relatively small number of amino acids. Examples are salmine (in salmon) and sturine (in sturgeon). See also Appendix 9.

Protease inhibitor. A substance that has the ability to inhibit the proteolytic activity of certain enzymes. It is found throughout the plant kingdom, particularly among the legumes. *Trypsin inhibitor* is found in soybeans, lima beans, and mung beans. *Chymotrypsin inhibitor* is found in cereal grains and potato. Protease inhibitors are destroyed by heating.

Protein. Complex organic compound essential to all living organisms. It is a polymer of *amino acids* linked together by peptide bonds. This forms the *primary structure,* and the sequencing or order of the amino acid chain determines its function and tertiary structure. Hydrogen bonds and disulfide, ester, and salt bridges between polypeptide chains result in the *secondary structure* of proteins. The folding of the amino acid chain and its shape (globular, coiled or spiral, etc.) is its *tertiary structure.* The grouping of units of protein molecules not joined by peptide bonds is its *quarternary* structure. An amino acid which is the backbone of proteins always contains carbon, hydrogen, oxygen, and nitrogen, and occasionally phosphorus, sulfur, zinc, copper, and iron. The nitrogen content distinguishes protein from fat and carbohydrate and is responsible for its unique physiologic functions (See under *Protein, functions*). Native protein in solution is colloidal because of its high molecular weight (6000 to several million). Protein is easily denatured, acts as an electrolyte, forms zwitterions, hydrates with water, and precipitates at its isoelectric point. Enzymes which are protein in nature are inactivated by heat. See also *Amino acid.*

Protein, absorption. See *Absorption, nutrients.*

Protein-bound iodine (PBI). Thyroxine-binding globulin. This is the form in which the thyroid hormone, bound to a plasma protein, is transported in the blood. The normal concentration is about 5 μg/dl of plasma or serum. It increases to about 8 μg/dl in hyperthyroidism. The PBI determination provides a good index of thyroid function and is useful in measuring basal metabolism.

Protein-calorie malnutrition (PCM). See *Marasmus* and *Protein-energy malnutrition.*

Protein classification. The chemistry and physiology of proteins are so complex that a single scheme of classification is not sufficient. Proteins are classified according to *composition and chemical properties* (simple, conjugated or compound, and derived), *nutritional quality* (complete, partially complete, and incomplete), *structure* (fibrous or globular), and *solubility* (in water, acid, or alcohol). See *Protein quality* and Appendix 9.

Protein deficiency. Lack of protein results in stunted growth and development, poor musculature, skin lesions, thin and fragile hair, hormonal imbalances, and edema due to hypoalbuminemia. In developing countries where good-quality protein is scarce and food intake is insufficient, prolonged protein deficiency accompanied by low intake of calories results in *protein-energy malnutrition.*

Protein-efficiency ratio (PER). Biologic method of evaluating *protein quality* in terms of weight gain per amount of protein consumed by a growing animal. Feeding, usually for a month, is ad libitum, with a diet that contains 10 gm protein/100 gm food. Casein is often used as a control protein. PER is calculated as follows:

$$PER = \frac{\text{Weight gain (gm)}}{\text{Protein consumed (gm)}}$$

Protein-energy malnutrition (PEM). Preferred name for protein-calorie malnutrition (PCM). A complex disorder caused by lack of protein and caloric intakes. Characterized by a broad array of clinical conditions ranging from mild to very serious physiological effects; manifested as poor growth or weight loss in mild PEM, to kwashiorkor and marasmus in more serious cases, with the latter having high fatality rates among children. For further details, see *Kwashiorkor* and *Marasmus.*

Protein-energy malnutrition in hospitals. It has been reported that nearly half of the patients admitted to hospitals are malnourished in varying degrees. About 25-30% more are likely to become malnourished sometime during their confinement. The malnutrition may be from poor appetite and inadequate total food intake or it may be stress-related. Total lymphocyte count, albumin, and transferrin are at low levels. *Dietary management:* provide a diet high in protein (1.5 gm/kg/day) and calories (40 kcal/kg/day). Supplementary vitamins and minerals are beneficial for effective utilization of calories and protein.

Protein food mixtures. Products that are specially formulated to provide cheap sources of protein in areas of the world where animal protein sources are expensive or scarce.

Made from local vegetables such as legumes, nuts, cereals, and leaves, and may have added skim milk powder, vitamins, and minerals. For protein food mixtures in the world, see Appendix 36.

Protein, food sources. Animal protein foods are excellent sources for complete proteins. Legumes and nuts are good sources, especially for vegetarian diets, but can be improved with supplementary mixtures of other protein foods. Examples of these are given in Appendix 36. See Appendix 5 for a list of the basic food groups in planning for dietary protein adequacy.

Protein, functions. The biologic role of protein is so unique that it merits its name, which originated from a Greek word, *proteios,* meaning "to take first place." An important function of protein is tissue synthesis. It is a *structural component* of all living cells and is found in muscles, nerves, bone, teeth, skin, hair, nails, blood, and glands. Almost all body fluids contain protein, with the exception of urine, sweat, and bile. All enzymes and some hormones are composed of protein. Thyroid hormones (triiodothyronine and thyroxine) and insulin are examples. Many inborn errors of metabolism are caused by lack of specific enzymes. As a *source of energy,* protein yields 4 kcal/gm; this function should be spared by fat and carbohydrate so that protein is used for building and repairing tissues, which is its primary role. Protein is a *regulator* of blood pH, osmotic pressure, and water balance. As a buffer, protein can accept or donate hydrogen ions so that blood pH is maintained within 7.35 to 7.45. Because of their larger size, protein particles cannot move from capillary beds into the tissues, which accounts for the oncotic force (osmotic pressure) exerted by protein, thereby keeping the body fluid in the bloodstream and counteracting the force of blood pressure. If a person has reduced blood albumin and globulin levels, as in protein deficiency, osmotic pressure is reduced and fluid is drawn out from the blood vessels to the extracellular or interstitial spaces, resulting in edema. Beta-lymphocytes form specific proteins called *antibodies* which aid in combating infections by producing antibody-antigen complexes. Other specific functions of protein are attributable to certain component amino acids such as *tryptophan* for vitamin synthesis, *methionine* as a lipotropic agent, and *phenylalanine* and *tyrosine* for neurotransmitter formation. Protein can form glucose, a process called "gluconeogenesis," which is an important process during starvation. This is critical for the brain, which uses glucose as its energy source. The brain uses about one-third of the total body needs for energy at rest (resting energy expenditure) in the form of glucose. See also *Nutrient* and *Nutrient classification.*

Protein hydrolysate. A predigested protein that contains a mixture of amino acids and peptides. It is useful for oral or parenteral feeding of patients with poor or impaired digestion, as seen in pancreatic diseases, postoperative cases, and severe burns.

Protein measurement. The quantity of protein can be estimated by a number of techniques, including colorimetry, microbiologic assay, isotope dilution, countercurrent distribution, the enzymatic method, and chromatography. For practical purposes, the *Kjeldahl method* for nitrogen determination is most commonly used, since proteins contain an average of 16% nitrogen. Thus % nitrogen $\times$ 6.25 = % protein. See also *Proximate analysis.*

Protein quality. An attribute of a protein that depends on the kinds and amounts of *amino acids* present relative to body needs. No two food proteins are alike in their efficiency for tissue synthesis. In general, plant proteins are lacking or "limiting" in the essential amino acids: lysine, methionine, threonine, and tryptophan. Animal proteins are of high quality or are said to be complete proteins. A *complete* protein contains all the essential amino acids in amounts sufficient for growth and life maintenance, e.g., casein and egg albumin. A *partially complete* protein can maintain life but cannot support growth, e.g., gliadin. An *incomplete* protein cannot support life or growth, e.g., zein and gelatin. The last two classes of protein can be used effectively for anabolic processes by combining with small amounts of complete proteins, by adding the limiting amino acid in synthetic form, or by mixing incomplete proteins to obtain a complete assortment of amino acids in the amounts needed for tissue synthesis. For different methods of evaluating protein quality, see *Biologic value, Chemical score, Net protein utilization,* and *Protein-efficiency ratio.*

Protein requirement. Protein needs vary among individuals according to age, body size, physiologic condition (growth, pregnancy, and lactation), state of health, type of protein in the diet, and adequacy of caloric intake. See Appendix 1 on the recommended dietary allowance for protein. A practical guide for meeting daily protein needs is provided by the basic food groups. See Appendix 5. For estimating protein requirements in special conditions and selected disorders, see Appendix 24 and *Parenteral nutrients.*

Protein reserve. The body does not store protein in the same way or to the same extent that it stores fat and carbohydrate. To a limited extent, all organs and tissues store protein, which is more appropriately termed "labile tissue protein." The latter designation signifies that the protein reserve is in a dynamic state, being constantly broken down or resynthesized, and is at equilibrium with the metabolic pool of amino acids. Muscle protein is not as readily available as is protein stored in the liver, kidney, and other organs. The determination of plasma amino acid levels or the regeneration of blood constituents and protein in the liver is indicative of the extent of protein storage or depletion. See also *Serum albumin, Total lymphocyte count,* and *Transthyretin.*

Protein-sparing action. The ability of a substance to save protein from being catabolized to supply energy. Protein can then be used for its unique function of anabolism, or tissue synthesis. Fats and carbohydrates are protein sparers.

Protein-sparing modified fast (PSMF). A *very-low-calorie diet* that provides a liberal amount of protein to preserve lean body tissue while fasting in order to lose weight. Carbohydrate is prohibited and fat is restricted to that present in the protein source. The daily caloric intake ranges from 400 to 800 kcal/day. Most PSMF diets are mainly a liquid formula of complete protein with vitamins and minerals. This fasting regimen should be done under medical supervision with the support of a registered dietitian. See under *Diet, calorie-modified.*

Protein supplementary value. The ability of a protein to provide or add the "limiting" or missing amino acid of another protein so that the combination approximates a *complete protein,* e.g., the combination of rice or corn with nuts and legumes. See *Protein quality* and Appendix 36.

Protein synthesis. Building of protein as opposed to catabolism. A specific protein is synthesized according to the genetic code as governed by the DNA. The DNA in the nucleus uncoils and a strand of mRNA is formed. A complement mRNA carries the genetic message from DNA to the *ribosome,* the site of protein biosynthesis. Transfer RNA (tRNA) picks up amino acids that have been activated by adenosine phosphate in the cytoplasm and brings them to a specific site on the mRNA. The amino acids are added one at a time by means of a peptide bond until the complete protein is synthesized. Protein synthesis follows the *all-or-none law:* all amino acids (both essential and nonessential) needed according to the genetic code must be present at the same time at the site of protein synthesis. The absence of a single amino acid will prevent synthesis. See also *Nucleic acid.*

Proteinuria. Presence of protein in the urine as a result of faulty reabsorption from a damaged tubule or leakage of an excessive amount of protein through a damaged or inflamed glomerulus of the kidney.

Proteolysis. Enzymatic or hydrolytic conversion of protein into simpler substances such as polypeptide, proteoses, peptones, and amino acids. See Appendix 11.

Prothrombin. Protein in blood plasma needed for blood clotting. Prothrombin time is the length of time it takes for the plasma to clot. This reflects the intake of vitamin K.

Protoplasm. The organized colloidal material in the living cell that is the seat of vital functions such as digestion, metabolic activities, growth, and reproduction. The protoplasm contains water, organic compounds, and inorganic salts.

Provitamin. A vitamin *precursor,* e.g., carotene is the provitamin of vitamin A. A provitamin is chemically related to the preformed vitamin, but it has no vitamin activity unless it is converted to the biologically active form.

Proximate analysis. Also called the "Weende scheme"; named after the Weende Experimental Station in Germany, which established the analytic method in 1865. A method of analyzing food and biologic materials according to their molecular components, such as water, ash or minerals, protein, fat, and carbohydrate, by difference. The first four are determined as follows: the sample is dried, and the difference in weight before and after drying represents *moisture content* or water; a subsample of the dried material is extracted with ether, and the ether extract represents *crude fat;* another subsample is analyzed for nitrogen content using the *Kjeldahl method,* and the percentage of nitrogen multiplied by the factor 6.25 represents *crude protein;* the third subsample is boiled for 30 minutes in dilute sulfuric acid, filtered, and the residue boiled in sodium hydroxide. The insoluble residue is made of crude fiber and ash; when ignited, the remaining residue is *ash,* representing minerals, and the loss or difference in weight is taken as *crude fiber* or indigestible carbohydrate. The proximate analysis of food is the basis of food composition tables. It is the starting point for analyzing individual nutrients. See *Carbohydrate by difference.*

PSMF. Abbreviation for *protein-sparing modified fast,* a variety of very-low-calorie diet (VLCD).

Psoriasis. Skin disease with many varieties. It is characterized by scaly red patches on the extensor surfaces of the body, scalp, ears, genitalia, and bony prominences. Treatments include corticosteroid and methotrexate, a folic acid antagonist. A taurine-restricted diet may be beneficial. See *Diet, taurine-restricted.*

P/S ratio. Ratio of polyunsaturated to saturated fatty acids. A high P/S ratio (at least 1.0) is considered beneficial. Foods in this category include the oils of corn, cottonseed, linseed, safflower, sesame, soybean, and sunflower; almonds and walnuts. A medium P/S ratio (0.5) is provided by glandular organs, hydrogenated shortenings, solid margarines, peanut oil, peanut butter, and pecans. A low P/S ratio (0.3) is found in lard, olive and palm oils, pork fat, and veal. A very low P/S ratio (0.1) occurs in beef, butter, egg yolk, milk, and mutton.

PSRO. Abbreviation for *Professional Standards Review Organizations.*

Psychodietetics. The interrelationship between psychology and nutrition. It deals with the study of the connotative meanings of food, the attitudes and habits of people, the interaction of diet and behavior, and the emotional aspects of eating. See *Nutrition, emotional stability,* and *Nutrition, psychiatry.*

Psyllium. Dried, ripe seed of *Plantago psyllium* and related species. It is a rich source of soluble fiber which is effective in regulating the blood sugar level and in lowering blood cholesterol, especially low-density-lipoprotein cholesterol. Psyllium is also a bulk-forming laxative. Undesirable side effects of psyllium are anorexia, abdominal discomfort, flatulence, and early satiety. The absorption of riboflavin, iron, and other minerals may also be impaired.

Pteroylglutamic acid (PGA). Chemical name for *folic acid,* one of the B complex vitamins. It is a conjugated product containing para-aminobenzoic acid (PABA), pteridine, and one to seven molecules of glutamic acid. The metabolically active forms have reduced pteridine rings and several glutamic acids attached.

Puberty. Age at which reproductive organs become mature functionally and secondary sex characteristics develop. See *Nutrition, adolescence.*

Public health. Science and art of preventing diseases, promoting health, and prolonging life through organized community efforts. See *Nutrition, public health.*

PUFA. Abbreviation for polyunsaturated fatty acids. See *Fatty acid.*

Pulmocare. Brand name of a high-fat, low-carbohydrate product designed to reduce carbon dioxide production in the dietary management of respiratory insufficiency. It is also lactose-free and may be given as an oral supplement or in tube feeding. Contains sodium and calcium caseinates, sucrose, hydrolyzed cornstarch, and corn oil. See also Appendix 39.

Pulmonary embolus. A life-threatening disorder caused by a blood clot developed in another part of the body which has found its way to the lung. Main symptoms are cyanosis, shortness of breath, pallor, fainting, and sometimes edema. *Dietary management:* restore fluid balance and restrict sodium to 2 gm/day if edema is present. Follow general dietary principles for *chronic obstructive pulmonary disease.*

Purine. A nitrogenous ring structure widely distributed in nature, especially in *nucleic acids.* Examples are xanthine, hypoxanthine, adenine, guanine and uric acid. Purines in the body come from the breakdown of nucleic acids (endogenous source) and from purines ingested in food (exogenous source). See *Diet, purine-restricted* and *Gout.*

Pyelonephritis. Inflammation of both the kidney and its pelvis. It is caused by bacterial invasion from the urinary tract, bloodstream, or periureteral lymphatics. *Dietary management:* an *acid-ash diet* is beneficial to increase the acidity of the urine and inhibit bacterial growth. See under *Diet, ash.* See also *Nephritis.*

Pyloric. Pertaining to the opening between the stomach and duodenum. *Pyloric stenosis* is a narrowing of the pyloric orifice (pylorus).

Pyrazinamide. A synthetic antituberculosis agent. It can induce vitamin B_6 deficiency. Neuritis and anemia due to pyrazinamide have been reported. This can be prevented by giving a vitamin B_6 supplement.

Pyridoxal. The aldehyde form of vitamin B_6.

Pyridoxal phosphate (PLP). Also called "codecarboxylase"; a coenzyme that contains vitamin B_6. It is important in many reactions, including amino acid metabolism involving transamination, deamination, decarboxylation, and desulfuration; formation and metabolism of tryptophan and the conversion of tryptophan to niacin and serotonin; hemoglobin synthesis and antibody formation; carbohydrate metabolism, particularly the breakdown of glycogen to glucose; fatty acid metabolism, particularly the conversion of linoleic acid to arachidonic acid; and syntheses of cholesterol and other sterols.

Pyridoxamine. The amine form of *vitamin B_6.*

Pyridoxamine phosphate (PMP). Coenzyme of vitamin B_6 that participates only in transamination reactions.

Pyridoxic acid. Metabolite of pyridoxine that is excreted in the urine. It is used to assess vitamin B_6 nutriture.

Pyridoxine. The alcohol form of vitamin B_6. It is also the collective name given to the three chemically related forms of vitamin B_6: aldehyde (pyridoxal or PL) amine (pyridoxamine or PM), and alcohol (pyridoxine, pyridoxol, or PN). These forms are converted in the liver, erythrocytes, and other tissues to *pyridoxal phosphate* and *pyridoxamine phosphate.* See also *Vitamin B_6.*

Pyridoxol. Former name given to the alcohol form of *vitamin B_6.* The new accepted name is *pyridoxine.*

Pyrimethamine. An antimalarial drug that inhibits dehydrofolate reductase and can produce folic acid deficiency and megaloblastic anemia when given in large doses. It may also decrease serum vitamin B_{12} and may cause loss of appetite, nausea, vomiting, and stomatitis. Excreted in breast milk. Brand names are Daraprim and Fansidar.

Pyrimidine. A six-membered ring compound with the two nitrogen atoms separated by a carbon atom. Pyrimidine bases are found in nucleic acids. Examples are cytosine, thymine, and uracil. See also *Nucleic acid.*

Pyrithiamin. Pyridine analog of *thiamin* that is antagonistic to the vitamin.

Pyruvic acid. Also called "ketopropionic acid"; an important compound in the intermediary metabolism of carbohydrate, protein, and fat. Pyruvate is the negatively charged ion and is the key substance or starting point of many reactions, including (1) complete oxidation to carbon dioxide and water, providing energy via the Krebs cycle; (2) oxidative decarboxylation, supplying acetyl CoA, the starting point for lipid metabolism; (3) reversible reduction to lactic acid, i.e., the Pasteur effect; (4) transamination to alanine, an amino acid; and (5) glycogenesis, or the storage of glycogen in the liver and other tissues.

PZI. Abbreviation for protamine zinc insulin.

Q

QAP. Abbreviation for *Quality Assurance Program.*

q.d. Or quotid. Abbreviation for the Latin phrase *quaque die,* meaning "every day."

Q enzyme. Factor isolated from potatoes that catalyzes the formation of branching linkages of the alpha-1,6 type in starches.

q.h. Abbreviation for the Latin phrase *quaque in hore,* meaning "every hour."

q.i.d. Abbreviation for the Latin phrase *quater in die,* meaning "four times a day."

Q. Symbol for quantity or blood volume.

QO₂. Oxygen consumption per milligram of tissue (dry weight); the amount of oxygen is expressed in microliters at standard pressure and temperature. It is a measure of the rate of respiration of different tissues.

Q substance. Term applied to a giant molecule complex of cholesterol with proteins and lipids that may be associated with the development of atherosclerosis.

Quackery. The actions, claims, or methods of a quack. A *quack* is an untrained person who practices with deception. *Food quackery,* like food faddism, leads people to believe that a particular food has miraculous properties to cure diseases. It makes use of vague, meaningless terms such as "health foods" and "cure-alls" that have scientific overtones and emotional appeal to gullible people.

Quadriplegia. A disorder characterized by paralysis of the four extremities and the trunk below the fifth and seventh vertebrae. The spinal cord injury is usually a result of an automobile or sports accident. Symptoms include loss of sensation and power in the affected areas, reduced peristalsis, bradycardia, flaccid arms and legs, cardiovascular impairment, and even respiratory failure which is fatal. Feeding problems are obvious from the severity of the symptoms and the resulting paralysis.

Quality Assurance Program (QAP). A systematized method of evaluating the quality of medical care given patients, based on acceptable standards. In health care facilities, a quality assurance director coordinates the various methods used by the different departments and follows a schedule for auditing or review for compliance. Actual results are compared with established standards, and deficiencies are identified for correction. Common quality assurance programs include appropriateness of diet order for the diagnosis; timeliness of nutritional screening and assessment; duration of clear liquid diets; isolated tray techniques; patient tray accuracy in terms of the kinds and amount of foods for modified diets; and recognition of drug-nutrient interactions.

Quercetin. A yellow pigment which is a flavone derivative; found in onion skin, tea, red rose, asparagus, the bark of the American oak, and lemon juice. It is used to reduce abnormal capillary fragility.

Quetelet index. See *Body mass index.*

Quinic acid. An acid that is incompletely oxidized in the body; it forms hippuric acid and is excreted in the urine. Found in large amounts in plums, prunes, and cranberries.

Quinolinic acid. One of the intermediary products formed in the metabolism of tryptophan. The level of its excretion in the urine is a measure of the extent of tryptophan utilization in the body.

Quinone. 1. A substance obtained by the oxidation of quinic acid. 2. Any benzene derivative in which two hydrogen atoms are replaced by two oxygen atoms. Vitamin K is a quinone derivative.

R

Rachitic. Pertaining to or affected with rickets. *Rachitic rosary* is a descriptive term used for the costochondral beading (appearance of nodules or bead-like swelling) on the ribs at the junction with the cartilage often seen in children with rickets. See also *Rickets.*

Radiation. Emission of electromagnetic waves such as those of light or particulate rays, e.g., alpha, beta, and gamma rays. Radiation treatment (e.g., for patients with buccal, esophageal, and gastric cancers) produces loss of taste acuity, decreased appetite, nausea, and vomiting.

Radioallergosorbent test (RAST). Diagnostic test for food allergy. It detects specific antibodies against foods by indicating the presence of a type I allergic reaction (IgE-mediated). It is useful for patients in whom the skin test technique is not recommended. However, it is more expensive and may cause adverse reactions in some individuals.

Radioisotope. A radioactive *isotope.* Used as a tracer or labeled substance incorporated in a compound to follow the course of the latter in a series of reactions; also used in the diagnosis and treatment of certain types of tumors, cancers, and thyroid gland disorders. An example is iodine-131, a radioactive isotope of iodine used as a tracer in thyroid studies and as therapy in hyperthyroidism and thyroid cancer.

Raffinose. Naturally occurring trisaccharide composed of a unit each of glucose, galactose, and fructose. It is found in sugar beets, roots and underground stems, cottonseed meal, and molasses. It is only partially digestible and not well utilized by humans, but it can be hydrolyzed by enzymes of the gastrointestinal bacteria in herbivorous animals.

Ranitidine. A histamine H_2 inhibitor used for relief of symptoms associated with active peptic ulcer. Its action reduces gastric acid secretion under daytime and nocturnal basal conditions and also when stimulated by food. It has a bitter taste and may cause transient diarrhea. It may also decrease iron absorption and induce vitamin B_{12} depletion, especially if taken by vegans for an extended period of time. It also increases the risk of bleeding associated with warfarin-induced vitamin K deficiency. The brand name is Xantac.

RBC. Abbreviation for *red blood cell.* See *Erythrocyte.*

RBP. Abbreviation for *retinol-binding protein.*

RDA. Abbreviation for *recommended dietary allowances.* See Appendix 1.

RDS. Abbreviation for *respiratory distress syndrome.*

RE. Abbreviation for *retinol equivalent.*

Reabilan. Brand name of a monomeric liquid formula containing peptides, maltodextrin, tapioca starch, soy oil, and MCT oil. Also available in a higher calorie and protein concentration as Reabilan HN. See Appendix 39.

Recommended dietary allowances (RDA). These are "levels of intake of essential nutrients that, on the basis of scientific knowledge, are judged by the *Food and Nutrition Board* to be adequate to meet the nutrient needs of practically all healthy persons." The latest RDA, revised in 1989, is given in Appendix 1. The term "allowance" is used to avoid the implication that these are absolute standards and to emphasize that the levels of nutrient intake recommended are based on a consensus of scientific opinion that should be reevaluated periodically as new information becomes available. Dietary allowances are designed to maintain good nutrition in healthy persons and are based on the average body sizes of adult men and women at different levels of activity, pregnant and lactating women, and children and adolescent boys and girls grouped according to age. It should be noted that dietary allowances are higher than physiologic requirements in order to allow for a safety factor which considers bioavailability of the nutrients and to allow for individual variations. The amount added differs for each nutrient because of variability in the body's ability to absorb and store the nutrient, the range of observed requirements among U.S. population groups, the criteria established for assessing requirements, and the possible hazards of excessive intake of certain nutrients.

Rectal surgery. Any surgical operation done in the rectum, as in rectal cancer or hemorrhoidectomy, requires a clear liquid diet which has no residue immediately before and after surgery. After 2 days, the postsurgical regimen is a monomeric formula or minimal-residue diet to permit wound healing and avoid infections. Depending on the type of surgery and the progress of recovery, gradual resumption of the normal diet is encouraged to provide fiber.

Rectum. Distal portion of the large intestine, from the sigmoid flexure to the anal canal. It is about 12 to 13 cm long. It stores the fecal matter until it is ready for excretion by the defecation reflex.

Red blood cell (RBC). See *Erythrocyte.*

REE. Abbreviation for *resting energy expenditure.*

Refeeding syndrome. Severe fluid and electrolyte imbalances and other complications resulting from the rapid refeeding (either orally, enterally, or parenterally) of individuals who have been malnourished or starved. The characteristic symptoms are severe hypophosphatemia, hypokalemia, hypomagnesemia, thiamin deficiency, hyperglycemia, fluid overload, cardiac dysfunction, and pulmonary and neurologic complications. Patients at great risk for refeeding syndrome include those with chronic alcohol abuse, anorexia nervosa, cachexia due to starvation or marasmus, prolonged fasting, and patients who have not been fed for

7-10 days. *Dietary management:* slow refeeding with gradual increases in calories and protein to allow the body to adjust to changes in metabolic load. Estimate the previous intake of calories and start refeeding with this amount or allow about 20 kcal/kg body weight. Gradually increase calories and protein every day during the first week. If there are no complications, continue with modest food increases to attain the desired weight and to replenish body protein stores. Allow 35 kcal/kg and 1.2-1.5 gm protein/kg of body weight.

Reflux esophagitis. Condition characterized by heartburn (pyrosis), which may be severe, often accompanied by regurgitation of the acid contents from the stomach into the lower part of the esophagus. It may occur after meals but is typically associated with a change in posture (e.g., bending, lifting, or straining) that produces a rise in intra-abdominal pressure. A hiatal hernia may not be present, although there may be malfunctioning of the gastroesophageal sphincter. *Dietary management:* weight reduction of obese individuals lessens the occurrence of this disorder. Use of antacids, avoidance of heavy meals, and proper postural positions after meals (head and chest upright) are preventive measures.

Refsum's disease. Rare genetic disorder due to a defect in the enzyme system for the metabolism of *phytanic acid,* which accumulates in the cerebrospinal fluid, liver, kidney, and blood. The main clinical features are peripheral neuropathy, cerebral ataxia, cataracts, nerve deafness, and skin changes. Since phytanic acid comes from exogenous sources, the treatment involves restriction of foods containing phytanic acid and its precursors. See *Diet, phytanic acid-restricted.*

Regimen. A systematic course or plan, including food and medication, to improve health. For specific dietary regimen, see *Diet.*

Regional enteritis. One of the two types of inflammatory bowel disease (IBD). See *Crohn's disease.*

Regurgitation. 1. Backflow of food from the stomach to the mouth without the effort of vomiting. 2. Return of blood through a defective heart valve.

Rehydralyte. Brand name of an oral electrolyte solution containing dextrose and 30 mEq citrate/liter. See Appendix 38.

Relapse. Return of symptoms after a disease seems to have been cured. The relapse-response-relapse method is one of the criteria for determining the nutritional essentiality of a substance. For example, deficiency signs of a specific nutrient disappear when the nutrient is administered; withdrawal of the nutrient leads to recurrence of the signs, and therapeutic supplementation again alleviates the deficiency signs. Thus the proof of essentiality is a series of alternate relapse-response-relapse reactions to the nutrient.

Renal. Pertaining to the *kidney.*

Renal acidosis. Reduction or lack of alkali reserve caused by the inability of the kidney to conserve base while excreting acid. See *Acidosis.*

Renal calculi. See *Urinary calculi or urolithiasis.*

Renal diabetes. Type of diabetes characterized by the presence of sugar in the urine even with a normal or below-normal blood sugar level. The condition is not associated with a disturbance in carbohydrate metabolism. It is ascribed either to a low renal threshold for sugar or to a defective reabsorption process in the kidney tubules, allowing glucose to find its way into the urine. This condition is more appropriately called *renal glycosuria.* See also *Phlorizin.*

Renal dialysis. The removal of toxic materials from metabolism from the blood and body fluids by mechanical means. Peritoneal dialysis uses the peritoneal membrane, while hemodialysis uses an artificial kidney and an extracorporeal dialysis method. Self-dialysis methods used at home are *continuous ambulatory peritoneal dialysis (CAPD)* and *continuous cyclic peritoneal dialysis (CCPD).* Hemodialysis is still the more effective method for end-stage renal failure. The comparative nutritional effects of hemodialysis (HD) and peritoneal dialysis (PD) are as follows: HD has no protein loss into the dialysate, while in CAPD, about 9 gm protein/day is lost; however, there is less loss of amino acids in PD (2 to 4 gm/day) compared to 5 to 8 gm/day in HD. With both methods, water-soluble vitamins are lost. For further details on dietary management, see *Hemodialysis* and *Peritoneal dialysis.* See also *End-stage renal disease* and *Renal failure.*

Renal erythropoietic factor (REF). An enzyme released by the kidney that acts on the plasma protein globulin to split off erythropoietin, which in turn acts on the bone marrow to stimulate red blood cell production.

Renal failure. Disorder of the kidney with severe loss of its functions, especially of its glomeruli and tubules. See *Acute renal failure* and *Chronic renal failure.*

Renal hypertension. Elevation in blood pressure as a result of reduction of blood flow to the kidney, as in ischemia. The ischemic kidney liberates into the blood an enzyme, *renin,* that splits angiotensin I from angiotensinogen, an alpha globulin formed in the liver. An enzyme present in the plasma acts on angiotensin I to form angiotensin II, which is a powerful pressor agent. However, the kidney tissues also contain a dipeptidase enzyme, angiotensinase, that destroys angiotensin II.

Renal solute load (RSL). The amount of urea, sodium, potassium, and chloride in the urine. If the renal solute load is too high and fluids are restricted, hypertonic dehydration will occur. The kidneys of a normal adult have the ability to concentrate urine to 1200–1400 mOsm/liter. In kidney disease or in immature infants, the kidneys need a higher fluid requirement for an equivalent RSL. A person with hypercatabolism has an increased RSL. Each gram of dietary protein contributes about 4 mOsm of renal solute, and each milliequivalent (mEq) of Na, K and Cl contributes 1 mOsm. To calculate the RSL, the following equation is used:

$$RSL = (gm\ protein \times 4) + [Na(mEq) + K\ (mEq) + Cl\ (mEq)]$$

Renal threshold. Concentration of a substance in plasma above which the substance appears in the urine. Various substances in plasma, such as glucose, do not appear in the urine until their plasma concentrations rise to certain values. Such substances are referred to as *threshold substances.* The renal threshold of glucose in the adult varies between 140 and 170 mg/dl.

Renal transplant. See *Kidney transplantation.*

RenAmin. Registered name of a 6.5% amino acid solution for total parenteral nutrition; has no electrolytes and contains 60% essential and 40% nonessential amino acids. Designed for use in renal disease and hepatic encephalopathy. See Appendix 40.

Renin. Proteolytic enzyme formed in the kidney and released into the blood. It liberates angiotensin I from its inactive precursor, angiotensionogen. See *Renal hypertension.*

Rennet. Enzyme preparation containing pepsin and rennin obtained from the stomach lining of a calf or lamb. Used in making cheese and junket.

Rennin. Enzyme present in the gastric juice of infants and young animals that is primarily responsible for the coagulation of milk (casein). It is capable of clotting about 10 million times its weight of milk at 37°C in 10 minutes. The process of clotting involves a change in the casein molecules to *paracasein,* which then forms calcium paracaseinate, or the milk clot.

Replena. Brand name for a high-calorie, low-protein, low-electrolyte, low-fluid formula designed for nondialyzed renal patients or as supplemental nutrition for hemodialyzed patients. Can be taken orally or by tube feeding. See Appendix 39.

RES. Abbreviation for *reticuloendothelial system.*

Reserpine. A rauwolfia alkaloid used in the treatment of hypertension. It may cause sodium and fluid retention with edema and weight gain, especially if the drug is not taken with a diuretic. It may also cause dry mouth, increased hunger, increased gastric secretion, and intestinal cramping. Brand names are Releserp, Sandril, Serpate, Serpalan, and Serpasil.

Residue. The remainder; the portion remaining after a part has been removed. In nutri-

tion, it refers to the amount of bulk remaining in the intestinal tract following digestion. It is composed of undigested and unabsorbed food, as well as metabolic and bacterial products. See also *Diet, residue-modified.*

Resol. Brand name of an oral electrolyte solution for infants. See Appendix 38.

Resource. Brand name of a liquid lactose-free, low-residue formula for oral supplementation or tube feeding. Contains sodium and calcium caseinates, soy protein isolates, maltodextrin, sucrose, and corn oil. Also available in a 1.5 kcal/ml concentration (Resource Plus). See Appendix 39.

Respiration. Commonly used to mean "external" respiration or *breathing,* which consists of two acts: *inspiration,* or taking in atmospheric air (i.e., consumption of oxygen), and *expiration,* or expulsion of modified air (i.e., elimination of carbon dioxide). "Internal" respiration refers to the exchange of gases at the cellular level between the systemic blood and the tissues. See *Physiologic oxidation.*

Respiration calorimeter. See *Respirometer.*

Respiratory carriers. Group of electron carriers, including coenzymes I and II (nicotinamide adenine dinucleotide and nicotinamide adenine dinucleotide phosphate), the flavoproteins (flavin mononucleotide and flavin adenine dinucleotide), coenzyme Q, and the cytochrome systems (cytochrome a_1, a_3, b, and c). They convey electrons from the dehydrogenated substrates to oxygen, harnessing free energy in the course of the reaction for the synthesis of adenosine triphosphate (ATP), a form of energy utilized in the endergonic processes of a living cell.

Respiratory distress syndrome (RDS). A secondary lung condition resulting from pulmonary edema, sepsis, shock and other trauma, or critical illnesses. Specifically among infants, RDS refers to an acute lung disorder caused by a deficiency of pulmonary surfactant resulting in inelastic lungs, distended alveoli, and severe hypoxemia, hence its other name, "live membrane disease." RDS occurs in low-birth-weight infants and in babies of diabetic mothers.

Dietary management: see under *Low-birth-weight infant.*

Respiratory enzymes. Enzymes found in the *mitochondria* that catalyze a series of reactions involved in the cellular oxidation of substrates, resulting in their complete oxidation to carbon dioxide and water. Electrons removed from the substrates are passed on to a highly ordered array of *electron* or *respiratory carriers* and thence to oxygen, forming water. The principal types of respiratory enzymes are the *oxidases* and *dehydrogenases.*

Respiratory quotient (RQ). Ratio of the volume of carbon dioxide eliminated to the volume of oxygen used. One gram molecule of carbon dioxide has the same volume as one gram molecule of oxygen. The complete oxidation of carbohydrate gives a respiratory quotient of 1. Oxidation of fat and oxidation of protein give approximate respiratory quotients of 0.7 and 0.8, respectively. Since the three foodstuffs are metabolized simultaneously, the respiratory quotient is always a result of the three. It is about 0.85 on an ordinary mixed diet. See also *Metabolic cart.*

Respirometer. Also called "respiration calorimeter"; an apparatus designed to measure the extent of respiration in humans, which is regarded as a function of two factors: food ingestion and metabolism. Many respirometers have been designed based on the principle of either direct or indirect *calorimetry.* Examples are the Atwater-Rose-Benedict respiration calorimeter and the Kofranyi-Michaelis respirometer.

Resting energy expenditure (REE). The energy expended by a person at rest under conditions of thermal neutrality. Unlike *basal metabolic rate (BMR),* REE is not measured soon after wakening in the morning after at least a 12-hour fasting. Therefore, REE may include the thermal effect of the previous meal. Since BMR and REE differ by less than 10%, the terms are used interchangeably. REE correlates directly with measures of lean body mass and is the largest component of total energy expenditure in normal activities.

Reticulocyte. Immature erythrocyte with a delicate interior network, or reticulum, that stains with basic dyes. Normally present in the blood in small numbers (0.5 to 1.5% of total erythrocytes), its presence in greater number (reticulocytosis) indicates stimulation of erythropoiesis, as seen in response to vitamin B_{12} injections in pernicious anemia.

Reticuloendothelial system (RES). Group of cells (except for leukocytes) with phagocytic properties. They are distributed throughout the body, particularly in the spleen, bone marrow, liver, and lymph nodes. These cells have the property of engulfing and digesting foreign particles or cells harmful to the body. The reticuloendothelial system also removes red blood cells on their destruction. Protein and iron are recovered for formation of new erythrocytes, and the heme portion is converted to *bile pigments.* See also *Hemopoiesis.*

Retina. Photosensitive portion of the eye; the innermost of the three coats of the eyeball and the terminal expansion of the optic nerve. It consists of several layers, including the pigmented epithelium, photoreceptors (rods and cones), associated cells, and ganglion cells. The retina receives light sensation and transforms it into nervous impulses via the optic nerve, which transmits the impulses to the brain for translation into a visual experience.

Retinaldehyde. Name now used for vitamin A aldehyde, retinal, or retinene.

Retinitis. Inflammation of the retina, which interferes with normal vision. Caused by a number of conditions such as diabetes, leukemia, kidney disease, and syphilis.

Retinoic acid. Name for vitamin A_1 acid, formed by the oxidation of vitamin A aldehyde. It has no activity in the visual process or the reproductive system and cannot be stored in the body.

Retinoids. A group of compounds consisting of four isoprenoid units and containing five conjugated double bonds. It is the collective term for the various forms of vitamin A activity (*retinol, retinaldehyde,* and *retinoic acid*) and a large number of synthetic analogs, with or without vitamin A activity. Retinoids vary qualitatively as well as quantitatively in vitamin A activity.

Retinol. Vitamin A₁ alcohol. Its corresponding aldehyde and acid are called "retinaldehyde" and "retinoic acid," respectively. Retinol and retinaldehyde can be reversibly oxidized and reduced, but retinoic acid cannot be converted back to the other two. Retinol circulates in the blood as a complex with retinol-binding protein (RBP) and transthyretin (TTR).

Retinol-binding protein (RBP). A plasma protein that binds and transports vitamin A, in the form of trans-retinol, from the liver to extrahepatic tissues. The binding of vitamin A to the protein serves to solubilize vitamin A and protect it against oxidation. RBP has a half-life of only 12 hours. The normal range in plasma is 30–70 mg/liter. It is decreased in vitamin A deficiency, liver disease, trauma, acute catabolic states, hyperthyroidism, and after surgery; it is increased in renal failure due to impaired glomerular filtration and decreased renal metabolism.

Retinol equivalent (RE). A measure of the total vitamin A activity. It takes into account the amount of absorption of the carotenes, as well as the degree of conversion to vitamin A. One RE equals 1 μg retinol, 6 μg beta-carotene, and 12 μg of other provitamin A carotinoids. See *Vitamin A* and also Appendix 1.

Retinopathy. Noninflammatory disease of the retina; characterized by retinal detachment, a waxy discharge, and a tiny amount of hemorrhaging. The nonproliferative type of retinopathy is more common and is confined to the retina. The proliferative type, which may occur in about 10% of diabetics, is characterized by the retinal capillaries extending into the vitreous, whereby the person's sight is impaired, eventually leading to blindness.

Retrolental fibroplasia (RLF). Also called "retinopathy of prematurity." A form of vitamin E deficiency to which premature or low-birth-weight infants are prone, with an incidence of about 10% in these infants. The occurrence is reduced with daily doses of vitamin E. The anemia seen among premature babies due to lack of body stores can be treated with vitamin E, iron, and folic acid.

Rheumatic fever. Acute or chronic inflammatory process that comes as a sequel to hemolytic streptococcal infection, usually after 3 to 4 weeks. It occurs most frequently in children and tends to recur. The inflammatory process initially affects connective tissues, but may spread to many organs, and when pronounced, conditions such as myocarditis and arthritis occur. *Acute rheumatic fever* is characterized by a sudden onset, with high fever and swelling and pain in the joints. Recurring episodes of rheumatic fever leads to damage of the heart muscle and heart valves, a disorder called "rheumatic heart disease". *Dietary management:* follow guidelines for *fevers.* If edema is present and/or adrenocorticotropic hormone (ACTH) is given, restrict sodium to 2 gm/day.

Rheumatism. Generally indicates diseases of the connective tissue, especially joints and muscles, accompanied by physical incapacity and discomfort. It includes such diseases as acute rheumatic fever, osteoarthritis, rheumatoid arthritis, gout, and bursitis. See *Arthritis.*

Rheumatoid arthritis. Also called "arthritis deformans" and "atrophic arthritis"; a painful, chronic condition common among women over the age of 30 and characterized by swelling, stiffness, and eventual deformity of the joints. Its cause is not known, although the condition is often associated with cold, damp weather and a variety of stress factors such as infection and psychologic shock. *Dietary management:* drug therapy is the primary approach, and diet modification is secondary. The joint deformity, particularly of the fingers, wrists, and elbows, may be quite serious, causing the person to need help in feeding. Damage of the temporomandibular joint hinders chewing. There may be dysphagia and decreased salivary secretion. Self-help devices are now available to encourage patients to feed themselves. The main goal of nutrition therapy is to prevent malnutrition and encourage the person to eat adequately. Monitor the side effects of drugs (nutrient-drug interactions).

Rhodopsin. Formerly called "visual purple"; the pigment in the rods of the retina that contains vitamin A. On exposure to light, it is bleached through a series of products, forming at the end opsin and another pigment known as "retinaldehyde (visual yellow)." As a result of these changes, images are transmitted to the brain through the optic nerve. Vitamin A is required for the regeneration of rhodopsin.

Riboflavin. Also called "vitamin B_2"; one of the water-soluble B complex vitamins. It was isolated from milk (lactoflavin), eggs (ovoflavin), and liver (hepatoflavin) and identified with Warburg's yellow enzymes. Riboflavin is associated with the health of the skin and eyes. As an essential component of two flavoprotein coenzymes, flavin mononucleotide (FMN) and flavin adenine dinucleotide (FAD), it participates in biologic oxidation as a hydrogen acceptor in aerobic dehydrogenases. Riboflavin is also involved in the activation of vitamin B_6 and the conversion of folic acid to its coenzymes. Deficiency in the vitamin results in *ariboflavinosis*, which is characterized by burning and itching of the eyes, photophobia, corneal vascularization, generalized seborrheic dermatitis, cheilosis, angular stomatitis, and glossitis with a characteristic magenta color of the tongue. It is rare to find riboflavin deficiency as an isolated and pure deficiency state. Because riboflavin is essential to the functioning of vitamins B_6 and niacin, some symptoms attributed to riboflavin deficiency are due to the failure of systems requiring these vitamins. Manifestations of riboflavin deficiency in animals vary with the species. Riboflavin is widely distributed in foods, but in small amounts. The richest food sources are milk, egg, meats, poultry, and fish; green vegetables like broccoli, spinach and turnip greens, and enriched grains and cereals are other good sources. It occurs in bound form in plant and animal tissues and is not made available unless binding is liberated by cooking. The vitamin is stable in heat and only slightly soluble in water but is readily destroyed in the presence of light and alkali. It is absorbed in the proximal small intestine and transported either attached to protein or linked with a phosphate molecule. There is little storage in the body, and the amount stored depends on the saturation of protein. No cases of toxicity from ingestion of riboflavin have been reported; toxicity may occur if it is given in massive doses by injection.

Ribonucleic acid (RNA). Also called "ribose nucleic acid"; one of the two main types of *nucleic acid*, with ribose as the pentose constituent. It is present in the cell cytoplasm and nucleolus and plays an important role in protein synthesis. Three distinct types of RNA are involved in *protein synthesis*, with varying size, shape, origin, and function.

Messenger RNA (mRNA). Also called "template RNA" or "informational RNA"; conceived to be a complementary copy of DNA, thus containing the genetic "information" for protein synthesis. mRNA functions at the site of protein synthesis and carries the genetic message from DNA to the *ribosome*, the site of protein synthesis.

Ribosomal RNA (rRNA). Ribonucleic acid in the ribosome, which is believed to direct the arrangement of the amino acids of proteins into their proper sequence within the polypeptide chain.

Transfer RNA (tRNA). Also called "soluble RNA" or "acceptor RNA." It occurs free in the cytoplasmic fluid and transfers the activated amino acid to a specific site on the ribosomal RNA template, resulting in an alignment of amino acids in a particular sequence to form the primary structure of a protein.

Ribose. Pentose sugar of significant physiologic importance. It is a constituent of ribonucleic acid, of the coenzymes nicotinamide adenine dinucleotide (NAD) and nicotinamide adenine dinucleotide phosphate (NADP), and of adenosine triphosphate (ATP). Any glycoside containing ribose as the sugar component is called a *riboside.*

Ribosome. Site of protein synthesis within the cells; contains 80 to 90% of the ribonucleic acid within the cell. As seen by electron microscopy, it appears as a delicate network of membranous tubules attached to numerous dense, spherical granules with diameters of 100 to 150 Å.

Ricinoleic acid. A monohydroxy monounsaturated fatty acid containing 18 carbon atoms; found in castor oil.

Rickets. A nutritional deficiency disease occurring in infancy and early childhood due to a lack of vitamin D or a disturbance in calcium-phosphorus metabolism. It is more likely to develop in dark, overcrowded sections of large cities where the ultraviolet rays of sunshine, especially in the winter months, cannot penetrate the fog, smoke, and soot. Rickets is essentially a disease of defective bone formation. The characteristic symptoms are delayed closure of the fontanelles; poor muscle tone, resulting in a "pot-belly" appearance of the abdomen; soft, fragile bones, leading to bowing of the legs; costochondral beading at the junction of the rib joints, forming the "rachitic rosary"; and projection of the sternum, giving the appearance of a "pigeon breast." Conditioned rickets may occur as a secondary result of other diseases, as in fat malabsorption of celiac disease, in renal failure, and in certain genetic disorders such as familial hypophosphatemia or vitamin D-refractory rickets.

RLF. Abbreviation for *retrolental fibroplasia.*

RNA. Abbreviation for *ribonucleic acid.* Abbreviations for the three types of RNA are mRNA, rRNA, and tRNA for messenger RNA, ribosomal RNA, and transfer RNA, respectively.

Ross RCF. Brand name of a carbohydrate-free soy protein formula base for feeding infants with carbohydrate intolerance. A source of carbohydrate that is tolerated (e.g., dextrose, polycose) is added to the formula to provide the calories required. See Appendix 37.

Ross SLD. Brand name of a powdered mixture of eggwhite solids, sucrose, and hydrolyzed cornstarch; readily soluble in water and suitable as a protein source for patients on a clear liquid diet. See also Appendix 39.

Rotation diets. Meal plans for 4 to 5 days to test for relief from food allergies. The meal plans rotate food items rather than completely eliminating suspected allergens. See *Diet, elimination.*

Roughage. Now called "insoluble dietary fiber." Indigestible carbohydrate material in plants; it passes through the intestines unchanged but absorbs and holds water, thus acting as a laxative. Usually composed for the most part of cellulose, an indigestible polysaccharide. See also *Dietary fibers* under *Fiber.*

R-protein. Protein produced by the salivary glands found to enhance the absorption of vitamin B_{12}.

RQ. Abbreviation for *respiratory quotient.*

S

S. Chemical symbol for sulfur.

Saccharin (Saccharine). Artificial sweetener about 700 times sweeter than cane sugar or sucrose. It has no caloric value, but some find a bitter aftertaste; possibly a carcinogenic substance, but it is still allowed to be used in the United States until May 1992, when it will be reevaluated. Sold under the brand names Sweet & Low and Sugar Twin.

Saliva. Secretion of the *salivary glands* in the mouth. It serves to moisten and hold particles of food together, thus aiding chewing and swallowing. It contains an enzyme, *salivary amylase,* that helps to digest starch. The salivary secretion also has some bacteriostatic properties.

Salivary amylase. Formerly called "ptyalin." It is the principal enzyme of human saliva, acting on starches, with oligosaccharides and maltose as the end products. It requires chloride ion and an optimum pH of 6.6 to 6.8 for its action. Digestion in the mouth is not appreciable, since food stays in contact with the enzyme for only a short time. Salivary amylase is easily inactivated at a pH of 4.0 or less, and its action ceases when food enters the stomach.

Salt. 1. Common table salt or sodium chloride ($NaCl$). 2. Class of compounds formed when the hydrogen atom of an acid radical is replaced by a metal or metal-like radical, as in neutralization reactions. See also *Sodium* and *Sodium-restricted diet* under *Diet.*

Saturation. 1. Point beyond which a solution can no longer dissolve a given substance. 2. Property of having all the chemical affinities satisfied. For example, in *saturated fatty acids,* all the carbons in the chain have all the hydrogen linked to carbon.

Saturation test. See *Load test.*

Schilling test. Procedure used in the differential diagnosis of macrocytic anemias to determine an individual's ability to absorb vitamin B_{12}. After an oral dose of radioactive vitamin B_{12} is given, the urinary excretion of the vitamin is low in patients with *pernicious anemia.* When the same test is repeated with intrinsic factor also given orally, the urinary excretion becomes almost normal in these patients because the vitamin is absorbed; it remains low in vitamin B_{12} deficiency due to other causes, such as malabsorption syndrome and intestinal resection.

School Breakfast Program. Established in 1966 as part of the *Child Nutrition Act.* In some schools, breakfast is served to children who are poor or who have traveled a long distance from home.

School Lunch Program. More appropriately called the "National School Lunch Program." A practical nutrition program designed to train schoolchildren in proper food habits and to improve their dietary intake of nutrients. The National School Lunch Act became a law in 1946 (and is the largest of the Child Nutrition Programs). A participating school is given financial and technical assistance to enable it to serve *free* and *reduced-price* lunches to children unable to pay the full price for nutritious, hot lunches.

Scleroprotein. Group of simple proteins that are insoluble in water and neutral solvents and resistant to digestive enzymes. They include the *collagen* of skin, tendons, and bones and the elastic proteins known as *elastin* and *keratin.* Scleroproteins have protective and supportive functions in bones, cartilage, ligaments, tendons, and other tough parts of the animal body. See Appendix 9.

Sclerosis. Hardening of a part of the body due to the growth of tough, fibrous tissues.

The term is more commonly used to describe a disorder of the nervous system characterized by hardening of the tissues as a result of hyperplasia.

SCP. Abbreviation for *single-cell protein.*

Scurvy. Deficiency disease caused by a lack of vitamin C. It tends to affect either the very young or the elderly. In *infantile scurvy,* the onset is usually in the second half of the first year. There is pain, tenderness, and swelling of the thighs and legs; the infant assumes the "pithed frog" position, with the legs flexed at the knees. Enlargement of the costochondral junction produces the scorbutic rosary, which has a sharper feel than that due to rickets (rachitic rosary). If the teeth have erupted, the gums may be swollen, spongy, and prone to bleeding. *Adult scurvy* may occur after several months on a diet devoid of vitamin C. Early symptoms are weakness, easy fatigue, and listlessness, followed by shortness of breath and aching in bones, joints, and muscles, especially at night. Perifollicular hemorrhages are common in the thorax, forearms, thighs, legs, and abdomen. In advanced scurvy the slightest injury produces excessive bleeding, and large hemorrhages may be seen beneath the skin; the gums are friable and bleed easily. Scurvy responds within a few days to administration of 100 to 200 mg vitamin C given in synthetic form or as orange juice.

SDA. Abbreviation for *specific dynamic action.*

Se. Abbreviation for selenium.

Seborrheic dermatitis. Skin lesion characterized by greasy scaling, especially on the nasolabial folds and around the eyes and ears. Hard sebaceous plugs also form over the bridge of the nose. The condition may be a result of various factors, such as oily skin, hormonal imbalance, emotional disturbance, and nutritional deficiency (as in riboflavin and pyridoxine deficiencies).

Secretin. Hormone secreted by the intestinal mucosa when gastric acid or chyme reaches the intestine. It is carried by the bloodstream to the pancreas and stimulates it to secrete the pancreatic juice.

Selenium (Se). Trace mineral essential to humans, animals, and plants. It is an active component of glutathione peroxidase, an enzyme that catalyzes the breakdown of hydroperoxide. In this manner, selenium protects membrane lipids from oxidant damage. A functional interrelationship exists between selenium and vitamin E; a deficiency in one can be partially corrected by supplementation with either nutrient. Selenium also protects against the toxicity of mercury, cadmium, and silver, and there is some evidence suggesting that selenium may reduce the incidence of cancer. Deficiency in humans has been described in severely malnourished children and in patients maintained on prolonged total parenteral nutrition unsupplemented with selenium. Characteristic signs are a low blood selenium level, abnormal nail beds, growth retardation, and muscle cramps; heart enlargement and varying degrees of heart insufficiency are seen in severe deficiency. Seafoods, liver, meats, and whole grains are good food sources; fruits and vegetables generally contain little selenium. The average daily intake is about 50-200 μg/day, and absorption is about 80% or more. Selenium is transported to various tissues bound to very-low-density and low-density lipoproteins and is taken up by the red blood cells, liver, heart, spleen, nails, and tooth enamel. Selenium is toxic beginning at levels 20-30 times the requirement. Signs of intoxication include loss of hair and nails, dental caries, dermatitis, peripheral neuropathy, irritability, and fatigue. Chronic selenium toxicity occurs in many seleniferous areas in the Americas, South Africa, Australia, New Zealand, and China. Intoxication from dietary selenium supplements has also been reported. The indiscriminate use of selenium self-supplementation should be avoided. See Appendix 1 for the recommended daily allowances. See also *Keshan disease.*

Self-feeding problems. Obstacles encountered by patients who are either blind or have problems in chewing, swallowing, and coordination, as well as physical handicaps with feeding. *Dietary management:* independence in self-feeding, where appropriate, should be encouraged. Provide adaptive feeding equipment such as special plates and utensils, special straws, plate guards, and tray rails. Alter feeding position if necessary. If there is a problem with chewing and swallowing, provide pureed, ground, or chopped foods. Soft foods such as cottage cheese, eggs, milk, and mashed fruits and vegetables are recommended. See also *Diet, dysphagia* and *Diet, supraglottic.*

Senna. An anthraquinone glycoside stimulant laxative obtained from the dried leaves of *Cassia angustifolia.* Abuse of this drug can cause potassium depletion and malabsorption with weight loss. Brand names are Gentlax and Senokot.

Sepsis. Infection that may be the result of fungal or bacterial agents. When it has spread from one part of the body to other areas via the circulatory system, it is called *septicemia* or, more colloquially, "blood poisoning." The presence of pathogenic bacteria and their toxins in the blood is accompanied by chills, excessive perspiration, intermittent fever, and weakness. In severe form, the body is in a hypercatabolic state which needs immediate nutrition intervention. *Dietary management:* because of the high fever, the resting energy expenditure is increased as much as 75%, which requires an increase in the patient's caloric intake to about 40–45 kcal/kg/day. Increased protein losses due to hypercatabolism should be replaced by providing protein of high biologic value and a daily protein intake of 1.2–1.7 gm/kg/day. Branched-chain amino acids, arginine, and taurine may be beneficial in supplementing enteral feedings.

Serine (Ser). Alpha-amino-beta-hydroxypropionic acid, a nonessential amino acid first obtained from the silk protein sericin. It is converted to glycine and one carbon (1-C) fragment, with *tetrahydrofolic acid* as the acceptor. The 1-C fragment becomes the source of methyl groups needed in the biosynthesis of many compounds.

Serotonin. 5-Hydroxytryptamine (5-HT), a *tryptophan* derivative. It is found in the serum and in a number of tissues, including the gastrointestinal tract, blood platelets, brain, and nerve tissues. Serotonin is a powerful vasoconstrictor and plays a role in brain and nerve function, gastric secretion, and intestinal peristalsis. It is also believed to influence the regulation of food intake by the brain. Metabolism of serotonin yields 5-hydroxyindole acetic acid (5-HIAA). See also *Diet, serotonin test.*

Serum. Clear liquid left after protein has clotted; refers to both blood and milk serum. The serum from milk is called *whey;* it contains lactose, proteins, water-soluble vitamins, and minerals. Blood serum is plasma *without* its fibrinogen. See also *Plasma.*

Serum albumin. The most abundant protein in human plasma. Serum albumin is commonly used as an indicator of visceral protein nutriture. The normal range is 3.5–5.0 gm/dl. Values of 2.8–3.4 gm/dl are indicative of mild depletion; 2.1–2.7 gm/dl of moderate depletion; and less than 2.1 gm/dl of severe depletion. However, serum albumin is a poor indicator of acute changes in nutritional status due to its long half-life (about 20 days) and large body pool size (about 5 gm/kg body weight). Mobilization of albumin from the extravascular pool during periods of protein depletion ensures that the serum concentration does not decline immediately. Measurement of albumin also cannot be used to reflect the nutritional status of protein in patients with chronic liver disease. Albumin is synthesized by the liver and constitutes as much as 50% of the liver's total protein production.

Serum creatinine. A useful index of renal function. The normal serum creatinine level is 0.6 to 1.5 mg/dl. It is increased in diseases of the kidney when a sufficient number of glomeruli are damaged. A value over 5 mg/dl is of serious significance.

Serum enzymes. Enzymes present in the blood plasma resulting from the breakdown of body cells. Examples are serum glutamic pyruvic transaminase (SGPT), serum glutamic oxalacetic transaminase (SGOT), and lactic dehydrogenase (LDH). The levels of subgroups of these enzymes provide diagnostic and clinical information on specific tissue damage.

SGOT. Abbreviation for serum glutamic oxalacetic transaminase; also called "aspartate aminotransferase (AST)." This *serum enzyme* is widely distributed in all body tissues (except bone), but its levels are highest in the heart muscle, skeletal muscle, liver, kidney, and brain. The normal level ranges from 5 to 40 units. Activity is high in myocardial infarction, infectious hepatitis, extrahepatic biliary obstruction, and liver damage from toxic agents. It is moderately increased in rheumatic fever and in disorders involving necrosis of the heart, liver, or muscle.

SGPT. Abbreviation for serum glutamic pyruvic transaminase; also called "alanine aminotransferase (ALT). A *serum enzyme* found in higher concentration than SGOT in the liver. It is also found in heart muscle, but in lower concentration than SGOT. This concentration difference between the two enzymes provides a more accurate diagnosis of myocardial infarction and liver disease.

Short-bowel syndrome (SBS). Set of symptoms resulting from massive resection of the small intestine which is life-threatening, especially if over 50% of the organ is removed. The patient undergoes three postsurgical phases: (1) severe diarrhea, fluid losses, and electrolyte imbalance; (2) 2 months or more of anorexia, mild diarrhea, steatorrhea, and weight loss; and (3) anemia, osteomalacia, gallstone formation, gastric hyperacidity, and nutritional deficiencies. *Dietary management:* during the first phase, intravenous and total parenteral nutrition feedings are needed. This can continue in the second phase, and after several weeks or so, a transition diet consisting of tube feeding that is lactose-free and low in residue is started before oral feedings are resumed. Provide 1.5 gm protein/kg/day and 45 kcal/kg/day or caloric intake of basal energy expenditure $\times$ 1.5.

Si. Chemical symbol for silicon.

Sialic acid. Acetyl derivative of an amino sugar acid; present in saliva, glycoproteins, lipids, and polysaccharides.

Siderophilin. Also called "transferrin," an iron-carbonate-protein complex circulating in the blood plasma.

Siderosis. The presence of excess iron in the body. This may be the result of hemolysis, excess intake of iron, multiple blood transfusions, or failure to regulate iron utilization.

Silicon (Si). An essential trace element in chickens and rats. Silicon deficiency results in growth retardation and incomplete development of the skeleton. It is believed to function in the metabolism of connective tissue, formation of collagen, calcification of bones, and maintenance of elastic tissue integrity. There is some evidence indicating that silicon may also be essential in humans. Of interest is its role in the development of atherosclerotic vascular disease. There is an inverse relationship between the silicon content of the arterial wall and the degree of atherosclerosis present, and some studies have reported blood lipid-lowering effects of silicates in the drinking water. Silicon may also be involved in osteoarthritis, hypertension, and the aging process. The minimum requirement for silicon has not been ascertained in animals, and nothing is known about the possible human requirement. Silicon is supplied by many foods, especially unrefined grains, cereal products, and root vegetables; foods of animal origin are low in silicon. When taken orally, silicon is essentially nontoxic. Magnesium silicate, an over-the-counter antacid, and other silicates in food additives used as anticaking or antifoaming agents have been used by humans without obvious harmful effects.

Similac. Brand name of a line of milk formulas for infant feeding; contains skim milk with added lactose, soy oil, coconut oil, and vitamins, with or without added iron. Similac 20 is designed for normal, full-term infants; Similac 13 for infants who have not been fed for several days or weeks and for whom a dilute formula is desired; Similac 24 for premature infants with a limited intake or for infants with increased energy needs; and Similac 27 for premature infants with increased growth needs. See also Appendix 37.

Similac PM 60/40. Brand name of an infant formula made with whey protein concentrate, sodium caseinate, lactose, corn oil, and coconut oil. It has a 60:40 whey/casein ratio that resembles that of human milk. It is also low in sodium, potassium, and renal solute load, which is beneficial for infants who have impaired renal or cardiovascular function. See also Appendix 37.

Similac Special Care. Brand name of a feeding formula designed for premature and low-birth-weight infants. Contains demineralized whey, cow's milk, lactose, polycose, glucose polymers, MCT oil, and coconut and soy oils. Provides 20 kcal/oz (Similac Special Care 20) and 24 kcal/oz (Similac Special Care 24). See also Appendix 37.

Simmonds' disease. Also called "hypopituitary cachexia"; a condition caused by a wasting away of the *adenohypophysis.* It results in premature aging, severe weight loss, mental disturbance, low basal metabolic rate, and low body temperature.

Simplesse. Brand name for a fat substitute made from egg white and milk protein with only 1.5 kcal/gm. It is usually used in dressings, butter, ice cream, and other foods that do not require cooking.

Single-cell protein (SCP). Protein produced by the growth of single-cell organisms such as algae, bacteria, yeasts, and fungi.

Sitosterol. Plant sterol similar to cholesterol but having an extra methyl group. Large doses can lower blood cholesterol and beta-lipoprotein levels. High intakes, however, produce toxic effects such as anorexia, diarrhea, and cramps.

Skatole. The substance that gives the characteristic foul odor to feces. It is a product of tryptophan deamination in the intestines.

Skeletal system. The bony framework of the body that gives support and structure. The human *skeleton* is composed of two parts:

the *axial part,* or bones of the trunk, which include the skull, vertebral column, ribs, and sternum, and the *appendicular part,* or bones of the extremities. The tendons attach the muscles to the skeleton. This aids in locomotion. See also *Nutrition, bone.*

Skin. Also called "integument"; the outermost covering of the body, consisting of a double-layered, tough, resilient epithelium averaging 1.7 m^2 of surface area. The outer layer, or *epidermis* (cuticle or scarf skin), produces the pigment *melanin.* The inner layer, or *dermis,* is the true skin, sometimes called the "corium." It is highly vascular and well supplied with nerve endings, sweat and sebaceous glands, and hair follicles. The skin protects the underlying tissues from mechanical injury, helps regulate body temperature, synthesizes vitamin D, and is sensitive to sensations of pain, touch, and temperature. The general condition of the skin is taken as an index of health and the state of nutrition (e.g., pallor of anemia, petechiae of vitamin C deficiency, follicular keratosis of vitamin A deficiency, and pellagrous dermatitis of niacin deficiency). See also *Nutrition, dermatology.*

Skinfold measurement. Also called the "pinch test"; measurement of the thickness of a fold of skin at selected body sites where adipose tissue is normally deposited, as in the biceps, triceps, subscapular, suprailiac, thigh, and calf muscles. The skinfold is measured with a *caliper* and gives an estimate of the degree of fatness of an individual. The most commonly measured skinfold is the triceps. See *Triceps skinfold* and Appendix 23.

SMA. Brand name of an infant formula that is low in sodium, potassium and renal solute load; used for infants with impaired renal or cardiovascular function. Contains demineralized whey, nonfat cow's milk, lactose, coconut oil, and soy oil. The protein and mineral contents are comparable to those of breast milk. See also Appendix 37.

Sn. Chemical symbol for tin.

Society for Nutrition Education (SNE). Professional organization formed to promote good nutrition among the public by making sound nutrition education more available and effective; provides technical assistance and consultation for interested groups; develops extensive bibliographies with evaluated annotations of content; and maintains the National Nutrition Education Clearing House. It publishes the *Journal of Nutrition Education.*

Sodium (Na). A major mineral essential to life. About 50% of the body's sodium is in extracellular fluids, 40% in bones, and the rest inside the cells. Sodium is the chief cation in the extracellular fluids. It regulates water and acid-base balance, osmotic pressure, contraction of muscles, and conduction of nerve impulses. Almost all foods contain sodium, either naturally or as an ingredient added during processing or cooking. The main sources are sodium chloride and sodium bicarbonate, and the average daily intake is about 4 gm sodium (10 gm salt). Normally, the quantity of sodium ingested daily equals the amount excreted, so that a state of sodium balance is maintained. Aldosterone, a hormone secreted by the adrenal cortex, controls the regulation of sodium balance. When sodium intake is high, the aldosterone level decreases and the urinary sodium level increases. When the sodium level is low, the aldosterone level increases and urinary sodium excretion decreases. Dietary sodium deficiency does not normally occur, even among those on very-low-sodium diets. Sodium depletion is usually the result of excessive loss from diuretic therapy, persistent diarrhea or vomiting, profuse sweating, and other disorders marked by loss of body fluids or inability to retain sodium. Symptoms of deficiency include weakness, muscle cramps, fatigue, and dizziness. In severe cases, there may be a drop in blood pressure, leading to confusion, fainting, and palpitations. Excessive sodium intake is thought to be a contributory factor in hypertension. In persons whose blood pressure is high, excessive sodium may increase the risk of heart disease, stroke, and kidney damage. The American Heart Association believes that epidemiologic evidence supports the recommendation that sodium intake not exceeding 3 gm/day is probably useful in the prevention of high blood pressure. See also *Diet, sodium-restricted.*

Sodium pump. Mechanism that mediates the active transport of sodium across cell membranes whereby sodium is pumped out in exchange for potassium. The operation of this pump requires cellular adenosine triphosphate and adenosine triphosphatase.

Somatic. Pertaining to the body framework as distinguished from the viscera.

Somatomedin C. One of a family of insulin-like peptides that have anabolic actions on fat, muscle, cartilage, and cultured cells. It has a very short half-life (3 to 7 hours) and may be a sensitive indicator of recent protein and calorie intake and deprivation. Plasma levels (normal range, 0.55-1.4 IU/ml) fall rapidly with fasting and quickly recover during refeeding; low values are also seen in hypothyroidism and with estrogen administration.

Somatostatin. A hormone secreted by the delta cells of the pancreas which inhibits the release of both *insulin* and *glucagon*. It is also secreted by the hypothalamus to inhibit the release of growth hormone and thyroid stimulating hormone.

Somatotrophin (somatotropic hormone). Growth hormone secreted by the anterior lobe of the *pituitary gland.* Its main action is to stimulate the growth of the epiphyseal cartilages of long bones. It also increases nitrogen retention, facilitates the transfer of amino acids from extracellular to intracellular compartments of the body, influences carbohydrate metabolism by its insulin-like effect, and causes lowering of the fat content in the body.

Sorbitol. A 6-carbon sugar alcohol formed by the reduction of glucose or fructose. It is a nutritive sweetener having the same caloric value as glucose (4 kcal/gm). However, sorbitol is slowly absorbed and delays the onset of hunger. It is only 50% as sweet as sucrose and is used in dietetic candies, gums, and ice creams. It can be converted to utilizable carbohydrate in the form of glucose. Excessive use may cause gastrointestinal distress and diarrhea.

Soyacal. Brand name of an intravenous fat emulsion with 10% or 20% soybean oil for total parenteral nutrition. See Appendix 41.

Specific dynamic action (SDA). See *Thermal effect of food.*

Specific fuel factor (value). Coefficient of digestibility and particular caloric contribution of foods coming from similar sources. For example, the coefficient of digestibility of proteins in milk, egg, and meat is 97%, whereas that of cornmeal protein is only 60%. Thus the caloric value per gram of protein would be much less for corn protein than for proteins in milk, egg, and meat. Specific fuel factors (values) for estimating calories from various foods have been established.

Specific gravity. Weight of a substance compared with that of an equal volume of another substance taken as a standard (water for liquids and solids, hydrogen for gases). The specific gravity of water is 1 (i.e., 1 gm/ml); it is less than 1 for fats.

Specificity. The ability of an enzyme to catalyze a single reaction or a limited range of reactions. Specificity is the main distinction between enzymes and inorganic catalysts like minerals, which are nonspecific.

Sphingomyelin. Complex *phospholipid* composed of 4-sphingenine (sphingosine), fatty acids, phosphoric acid, and choline. It is a part of cell structures and is found primarily in brain and nervous tissue as a constituent of the myelin sheath.

Spirometer. Also called "respirometer"; an apparatus that measures air taken into and from the lungs. It is used in indirect calorimetry. See *Respirometer* and *Calorimetry.*

Spironolactone. A synthetic steroid aldosterone antagonist; a potassium-sparing diuretic used for edema and hypertension. It may cause hyperkalemia, especially in patients with renal insufficiency. Dehydration and hyponatremia manifested by low serum concentration, dry mouth, thirst, and men-

tal confusion may occur. Brand names are Aldactone and Spiractone.

Spleen. Ductless organ situated in the upper part of the abdomen just below the diaphragm and to the left of and behind the stomach. It is composed of a mass of sinuses with various openings. The spleen is an organ of the *reticuloendothelial system.* It also serves as a reservoir for the storage of blood and is capable of increasing and decreasing its volume to maintain normal blood cell levels in active circulation.

Sports' anemia. Also called "runners' anemia." Observed in some athletes who have decreased ability to carry oxygen (in the red blood cells) caused by excessive iron loss through perspiration or increased red blood cell destruction from intense physical activity.

Sprue, nontropical. See *Celiac disease.*

Sprue, tropical. A malabsorption syndrome that is endemic in tropical and subtropical countries. The exact etiology is unknown. It is most likely due to a combination of nutritional deficiencies and infections. It responds well to antibiotics and a feeding regimen of adequate calories and protein, with vitamin and mineral supplementation.

Squalene. Unsaturated hydrocarbon formed by four molecules of acetic acid. It is an intermediate step in the synthesis of *cholesterol.*

Stachyose. Tetrasaccharide containing glucose, fructose, and two molecules of galactose. It is found in tubers, peas, lima beans, and beets.

Stapling, gastric. See under *Gastric bypass (stapling).*

Starch. Storage form of carbohydrates in plants. It is a polysaccharide composed of many glucose units linked in a straight line (amylose) or with branches (amylopectin). Starch is the principal source of energy and the basic staple of the daily diet. Chief food sources are cereals and cereal products, root crops such as potatoes and yams, tapioca, legumes, and starchy vegetables. See Appendix 8.

Starvation. A condition resulting from prolonged deprivation of food, hence the lack of calories and nutrients. The starved body suffers from physiologic malfunctions. Energy expenditure continues during starvation thus, the body mobilizes nutrients from body fuel reserves. Glycogen stores are depleted fairly early in starvation, after which the body adjust by hydrolyzing skeletal muscle protein and using the amino acids as sources of glucose. In the early days of starvation, the urinary excretion of nitrogen is about 12 gm/day (equal to 75 gm protein or 360 gm lean tissue). As much as 500 gm protein, or 5% of total body intracellular protein, may be lost in 7 days of starvation. During prolonged starvation, the adipose tissue becomes the principal source of energy. Production of ketone bodies from fatty acids is accelerated, and the brain and other tissues begin to use ketones as an energy source. Muscle protein continues to be catabolized but at a reduced rate, with protein loss decreasing to 20 gm/day. At the same time, the body reduces its energy needs by slowing the metabolic rate. *Dietary management:* rehabilitation of the starved, hypometabolic patient should be gradual. Suggested daily caloric progressions are as follows: basal energy expenditure (BEE) × 0.8 on days 1 and 2; BEE × 1.0 on days 3 and 4; BEE × 1.2 on days 5 and 6; and BEE × 1.5 on day 7 and thereafter. Increase the calories to BEE × 2 if weight gain is desired. Protein intake should be 1.2–1.5 gm/kg body weight, depending on the degree of repletion required. Supplemental vitamins and minerals are recommended.

Stearic acid. Long-chain saturated *fatty acid* with 18 carbon atoms. It is present in most animal and vegetable fats as the triglyceride *stearin.*

Steatorrhea. Presence of fat in stool. It may be caused by defective fat absorption, lack of bile, or lack of lipase. Fatty stools are seen in celiac disease and other malabsorption syndromes.

Steroids. Large group of cyclic lipid compounds. Included in this group are the *sterols, sex hormones, adrenocortical hormones,* *bile acids, vitamin D, saponins,* and *sterol glycosides.*

Sterols. Class of *steroids* that are complex monohydroxy alcohols universally found in both plants and animals. Mycosterols are found in yeasts and fungi; the most important one is *ergosterol,* a precursor of vitamin D. Phytosterols, or plant sterols, include *sitosterol,* which is found in oils of higher plants, especially wheat germ oil. *Cholesterol* is the most familiar sterol; it is present only in animal sources.

STH. Abbreviation for *somatotropic hormone.* See *Somatotrophin.*

Stomach. Also called the "gastric gland"; the most dilated part of the alimentary canal, situated below the diaphragm. It is composed of three parts: the *cardia,* or the upper part; the *fundus,* which secretes digestive juices and stores food temporarily; and the *antrum,* which provides powerful mixing movements. Three types of cells in the stomach secrete the gastric juice: *mucous cells,* which secrete mucin; *parietal cells,* which secrete hydrochloric acid; and *zymogenic* or *chief cells,* which secrete the enzymes pepsin, the intrinsic factor, rennin, and lipase. See also *Gastrectomy, Gastric by-pass* and *Gastritis.*

Stomatitis. Inflammation of the oral mucosa or soft tissues of the mouth. In *angular stomatitis,* the inflammation occurs at the angles of the mouth. See also *Nutrition, tongue and mouth conditions.*

Stress. 1. Time of extreme pressure or a trying period. 2. Any stimulus that disrupts the homeostasis of the organism. Stress factors that alter nutrient needs are *physiologic stresses,* as in growth, pregnancy, and lactation; *pathologic stresses* such as fever, infection, and disease; *physical stresses* such as heavy labor, strenuous exercise, and severe environmental conditions; and *psychological stresses* such as anorexia nervosa and psychic overeating. See *Nutrition, stress.*

Stresstein. Brand name of a nutritional product containing free amino acids (44% branched-chain amino acids plus essential amino acids), maltodextrin, MCT oil, and soy oil; used in severe metabolic stress and trauma. See also Appendix 39.

Stroke. 1. A sudden and severe attack of a disease. 2. Common term for *apoplexy,* a symptom complex caused by hemorrhage of the brain or thrombosis of the cerebral vessels. See *Cerebrovascular accident.*

Strontium. A metallic element that is present in various compounds, seawater, marine plants, and food. It is also found in the body, although it is not established as essential to humans. It is metabolized in a manner similar to that of calcium and has the ability to replace calcium in bone formation. There are several radioisotopes of the element, of which strontium 90 is of public health importance. It is produced in nuclear fission reactions and is present in the fallout from nuclear bomb explosions. Of major concern is the possibility of ingesting radioactive strontium 90 by drinking milk from cows fed grass and hay that have absorbed the element from the soil or the atmosphere as radioactive fallout. Strontium 90 emits radiation for a long time (half-life of 28 years) and accumulates in the bone, where the radiation may cause leukemia and/or bone tumors.

Struvite. Compound of magnesium ammonium phosphate, a common constituent of urinary tract stones. Usually associated with chronic urinary tract infections, neurogenic bladder, and paraplegia.

Substance abuse. Chronic use of alcohol and drugs resulting in physiologic, social, emotional, and occupational problems. Recent studies show that persons with substance abuse have abnormal metabolism of dopamine, serotonin, and norepinephrine. See *Alcoholism* and *Nutrition, chemical dependency.*

Sucaryl. Brand name for *cyclamate,* an artificial sweetening agent. See also *Alternative sweeteners.*

Succus entericus. The intestinal juice. It is slightly alkaline and contains mucin, amylase, lipase, peptidases, disaccharidases, and other enzymes. Its composition and volume throughout the intestines vary.

Sucralose. Also called "chlorosucrose." A noncaloric sweetener under study; has high-intensity sweetening power (600 times that of sucrose).

Sucrose. Table sugar; made from cane or beet sugar. It is a *disaccharide* consisting of glucose and fructose. Sucrose is easily hydrolyzed by acid or the enzyme invertase to form *invert sugar.* Intestinal *sucrase* readily splits sucrose into glucose and fructose.

Sucrose intolerance. Condition characterized by watery diarrhea associated with the malabsorption of sucrose. It is due to a genetic defect in which the enzyme sucrase-isomaltase, required in the hydrolysis of sucrose, is absent or deficient. See *Diet, sucrose-restricted.*

Sucrose polyester (SPE). A fat substitute under study, made by replacing the glycerol of the fat with sucrose. It is totally nonabsorbable and noncaloric.

Sugar. 1. Any sweet, soluble, crystalline organic compound belonging to the carbohydrates. 2. Specifically refers to sucrose extract from sugar cane and sugar beet. See *Sweetener.*

Sulfasalazine. A sulfonamide derivative used in the treatment of ulcerative colitis and Crohn's disease. It inhibits intestinal transport of folate and may induce folate deficiency. It may also decrease the intestinal synthesis of vitamin K and increase the urinary excretion of protein and ascorbic acid. Adverse gastrointestinal effects include anorexia, nausea, vomiting, gastric distress, and diarrhea. It is excreted in breast milk and known to have adverse effects on the infant. Brand names are Azaline and Azulfidine.

Sulfinpyrazone. A uricosuric agent used in the treatment of gouty arthritis and tophaceous gout. It reduces the amount of uric acid in the blood by increasing the amount excreted in the urine. Maintenance of a large volume of alkaline urine reduces the risk of stone formation in the kidneys. The brand name is Anturane.

Sulfites. Oxides of sulfur widely used in the food industry and in restaurants: as sanitizing agents for food containers and equipment; in wine and beer to stop fermentation; on seafoods, vegetables, and fruits (fresh or dried) to prevent discoloration or spoilage; and in salad bars to keep vegetables and fruits looking fresh. Some asthmatics experience acute reactions to foods treated with sulfites; these include wheezing, flushing, weakness, and tightness in the chest. Severe reactions, which have resulted in death, prompted the Food and Drug Administration to issue a labeling regulation requiring manufacturers to declare sulfite on the label of any food containing sulfite at a level of 10 ppm or more. Sulfite used as a preservative must be declared on the label regardless of the amount in the finished product. There is another regulation that bans the use of sulfites on fruits and vegetables intended to be served or sold raw to consumers.

Sulfonamides. Also called "sulfa drugs"; a group of antibacterial drugs used mainly to treat urinary tract infections. Sulfonamides interfere with the utilization of para-aminobenzoic acid and thus inhibit the biosynthesis of folic acid by colonic bacteria. Possible adverse effects include diarrhea, anorexia, stomatitis, and gastritis. Brand names include Bactrim, Gantanol, Gantrisin, Renoquid, and Thiosulfil.

Sulfonylurea. Class of chemical compounds that includes the oral hypoglycemic agents *acetohexamide, chlorpropamide, glipizide, glyburide, tolazamide,* and *tolbutamide.* These drugs stimulate the synthesis and release of insulin from the beta cells of the pancreas and are used to treat patients with noninsulin-dependent diabetes mellitus. They have no hypoglycemic effects on patients with insulin-dependent diabetes mellitus who have nonfunctional beta cells and cannot produce insulin.

Sulfur (S). Also spelled "sulphur." Mineral that is present in all cells, especially in cartilage and keratin of skin and hair. It occurs principally as a constituent of the amino acids cystine, cysteine, and methionine; it is also a constituent of insulin, thiamin, biotin, heparin, glutathione, coenzyme A, and other coenzymes. All protein foods provide sulfur, and the need for this mineral is met when the protein supply is adequate.

Sumacal. Brand name of a powdered carbohydrate (maltodextrin) supplement that is protein-free and low in electrolytes; provides 3.8 kcal/gm. See Appendix 39.

Supplementary feeding. The giving of food in addition to the regular meals to increase or supplement nutrient intake.

Suprarenal glands. The *adrenal glands.* The term "suprarenal" means lying above the kidneys.

Surgery. Treatment of disease by manual or instrumental operations. The patient's nutritional status is affected directly or indirectly, depending on the part of the body that undergoes surgery. For example, gastric resection results in decreased gastric acid production and the dumping syndrome; intestinal resection causes general malabsorption of all nutrients; and pancreatic resection leads to diabetes mellitus and malabsorption; other surgical procedures place the patient under physiologic and psychological stresses. The patient's weight, blood glucose, albumin, blood count, and electrolytes should be assessed and monitored regularly. *Dietary management:* if surgery is elective and the patient is overweight or obese, a weight reduction regimen is recommended. The undernourished patient should be rehabilitated with a diet high in protein, carbohydrate, and calories to build up tissue and glycogen reserves. Immediately before and after surgery, nothing is given by mouth to avoid vomiting and aspiration during surgery and postoperatively while recovering from anesthesia. Initially, intravenous glucose is the main source of energy. Depending on the patient's recovery and type of surgery, progressive oral feeding of clear to full liquids, followed by soft to regular foods, is often tolerated within a few hours or the next few days. The postoperative nutritional approach depends on whether the patient is hypometabolic or hypermetabolic. Because of the risk of hypophosphatemia and heart failure on refeeding, nutritional support for the nonstressed, hypometabolic, starved patient should be increased cautiously and gradually, taking up to a week to reach the final caloric goal. This allows the patient to adapt to the high caloric and glucose loads. If the intravenous route is required, one-third or more of the calories should be provided as lipid to reduce the glucose load. With either type of feeding, blood phosphorus levels should be assessed before repletion and monitored daily during the initial period of refeeding. In the hypermetabolic, stressed patient, nutritional support should be more aggressive. It is possible to reach the goal for calorie and protein intake within 2 to 3 days of initiating enteral or parenteral feeding. See *Refeeding syndrome.*

Sustacal. Brand name of a high-protein, lactose-free product for tube feeding or oral supplementation; contains sodium and calcium caseinates, soy protein isolates, corn syrup solids, sucrose, and soy oil. Also available as Sustacal HC (high-calorie) and with fiber (5.6 gm dietary fiber/liter). Sustacal Pudding and Sustacal Nutritional Powder are brand names for products containing milk and lactose, available in different flavors, for use as high-protein oral supplements. See also Appendix 39.

Sustagen. Brand name of a high-protein, high-calorie, low-fat oral supplement; contains whole and nonfat milk, calcium caseinate, corn syrup solids, and dextrose. See Appendix 39.

Sweetener. A substance that gives a sweet taste; may be *nutritive* (supplies calories) or *non-nutritive* (supplies no calories). Sucrose is the most common sweetener and is used as the standard (100%) for comparing the sweetness of other agents. The relative sweetnesses of natural agents are as follows: fructose, 173%; glucose, 74%; maltose, 33%; lactose, 16%; glycerol, 60%; sorbitol, 60%; and glycine, 70%. See also *Artificial sweeteners.*

Sympathetic nervous system. One of two parts of the autonomic nervous system. Its actions are opposite to those of the other part, the parasympathetic nervous system. For example, heart action is accelerated by the sympathetic system but decelerated by the parasympathetic system; intestinal peristalsis is decreased by the sympathetic system and increased by the parasympathetic system.

Symptom. The manifestation or expression of a disease as the patient experiences it, in contrast to the *sign,* or the manifestation of a disease as the examiner perceives it. Headache is a symptom; rapid pulse is a sign.

Syndrome. Set of symptoms and signs that occur together and characterize a particular disease or condition.

Synergism. Joint action of agents so that their combined effect is greater than the sum of their individual effects. Malnutrition lowers resistance to infection, and infectious diseases tend to magnify an existing malnutrition. The simultaneous presence of malnutrition and infection results in an interaction with an enlarged effect that is more serious than would be expected if malnutrition or infection acted separately.

T

T. Symbol for temperature.

T₃. Abbreviation for *triiodothyronine,* a thyroid hormone. See *Thyroid gland.*

T₄. Abbreviation for *tetraiodothyronine* or *thyroxine.* See *Thyroid gland* and *Thyroxine.*

Tachycardia. Rapid heartbeat. The term is usually applied to a pulse rate above 100/min; the rapid stimulus of heart action is associated with several causes, varieties, and sites in the heart.

Tachysterol. An isomer of ergosterol produced by irradiation, as is calciferol. It has no antirachitic activity unless reduced to dihydrotachysterol.

Tangier disease. A rare inherited disorder of lipid metabolism characterized by enlarged, orange-colored tonsils and storage of large amounts of cholesterol esters in foam cells; the mucosa of the colon and rectum also frequently has an orange color. The most striking feature is the almost complete absence of high-density lipoprotein. Plasma triglycerides may be elevated by the presence of chylomicrons and raised levels of low-density-lipoprotein. The condition is probably due to the absence of an apoprotein involved in the metabolism of lipoproteins. There is no specific treatment. Partial alleviation of symptoms occurs with a low-cholesterol diet, thereby reducing the storage of dietary cholesterol and cholesteryl esters. A low-fat diet is unnecessary, as fat transport appears to be normal. Since diabetes mellitus may develop in old age, weight control from an early stage is advisable.

Tartrazine. An alternate name for the yellow color FD & C Yellow No. 5, which is approved for use in foods, drugs, and cosmetics. Tartrazine may cause allergic reactions, including bronchial asthma, in susceptible individuals.

Taurine. B-aminoethanesulfonic acid; a sulfur-containing amino acid found in biologic fluids and most tissues, especially in the developing central nervous system, muscles, and platelets. It is a component of bile acids and is involved in many biologic activities, including the regulation of heartbeat, platelet aggregation, and maintenance of membrane stability. It is synthesized from methionine and cysteine, although humans have poor synthetic ability. Dietary intake and biosynthesis contribute to the concentration of taurine in the body. Under normal physiologic conditions, dietary taurine is generally not considered essential. It is found in meat and fish in high concentrations but is virtually absent from the diet of strict vegetarians and from most enteral and parenteral preparations. There is concern that adults and infants, especially the premature, receiving long-term parenteral nutrition have low plasma and urinary taurine concentrations. Reduced body pools of taurine are associated with retinal degeneration. While research on the essentiality of dietary taurine continues, it may be wise to include it in the diet. Most infant formulas are now supplemented with taurine to provide concentrations similar to that in human milk. Two parenteral solutions containing taurine are *TrophAmine* and pediatric *Aminosyn.*

TBA. Abbreviation for *thyroxine-binding albumin.*

TBPA. Abbreviation for *thyroxine-binding prealbumin.*

Ten-State Nutrition Survey. Originally called the National Nutrition Survey; conducted between 1968 and 1970, covering about 40,000 persons in California, Kentucky, Louisiana, Massachusetts, Michigan, New

York, South Carolina, Texas, Washington, and West Virginia. Nutritional status was evaluated using physical and dental examinations, anthropometric measurements, biochemical analysis for hematocrit and hemoglobin, and dietary data. Details of the findings are available from the U.S. Department of Health and Human Services or have been published in books and journals. See also *National Health and Nutrition Examination Survey (NHANES)*.

Tetany. Syndrome characterized by intermittent bilateral spasms, muscle twitchings, cramps, and sharp flexion of the wrist and ankle joints. Causative factors include alkalosis or excessive ingestion of alkaline salts, parathyroid hypofunction, abnormal calcium metabolism, and vitamin D deficiency.

Tetracycline. A group of antibiotics used to treat specific conditions including acne, bronchitis, syphilis, gonorrhea, and certain types of pneumonia. Milk and dairy products and foods high in calcium, iron, magnesium, and zinc inhibit drug absorption and should not be taken 2 hours before or after oral drug administration. Tetracycline decreases the synthesis of vitamin K by intestinal bacteria and increases the urinary excretion of vitamin C, riboflavin, folic acid, and niacin. Frequent gastrointestinal effects include nausea, vomiting, diarrhea, bulky loose stools, anorexia, stomatitis, glossitis, dysphagia, and epigastric burning. Tetracycline is excreted in breast milk and can have adverse effects; it may also discolor developing teeth. Brand names are Achromycin, Declomycin, Minocin, Mysteclin F, Panmycin, Rondomycin, Sumycin, Terramycin, and Vibramycin.

Tetrahydrofolic acid (THFA). Designated name for the compound tetrahydropteroylglutamic acid or tetrahydrofolacin; the most active form of *folic acid*. It acts as a carrier of 1-carbon fragments that are important for the synthesis of *purines* and *pyrimidines* and for methylation reactions.

Tetraiodothyronine (T₄). See *Thyroxine*.

Textured vegetable protein (TVP). Fabricated food product made from vegetable protein sources such as peanuts, sesame seeds, soybeans, and wheat and suitably flavored, colored, and textured to simulate commonly used foods such as bacon, beef, and chicken. Useful for select vegetarians and for food allergies.

Theine. Alkaloidal stimulant in tea chemically identical to caffeine.

Theobromine. Alkaloidal stimulant in cocoa beans; also occurs in tea leaves and cola nuts. It is closely related to caffeine and used as a diuretic, an arterial dilator, and a myocardial stimulant.

Thermal effect of food. Also known as "thermogenic" or "thermic effect of food." Formerly called "specific dynamic action (SDA) of food." Energy expended when food is digested, absorbed, and metabolized. It refers to an increase in metabolism after eating, which varies with the quantity and type of food consumed. The thermic effect of protein is about 30%; fat, 13%; and carbohydrate, 5%. For a mixed diet, the thermic effect is about 5 to 10% of total calories needed for basal metabolism and physical activity. See *Energy requirement.*

Thermogenesis. The reaction of the body to produce extra heat by shivering or by increasing the metabolic rate.

THFA. Abbreviation for *tetrahydrofolic acid.*

Thiamin (thiamine). Vitamin B₁, one of the water-soluble B complex vitamins. It was formerly called "aneurine," "antiberiberi vitamin," "antineuritic factor," "vitamin F," "oryzamine," and "morale vitamin." As a component of the coenzyme *thiamin pyrophosphate,* it functions in oxidative decarboxylation of keto acids and in the transfer of glycolaldehyde in the pentose phosphate pathway. Thiamin also helps maintain normal nervous system activity and regulates the muscle tone of the gastrointestinal tract. Early signs of thiamin deficiency include loss of appetite, irritability, depression, gastrointestinal disturbances, and easy fatigability. A severe deficiency is clinically recognized as *beriberi,* whose primary symptoms involve the nervous and cardiovascular systems. The causes of the deficiency are several and include inadequate intake due to diets dependent on milled and unenriched grains such as rice and wheat; ingestion of raw fish containing microbial *thiaminase,* which destroys the vitamin; chronic alcoholism, in which there is not only a low intake of thiamin (and other B vitamins) but also impaired absorption and increased requirement; and thiamin-responsive inborn errors of metabolism. Other persons at risk are patients undergoing long-term renal dialysis or intravenous feeding and those with chronic febrile infections. Good food sources are brewer's yeast, unrefined or enriched cereal grains, organ meats, lean pork, legumes, and nuts. The vitamin is very soluble in water. Cooking losses are high if the cooking liquid is discarded and if high temperature and prolonged heating are employed. It is absorbed primarily from the duodenum. The body is incapable of storing the vitamin; excess quantities are excreted in the urine. There is no evidence of thiamin toxicity by oral administration, although there is some toxicity from large doses given parenterally. See Appendix 1 for the recommended dietary allowances.

Thiaminase. An enzyme that splits the thiamin molecule, thereby inactivating it and causing a thiamin deficiency. It is present in bracken fern, raw fish, and a variety of fruits and vegetables. Cooking inactivates thiaminase.

Thiamin pyrophosphate (TPP). Also called "cocarboxylase"; the thiamin-containing coenzyme that participates in the oxidative decarboxylation of alpha keto acids and in the formation of alpha ketols.

Thioridazine. A phenothiazine antipsychotic agent. It may induce riboflavin depletion, alter glucose tolerance, and increase serum cholesterol. It may also cause weight gain due to fluid retention. Liquid preparations are incompatible with enteral formulas and can block nasogastric tubes if given during formula administration. Adverse gastrointestinal effects include anorexia, constipation, dry mouth, and stomatitis. The brand name is Mellaril.

Thiouracil. Antithyroid pyrimidine derivative that interferes with the formation of thyroxine; used in the treatment of thyrotoxicosis.

Thiourea. Also called "thiocarbamide"; an antithyroid substance used in the treatment of thyrotoxicosis. It inhibits the production of thyroxine by interfering with the incorporation of inorganic iodine into the organic form.

Threonine (Thr). Alpha-amino-beta-hydroxybutyric acid. An *essential amino acid* that participates in many of the reactions involving glycine and is important in purine synthesis and methylation reactions. Its metabolism is similar to that of serine, and both act as phosphate carriers in phosphoproteins.

Thrombin. Enzyme that hastens the conversion of fibrinogen to fibrin, forming a blood clot. It exists in shed blood as an inactive precursor, *prothrombin,* which is changed to active thrombin by the action of thromboplastin and calcium ions. See *Blood clotting.*

Thrombocyte. Also called "blood platelet"; one of the three formed elements of the blood. See *Blood.*

Thromboplastin. Enzyme that accelerates the conversion of prothrombin to thrombin; a cephalin-protein complex.

Thrombosis. Formation of an intravascular clot, or thrombus. It is likely to occur when there is slowing or stasis of the blood current as a result of circulatory or cardiac disorders or secondary to certain infections. If a thrombus or any part of it is dislodged, it may be carried through the bloodstream as an *embolus.*

Thymus. Ductless gland-like body located behind the sternum at the base of the throat and upper mediastinum just above the heart. It is developed early in fetal life, increases in size and weight shortly after birth, and then retrogresses by fatty metamorphosis after puberty. The thymus gland is believed to influence the maturation and proliferation of lymphoid cells involved in cell-mediated immunity and general host resistance. Other possible functions include its roles in malignant growth, reproduction, and calcium and phosphorus metabolism.

Thyrocalcitonin. Also called "calcitonin." Thyroid hormone having a significant effect on the calcium content of blood and bone. It is secreted in response to an elevated plasma calcium level and acts principally on bone, causing inhibition of bone resorption. Thyrocalcitonin is a polypeptide composed of 32 amino acids.

Thyroglobulin. Gelatinous iodine-containing protein synthesized by the *thyroid gland.* Hydrolysis of thyroglobulin yields *thyroxine* and other iodinated amino acids.

Thyroid gland. Butterfly-shaped endocrine gland consisting of two major lobes connected by a central isthmus. It is located in the neck just below the larynx. The thyroid gland has a unique ability to remove and concentrate blood iodide. This activity is influenced largely by the *thyrotropic hormone* and other chemical substances such as thiouracil, thiourea, thiocyanates, sulfonamides, and goitrogens. The chief function of the thyroid gland is to elaborate the thyroid hormones thyroxine, mono-, di- and triiodothyronine. Thyroxine and triiodothyronine are the most active biologically. The thyroid hormones regulate metabolism by stimulating oxygen consumption. For the effects of hypo- and hyperfunction of the thyroid gland, see *Cretinism, Goiter, Hyperthyroidism, Hypothyroidism, Myxedema,* and *Thyrotoxicosis.*

Thyronine. An amino acid that occurs in proteins only in the form of iodinated derivatives (iodothyronines), such as thyroxine. See *Thyroid gland.*

Thyrotoxicosis. Hyperactivity of the thyroid gland resulting from excessive secretion of thyroxine, tumor formation, or toxins that have entered the thyroid gland. See *Goiter* and *Hyperthyroidism.*

Thyrotropic hormone. Thyroid-stimulating hormone (TSH) or thyrotropin; a hormone secreted by the anterior lobe of the pituitary gland. It stimulates the thyroid gland to oxidize iodide to iodine and to release the thyroid hormones into the circulation.

Thyroxine. Also called "tetraiodothyronine"; the principal hormone of the thyroid gland. It is secreted into the blood bound to plasma protein (PBI) for transport to the tissues. Thyroxine regulates the rate of oxygen consumption in cells. It is also involved in growth and differentiation of the tissues.

Thyroxine-binding albumin (TBA). A thyroid hormone (triiodothyronine and thyroxine), a carrier protein of blood plasma.

Thyroxine-binding prealbumin (TBPA). A protein that binds the retinol-binding protein complex in the plasma and serves to carry vitamin A to the eye. It also binds the thyroid hormones, thyroxine and triiodothyronine. See *Transthyretin.*

Tin (Sn). An ultra trace element; possibly essential based on its growth-enhancing effect when added to the purified diet of rats. The human body contains about 0.2 ppm of tin, or about 12 mg/60 kg body weight, with the highest concentrations in liver and spleen. Naturally occurring tin deficiency is unknown either in animals or in humans. The average intake is about 3-4 mg/day, mostly in inorganic form. Ingested tin is poorly absorbed and is excreted mainly in the feces. There is no evidence of human toxicity from inorganic tin in foods; however, the widespread use of unlacquered tin and tin foil in cans and in packaged foods presents a potential hazard. Very high intakes of tin in experimental animals have produced changes in zinc and iron metabolism, with decreased hematocrit, hemoglobin, and serum iron. In humans, inhalation from the industrial environment may cause a mild lung condition called "pneumoconiosis."

TLC. Abbreviation for *total lymphocyte count.*

T lymphocytes. Type of white blood cells, or lymphocytes, traced from thymus-derived cells, which in turn come from the bone marrow. They are important cells for the immune system of the body.

Tocopherol. A generic name for all mono-, di-, and trimethyl tocols, which are complex alcohols of the chromanol type. Several tocopherols have been isolated, but only four forms have vitamin E activity (alpha-, beta-, gamma-, and delta-tocopherol). Alpha-tocopherol is the most potent biologically, and delta-tocopherol is the most active antioxidant. Tocopherols occur naturally in certain plant oils, particularly in wheat germ; they can also be produced synthetically. See *Vitamin E.*

Tolazamide. A *sulfonylurea* oral hypoglycemic agent used in the management of noninsulin-dependent diabetes mellitus. It is five times as potent as *tolbutamide.* Concomitant use with alcohol may cause disulfiram-like reactions. The drug is bound to plasma proteins. In protein malnutrition with hypoalbuminemia, more drug is available for a hypoglycemic effect. Hypoglycemia may also occur with inadequate food intake, with prolonged exercise without caloric supplementation, or with alcohol consumption. Excreted in breast milk. The brand name is Tolinase.

Tolbutamide. A *sulfonylurea* oral hypoglycemic agent used in the treatment of noninsulin-dependent diabetes mellitus. Concomitant use with alcohol may cause disulfiram-like reactions. There is a risk of hypoglycemia, although less than with *chlorpropamide* and *tolazamide.* Excreted in breast milk. The brand name is Orinase.

Tolbutamide test. Blood sugar determination before and 20 minutes after the intravenous administration of a solution containing 1 gm tolbutamide. A fall in blood sugar level by more than 89% in 20 minutes is diagnostic of diabetes mellitus.

Tolerance. 1. Limit to which substances can be ingested, absorbed, and metabolized with no deleterious physiologic effect. 2. Maximum limit established by the Food and Drug Administration to which additives may be incorporated in food.

Tolerex. Brand name of an elemental formula consisting of free amino acids, glucose oligosaccharides, and safflower oil. See Appendix 39.

Tongue. Movable muscular organ in the mouth that aids in mastication, swallowing, speech, and taste perception. It is covered by a mucous membrane and has numerous pa-pillae, minute nipple-like projections containing the taste buds. Color changes and lesions in the tongue are indicative of certain disorders, including nutritional deficiencies. See *Nutrition, tongue and mouth conditions.*

Tonsillectomy and adenoidectomy (T&A). Surgery performed to remove diseased tonsils and/or to correct adenoidal impairment. *Dietary management:* postoperatively, ample cold fluids may be administered, but avoid milk products, which tend to produce mucus. Gradually introduce soft foods. Supplement with vitamin C if juices cannot be taken by the patient. See also *Cold semi-liquid diet* under *Diet, liquid.*

Tooth. One of the calcified structures supported by the gums of both jaws. It is important for biting and chewing, supports the facial contour, and helps in articulation of sounds (speech). Several nutrients are essential for proper tooth formation and calcification. Protein influences matrix formation in the enamel and dentin of the developing tooth. The presence of vitamin A affects the formation of the enamel matrix and the maintenance of the epithelium of the periodontal tissue. Vitamin C influences the formation of the collagen matrix in dentin, cementum, and the periodontal membrane. Vitamin D, calcium, and other minerals are needed for the calcification of enamel, dentin, and cementum. Deficiencies and excesses of several minerals (fluoride, calcium, phosphorus, etc.) affect the composition of the calcified tissues. See *Nutrition, dental health.*

Tophus. Pl. "tophi." Mineral deposit in the joints, ear, or bone, such as sodium urate in gout.

TOPS. Abbreviation for *Take Off Pounds Sensibly.* A noncommercial self-help group concerned with the management and problems of obesity. See *Nutrition, weight control.*

Total arm length (TAL). Useful measurement to estimate the height of bedridden patients or persons with kyphosis or bone deformities (bowlegged, curved spine, bent knee gait, etc.). Using a nonstretchable tape, measure from the tip of the acromial process of the scapula at the shoulder to the end of the arm at the styloid process of the ulna at the wrist.

Total body electrical conductivity (TOBEC). A method of measuring body composition based on the principle of differences in electrical conductivity of fat, muscle and bone. Used to monitor weight loss, fitness of athletes, and to analyze fat content of tissues and food. See also *Bioelectrical impedance analysis* (BIA).

Total iron binding capacity (TIBC). A measure of the concentration of serum iron that is equal to the sum of the iron bond to *transferrin* and the unsaturated binding capacity. TIBC is often increased in iron deficiency, in the third trimester of pregnancy, and in hypoxia. It is decreased during infections and in iron overload, cancer, protein-calorie malnutrition, chronic diseases, and conditions associated with loss of protein. See also *Iron-binding capacity.*

Total lymphocyte count (TLC). An indicator of visceral protein stores. Determined from the formula:

$$TLC = \text{Total white blood cell count} \times \% \text{ lymphocytes.}$$

A TLC of 1200–1500/mm^3 indicate depressed immune competence associated with mild protein depletion; 800–1200/mm^3, moderate depletion; and less than 800/mm^3, severe protein depletion. TLC is not always useful in detecting malnutrition. It shows marked fluctuations daily and is affected by other factors such as blood dyscrasias, infection, chemotherapy, and immunosuppressive therapy.

Total parenteral nutrition (TPN). Feeding of a nutritionally adequate solution into the veins. There are two routes: through the subclavian or internal jugular vein that leads to the large central vein (called "central parenteral nutrition or CPN") and through the peripheral vein (called "peripheral parenteral nutrition or PPN"). Cyclic TPN refers to the intermittent infusion of intravenous solution over a specified period of time. It is useful for patients who need home TPN so that they can resume normal activities during periods when the TPN is not administered. Cyclic TPN is especially useful for cases of fatty liver. When a standard solution of all the nutrients needed for maintenance are not adequate due to increased demands of the patient, hypertonic solutions supplying more nutrients and calories (e.g., 3000 to 4000 kcal/day) are given by CPN which is sometimes called "parenteral hyperalimentation."

The decision to begin TPN is based on the presence or absence of malnutrition and on the attending medical problems. Indications when TPN should be used include: patients whose gastrointestinal tract are totally unavailable, those undergoing high-dose chemotherapy, radiation or bone-marrow transplantation; persons who are unable to absorb nutrients via the gastrointestinal tract (e.g., severe diarrhea, massive small bowel resection, severe enteritis, acute pancreatitis); severely malnourished patients in the presence of a nonfunctional gastrointestinal tract; patients who cannot receive adequate nutrition by enteral feedings within 7 days (e.g., severe mental state or comatose state); and those who require increased nutrients due to severe catabolism and whose gastrointestinal tract has been nonfunctional for 5 to 7 days (e.g., severe trauma, major surgery, extensive body surface burns). Clinical settings where TPN should not be used include: patients who have functional gastrointestinal tract capable of absorbing adequate nutrients; patients whose prognosis does not need aggressive nutritional support; and cases when the risks of TPN outweigh potential benefits, and the patient or legal guardian is against aggressive nutrition support.

The main problems attending TPN are sepsis or infection and metabolic complications. The latter group includes hyper- or hypoglycemia, electrolyte imbalance, excess or lack of certain trace elements or vitamins, anemia, bleeding, amino acid imbalance, essential fatty acid deficiencies, and others. See also *Parenteral nutrition.*

Toxemia. 1. Condition in which blood contains toxic or poisonous substances either produced by the body or elaborated by microorganisms. 2. Collective term for toxemias of pregnancy. The preferred designation is *pregnancy-induced hypertension.* See also *Eclampsia* and *Preeclampsia.*

TPN. Abbreviation for (1) *total parenteral nutrition.* (2) archaic term for *triphosphopyridine nucleotide* or coenzyme II, currently called "nicotinamide adenine dinucleotide phosphate."

TPP. Abbreviation for *thiamin pyrophosphate.*

Trace mineral. An element that is an essential nutrient but is required only in minute amounts (milligrams or micrograms per day) for humans. Examples are chromium, copper, manganese, and zinc. See *Mineral.*

Tracer technique. Research method that uses a radioactive element to follow the fate of a substance or its reactions. Compounds containing tracer elements are said to be "tagged" or "labeled."

Transamination. Transfer of an amino group from one compound to another, with *pyridoxal phosphate* acting as the intermediate amino carrier. The reaction is catalyzed by the enzyme *transaminase.* By this process the body is able to use ammonia and synthesize the nonessential amino acids.

Transcobalamin. Vitamin B_{12} bound to a protein; the transport form of the vitamin. There are three different cobalamin-binding proteins: transcobalamin I, II, and III.

Transferrin. A beta-globulin which transports iron in plasma. It is synthesized by the liver and has a half-life of 8 to 10 days. The normal range for serum transferrin is 250-300 mg/dl; values of 150-200 mg/dl indicate mild depletion; 100-150 mg/dl, moderate depletion; and less than 100 mg/dl, severe depletion. Transferrin is decreased in acute catabolic states, protein-losing enteropathy and nephropathy, chronic infections, and uremia. It is increased during pregnancy, estrogen therapy, iron deficiency, and acute hepatitis. Serum transferrin is measured by radial immunodiffusion, but a close estimate can be obtained from the more widely available measurement of total iron-binding capacity (TIBC), using the following formula:

$$Transferrin = (0.8 \times TIBC) - 43$$

Transketolase. Enzyme found in blood cells, liver, and other tissues; necessary for the synthesis of the 5-carbon sugars found in DNA and RNA. It requires thiamin pyrophosphate as a coenzyme.

Transmanganin. Protein carrier that transports manganese in the blood. See *Manganese.*

Transmethylation. Transfer of a methyl radical ($-CH_3$ group) from one compound to another. This reaction is important in intermediary metabolism, particularly in fat, sulfur, and creatine metabolism. Vitamin B_{12} and folic acid are involved in the synthesis of methyl groups. Methionine is considered the primary methyl donor in transmethylation reactions. Choline and betaine are also methyl donors.

Transthyretin. Also called "thyroxine-binding prealbumin (TBPA)." A plasma protein that serves as a secondary carrier of thyroxine and exists as a complex with *retinol-binding protein.* The very short half-life of this protein (2 days) makes it extremely sensitive to a decreased protein and energy intake of a few days duration. It declines in 3 days in response to a lowered energy intake, even when protein intake is adequate. Normal ranges are between 16-36 mg/dl. Values of 5-10 mg/dl are indicative of moderate depletion; less than 5 mg/dl, severe protein depletion.

Trauma. Severe injury caused by an accident or injury of the central nervous system and heart affected by shock. Trauma is also classified according to etiology as thermal (burns), neurologic (central nervous system or brain), severe emotional shock, chemical (toxic agent), and physical (as in multiple fractures and major surgery). Internal risk factors include the nutritional status of the person. The immediate reaction to trauma is a high plasma level of catecholamines, glucocorticoids, and glucagon. Blood glucose is elevated due to impaired utilization or insulin resistance by muscles; protein and fat catabolism is increased; and the electrolyte/water balance is affected. *Dietary management:* specialized nutrition support is needed, usually by *tube feeding,* if the gastrointestinal tract is functional. Provide adequate hydration and monitor serum levels of protein, electrolytes, and glucose. In severe cases, as in serious head injuries, intravenous feeding is a more effective method. Return to oral feedings only when there is no vomiting and the patient can gradually resume normal digestion and absorption. See also *Burn* and *Surgery.*

Traumacal. Brand name of a high-nitrogen, restricted-carbohydrate formula for stressed patients with hyperglycemia. Contains branched-chain amino acids (23%) plus essential and nonessential amino acids, corn syrup, sucrose, MCT oil, and soy oil. See also Appendix 39.

Traum-Aid HBC. Brand name of a chemically defined formula high in branched-chain amino acids (50%) plus essential amino acids. For oral or tube feeding of hypercatabolic patients and in hepatic insufficiency. See also Appendix 39.

Travasol. Brand name of an amino acid solution for total parenteral nutrition. Contains both essential and nonessential amino acids in 3.5, 5.5, 8.5, and 10% concentrations, with and without electrolytes. See also Appendix 40.

Travasorb. Brand name of a line of products for specialized nutritional support by tube feeding or as an oral supplement. Travasorb Hepatic contains amino acids as a protein source, high in branched-chain amino acids (50%) and low in aromatic amino acids (2%) for oral supplementation in liver failure; Travasorb MCT contains medium-chain triglycerides, with a high ratio of medium- to long-chain triglycerides (80:20 w/w); Travasorb Renal is a low-protein (from amino acids), high-calorie, electrolyte-free powder for use in renal failure; Travasorb STD and Travasorb HN contain peptides from enzymatically hydrolyzed lactalbumin in soluble powder form. See also Appendix 39.

Triamterene. A potassium-sparing diuretic which is structurally related to folic acid. Used in the treatment of edema associated with congestive heart failure, liver cirrhosis, or nephrotic syndrome. It is a folic acid antagonist and can cause folate depletion; it may cause hyperkalemia, decrease serum vitamin B_{12}, and increase urinary excretion of calcium, sodium, and chloride. Possible gastrointestinal effects are dry mouth, nausea, vomiting, diarrhea, and gastric distress. Excreted in breast milk. The brand name is Dyrenium.

Tricarboxylic acid (TCA) cycle. Krebs cycle or citric acid cycle; the final common pathway of energy metabolism for carbohydrate, protein, and fat. See *Krebs cycle.*

Triceps skinfold (TSF). Anthropometric measurement to estimate subcutaneous fat indirectly. Together with mid-arm muscle circumference, it also gives an estimate of skeletal muscle mass. Measurement of a skinfold is taken at the midpoint between the acromion of the scapula and the olecranon of the ulna. A decrease in triceps skinfold thickness reflects a chronically inadequate nutritional intake. Measurements greater than the 50% percentile are acceptable; 40th–50th percentile indicate mild depletion; 25th–39th percentile, moderate depletion; and below the 25th percentile, severe fat depletion. See Appendix 22.

Triglyceride. Also called "triacylglycerol." *Fat* in which the glycerol molecule has three fatty acids attached to it. Chemically, triglycerides comprise about 95% of dietary fats and have been used interchangeably in practical dietetics; for example, a fat-restricted diet is referred to by some clinicians as a "low-triglyceride" diet. Circulating triglyceride levels are influenced by genetics, dietary factors (calories, fat, carbohydrate, alcohol intake), and disease (diabetes mellitus, pancreatitis, fatty liver). See *Hyperlipoproteinemia* and *Diet, fat-modified.*

Trigonelline. An inactive form of *niacin* that is found in seeds and nuts. Roasting coffee beans activates this substance.

Triidothyronine (T₃). A thyroid hormone that exerts the same effects as thyroxine, but is present in much smaller amounts. See *Thyroid gland.*

Trimethoprim. A synthetic folate antagonist antibacterial used in the treatment of urinary tract infections caused by susceptible organisms. High doses for prolonged periods (more than 6 months) can cause folate deficiency, especially in geriatric, malnourished, alcoholic, pregnant, or debilitated patients; in patients receiving other folate antimetabolites, like the phenytoin anticonvulsants; and when the dietary folate intake is low. Supplementation with folic acid may be necessary. Brand names are Bactrim, Bethaprim, Proloprim, Septra, and Sulfatrim.

Triose. A sugar that contains 3 carbon atoms. It is an intermediate product of metabolism and does not occur naturally. *Glyceraldehyde* is a triose.

Trisaccharide. An oligosaccharide containing three monosaccharide units. Examples are *raffinose* (has fructose, glucose, and galactose) and *melezitose* (has two molecules of glucose and one molecule of fructose). See Appendix 8.

Tritium. The hydrogen isotope with a mass of 3. It is radioactive and has a half-life of 31 years. Tritium is used in tracer studies and body water determination.

TrophAmine. Brand name of a 6% amino acid solution especially formulated for pediatric total parenteral nutrition. Contains taurine, high in branch-chain amino acids and low in phenylalanine, methionine, and glycine. See also Appendix 40.

Trypsin. Proteolytic enzyme of the pancreas secreted as the inactive precursor *trypsinogen.* It is an endopeptidase and catalyzes the hydrolysis of peptide linkages containing the carboxyl group of lysine and arginine, yielding polypeptides with C-terminal lysine and arginine groups.

Trypsin inhibitor. A substance capable of reducing the activity of the proteolytic enzymes in the digestive juices; it can also slow down the absorption of some amino acids, either by reducing the utilization of nitrogenous material in food or by increasing the needs of the organism for certain amino acids. It is found in raw egg white, soybeans, peanuts, peas, beans, and lentils.

Tryptophan (Try). Alpha-amino-beta-indolyl-propionic acid. An *essential amino acid* for humans and animals. It is frequently a limiting amino acid for tissue synthesis. Tryptophan is the only amino acid with an indole nucleus; it can be converted to nicotinic acid, serotonin, and melatonin.

TSF. Abbreviation for *triceps skinfold.*

TSH. Abbreviation for *thyroid-stimulating hormone.* See *Thyrotropic hormone.*

Tube feeding (TB). Introducing food through a tube to persons with a functional gastrointestinal tract as supplemental nourishment or as the only source of nutrient intake. Indicated for patients who cannot eat solid foods orally and cannot retain foods in the stomach or who are unwilling or unable to eat enough by mouth. Patients may include those with head and neck injuries; anorexia nervosa; hypercatabolic states like sepsis, burns, and multiple trauma; acute pancreatitis; inflammatory bowel disease; short bowel syndrome; cancer; AIDS; upper gastrointestinal surgery; severe dysphagia; and disorders of the central nervous system like cerebrovascular accident or stroke. The tube feeding routes are nasogastric, orogastric, nasoduodenal, nasojejunal, esophagostomy, gastrostomy, and jejunostomy. The choice of the route, kinds of tubes and pumps, rate of administration, and nutritional formula have to be individualized according to the disorder(s) and capabilities of the patient. With regard to formulas, many are available commercially (see Appendix 39). The type of feeding (e.g., blenderized, polymeric, monomeric, or special formula), dilution and total volume/day, osmolality, and nutrient density needed (especially for calories and protein) are important considerations in choosing the right formula. The formula consumed daily has to be monitored for adequacy of nutrient intake. Some of the nutritional problems of tube feeding include glucose intolerance, electrolyte imbalance (hypo- or hyperkalemia, hypo- or hypernatremia, hypo- or hyperphosphatemia), essential fatty acid deficiencies, and trace mineral deficiencies. Possible gastrointestinal problems may arise, such as nausea and vomiting, diarrhea, constipation, lactose intolerance, reduced gastrointestinal motility, nutrient-drug interactions, and malabsorption.

Tuberculosis. An infectious disease caused by the tubercle bacillus, *Mycobacterium tuberculosis,* which invade the lungs. Characterized by inflammation of lung tissues, high fever, tissue wasting, coughing and expectoration, general weakness and *hemoptysis.* In recent years, the incidence of tuberculosis has increased, especially among AIDS patients. Good nutrition and sanitation are preventive factors. *Dietary management:* provide a liberal intake of protein (1.2 to 1.5 gm/kg to restore plasma protein and promote wound healing) and a high caloric level (1.5 times more than the individual's needs) due to fever. Supply adequate minerals, especially calcium to help in the calcification of the lesions, and iron, plus other hematopoietic nutrients in case of hemorrhaging. If the drug used is isoniazid, increase vitamin B_6 (isoniazid is an antagonist for pyridoxine) and folic acid.

Two Cal. Brand name of a high-calorie, high-protein supplement for severely hypermetabolic and stressed patients on fluid restriction. Provides 2 kcal/ml and contains sodium and calcium caseinates, soy protein isolates, hydrolyzed corn starch, sucrose, corn oil, and MCT oil. See also Appendix 39.

Tyramine. A pressor amine similar in action to epinephrine; found mainly in foods and beverages that have undergone bacterial decomposition during the process of fermentation, aging, pickling, or spoiling. It is normally degraded in the body by the enzyme monoamine oxidase (MAO). Inhibitors of this enzyme interfere with this process, causing the release of norepinephrine, a powerful vasoconstrictor. The concomitant ingestion of tyramine-rich foods and MAO inhibitors can trigger a hypertensive crisis. See *Monamine oxidase* and *Diet, tyramine-restricted.*

Tyrosinase. Copper-containing enzyme that oxidizes tyrosine and other phenolic compounds, forming brown to black pigments. Lack of this enzyme results in *albinism.*

Typhoid fever. Food-borne infection caused by *Salmonella typhosa.* It occurs endemically wherever sanitation is poor and the water supply is likely to be contaminated with sewage. The organism is transmitted through polluted water and food, especially milk, shellfish, and raw vegetables. *Dietary management:* see guidelines under *Fever.* See also *Food poisoning.*

Tyrosine (Tyr). Alpha-amino-beta-hydroxy-phenylpropionic acid. A nonessential amino acid that has some sparing action on the essential amino acid phenylalanine. It participates in transamination reactions and is the starting material for the synthesis of melanin, thyroxine, and epinephrine.

Tyrosinemia. An inherited disorder characterized by an elevated blood tyrosine level due to an enzyme deficiency in tyrosine metabolism. Type I tyrosinemia, or *tyrosinosis,* affects predominantly the liver and kidneys; it is due to a deficiency in the enzyme fumarylacetoacetase. Type II tyrosinemia affects the eye and skin, resulting in keratitis and ocular lesions; it is due to tyrosine aminotransferase deficiency. Dietary treatment is by protein restriction or a diet low in tyrosine and phenylalanine to reduce plasma tyrosine level down to 1 mmol/liter. See *Product 3200AB.*

U

U. Abbreviation for Unit, as in IU. (International Unit).

u. Symbol for micro-; often written as μ.

UAC. Abbreviation for *upper arm circumference.*

UAMA. Abbreviation for *upper arm muscle area.*

Ubiquinone. General term for a group of related quinones with variable numbers of isoprene residues. Ubiquinone is found in the mitochondria and serves as an electron transport agent. See *Coenzyme Q.*

UFA. Abbreviation for unsaturated fatty acid.

Ulcer. An eroded lesion or an excavated sore. See *Decubitus ulcer, Peptic ulcer disease,* and *Ulcerative colitis.*

Ulcerative colitis. A chronic inflammatory disease of the large intestine, or colon and rectum, characterized by diarrhea, fever, abdominal cramps, anemia, and weight loss. The mucosal and submucosal tissue layers of the large intestine are usually inflamed for brief periods. *Dietary management:* in the acute stage, use a minimal-residue diet to avoid undue irritation to the colon. A semisynthetic fiber-free diet is available commercially. In intractable cases, total parenteral feeding is needed. As the patient improves, oral feeding is resumed, using a fiber-restricted diet high in protein and calories. Use preparations high in medium-chain triglycerides for better fat digestion and utilization. Vitamin and mineral supplements, particularly chromium, copper, selenium, and zinc, are recommended. See also *Crohn's disease* and *Inflammatory bowel disease.*

Ultra-. A combining form meaning "beyond a certain limit or more than the normal range."

Ultracal. Brand name of a fiber-containing formula for tube feeding; has a fiber content of 13.6 gm/liter. It is lactose-free and isotonic, and contains calcium and sodium caseinates, MCT oil, and a blend of oat and soy fibers. See Appendix 39.

Undernutrition. A form of *malnutrition.* A deficiency state due to lack of calories and/or one or more of the essential nutrients. For examples of undernutrition, see *Anorexia nervosa, Kwashiorkor, Marasmus,* and *Nutrition, starvation.*

Underweight. Term applied to individuals whose body weight is more than 10% below the established standard for individuals of the same age, sex, and height. *Dietary management:* theoretically, an excess of 500 kcal/day results in a weekly gain of 1 lb. A gradual gain of 1–2 lb/week is a desirable rate. A high-calorie, high-protein diet is best given in six to eight feedings per day. Supplemental vitamins and minerals may be necessary. See *Weight control.*

UNESCO. Abbreviation for United Nations Educational, Scientific, and Cultural Organization. An organization that aims to eliminate illiteracy and to help people, through education, to use science and understand cultural forces for the improvement of their lives.

UNICEF. Abbreviation for United Nations International Children's Emergency Fund. An organization that aims to help children all over the world by eradication of disease, improvement of health, and provision of emergency relief rations by milk distribution and school feeding programs and through the establishment of maternal and child health care centers.

United States Department of Agriculture (USDA). A department of the federal government whose goals are to improve farm income and develop markets for agricultural products; to reduce and cure poverty, hunger, and malnutrition; to ensure standards of food quality through inspection and grading services; and to conduct research and nutrition programs. Examples of the last are the Food Stamp Program, the National School Lunch Program, the Child Care Food Program, the WIC Program, the Special Milk Program for Children, the School Breakfast Program, and the Commodity Supplemental Food Program. The divisions directly concerned with nutrition include the Extension, Human Nutrition Center, Food and Nutrition Service (FNS), Food Safety and Quality Service (FSQS), Agriculture Research, Cooperative Research, and Technical Information Service.

United States Department of Health, Education and Welfare (USDHEW). Created on April 11, 1953, it was renamed the Department of Health and Human Services (DHHS) on October 17, 1979.

United States Department of Health and Human Services (USDHHS). The goals of this department are to serve people ranging from newborn infants to the oldest citizens; to advise the president on health, welfare, and social security plans; and to form policies related to human development, general health, and welfare. Some of the offices *directly* concerned with nutrition are the Administration on Aging (AOA), Administration for Children, Youth, and Families (ACYF), Administration for Native Americans (ANA), Public Health Service (PHS), President's Council on Physical Fitness and Sports, National Center for Health Statistics, Centers for Disease Control (CDC), Food and Drug Administration (FDA), National Institutes of Health (NIH), National Cancer Institute (NCI), National Heart, Lung, and Blood Institute (NHLBI), and the Alcohol, Drug Abuse, and Mental Health Administration.

United States Pharmacopeia (USP). The standard weight reference for nutrients in the United States. The USP standards for ascorbic acid, calcium pantothenate, choline, chloride, nicotinamide, nicotinic acid, pyridoxine hydrochloride, riboflavin, thiamin hydrochloride, essential amino acids, and vitamins A and D are available to the public. When an international standard exists, the USP standard is compared and brought as closely as possible into agreement. A USP unit is therefore equal to an international unit.

Unsaturated fatty acid (UFA). See under *Fatty acid.*

Upper arm circumference (UAC). Also called "mid-arm circumference (MAC)." Combination of muscle mass, bone size, and subcutaneous fat deposits. Measurement is taken midway between the tip of the acromial process of the scapula and the olecranon process of the ulna. UAC measures skeletal mass and fat stores but is not a sensitive method by itself; it is used in formulas for other anthropometric measurements.

Upper arm muscle area (UAMA). A reliable indicator of lean body mass and skeletal protein reserves. Useful in evaluating protein-energy malnutrition. It is determined from the following formula:

$$\text{UAMA (mm}^2) = \frac{(\text{MAC,mm} - \text{TSF,mm} \times 0.314)^2}{4 \times 0.314}$$

where MAC is *mid-arm circumference* and TSF is *triceps skinfold* measurement. To measure the bone-free arm muscle area, subtract 10 (for males) and 6.5 (for females) from the results of this formula.

Urate. A salt of uric acid. An increased amount of urates in the urine is called "uraturia." Urates may be deposited as crystals in body joints or as calcareous deposits in tissues. See also *Gout.*

Urea. The diamide of carbonic acid. It is the major end product of human nitrogen (protein) metabolism and the chief nitrogenous constituent of *urine.* Urea formation occurs chiefly in the liver.

Urea clearance test. Test that measures the quantity of blood "cleared" of urea per minute to determine renal function.

Urea cycle. The overall reactions of the urea cycle proceed as follows: the combination of CO_2, NH_3, and adenosine triphosphate forms carbamyl phosphate, which combines with ornithine to form citrulline. The latter combines with aspartic acid to form argininosuccinic acid, which is broken down to arginine and fumaric acid. The last reaction of the urea cycle is the hydrolytic cleavage of arginine to yield urea and ornithine.

Urease (urase). Specific enzyme that decomposes urea, forming ammonia and carbon dioxide.

Uremia. Excessive retention of urinary constituents in the blood. It is a toxic condition and the terminal manifestation of *renal failure* or end-stage renal disease. The clinical features include nausea and vomiting, anorexia, dizziness, anemia, convulsions, and coma. *Dietary management:* protein is restricted to 15 to 20 gm/day, supplied mainly by one egg and 4 to 6 oz milk. Provide sufficient calories to prevent breakdown of body tissues. Nonprotein calories should come from fats, sugars, fruits and vegetables, and special low-protein, high-calorie commercial products. See *Diet, minimal-protein,* under *Diet, protein-modified.*

Ureterolithiasis. Formation of a stone, or calculus, in the ureter, which is a long, narrow tube that conveys the urine from the pelvis of the kidneys to the bladder. The surgical removal of a stone in the ureter is called *ureterolithotomy.* See also *Urinary calculi.*

Uric acid. The end product of purine metabolism in humans and of protein metabolism in birds and some reptiles. In humans, uric acid is excreted in the urine in the free state and as the urates of sodium, potassium, and ammonium. It is formed in part from purines taken in food (exogenous uric acid) and in part from body purines as a result of the breakdown of nucleic acids (endogenous uric acid). Abnormal metabolism of uric acid is characteristic of *gout.*

Urico-. A combining form meaning "pertaining to uric acid."

Uridine. Nucleoside that consists of uracil and ribose. This is obtained by the removal of phosphate from uridylic acid.

Uridine diphosphate glucose (UDPG). The glucose ester of uridine diphosphate formed from glucose-1-phosphate in the presence of a pyrophosphorylase. It is the prosthetic group of the enzyme responsible for the conversion of galactose to glucose.

Uridylic acid. Nucleotide containing ribose, phosphoric acid, and the pyrimidine uracil. The nucleotides of uridine monophosphate, uridine diphosphate, and uridine triphosphate function as coenzymes in a wide variety of reactions.

Urinalysis. Physical, chemical, and microscopic analyses of the urine. These include a description of color and clarity or turbidity; the determination of pH and specific gravity; and the observation of the presence or absence of abnormal constituents such as proteins (albumin), sugar, ketone bodies, casts, bacterial cells, pus, and blood cells. See Appendix 31.

Urinary calculi (urolithiasis). Insoluble constituents in the urine that precipitate as stones in the urinary passages. Variable in composition, these may contain urates, cystine and calcium oxalates, phosphates, carbonates, and *struvite.* Urinary calculi formation is the result of a number of factors, including hyperfunction of the parathyroid glands; vitamin A deficiency; systemic infections; inadequate fluid intake; metabolic disturbances; prolonged bed rest; and obstruction in the renal flow, producing stasis of the urine. *Dietary management:* a liberal fluid intake to dilute the urine and prevent concentration of "stone-forming" substances is the main guideline. Control of urinary pH and foods to avoid will depend on the composition of the stone. See *Diet, ash; Diet, calcium-phosphorus-restricted;* and *Diet, oxalate-restricted.*

Urinary tract infection (UTI). Infection usually caused by gram-negative bacteria in one or more of the organs in the urinary tract (kidneys, ureter, bladder, urethra). Characterized by a burning sensation during urination, pain, frequent urination, and sometimes visible blood and pus in the urine. Treatment is by drug therapy, liberal fluid intake, and control of urinary pH. See also *Diet, ash.*

Urine. Fluid excreted by the kidneys. The quantity excreted in 24 hours varies with the amount of fluid consumed but averages between 1000 and 1500 ml. It is slightly acidic in reaction (pH 4.6 to 7) and has a specific gravity of 1.005 to 1.030. The amount of solids varies with the diet and with renal function, although urine collection normally contains 40 to 75 gm solids/24 hours. Urine formation is the result of three processes that occur in the nephron: filtration through the glomerular capillaries; reabsorption of fluid and solutes in the proximal tubule, the loop of Henle, and the distal tubule; and secretion into the lumen of the distal tubule. Urinalysis is an important biochemical method of *nutritional assessment* and aids in diagnostic testing. See also Appendix 31.

Urobilin. Also called "stercobilin"; a brownish pigment derived from the oxidation of urobilinogen, a derivative of the bile pigment bilirubin. This is found in the feces and sometimes in the urine after exposure to air. It is primarily responsible for the brown color of the feces.

Urochrome. The chief yellow pigment of the urine. Other pigments are uroerythrin and uroporphyrin.

Urogastrone. A substance found in the urine similar to enterogastrone. It also inhibits gastric secretion and motility.

Urokinase. An enzyme produced in the kidney and found in the urine. As a drug preparation, it is used to treat pulmonary embolism.

Urolith. A stone, or calculus, in the urine. The formation of urinary calculi is called *urolithiasis,* and the removal of a calculus from the urinary tract is called *urolithotomy.* See *Urinary calculi (urolithiasis).*

Uroporphyrin. A porphyrin found in small amounts in the urine. It is excreted in abnormally large amounts in lead poisoning, congenital prophyria, and prophyrinuria.

USDA. Abbreviation for *United States Department of Agriculture.*

USP. Abbreviation for *United States Pharmacopeia.*

Uterus. The womb; a pear-shaped, hollow, muscular organ in the female that receives and nourishes the fertilized ovum during its fetal development. It is about 3 inches long, 2 inches wide, and 1 inch thick, and includes the fundus (the upper and broad portion) and the body, which gradually narrows down to the cervix and extends down to the vagina. It weighs only about 40 gm in a normal adult. During pregnancy, the uterus expands many times its normal size by cellular hypertrophy.

UTI. Abbreviation for *urinary tract infection.*

V

V. Chemical symbol for vanadium.

Vagotomy. Cutting of certain branches of the vagus nerve, often accompanied by gastrectomy. Usually performed to reduce the recurrence of a gastric ulcer. Dietary management is the same as for *gastrectomy*.

Vagus. The 10th and largest cranial nerve, originating from the brain and carrying impulses to many organs in the head, neck, chest, and abdomen. Resection of the vagus nerve is called *vagotomy*.

Valine (Val). Alpha-aminoisovaleric acid; an *essential* amino acid necessary for growth and maintenance of tissues. Deficiency in rats causes hyperesthesia and muscular incoordination.

Valproic acid. A derivative of carboxylic acid that is used alone or with other anticonvulsants in the management of seizures. It may cause hyperglycinemia and carnitine deficiency with hyperammonemia; it may also cause nausea, vomiting, diarrhea, and stomach cramps. It is excreted in breast milk; infants must be observed for drowsiness. Brand names are Depakene and Depakote.

Vanadium (V). Trace element found in the human body; the concentration in human blood is about 100 μg/ml. It is probably essential and may have a role in the regulation of the sodium pump and the metabolism of bones, glucose, and lipids. Vanadium at pharmacologic levels can inhibit cholesterol synthesis in the liver and lower plasma cholesterol and triglycerides. There has been no report of vanadium deficiency. It is found in small amounts in most foods. The typical American diet probably provides 25 μg daily. Vanadium can also be absorbed through inhalation. Potential toxicity from exposure in industry has been a concern because vanadium is rapidly absorbed through the lungs and skin. The use of vanadium in various industrial processes and its release into the environment have resulted in many cases of vanadium toxicity in humans. Signs of intoxication include sore eyes, diarrhea, dermatitis, depressed food intake, elevated tissue vanadium level, and death. An interesting aspect of vanadium toxicity is its depletion of ascorbic acid and the counteraction of vanadium toxicity by this vitamin. Toxicity from the diet is rare, although vanadium is toxic in relatively low doses.

Vanillylmandelic acid (VMA). Also spelled "vanylmandelic acid." An end product in the metabolism of epinephrine and norepinephrine. It is excreted in urine in the free form and is frequently increased in *pheochromocytoma*. The reference range for VMA is 1.8-7.1 mg/day. See also *Diet, VMA test*.

Vascular. Relating to blood or lymphatic vessels and ducts. Most often refers to blood vessels. The vascular bed is the total blood supply (i.e., arteries, capillaries, and veins) of an organ or region.

Vasoconstriction. Constriction of the blood vessels, especially the arterioles, leading to a decrease in the caliber of the vessels and a reduced blood supply. This is brought about by a *vasoconstrictor agent*.

Vasodilation. Dilation or increase in the caliber of a blood vessel, especially the arterioles, leading to an increased blood supply. This effect is brought about by a *vasodilator agent*.

Vasomotor. Regulating the movements of the walls of the blood vessels, i.e., their contraction (vasoconstriction) and expansion (vasodilation).

Vasopressin. A posterior pituitary hormone that exerts both pressor and antidiuretic actions. Its *pressor* action is a result of peripheral vasoconstriction in the systemic arterioles and capillaries. There is also constriction of the coronary and pulmonary vessels but dilation of the cerebral and renal vessels. The *antidiuretic effect* is exerted by increasing the rate of reabsorption of water in the renal tubules, resulting in relatively concentrated urine. A lack of this hormone results in *diabetes insipidus.* This is characterized by excessive renal loss of water and excessive thirst. Release of vasopressin is stimulated by a variety of neurogenic stimuli such as pain, trauma, and emotional stress.

Vegan. A *vegetarian* who excludes from the diet all foods of animal origin.

Vegetable protein mixtures. Blend of processed vegetable protein foods with or without skim milk powder and with or without added vitamins and minerals. They can be cheap sources of protein-rich food in countries where animal protein foods are expensive or unavailable. See Appendix 36.

Vegetarian. A person subsisting entirely or largely on foods of plant origin; intake of food of animal origin is restricted or not allowed. A vegetarian follows one of several patterns. A *pure vegetarian* (or vegan) is one who eats only foods of plant origin, without specific restrictions as to kind. A *fruitarian* is one who restricts the variety of plant foods eaten to fresh and dried fruits, nuts, honey, and sometimes olive oil. A *lactovegetarian* eats plant foods plus milk and other dairy products. An *ovovegetarian* includes eggs as the only source of animal protein. A *lactoovovegetarian* consumes milk, dairy products, and eggs, in addition to plant foods. A *pescovegetarian* includes fish, and a *pollovegetarian* includes poultry in the diet. Other people who also consider themselves vegetarians are the *red meat abstainers,* who eat any animal product except red meat, and the semivegetarians, who exclude some animal food groups. See also *Nutrition, vegetarianism* and *Diet, Zen macrobiotic.*

Verdohemoglobin. Also called "choleglobin". Intermediate compound formed in the breakdown of hemoglobin. It is a biliverdin-iron-protein complex that has a green color.

Very-low-calorie diet (VLCD). See *Diet, calorie-modified.*

Very-low-density lipoprotein (VLDL). A plasma protein that has a density of 0.95-1.006 gm/ml; classified as the pre-beta fraction on the basis of electrophoresis and contains about 10% protein, 18% phospholipid, 22% cholesterol, and 50% triglycerides. VLDL is involved in the transport of triglycerides from the intestinal tract and liver to adipose tissues and muscles. An increase in the concentration of VLDL is believed to be linked to an increase in the incidence of atherosclerosis.

Villi. Small, finger-like projections on the surface of a mucous membrane, as in the walls of the small intestine, where absorption takes place.

Vincristine. An antineoplastic drug that interferes with amino acid metabolism and inhibits nucleic acid and protein synthesis. It is used alone or in combination with other chemotherapeutic agents in the treatment of Hodgkin's disease and other lymphomas. Its adverse effects are dose related and may cause nausea, vomiting, diarrhea, stomatitis, oral ulcerations, hyponatremia, anorexia, and weight loss. The brand name is Oncovin.

Viral hepatitis. Inflammatory liver disease caused by a hepatitis virus (type A, B, non-A, or non-B). Clinical signs include anorexia, fever, nausea and vomiting, jaundice, malaise, diarrhea with clay-colored stools, and pain over the liver area. The severity of symptoms and the course of the illness depend on the kind and strain of the virus. Prolonged infection, observed especially with hepatitis B, may result in cirrhosis, hepatic coma, and even death. *Dietary management:* liberal fluid intake plus a high-calorie diet that is high in protein and carbohydrate and moderate in fat is used. High-fat foods are not restricted unless the patient finds them difficult to tolerate. At least six small feedings a day are encouraged. Avoidance of alcohol is recommended.

Virus. Disease-producing agent smaller than the ordinary germ; consists of a nucleic acid, either RNA or DNA, enclosed in a protein layer. It is a living pathogen that can multiply only in the presence of living, healthy host cells. Some viruses are visible under the ordinary microscope; others, the ultraviruses, are visible only under the ultramicroscope. Some can pass through porcelain filters; the nonfilterable viruses, however, cannot.

Viscera. Organs enclosed within the four great cavities: the cranium, thorax, abdomen, and pelvis. Pertains most commonly to the digestive organs within the abdominal cavity.

Viscosity. Resistance of a liquid to flow. The viscosity of a liquid is measured by an instrument called a *viscosimeter.*

Visual process. The eyes contain two kinds of light receptors (rods and cones) located in the retina. The rods are involved in vision in dim light, and the cones function in vision in bright light. The light sensitivity of these two receptors comes from two photosensitive pigments, *rhodopsin* (in the rods) and *iodopsin* (in the cones), which are protein complexes of vitamin A. The prosthetic group in both of these pigments is vitamin A in the form of retinaldehyde, although the proteins to which the aldehyde is attached are different. On exposure to light, rhodopsin is bleached through a series of intermediate compounds, giving as end products *opsin* (a protein) and retinaldehyde (vitamin A aldehyde). These changes initiate a nerve impulse that is transmitted to the brain by way of the optic nerve. Regeneration of rhodopsin occurs in the dark, but some retinaldehyde is lost in each cycle, so that a constant supply must be present in the blood to recombine with opsin to regenerate rhodopsin.

Visual purple. Also called "rhodopsin"; a conjugated protein containing vitamin A. It is a photosensitive pigment in the retina of the eye that is bleached to visual yellow by light.

Visual threshold. Minimal light intensity required to evoke a visual sensation.

Visual violet. Also called "iodopsin"; a photosensitive pigment of the cones in the ret-ina of the eye that is important for vision. It contains vitamin A.

Visual yellow. Colorless substance formed in the retina when visual purple (rhodopsin) is exposed to light. It is a mixture of retinaldehyde and a protein, opsin.

Vital HN. Brand name of a low-residue product for oral or tube feeding; it is also lactose-free and low in electrolytes. Contains partially hydrolyzed whey, meat and soy protein hydrolysates, sucrose, hydrolyzed cornstarch, MCT oil (40%), and safflower oil (60%). See also Appendix 39.

Vital statistics. Figures on births, deaths, longevity, disease rates, and other data that indicate the state of health of a population.

Vitamer. 1. Substance structurally related to a vitamin and capable of producing the same biologic activity. 2. One of the early names given to vitamins.

Vitamin. General term given to a group of organic substances that are present in food in minute quantities but are distinct from carbohydrates, lipids, and proteins; essential for normal health and growth; cause a specific deficiency diseases when not adequately supplied by the diet or improperly absorbed from the food. See *Vitamin nomenclature.*

Vitamin A. Formerly called "axerophthol" and "antixerophthalmic vitamin"; a group of fat-soluble compounds which occur in several isomeric forms and occur preformed only in foods of animal origin. It exists in two forms: *retinol,* or vitamin A_1, which predominates in mammals and saltwater fish, and *dehydroretinol,* or vitamin A_2, which predominates in freshwater fish. It is present in yellow and green leafy plants as provitamin A, of which there are several forms; the most important ones in human nutrition are the *carotenoids* alpha- and beta-carotene and cryptoxanthin. These are converted to the active vitamin in the intestinal wall and liver. The richest sources of preformed retinol are fish liver oils, egg yolk, and fortified milk. Biologically active carotenoids are found in dark green leafy vegetables and yellow fruits and vegetables such as squash and carrots. The color intensity of a fruit or vegetable is not a reliable indication of its content of provitamin A, since many other yellow and orange carotenoids in plants are not readily converted to the vitamin. Vitamin A is necessary for normal growth and development, maintenance of normal epithelial tissue structure, integrity of the immune system, and other physiologic functions, including vision and reproduction. Vitamin A deficiency is usually due to inadequate dietary intake; deficiency also occurs as a result of chronic fat malabsorption. Symptoms of deficiency vary with the animal species. In humans the most common signs are poor growth, lowered resistance to infection, night blindness, and rough, scaly skin. Severe deficiency leads to *keratomalacia* and *xerophthalmia.* Vitamin A is not normally excreted and can accumulate in the body. Excessive intake (hypervitaminosis A) causes headache, dry skin, loss of hair, softening of bones, and liver damage. A high incidence of spontaneous abortions and birth defects has been reported in women ingesting large doses of *isotretinoin* (13-cis retinoic acid) during the first trimester of pregnancy. Carotenoids are not toxic but can color adipose tissue stores and make the skin look yellow when taken in large doses over several weeks; the yellow coloration disappears gradually when the high intake is discontinued. See Appendix 1 for the recommended dietary allowances for vitamin A.

Vitamin B complex. Group of water-soluble vitamins generally found together in nature and somewhat related in function, although unrelated chemically. These include vitamin B₁ (thiamin), vitamin B₂ (riboflavin), the vitamin B₆ group (pyridoxine, pyridoxal, and pyridoxamine), the vitamin B₁₂ group (the cobalamins), nicotinic acid (niacin), folic acid (pteroylglutamic acid or PGA), pantothenic acid, and biotin.

Vitamin B₁. Also called *thiamin;* originally designated "water-soluble vitamin B" or the "antiberiberi vitamin" or "antineuritic factor" found in rice polishings. It was given the subscript number 1 when the B vitamin was discovered to be not a single factor but a complex composed of several factors. The vitamin was identified and synthesized by R. R. Williams and coworkers, who coined the word "thiamine" to indicate its structure, containing both sulfur (thio group) and an amino group. See *Thiamin.*

Vitamin B₂. Also called *riboflavin;* name given to the heat-stable fraction of vitamin B to differentiate it from the heat-labile fraction, designated "vitamin B₁." It was recognized to be a yellowish-green fluorescent pigment belonging to a group of compounds known as "flavin" and given the names Warburg's "yellow enzyme," "vitamin G," and "lactoflavin," "ovoflavin," "hepatoflavin," or "verdoflavin," since it was isolated from milk, egg, liver, and grass. The compound was later called "riboflavine" because it contains a ribose conjugated to a protein plus a pigment, flavin. The final "e" was dropped from the spelling because the vitamin is not really an amine. See *Riboflavin.*

Vitamin B₆. A group of chemically related compounds that are metabolically interchangeable: pyridoxine (alcohol form), pyridoxal (aldehyde form), and pyridoxamine (amine form). The three forms are all widely distributed in low concentrations in all animal and plant tissues. Good food sources are muscle meats, liver, pork, egg, whole grain cereals, and soybeans. The vitamin is readily and completely absorbed from the gut, but the level in the blood is extremely low and storage is very limited. The biologic activity of the three forms is about equal; all can be converted in the liver, erythrocytes, and other tissues to *pyridoxal phosphate* and *pyridoxamine phosphate,* which function as coenzymes in transamination reactions. Pyridoxal phosphate is also involved in the degradation, decarboxylation, and racemization of amino acids; in the conversion of tryptophan to nicotinic acid; in urea production; and in the metabolism of essential fatty acids. It is used therapeutically to control nausea and vomiting of pregnancy and to alleviate the peripheral neuritis of isonicotyl hydrazide medication. Vitamin B₆ deficiency in adults rarely occurs alone, but it is seen in persons with multiple vitamin deficiencies and during long-term use of certain drugs, such as oral contraceptives, isoniazid, levodopa, and hydralazine. Signs of deficiency include seborrheic dermatitis, nausea and vomiting, stomatitis, and depression. In infants, vitamin B₆ deficiency has been induced with milk formulas deficient in the vitamin, causing hyperirritability, poor growth, and convulsions. The vitamin is relatively safe in oral doses of up to 50 times the recommended dietary allowance. A transient dependency state, consisting of ill-defined symptoms including nervousness, and tremulousness, is induced when pharmacologic doses are given for several weeks and then suddenly withdrawn. See Appendix 1 for the recommended dietary allowances.

Vitamin B₁₂. Also called "cobalamin"; the antipernicious anemia factor found to be identical to the extrinsic factor of Castle, erythrocyte maturation factor, animal protein factor, and zoopherin. It has a characteristic red color and contains cobalt as an essential mineral constituent. As a constituent of two coenzymes, methylcobalamin and 5-deoxyadenosylcobalamin, vitamin B₁₂ functions in the stimulation of red blood cell formation; synthesis of nucleic acids and nucleoproteins; and metabolism of nervous tissue, folate, sulfur-containing amino acids, carbohydrate, fat, and protein. It is present only in animal foods; plant foods are practically devoid of the vitamin. Good food sources are liver, eggs, milk, meat, and fish. The average intake is about 0.6 μg/day. Cyanocobalamin is the commercially available form of vitamin B₁₂ used in pharmaceuticals and vitamin pills. The primary absorption of the vitamin involves cleavage from dietary protein by gastric acid and binding to the intrinsic factor of Castle secreted by the gastric mucosa. A small amount of the vitamin (1–3%) may be absorbed by simple diffusion. The vitamin is present in blood bound to three different proteins as transcobalamins and is transported to the liver and other tissues. There is unusual storage in the liver; the amount stored may last for 3 to 4 years in the absence of any additional supply. Dietary deficiency is rare but may be seen in strict vegetarians. However, symptoms of deficiency have been observed in some breast-fed infants of women who are strict vegetarians. Vitamin B₁₂ deficiency is nearly always the result of inadequate absorption due to absence of intrinsic factor, which may be an inherited condition or a result of surgical resection of the stomach or the absorbing surfaces of the ileum. Small bowel diverticula, intestinal infestations, sprue, and other malabsorption syndromes may also induce a deficiency state. Manifestations of deficiency include sore tongue, general weakness, macrocytic anemia, and neurologic symptoms due to demyelination of the spinal cord, brain, and optic and peripheral nerves. Correction of a deficiency resulting from inadequate absorption requires injection of 100 μg/month of vitamin B₁₂. There has been no report of toxicity with excessive intakes. See Appendix 1 for the recommended dietary allowances.

Vitamin B₁₃. A compound from distillers' dried solubles that was provisionally called "vitamin B₁₃"; later identified as orotic acid, an intermediate in pyrimidine metabolism. Orotic acid is not recognized as a vitamin, since all amino acids are capable of contributing to the orotic acid pool.

Vitamin B₁₄. Crystalline compound isolated from wine and originally thought to be a metabolite of xanthopterin; claimed to check the growth of cancer cells.

Vitamin B₁₅. Pangamate (pangamic acid), a preparation marketed as a vitamin but not recognized as such by U.S. drug authorities. See *Pangamic acid.*

Vitamin B₁₇. A term used to describe laetrile and/or amygdalin. Not recognized as a vitamin by United States drug authorities. See also *Laetrile.*

Vitamin C. Formerly called "antiscorbutic vitamin" and "cevitamic acid"; a water-soluble vitamin that exists in several forms, of which the two most active are L-*ascorbic acid* and L-*dehydroascorbic acid.* It is synthesized from glucose or galactose by most animals except the human, monkey, guinea pig, Indian fruit-eating bat, and red-vented bulbul bird. Vitamin C functions in a wide variety of roles, such as formation and maintenance of the intercellular cementing substance; metabolism of phenylalanine, tyrosine, folic acid, and histamine; conversion of ferric to ferrous iron to facilitate absorption; and wound healing and immune response. It also acts as a good antioxidant and may prevent the formation of carcinogenic nitrosamines by reducing nitrites. The ingestion of fruits and vegetables rich in vitamin C has been associated with a reduced incidence of some cancers. Deficiency of the vitamin results in *scurvy,* anemia, delayed or incomplete wound healing, and reduced resistance to infection. The richest food sources are acerola and camu-camu; other good sources are green and red peppers, collard greens, broccoli, spinach, tomatoes, potatoes, strawberries, kiwi, oranges, and other citrus fruits. The dietary vitamin C is generally much lower than the calculated amount in foods because of its destruction during processing and loss in cooking water. It is the most unstable vitamin, and is easily oxidized on exposure to air and light and destroyed by high temperature, alkali, and copper. Absorption in the intestines is almost complete, although tissue storage is quite limited and deficiency can result readily when intake is inadequate. Much of the body's store is concentrated in cells and is found in greatest concentration in the adrenals, eye lens, and liver. Excess intake is readily eliminated in the urine after tissue saturation. Pharmacologic doses of ascorbic acid have been reported to reduce the frequency and severity of symptoms of the common cold and other respiratory illnesses and to lower serum cholesterol in some hypercholesterolemic individuals. However, there is no general agreement on the benefits obtained from large doses of

the vitamin for these conditions. A number of adverse effects with high intakes have been reported. See Appendix 1 for the recommended dietary allowances.

Vitamin C₂. See *Bioflavonoids.*

Vitamin D. Also called "calciferol"; a fat-soluble vitamin necessary for the formation of the skeleton and for mineral homeostasis. It was previously called the "sunshine vitamin," "antirachitic factor," and "rachitamin." Vitamin D is a group of several related sterols, but the two most important are vitamin D_2 (ergocalciferol or ercalciol), which is obtained from irradiation of the provitamin ergosterol found in plants, and vitamin D_3 (cholecalciferol or calciol), which is produced from the provitamin 7-dehydrocholesterol found underneath the skin on exposure to ultraviolet light from the sun. The vitamin is metabolized in the liver into 25-hydroxyvitamin D (25-hydroxycholecalciferol, 25(OH)D, 25HCC, or calcidiol) and then further hydroxylated in the kidney to the active metabolite 1,25-dihydroxyvitamin D (1,25-dihydroxycholecalciferol, 1,25(OH)₂D, 1,25-DHCC, or calcitriol). The active metabolite then returns to the intestinal mucosal cells, where it initiates the production of a calcium-binding protein which assists in the absorption of calcium from the intestines. It also helps to maintain plasma calcium regulation by increasing bone resorption synergistically with parathormone and by stimulating reabsorption of calcium by the kidney. Because of this action, vitamin D acts more like a hormone than a cofactor for an enzyme. Vitamin D is thus considered both a vitamin and a prohormone. The requirement for vitamin D can be met under normal conditions of exposure to sunlight. When sun exposure is restricted or limited, dietary intake may be important, especially in the elderly, whose capacity to synthesize the vitamin is approximately half that of younger people. Fish liver oil and foods fortified with vitamin D are the major dietary sources; smaller amounts are found in liver, egg yolk, sardines, and salmon.

Vitamin D deficiency is characterized by inadequate mineralization of the bone. Severe deficiency in children results in *rickets;* a deficiency in adults leads to *osteomalacia.* The vitamin is potentially toxic; excessive intake (hypervitaminosis D) causes anorexia, nausea, calcification of soft tissues, and renal damage. Although the toxic level has not been established for all ages, consumption of as little as 45 μg (1800 IU) of cholecalciferol per day has been associated with signs of hypervitaminosis D in young children. See Appendix 1 for the recommended dietary allowances.

Vitamin E. Originally known as the "antisterility vitamin." It is a fat-soluble vitamin required by humans and several species of animals. A derivative of chromanol, vitamin E includes eight naturally occurring forms of the tocopherol and tocotrienol compounds found in plants. The most active form, and the one most widely distributed in nature, is alpha-tocopherol. Vitamin E is a biologic antioxidant capable of protecting cellular membranes from oxidative damage by preventing lipid oxidation, especially the peroxidation of polyunsaturated fatty acids (PUFA) and cholesterol; it can also inhibit accumulation of ceroid pigment granules. Together with selenium, carotenoid, and ascorbic acid, vitamin E is the primary defense against potentially harmful oxidation. Major food sources are the vegetable and seed oils, especially those with polyunsaturated fatty acids, like soybean, corn, cottonseed, and safflower oils; however, various amounts of the vitamin in these oils are lost during production, storage, and refining processes. Meats, fish, animal fats, and most fruits and vegetables have little vitamin E. Absorption of the vitamin varies, depending on total lipid absorption and the presence of bile salts and pancreatic enzymes. The efficiency of absorption decreases as large amounts of tocopherol are consumed. Once absorbed, the vitamin is transported in plasma with the lipoproteins and taken up by most tissues, including the liver, lung, heart, skeletal muscle, and adipose tissue. But unlike other tissues, fat tissue can sequester and accumulate the vitamin. The results of vitamin E deficiency in animals are varied and include reproductive failure, muscular dystrophy, liver necrosis, and neurologic abnormalities. In humans the occurrence of vitamin E deficiency is rare, except in susceptible individuals like premature and very-low-birth-weight infants and those with steatorrhea and malabsorption problems associated with a variety of conditions such as biliary atresia, cystic fibrosis, chronic pancreatitis, and abetalipoproteinemia. Newborn infants delivered prematurely develop vitamin E deficiency because of limited storage at birth, intestinal malabsorption, and rapid growth rates that increase nutrient requirements in general. Some infant formulas also have marginal or low tocopherol contents relative to the amount of PUFA and iron present. A subclinical deficiency of vitamin E in humans is considered when the plasma or serum tocopherol level is below 0.5 mg/dl, accompanied by a low ratio of serum tocopherol to lipid and/or hemolysis of erythrocytes incubated in 2% hydrogen peroxide. There is no evidence of adverse effects with large intakes of vitamin E. See Appendix 1 for the recommended dietary allowances.

Vitamin K. Formerly called "antihemorrhagic factor" and "Koagulation vitamin"; a group of fat-soluble 2-methyl-1,4-naphthoquinone derivatives necessary for the prevention of hemorrhagic conditions. The naturally occurring vitamins K are vitamin K_1 (phylloquinone), found in plants, and vitamin K_2 (menaquinone), formed by bacterial synthesis in the intestine. Vitamins K_3 to K_7 are synthetic preparations, of which the most active is vitamin K_3 (menadione). Compounds with vitamin K activity are essential for the formation of prothrombin and other coagulation factors involved in the regulation of blood clotting. Vitamin K is also required for the biosynthesis of certain proteins, found in plasma, bone, and kidney, that bind calcium ions and probably function in bone crystal formation, photosynthetic phosphorylation, and the respiratory enzyme system. Deficiency of the vitamin results in a delayed blood clotting time and a hemorrhagic tendency. Because of its wide distribution in plants and intestinal synthesis by bacteria, deficiency resulting from dietary lack in human adults is rare. It may, however, occur in the presence of conditioning factors such as fat malabsorption, biliary obstruction, liver dysfunction, and prolonged treatment with broad-spectrum antibiotics and anticoagulants. Infants are susceptible to vitamin K deficiency because of small prenatal vitamin K storage and inadequate intestinal flora for its synthesis. Although vitamin K is fat-soluble, there are no known cases of toxicity in humans, except for the synthetic form, menadione, which can produce hemolytic anemia, hyperbilirubinemia, and kernicterus in the newborn with immature liver function. See Appendix 1 for the recommended dietary allowances.

Vitamin P. Name originally given to a group of factors that decrease capillary fragility. They were later identified as flavonoids but are now more commonly called *bioflavonoids* to indicate that they have biologic activity. It is no longer considered a vitamin.

Vitamine. Original spelling of *vitamin,* as proposed by Funk in 1911 to indicate that the *accessory food factor* necessary for life is a vital amine. The final letter, "e," was dropped when analysis of the chemical nature of several of these factors showed that not all of them are amines.

Vitamin-like substances. Substances that, on the basis of current information, fail to meet all the criteria necessary to be classified as vitamins but still have some properties of vitamins. In some cases, they are present in larger amounts than vitamins; in others, the body can synthesize sufficient amounts to meet its needs if precursors are present. Examples of these substances are *carnitine, inositol,* and *bioflavonoids.*

Vitamin nomenclature. As suggested by Osborne and Mendel and McCollum and Davis, vitamins were originally classified, according to their solubility, as fat-soluble A and water-soluble B. Successive letters were assigned to new vitamins as they were characterized and isolated. Later it became evident that vitamin B was not a single vitamin but a group of vitamins, and subscripts were added for identification. The nomenclature became confusing when new factors thought to be new vitamins were so named, only to be found to be duplicates of other vitamins already named. The present trend is to call the vitamins by their chemical names. To date we recognize 13 vitamins essential to human nutrition: 4 fat-soluble vitamins (A, D, E, and K) and 9 water-soluble vitamins (ascorbic acid, thiamin, riboflavin, nicotinic acid, pyridoxine, cobalamin, pantothenic acid, folic acid, and biotin). The *fat-soluble vitamins* have the following general properties: soluble in fat and fat solvents; not absolutely necessary in the diet every day; have precursors or provitamins; intake in excess of daily need is not excreted but stored in the body; and deficiencies are slow to develop. The *water-soluble vitamins* have the following general properties: soluble in water; must be supplied every day in the diet; generally do not have precursors; intake in excess of daily need is excreted in the urine, with minimal storage in the body; and deficiency symptoms often develop rapidly.

Vitaneed. Brand name of a lactose-free blenderized formula containing fiber for tube feeding and not intended for oral use. Made with beef puree, sodium and calcium caseinates, maltodextrins, pureed fruits and vegetables, and soy oil. See also Appendix 39.

Vitellin. Phosphoprotein found in egg yolk.

Vitreous humor. Transparent gel-like fluid that fills the posterior chamber of the eye; consists of hyaluronic acid within a protein framework called "vitrein."

Vivonex. Brand name of a line of monomeric (elemental) formulas containing crystalline amino acids, glucose oligosaccharides, and safflower oil for tube feeding and oral supplementation. They are lactose-free, have minimal residue, and are low in fat. Available in powder form as Vivonex Standard, Vivonex HN, and Vivonex T.E.N., which has added glutamine and is high in branched chain amino acids (33%) and low in aromatic amino acids. See also Appendix 39.

VLCD. Abbreviation for very-low-calorie diet. See *Diet, calorie-modified.*

VLDL. Abbreviation for *very-low-density lipoprotein.* See also *Blood lipids.*

Vomiting. Process of "throwing up" or expelling materials from the stomach through the esophagus and out of the mouth. Prolonged or persistent vomiting leads to nutritional deficiencies and is one factor considered in the initial screening and nutritional assessment of patients. If food cannot be retained and liquid intake is not adequate, dehydration and undernutrition can be avoided by using methods other than oral feeding. See *Parenteral feeding.* See also *Hyperemesis.*

von Gierke's disease. Type I glycogen storage disease; an inborn error of metabolism due to a deficiency in the enzyme glucose-6-phosphatase, which is required for the conversion of glycogen to glucose. This results in the accumulation of glycogen in the liver, which becomes enlarged, and in hypoglycemia, which may be frequent, severe, and even fatal. Excessive glycogen accumulation, accompanied by acute and chronic hypoglycemia, causes liver damage and growth retardation. *Dietary management:* small, frequent feedings of glucose as the carbohydrate source, including interruption of sleep for feeding, to prevent hypoglycemia. Nasogastric or gastrostomy feeding or even intravenous administration of glucose may be necessary at times. Both sucrose and lactose should be avoided because their end products, fructose and galactose, are readily converted to glycogen in the liver. Thus, milk and sugar-containing foods are to be avoided. Starches are not restricted unless they contain forbidden sugars. Acceptable infant formulas and oral supplements include Isomil, Nutramigen, and Pregestimil.

Vulnerability. Susceptibility to injury or contagion. In nutrition, the phrase *vulnerable group* refers to infants, children, pregnant or lactating women, and elderly people, groups particularly prone to develop nutritional disorders.

W

Waist-hip ratio (WHR). An anthropometric measurement to determine body shape; used as an index for healthy weight. Estimated by measuring around the waist where it is smallest and around the hip where it is largest and use the equation given below:

$$\text{WHR} = \frac{\text{smallest waist measurement (cm or inch)}}{\text{largest hip measurement (cm or inch)}}$$

Ratios above 0.8 for women and 0.95 for men are linked to greater risk for several diseases. See also *Weight* and Appendix 20 A.

Warfarin. From Wisconsin Alumni Research Foundation; an anti-vitamin K compound used as a rat poison and therapeutically as an anticoagulant. Foods high in vitamin K may reduce its anticoagulant effect. Brand names are Athrombin-K, Coumadin, and Panwarfin.

Water (H_2O). One of the major nutrients needed by the body. It comprises about 50 to 80% of total body weight, depending on body fat content. It performs varied functions and is second only to oxygen in maintaining life. The body can live for several days, even months, without food but dies within 5 to 10 days without water. Loss of 20% of body water results in death. All chemical reactions in the body take place in the presence of water. It acts as a solvent for products of digestion, as a lubricant of moving parts, and as a regulator of body temperature. Blood is 90% water and urine is 97% water. Water is also important for the proper elimination of waste products. See also *Water, sources.*

Bound w. Portion of water in food and body tissues that is attached to the colloids and is therefore more difficult to release than *free water.*

Endogenous w. Also called "metabolic water"; water derived from the metabolism of food in the body.

Exogenous w. Water in the body coming from dietary sources either as liquid or as a food component.

Free w. The portion of the water in the body or food that is not closely bound by attachment to the colloids.

Metabolic w. Also called "water of combustion"; water in the body that is provided by the combustion of foodstuffs (i.e., carbohydrate, protein, and fat). Oxidation of 1 gm carbohydrate, protein, and fat yields approximately 0.60, 0.41, and 1.07 gm water, respectively.

Water balance. Balance between water intake and output. Water intake comes from fluids and beverages (free water), as a component of food, or as a product of the oxidation of foods in the body (metabolic water). The channels of water output are through the kidney (urine), the skin (sweat and insensible perspiration), the lungs (expired air), and the gastrointestinal tract (saliva and feces). Insensible water loss from lungs and skin accounts for 50% of the turnover of water, even without visible perspiration. Water intake must equal output, the difference resulting in edema or dehydration, depending on whether intake is greater or less than output. Water intake is controlled by the thirst center in the hypothalamus. Water output is controlled by the hormone *vasopressin* (also called "antidiuretic hormone or ADH"), which is secreted by the pituitary gland. Release of this hormone decreases water excretion by the kidney by increasing the rate of water reabsorption from the tubules. The urine is an important medium for the elimination of excess water.

Abnormal losses of water, however, may occur in diarrhea, excessive vomiting, and severe burns. See also *Balance study.*

Water compartment, body. Water inside the body exists in two main compartments: within the cells (intracellular water) or outside the cells (extracellular water). Water outside the cells is found within the blood vessels (intravascular water) or between the vascular spaces and the cells (interstitial water). Smaller amounts are found in cerebrospinal fluid, synovial fluid, aqueous and vitreous humors, and lymph.

Water determination, body. The two general methods of measuring body water are direct and indirect. The direct method is obviously feasible only in human autopsy studies. The indirect methods of estimating the volume of each of the various water compartments are essentially the same. A material, previously found to be distributed almost exclusively within the compartment to be measured, is given intravenously in known amounts. After a sufficient time for mixing, a plasma sample is obtained and the concentration of the administered material is measured. *Total body water* can be measured by the use of a substance such as heavy water or antipyrine, which passes freely through capillary walls, cell membranes, and the blood-brain barrier. Determination of this material in any available fluid (e.g., plasma or urine) indicates the amount of total body water. Determination of total *extracellular fluid* requires a substance such as inulin, thiocyanate, or thiosulfate that can cross capillary walls and distribute itself uniformly in the plasma and interstitial fluid without entering the cells. Estimation of plasma volume requires the administration of dyes or iodine 131 attached to albumin which will be retained only within the vascular spaces. The volume of the *interstitial water* is the difference between the volume of total extracellular fluid and plasma volume.

Water intoxication (water toxicity). Condition that results from excessive intake of fluids without an equivalent amount of salt, as in intravenous glucose administration to persons with inadequate renal function. The kidney cannot excrete the extra load, and the accumulated water enters all the fluid compartments, including the cells and tissues, which become waterlogged. Serious symptoms develop, including confusion, convulsions, coma, and even death.

Water requirement. Two vital needs of the body demand a continual expenditure of water: removal of body heat by vaporization of water through the skin and lungs, and excretion of urea and other products of metabolism in the urine. There is an obligatory daily loss of approximately 1500 ml water. Of this amount, about 600 ml is lost through the skin as insensible perspiration, 400 ml in expired air, and 500 ml in urine. Any excess in water intake over this obligatory water loss appears as an increase in urine volume, and any deficit under the obligatory water loss is taken at the expense of total body water, resulting in dehydration. The need for water is increased in hot climates; with excessive exercise because of the loss of water through sweat; and in burns, fever, and other pathologic conditions that increase the need for water above the normal requirement. A water allowance of 1 ml/kcal for adults is generally considered sufficient under average environmental conditions. Increasing the water requirement to 1.5 ml/kcal, allowing for variations in physical activity, perspiration loss, and solute load of the kidneys, is still safe from *water intoxication.* The water requirement for infants, however, needs special attention due to the higher percentage of water content of their bodies and their greater body surface area. Infants are more susceptible to severe *dehydration* and have a higher rate of water turnover. A daily intake of 1.5 ml/kcal during infancy is recommended. In pregnancy, the water requirement is increased compared to that of the nonpregnant state in order to supply the needs of the growing fetus, the increased extracellular fluid space, and the amniotic fluid. The extra water needed for lactation is for milk secretion. See also *Dehydration* and *Electrolyte balance.*

Water sources. The main form of water ingested to meet bodily requirements is water as such. The second category is in the form of beverages such as fruit juices, milk, coffee, tea, soft drinks, soups, and alcoholic beverages. For Americans, most of the water sources come from beverages and fewer from water as such. The rest of their water needs are supplied by the so-called solid foods, which vary in their water content from 95% in succulent fruits and vegetables to 65% in meats and fish. Butter and nuts contain 16% and 5% water, respectively. Water from exogenous sources, referred to as "preformed water," averages about 2000 ml/day. Water produced internally by oxidation or from metabolic processes amounts to about 300 ml/day.

Waxes. Simple lipids; esters of fatty acids with certain alcohols. Some waxes are sperm oil, beeswax, carnauba oil, and lanolin. See Appendix 10.

WBC. Abbreviation for *white blood cell.* See *Leukocyte.*

Wean. Gradual or abrupt stoppage of breast feeding when the infant is capable of taking substantial nourishment from sources other than breast milk. Early weaning may be indicated when there is insufficient breast milk or when the mother is in poor health or when she becomes pregnant again.

Weanling diarrhea. Diarrhea associated with weaning of malnourished infants. It is commonly seen in developing countries where the incidence of food-borne infections is high. Malnutrition lowers body resistance to disease, thus making these infants more susceptible to such infections.

Weight. Force with which a body is attracted to the earth. In reference to body weight, the word "weight," if used without qualification, means the *actual* body weight as measured on a weighing scale. *Standard weight* is the average weight for each sex for different statures at various ages. *Ideal weight* (taken as the standard weight at age 25) is the weight associated with the most favorable mortality. Standard weight tables imply that average weights are normal (see Appendix 19). Currently, the concept and

usage of ideal body weight have been replaced by that of healthy body weight. A healthy weight depends on how much of the body weight is fat, where fat is located in the body, and whether there is a weight-related medical problem. See Appendix 20-A.

Weight, computed. Useful equations to estimate body weight for persons who have bone fractures that need traction or casting; also for persons whose weight cannot be measured directly due to some specific illnesses. The formulas are given below:

Body weight for men (in kg)
$$= (0.98 \times \text{calf C}) + (1.16 \times \text{knee H})$$
$$+ (1.73 \times \text{MAC}) + (0.37 \times \text{subsc SF})$$
$$- 81.69$$

Body weight for women (in kg)
$$= (1.27 \times \text{calf C}) + (0.87 \times \text{knee H})$$
$$+ (0.98 \times \text{MAC}) + (0.4 \times \text{subsc SF})$$
$$- 62.35$$

The recumbent measurements are in centimeters for the calf circumference (calf C), knee height (knee H), midarm circumference (MAC), and sub-scapular skinfold thickness (subsc. SF), which is measured just posterior to the left scapula or shoulder blade.

Weight control. Process of adjusting variable factors that affect body weight, aiming at a desirable level considered optimum. As a result of the prevalence of obesity, weight control programs concentrate on reducing body weight using a multifaceted approach. See *Nutrition, weight control, Obesity, Overweight,* and *Underweight.*

Wernicke-Korsakoff syndrome. Disorder combining *Wernicke's encephalopathy* and *Korsakoff's* neurologic signs and symptoms. In severe alcoholism, both syndromes occur. Lack of vitamins, especially thiamin, is the main cause, in addition to the direct toxic effects of alcohol on the brain and peripheral nerves.

Wernicke's encephalopathy. Disease caused by an acute biochemical lesion in the brain due to *thiamin deficiency.* The syndrome was originally described by Wernicke among alcoholics and can be considered as the human counterpart of the encephalopathy produced in animals by acute deprivation of thiamin. It is characterized by paralysis or weakness of eye movements, ataxia, and mental disturbances. See *Thiamin.*

Wetzel grid. Technique for measuring and evaluating a child's growth. It consists of nine physique channels that range from the very fat to the very thin. The height-weight data of a child are plotted throughout the growth period. The rate of growth is thought to be a more accurate measure of nutritional status than one weight measurement. The grid can be used to detect children who are failing to develop normally.

Whey. "Milk serum," the liquid that remains after the curd and cream are removed from coagulated milk. It contains most of the lactose of the original milk but has little protein and almost no fat.

White blood cell (WBC). See *Leukocyte.*

WHO. Abbreviation for *World Health Organization.*

WHR. Abbreviation for *Waist-hip ratio.*

WIC. Abbreviation for *Women, infants,* and *children.*

Wilms' tumor. A highly malignant embryonoma of the kidney occurring mostly in young children. Symptoms include weight loss, anorexia, abdominal pain, anemia, fever, and hypertension. *Dietary management* is aimed at correcting these symptoms. A high-calorie, high-protein diet with mineral supplements is indicated. Sodium intake is controlled if hypertension exists.

Wilson's disease. Also called "hepatolenticular degeneration." Rare inherited disorder of copper metabolism characterized by a decrease in plasma *ceruloplasmin* concentration and excessive accumulation of copper in the liver, brain, cornea, and kidney. If untreated, it causes liver damage and progressive neurologic changes. Treatment of Wilson's disease is aimed at reducing copper absorption and mobilizing copper in the liver and other organs. A diet low in copper (1 to 2 mg/day) may be of value, although the mainstay of treatment is

D-penicillamine or other drugs that inhibit copper absorption or increase urinary copper excretion. Adequacy of vitamin B_6 intake should be monitored with D-penicillamine administration, as it is an antagonist of pyridoxine. Oral vitamin B_6 and zinc supplementation of about 25 mg zinc/day may be necessary. See *Diet, copper-restricted.*

Witch's milk. Lay term for milk secreted from the breasts of a newborn infant; milk secretion is stimulated by the lactating hormone circulating in the mother and passed on to the fetus.

Women, Infants, and Children (WIC) Program. An assistance program for women, infants, and children providing nutrition education and supplemental foods. Qualifications of participants are children under 5 years of age of mothers who meet certain income guidelines; women who are pregnant or have recently delivered a baby; and mothers, infants, and children who are identified nutritional risks by a health professional. They must live in a local WIC agency's service area to receive vouchers for purchasing specific nutritious foods.

World Health Organization (WHO). International organization that aims to eliminate all kinds of diseases. In the field of nutrition, WHO has been involved in developing and testing new protein-rich foods; combating protein-calorie malnutrition, nutritional anemias, vitamin A deficiency, endemic goiter, and rickets; assessing nutritional requirements; and developing coordinated applied nutrition programs and training personnel for them. WHO was created in 1948 with about 100 member countries and has its headquarters in Geneva, Switzerland.

Wound. Physical injury to the body tissues disrupting the normal continuity of structures. *Wound healing* involves tissue synthesis and needs good-quality protein ingested orally or intravenously, using amino acid supplements for the latter route. High protein intake is recommended, with liberal supply of vitamins and minerals, particularly vitamin C and zinc. Other nutrients required in wound healing include arginine, histidine, magnesium, selenium, and vitamin A.

Wrist circumference. A simple anthropometric measurement to estimate frame size. Determined by measuring the smallest part of the wrist distal to the styloid process of the ulna and radius. Frame size is based on a specific "R" value for a small, medium, or large body frame for men and women. See Appendix 21.

WSB. Wheat-soy blend; a mixture of 74% wheat flour and 24% soy flour with a protein concentrate, vitamins, and minerals. Distributed by U.S. government programs, it is used in developing countries as a dietary supplement.

X

Xanthine. An intermediate product in the catabolism of adenine and guanine. It is formed by the oxidation of hypoxanthine or by the hydrolytic deamination of guanine. Oxidation of xanthine by *xanthine oxidase* yields uric acid, the major end product of purine metabolism in humans and higher apes.

Xanthine oxidase. Flavoprotein enzyme found in liver and milk. It contains iron, molybdenum, and flavin mono- or dinucleotide as a prosthetic group. It catalyzes the oxidation of hypoxanthine to xanthine and of the latter to uric acid. It also catalyzes the oxidation of various aldehydes.

Xanthinuria. Hereditary disorder in humans resulting from a lack of xanthine oxidase and characterized by the excretion of xanthine in the urine. *Dietary management:* purine restriction and plenty of fluids. See *Diet, purine-restricted.*

Xanthoma. A deposit of lipid in the skin; usually yellow-orange in color due to the presence of lipid-soluble pigments such as carotene.

Xanthomatosis. Condition characterized by yellow lipoid deposits in the skin, tendon sheaths, and internal organs. The condition is associated with lipemia and hypercholesterolemia.

Xanthophyll. Yellow plant pigment occurring with carotene in green leaves and other vegetables. It is one of the *carotenoids* but has no vitamin A activity.

Xanthoproteic test. Test for the presence of tyrosine and tryptophan. A yellowish derivative formed with concentrated nitric acid turns orange on the addition of ammonia.

Xanthopterin. Yellow pigment present in the liver and urine that has folic acid activity in several animal species. It has antianemic activity in large doses.

Xanthosis. Yellowish discoloration of the skin due to the deposition of carotenoid pigment; often results from excessive intake of yellow fruits and vegetables such as carrots and squash. The skin discoloration is reversible.

Xanthurenic acid. Compound formed in the metabolism of tryptophan to niacin. It is excreted in large amounts in the urine in pyridoxine deficiency. Thus the *xanthurenic acid index* in the urine after administration of a standard dose of tryptophan is used to determine the degree of pyridoxine deficiency. A high index in pregnancy can be reduced by pyridoxine administration.

Xeroderma. Sometimes called "fish skin" or "alligator skin"; the skin becomes dry and rough and comes off in fine or branny scales. Sometimes a layer of "lacquer" appears on the surface that, on drying, breaks up into individual "islands" or patches of varying sizes. There is often desquamation from the borders of each island, while the intervening gaps become fissured. Xeroderma is often associated with vitamin A deficiency, although exposure to dirt and alternative heat and moisture often contribute to its causation.

Xerophthalmia. Dry, lusterless condition of the eyeball characterized by atrophy of the paraocular glands, hyperkeratosis of the conjunctiva, and finally, involvement of the cornea, which becomes dry and opaque. This is followed by cloudiness and infection, leading to ulceration, softening, and blindness. Xerophthalmia is associated with severe vitamin A deficiency; it may also follow chronic conjunctivitis and other diseases of the tear-producing gland.

Xerosis. Abnormal dryness of the skin, mucous membranes, or conjunctiva. In *conjunctival xerosis,* the bulbar conjunctiva is dry, thickened, wrinkled, and pigmented, due to a failure to shed the epithelial cells and consequent keratinization. The pigmentation gives the conjunctiva a peculiar "smoky" appearance. In *corneal xerosis,* the dryness spreads to the cornea, which takes on a dull, hazy, and lusterless appearance; ulceration and infection may occur, leading to softening of the cornea (keratomalacia) and blindness. The condition is associated with a deficiency in vitamin A but may also be due to other causes, such as long periods of exposure to glare, dust, and infections.

Xerostomia. Abnormal dryness of the mouth and lack of saliva due to a salivary gland dysfunction, affecting food intake. Associated with certain drugs, radiation therapy in the head and neck, paralysis of facial nerves, diabetes, acute infections, and Sjögren's syndrome. Encourage the intake of fluids between meals and serve foods that are moist. Use of sugar-free gums and artificial saliva may be beneficial.

Xylan. A hemicellulose of the pentosan type occurring in woody tissues, corncobs, peanut shells, and straw. Yields xylose on hydrolysis.

Xylitol. A sugar alcohol derived from *xylose* and commercially produced from birchwood chips, berries, leaves, and mushrooms. It tastes almost as sweet as sucrose (table sugar) and can be used as a sugar substitute. Xylitol is less cariogenic and less insulin dependent than sucrose.

Xylose. Wood sugar; a pentose obtained from the hydrolysis of *xylan.* It is used as a diagnostic aid for the detection of malabsorption. Urinary excretion of less than 4.5 gm in 5 hours following ingestion of a 25-gm load suggests decreased absorptive capacity.

Y

Yeast. Microscopic, unicellular, fungal plant extensively used by humans for fermentation processes and for bread making. In nutrition, yeast extract is a rich source of the B vitamins; it also contains protein and considerable ergosterol.

Yo-yo dieting. Layman's description of a dietary regimen resulting in fluctuations of body weight, usually due to calorie restriction periodically between periods of overeating or binging.

Z

Zeaxanthin. One of the carotenoid pigments in corn and egg yolk; used as a coloring agent and exhibits no vitamin A activity.

Zein. Protein from corn; an incomplete protein deficient in lysine and low in tryptophan. As the sole source of protein, zein can neither support growth nor maintain life.

Zen macrobiotic. See *Diet, Zen macrobiotic.*

Zinc (Zn). An essential trace mineral for humans, animals, and plants. As a cofactor in more than 100 different enzymes, zinc is involved in carbohydrate and energy metabolism, protein synthesis and degradation, nucleic acid synthesis, acid-base balance, carbon dioxide transport, and many other reactions; it is also important in wound healing, metabolism of vitamin A and collagen, cellular immunity, and development of the reproductive organs. The normal zinc intake is about 10-15 mg/day. Good food sources are meat, liver, eggs, and seafoods; cereals and whole grains provide moderate amounts. Almost 30% is absorbed from the gastrointestinal tract; absorption is influenced by the level of zinc in the diet and by the presence of interfering substances like phytate, calcium, fiber, and chelating agents. Zinc also competes with copper and ferrous iron for absorption. In the body, zinc is concentrated in the liver, kidney, bone, retina, prostate, and muscle; it is mainly bound to albumin in the plasma. Zinc deficiency is usually the result of poor intake associated with conditions that decrease absorption or increase loss, such as malabsorption syndrome, inflammatory bowel disease, liver cirrhosis, thermal burn and loss from exudates, and use of antimetabolites and antianabolic drugs. Primary zinc deficiency is also seen when inadequate zinc is supplied in solutions for total parenteral nutrition. Manifestations of deficiency are diverse, including hair loss, dermatitis and skin changes, growth retardation, impaired taste acuity, delayed wound healing, decreased dark adaptation, immunologic abnormalities, and delayed sexual maturation. Zinc toxicity has occurred as a consequence of severe pollution, inhalation of zinc oxide fumes, and prolonged storage of food and drink in galvanized containers that allow zinc to leach out. Contamination of dialysis water stored in a galvanized tank has been reported to increase plasma zinc concentrations and to produce nausea, vomiting, fever, and anemia. Prolonged intake of dietary zinc supplements also has adverse effects, such as induction of copper deficiency anemia, depressed levels of white blood cells, increased low-density lipoprotein and decreased high-density lipoprotein cholesterol, and decreased serum ferritin and hematocrit levels. Prolonged ingestion of zinc supplements exceeding 15 mg/day is therefore not recommended. See Appendix 1 for the recommended dietary allowances.

Zn. Chemical symbol for zinc.

Zollinger-Ellison syndrome. Tumor of the delta cells of the *islets of Langerhans.* Characterized by hypersecretion of the gastric acid and ulceration of the esophagus, stomach, and upper small intestine. Malabsorption and diarrhea are the main problems. *Dietary management:* correct diarrhea and electrolyte imbalance; restrict fat and use MCT oil; modify protein and fiber intakes according to the patient's needs.

Zwitterion. A dipolar ion containing both a positive and a negative charge and hence electrically neutral. Amino acids may form zwitterions in solution by migration of a hydrogen ion from the carboxyl group to the basic nitrogen atom of the amino group.

Zymase. 1. An enzyme. 2. A mixture of enzymes in yeast that results in alcoholic fermentation.

Zymogen. A proenzyme or the inactive precursor of an enzyme that is converted to its active form. The conversion of a zymogen to its active form is affected by various agents, such as hydrogen ions, specific enzymes, or proteolytic enzymes. In many instances the active enzyme, once formed, acts as an activator of its own zymogen.

Zymosterol. An intermediate in the biosynthesis of cholesterol and lanosterol.

Appendixes

Appendix 1
Recommended Dietary Allowances,[a] * Revised 1989

Designed for the maintenance of good nutrition of practically all healthy people in the United States

Category	Age (years) or Condition	Weight[b] (kg)	(lb)	Height[b] (cm)	(in)	Protein (g)	Fat-Soluble Vitamins				Water-Soluble Vitamins							Minerals						
							Vitamin A (µg RE)[c]	Vitamin D (µg)[d]	Vitamin E (mg α-TE)[e]	Vitamin K (µg)	Vitamin C (mg)	Thiamin (mg)	Riboflavin (mg)	Niacin (mg NE)[f]	Vitamin B₆ (mg)	Folate (µg)	Vitamin B₁₂ (µg)	Calcium (mg)	Phosphorus (mg)	Magnesium (mg)	Iron (mg)	Zinc (mg)	Iodine (µg)	Selenium (µg)
Infants	0.0–0.5	6	13	60	24	13	375	7.5	3	5	30	0.3	0.4	5	0.3	25	0.3	400	300	40	6	5	40	10
	0.5–1.0	9	20	71	28	14	375	10	4	10	35	0.4	0.5	6	0.6	35	0.5	600	500	60	10	5	50	15
Children	1–3	13	29	90	35	16	400	10	6	15	40	0.7	0.8	9	1.0	50	0.7	800	800	80	10	10	70	20
	4–6	20	44	112	44	24	500	10	7	20	45	0.9	1.1	12	1.1	75	1.0	800	800	120	10	10	90	20
	7–10	28	62	132	52	28	700	10	7	30	45	1.0	1.2	13	1.4	100	1.4	800	800	170	10	10	120	30
Males	11–14	45	99	157	62	45	1,000	10	10	45	50	1.3	1.5	17	1.7	150	2.0	1,200	1,200	270	12	15	150	40
	15–18	66	145	176	69	59	1,000	10	10	65	60	1.5	1.8	20	2.0	200	2.0	1,200	1,200	400	12	15	150	50
	19–24	72	160	177	70	58	1,000	10	10	70	60	1.5	1.7	19	2.0	200	2.0	1,200	1,200	350	10	15	150	70
	25–50	79	174	176	70	63	1,000	5	10	80	60	1.5	1.7	19	2.0	200	2.0	800	800	350	10	15	150	70
	51+	77	170	173	68	63	1,000	5	10	80	60	1.2	1.4	15	2.0	200	2.0	800	800	350	10	15	150	70
Females	11–14	46	101	157	62	46	800	10	8	45	50	1.1	1.3	15	1.4	150	2.0	1,200	1,200	280	15	12	150	45
	15–18	55	120	163	64	44	800	10	8	55	60	1.1	1.3	15	1.5	180	2.0	1,200	1,200	300	15	12	150	50
	19–24	58	128	164	65	46	800	10	8	60	60	1.1	1.3	15	1.6	180	2.0	1,200	1,200	280	15	12	150	55
	25–50	63	138	163	64	50	800	5	8	65	60	1.1	1.3	15	1.6	180	2.0	800	800	280	15	12	150	55
	51+	65	143	160	63	50	800	5	8	65	60	1.0	1.2	13	1.6	180	2.0	800	800	280	10	12	150	55
Pregnant						60	800	10	10	65	70	1.5	1.6	17	2.2	400	2.2	1,200	1,200	320	30	15	175	65
Lactating	1st 6 months					65	1,300	10	12	65	95	1.6	1.8	20	2.1	280	2.6	1,200	1,200	355	15	19	200	75
	2nd 6 months					62	1,200	10	11	65	90	1.6	1.7	20	2.1	260	2.6	1,200	1,200	340	15	16	200	75

[a] The allowances, expressed as average daily intakes over time, are intended to provide for individual variations among most normal persons as they live in the United States under usual environmental stresses. Diets should be based on a variety of common foods in order to provide other nutrients for which human requirements have been less well defined. See text for detailed discussion of allowances and of nutrients not tabulated.

[b] Weights and heights of Reference Adults are actual medians for the U.S. population of the designated age, as reported by NHANES II. The median weights and heights of those under 19 years of age were taken from Hamill et al. (1979) (see pages 16–17). The use of these figures does not imply that the height-to-weight ratios are ideal.

[c] Retinol equivalents. 1 retinol equivalent = 1 µg retinol or 6 µg β-carotene. See text for calculation of vitamin A activity of diets as retinol equivalents.

[d] As cholecalciferol. 10 µg cholecalciferol = 400 IU of vitamin D.

[e] α-Tocopherol equivalents. 1 mg d-α tocopherol = 1 α-TE. See text for variation in allowances and calculation of vitamin E activity of the diet as α-tocopherol equivalents.

[f] 1 NE (niacin equivalent) is equal to 1 mg of niacin or 60 mg of dietary tryptophan.

*National Research Council. Recommended Dietary Allowances. 10th ed. Washington, D.C., National Academy Press, 1989.

Appendix 2
Estimated Safe and Adequate Daily Dietary Intakes of Selected Vitamins and Minerals[a]*

Category	Age (years)	Vitamins	
		Biotin (μg)	Pantothenic Acid (mg)
Infants	0–0.5	10	2
	0.5–1	15	3
Children and	1–3	20	3
adolescents	4–6	25	3–4
	7–10	30	4–5
	11 +	30–100	4–7
Adults		30–100	4–7

Category	Age (years)	Trace Elements[b]				
		Copper (mg)	Manganese (mg)	Fluoride (mg)	Chromium (μg)	Molybdenum (μg)
Infants	0–0.5	0.4–0.6	0.3–0.6	0.1–0.5	10–40	15–30
	0.5–1	0.6–0.7	0.6–1.0	0.2–1.0	20–60	20–40
Children and	1–3	0.7–1.0	1.0–1.5	0.5–1.5	20–80	25–50
adolescents	4–6	1.0–1.5	1.5–2.0	1.0–2.5	30–120	30–75
	7–10	1.0–2.0	2.0–3.0	1.5–2.5	50–200	50–150
	11 +	1.5–2.5	2.0–5.0	1.5–2.5	50–200	75–250
Adults		1.5–3.0	2.0–5.0	1.5–4.0	50–200	75–250

[a] Because there is less information on which to base allowances, these figures are not given in the main table of RDA and are provided here in the form of ranges of recommended intakes.

[b] Since the toxic levels for many trace elements may be only several times usual intakes, the upper levels for the trace elements given in this table should not be habitually exceeded.

*National Research Council. Recommended Dietary Allowances, 10th ed. Washington, D.C., National Academy Press, 1989, p. 284. (reprinted with permission)

Appendix 3
U.S. Reference Daily Intakes (USRDI)
for Nutrition Labeling*+

Nutrient (Unit)	Adults‡/Child-ren over 4 yr	Children under 4 yr	Infants Birth-12 mo
Protein (g)	50	16	14
Vitamin A (µg, RE)	875	400	375
Vitamin D (µg)	6.5	10	9
Vitamin E (mg, α-TE)	9.0	6	3.5
Vitamin K (µg)	65	15	7.5
Vitamin C (mg)	60	40	33
Thiamin (mg)	1.2	0.7	0.4
Riboflavin (mg)	1.4	0.8	0.5
Niacin (mg, NE)	16	9	5.5
Vitamin B_6	1.5	1.0	0.5
Folate (µg)	180	50	30
Vitamin B_{12}	2.0	0.7	0.4
Biotin (µg)	60	20	13
Pantothenic acid (mg)	5.5	3.0	2.5
Calcium (mg)	900	800	500
Phosphorus (mg)	900	800	400
Magnesium (mg)	300	80	50
Iron (mg)	12	10	8
Zinc (mg)	13	10	5
Iodine (µg)	150	70	45
Selenium (µg)**	55	20	13
Copper (mg)	2.0	0.9	0.6
Manganese (mg)	3.5	1.3	0.6
Fluoride (mg)**	2.5	1.0	0.5
Chromium (µg)**	120	50	33
Molybdenum (µg)	150	38	26
Chloride (mg)	3150	1000	650

*Proposed regulatory amendment in the Federal Register, 55(139):29476-29486, July 19, 1990. (Food labeling: reference daily intakes and daily reference values, proposed rule, docket no. 90N-0134).

+Reference values were based on the 1989 revision of the Recommended Dietary Allowances (RDA) and other diet and health reports.

‡Separate RDIs are proposed for pregnant and lactating women.

**RDIs are proposed for selenium, fluoride and chromium only for the purpose of declaring nutrients naturally present in a food.

Appendix 4
Recommended Dietary Standards for Adults in Selected Countries and FAO/WHO

Country	Sex	Age (yr)	Wt (kg)	Activity	Calories	Protein (gm)	Calcium (mg)	Iron (mg)	Vitamin A (ug RE)	Thiamin (mg)	Riboflavin (mg)	Niacin (mg NE)	Ascorbic Acid (mg)
FAO/WHO[a]	M	18-30	65	MA	3000	37[b]	450[c]	7[d]	750	1.2	1.8	20[e]	30
	F	18-30	55	MA	2200	29[b]	450[c]	21[d]	750	0.9	1.3	14[e]	30
Australia[a]	M	18-35	70	FN[b]	2800	70	800	7	750	1.1	1.7	19[d]	30
	F	18-35	58	FN[b]	2000	58	800	14[c]	750	0.8	1.2	13[d]	30
Canada[a]	M	19-24	71	FN[b]	3000[b]	57	800	8	1000	1.2[c]	1.5[c]	22[c]	60
	F	19-24	58	FN[b]	2100[b]	41	700	14	800	0.8[c]	1.1[c]	15[c]	45
Caribbean[a]	M	20-39	65	MA	3000	53[b]	500	6	750	1.2	1.7	20	30
	F	20-39	55	MA	2200	41[b]	500	19	750	0.9	1.2	15	30
China[a]	M	18-44	63	MA	3000	90	800	12	800	1.5	1.5	15	60
	F	18-44	53	MA	2700	80	800	18	800	1.4	1.4	14	60
Czechoslo-vakia[a]	M	19-34	NS	MA	3000	105[b]	800	12	1000	1.2	1.8	20	60[b]
	F	19-34	NS	LA	2300	90[b]	800	14	900	1.1	1.6	17	50[b]
France[a]	M	Adult	NS	FN[b]	2700	81	800	10	1000	1.5	1.8	18	80
	F	Adult	NS	FN[b]	2000	60	800	18	800	1.3	1.5	15	80
Germany[a] (Dem Rep)	M	18-35	NS	MA	3000	85	600	10	800	1.5	1.8	20	45
	F	18-35	NS	MA	2400	75	600	15	750	1.2	1.4	16	45
Germany[a] (Fed Rep)	M	Adult	NS	SA	2600	0.9 g/kg	800	12	900	1.6	2.0	12[b]	75
	F	Adult	NS	SA	2200	0.9 g/kg	700	18	900	1.4	1.8	12[b]	75
Hungary[a]	M	19-30	70	MA	3200	94	800	12	1000	1.4	1.8	18	60
	F	19-30	60	MA	2400	70	800	18	800	1.3	1.5	15	60
INCAP[a]	M	19-40	63	MA	2900	60	450	9	750	1.2	1.6	19	30
	F	19-40	52	MA	2050	45	450	28	750	0.8	1.1	14	30
India[a]	M	Adult	NS	MA	2800	55	450[b]	24	750	1.4	1.7	19	40
	F	Adult	NS	MA	2200	45	450[b]	32	750	1.4	1.3	15	40
Indonesia[a]	M	20-39	55	FN[b]	2530	51	500	9	4000,IU	1.0	1.4	17[c]	30
	F	20-39	47	FN[b]	1880	40	500	28	3500,IU	0.8	1.3	12[c]	30
Israel[a]	M	18-25	NS	NS	33 kcal/kg	.8 g/kg	1200	10	1000	1.5	1.7	19	60
	F	18-25	NS	NS	31 kcal/kg	.8 g/kg	1200	15	800	1.1	1.3	15	60
Italy[a]	M	20-39	65	MA	3000	64	600	10	750	1.2	1.6	20	45
	F	20-39	54	MA	2160	53	600	18	750	0.9	1.2	14	45
Japan[a]	M	20-29	NS	LA	2500	70	600	10	2000,IU	1.0	1.4	17	50
	F	20-29	NS	LA	2000	60	600	12	1800,IU	0.8	1.1	13	50
Korea[a]	M	20-49	60	MA	2700	80	600	10	600	1.1	1.6	18	55
	F	20-49	52	MA	2000	70	600	18	500	1.0	1.2	13	50
Mexico[a]	M	18-34	65	NS	2750	83	500	10	1000	1.4	1.7	25	50
	F	18-34	55	NS	2000	71	500	18	1000	1.0	1.2	18	50
Netherlands[a]	M	19-22	NS	MA	2900	79	800[b]	10	1000	1.2	1.6	NS	70
	F	19-22	NS	MA	2250	60	800[b]	16	800	1.0	1.3	NS	70
Philippines[a]	M	20-39	56	MA	2570	60	500	12	525	1.3	1.3	25	75
	F	20-39	49	MA	1900	52	500	26[b]	450	1.0	1.0	18	70
Spain[a]	M	20-40	NS	FN[b]	3000	54	600	10	750	1.2	1.8	20	45
	F	20-40	NS	FN[b]	2300	41	600	18	750	0.9	1.4	15	45

Country	Sex	Age (yr)	Wt (kg)	Activity	Calories	Protein (gm)	Calcium (mg)	Iron (mg)	Vitamin A (µg RE)	Thiamin (mg)	Riboflavin (mg)	Niacin (mg NE)	Ascorbic Acid (mg)
Sweden[a]	M	19-30	70	MA	3150	75	600	10	1000	1.4	1.7	18	60
	F	19-30	60	MA	2500	62	800	18	800	1.1	1.3	14	60
Turkey[a]	M	19-39	65	NS	2700	65	500	7	750	1.1	1.6	15	50
	F	19-39	55	NS	2200	55	500	23	750	0.9	1.3	12	50
United Kingdom[a]	M	18-34	NS	MA	2900	72	500	10	750	1.2	1.6	18	30
	F	18-34	NS	FN[b]	2150	54	500	12	750	0.9	1.3	15	20
United States[a]	M	19-24	72	FN[b]	2900	58	1200	10	1000	1.5	1.7	19	60
	F	19-24	58	FN[b]	2200	46	1200	15	800	1.1	1.3	15	60
U.S.S.R.[a]	M	18-60	NS	MA	3050[b]	96[c]	800	18[d]	1500	1.8[e]	2.3[f]	19[g]	72[h]
	F	18-60	NS	MA	2500[b]	80[c]	800	18[d]	1500	1.4[e]	2.0[f]	16[g]	62[h]
Venezuela[a]	M	20-39	65	NS	3000	63	450	9	750	1.2	1.6	20	30
	F	20-39	55	NS	2200	48	450	28	750	0.9	1.2	14	30

FN = footnote; NS = not specified; LA = light activity; MA = medium or moderate activity; SA = sedentary activity

EXPLANATIONS:
The purpose for establishing a national dietary standard is not the same in all countries. Some variation in nutrient allowances from country to country should therefore be expected. The "reference" individual varies in different countries, and even in instances where presumed similar objectives exist among countries as to the purpose and usefulness of proposed dietary standards, the table shows that there is no uniform agreement as to the nutrient allowance that may be considered desirable.

FAO/WHO (1985)
[a]Handbook on Human Nutritional Requirements. FAO Nutritional Studies No. 28, WHO Monograph Series No. 61, Rome, 1974; Energy and Protein Requirements, Report of a Joint FAO/WHO Expert Group, Technical Report Series No. 724, 1985.
[b]Protein quality varies from country to country. The FAO/WHO standard is stated in terms of high-quality protein of milk or egg (protein score of 100). Protein recommendations are 46 gm for males and 36 gm for females for a protein score of 80; and 62 gm for males and 47 gm for females for a protein score of 60.
[c]Average of 0.4-0.5 gm calcium recommended for both males and females.
[d]Average of 5-9 mg iron for males, and 14-28 mg iron for females. The recommendations were based on the assumption that the upper limit of iron absorption is 10 percent if less than 10% of kilocalories come from foods of animal origin.
[e]Rounded to nearest whole number.

Australia (1987)
[a]Recommended Dietary Intakes for Use in Australia. National Health and Medical Research Council, Australian Government Publishing Service, Canberra, 1987.
[b]Basic activity level; [c]Average of 12-16 mg range; [d]Average of 18-20 mg range for males, and 12-14 mg range for women.

Canada (1983)
[a]Recommended Nutrient Intakes for Canadians. Department of National Health and Welfare, Canadian Government Publishing Center, Ottawa, Canada, 1983.

(continued)

Appendix 4 *(continued)*

[b]The figures for energy are estimates of average requirements for expected pattern of activity and can be expected to vary within a range of $\pm$ 30%.

[c]Figures represent amounts recommended: thiamin, 0.4 mg/1,000 kcal; riboflavin, 0.5 mg/1,000 kcal; and niacin, 7.2 mg NE/1,000 kcal.

Caribbean (1979)

[a]Recommended Dietary Allowances for Use in the Caribbean. Caribbean Food and Nutrition Institute, Kingston, Jamaica, 1979. The allowances are intended to provide amounts of nutrients sufficient for the maintenance of health in nearly all people in the Caribbean.

[b]Adjusted to NPU = 70 for average Caribbean diet.

China (1988)

[a]Chinese Nutrition Society. Recommended Dietary Allowances, Revised October, 1988. Acta Nutrimenta Sinica, Vol. 12:3, March 1990.

Czechoslovakia (1981)

[a]Institute of Hygiene and Epidemiology. Recommended Dietary Allowances, 1981.

[b]Protein and Vitamin C recommendations increase with calories for increasing degrees of activity.

France (1981)

[a]Apports Nutritionnels Conseilles du Centre National de Coordination des Etudes et Recherches sur l'Alimentation et la Nutrition (CNERNA), 1981. "Apports Nutritionnels Conseilles pour la population francaise". Technique et Documentation, Paris.

Germany, Democratic Republic (1980)

[a]Central Institute of Nutrition, Science Academy of the GDR and Nutrition Society of the GDR. Ketz, H.A. and M. Moehr, M.: Durchschnittswerte des physiologischen Energie - und Nährstoffbedarfs für die Bevölkerung der Deutschen Demokratischen Republik, Zentralinstitut für Ernährung der Akademie der Wissenschaften der DDR und der Gesellschaft für Ernährung in der DDR, Auflage, 1980.

Germany, Federal Republic (1975)

[a]German Nutrition Society (Deutsche Gesellschaft für Ernährung). "Empfehlungen für die Nährstoff-zufur - Emfehlungen der Deutschen Gesellschaft für Ernährung e. V." 4th ed. 1979, Umschau-Verlag, Frankfurt/Main.

Hungary (1988)

[a]Biro, G. and Karoly, L.: Tapanyagtablazat, Tapanyagszukseglet es Tapanyag-Osszetetel (Food Composition Tables. Requirements and composition of nutrients), 11th revised, enlarged edition. Medicina, Konyvkiado, Budapest, 1988.

INCAP (1973)

[a]Institute of Nutrition for Central America & Panama (Guatemala, Honduras, Nicaragua, El Salvador, Costa Rica, & Panama, Instituto de Nutricion). "Recommendaciones Dieteticas Diarias para Centro America y Panama", Publicacion INCAP E-709, 1973.

India (1981)

[a]Indian Council of Medical Research, National Institute of Nutrition. Recommended Dietary Intakes of Nutrients, 1981. Nutrition News, Vol. 2, No 3, Hyberabad.

[b]Average of 400-500 mg range for both males and females.

Appendix 4 *(continued)*

Indonesia (1980)
[a]Recommended Dietary Allowance (RDA), Indonesia. Nutr Abs Rev, Clinical Nutrition Series A, 53:972, 1983.
[b]RDA's "for good health in Indonesia". Activity level not specified.
[c]Figures were rounded: from 16.7 mg niacin for males, and 12.4 mg for females.

Israel (1990)
[a]Recommended Dietary Allowances. State of Israel Ministry of Health, Department of Nutrition, 1990. (Based on National Academy of Sciences USA 1989 and World Health Organization).

Italy (1978)
[a]Commissione "Ad Hoc" Della Societa Italiana di Nutrizione Umana, Istituto Nazionale Della Nutrizione, Ministero Dell'Agricoltura e Delle Foreste (1978).: "Livelli di Assunzione Raccomandati di Nutrienti per gli Italiani", Roma.

Japan (1984)
[a]Recommended Dietary Allowances, revised 1984. Ministry of Health and Welfare, Tokyo, Japan.

Korea (1980)
[a]Recommended Dietary Allowances (per person per day). 3rd ed, 1980. Nutr Abs Rev, Clinical Nutrition Series A, 53:975, 1983.

Mexico (1970)
[a]Bourges, H., Chavez, A. and Arroyo, P.: Recommendaciones de Nutrimentos para la Poblacion Mexicana. Publ. L-17, Instituto Nacional de Nutricion, 1970.

Netherlands
[a]Adviescollege van de Minister van Welzijn, Volksgezondheid en Cultuur en de Minister van Landbouw en Visserij inzake voeding en voedselvoorziening, Voedingsraad.

Philippines (1989)
[a]Food and Nutrition Research Institute, Department of Science and Technology. Recommended Dietary Allowances for Filipinos, 1989 edition.
[b]Cannot be met by the usual diet, thus supplementation is recommended.

Spain (1980)
[a]Institute of Nutrition, Madrid and Spanish Nutrition Society. Instituto de Nutricion (CSIC) Facultad de Farmaciaciudad Universitaria, Madrid (1980). "Ingestas Recomendadas de Energia y Nutrientes para la Poblacion Espanola".
[b]Energy for active work; subtract 10% for light work; add 20% for very active work.
[c]Protein NPU = 70

Sweden (1989)
[a]Swedish Nutrition Recommendations (Svenska naringsrekommendationer, SNR). 2nd edition. Statens livsmedelsverk, National Food Administration, Uppsala, Sweden, 1989.

Turkey (1972)
[a]Institute of Nutrition and Food Sciences, Hacettepe Universitesi, Ankara. "Recommended Dietary Allowances, 1972.

(continued)

United Kingdom (1979)

[a]Recommended Daily Amounts of Food Energy and Nutrients for Groups of People in the United Kingdom. Report by the Committee on Medical Aspects of Food Policy, Department of Health and Social Security, London, 1979 (as per third impression, 1985).

United States (1989)

[a]Recommended Dietary Allowances, 10th edition. National Research Council, National Academy Press, Washington, DC, 1989.

U.S.S.R. (1980)

[a]Institute of Nutrition, U.S.S.R. Academy of Medical Sciences, Moscow. Voroncova, I.M. and Mazurina, A.V.: "Spravochnik po Detskoy Dietetike". Second enlarged and revised edition (1980), Medicina, Leningrad. ("Guide in Children's Dietetics"); Vanhanen, V.D. et al.: Higiene Pitanija" (1980), Zdorovja, Kiev. ("Nutrition Hygiene").

[b-h]Dietary allowances shown are for people living "in cities with developed communal services". Figures shown are rounded averages. [b]Average for calories (2800-3300 for males, 2400-2600 for females); [c]Average for protein (92-99 gm for males, 77-84 gm for females); [d]Average for iron (15-20 mg for both males and females); [e]Average for thiamin (1.7-1.8 mg for males, 1.4-1.5 mg for females); [f]Average for riboflavin (2.2-2.4 mg for males, 1.9-2.0 mg for females); [g]Average for niacin (10-18 mg for males, 15-17 mg for females); [h]Average for vitamin C (70-75 mg for males, 60-65 mg for females).

Venezuela (1976)

[a]National Institute of Nutrition, National Council for Scientific Investigations & Technology. Instituto Nacional de Nutricion, Consejo Nacional de Investigaciones Cientificas y Technologicas (1976). "Requerimientos de Energia y de Nutrientes de la Poblacion Venezolana". Serie de Cuadernos Azules, publication no. 38. Republica de Venezuela.

Appendix 5
A Daily Food Guide for the Basic Food Groups

Food Group	Major Nutrients	Suggested Daily Servings

Milk & Dairy	Protein
	Calcium
	Phosphorus
	Riboflavin
	Vitamins A
	and D
		2-3 servings for children under 9
		3-4 servings for children over 9
		4 or more servings for adolescents
		2 or more servings for adults
		3-4 servings for pregnant women and
		  nursing mothers
		
		Equivalents in calcium of one serving:
		  1 cup milk - whole, skim, low fat
		  1 cup yogurt or cottage cheese
		  2-inch cube cheddar type cheese
		  2 ounces processed cheese

Meats & Legumes	Protein
	B vitamins
	Iron
	Phosphorus
	Zinc
		2-3 servings, with a daily total of about
		six ounces of cooked lean meat, poultry
		without skin or broiled fish.
		
		Count as 1 ounce of meat:
		  1 egg
		  1/2 cup cooked dry beans or peas
		  2 tablespoons peanut butter
		  1/4 cup nuts or seeds

Vegetables
& Fruits
	Vitamins A
	and C
	Folic acid
	Minerals
	Fiber
		3-5 servings of vegetables and 2-3 servings
		of fruits. Include daily one good source of
		vitamin C and a deep yellow or dark green
		vegetable at least every other day. Use dry
		beans and peas often, unpeeled fruits and
		vegetables, and those with edible seeds for
		fiber.
		
		Count as one serving:
		  1/2 cup cooked or chopped raw vegetables
		  1 cup of raw leafy vegetables
		  A fruit portion as ordinarily served, such
		    as 1 medium apple, orange, and banana;
		    grapefruit half; melon wedge
		  1/2 cup sliced fruit or juice
		  1/4 cup dried fruit

Grain Products	Carbohydrate
	Thiamin
	Niacin
	Riboflavin
	Iron
	Fiber
		6 or more servings. Include whole-grain and
		enriched breads, cereals, pasta, and rice.
		
		Count as one serving:
		  1 slice bread, small roll or biscuit
		  1/2 bun, bagel, or English muffin
		  1/2 cup cooked cereal, rice, or pasta
		  1 ounce dry breakfast cereal

Appendix 6
Food Grouping Systems in Different Countries*

	Number of groups	Milk	Cheese	Fish	Meat	Eggs	Pulses	Seeds	Nuts	Fats, oils	Bread	Cereals	Rice	Sugar, sweets	Tubers, roots	Potato	Vege-tables	Fruits, berries
Australia	5	1	1	2	2	2	2	—	2	3	4	4	—	—	5	5	5	5
Bulgaria	7	1	1	2	2	2	3	—	3	4	5	—	—	—	—	—	6	7
Canada	5	1	2	2	2	2	2	—	—	—	3	3	2	2	2	4	4	5
Central America[1]	3	1	1	1	1	1	2	—	—	2	2	2	2	2	2	2	3	3
China	5	1	1	2	1	1	2	—	—	3	4	4	4	3	4	4	5	5
Chile	4	1	1	2	2	2	3	—	—	3	3	3	3	3	—	4	4	4
Czechoslovakia	5	1	1	2	2	2	2	—	—	3	4	4	4	—	5	5	5	5
Denmark	6	1	1	2	2	2	3	—	—	4	3	3	3	—	5	5	5,6	6
Ecuador	4	1	1	2	2	2	3	3	3	3	3	3	3	—	4	4	4	4
Egypt	3	1	1	1	1	1	1	—	1	—	2	2	—	—	—	—	3	3
Finland	6	1	1	2	2	2	3	—	—	4	5	5	—	—	6	6	3	3
France	6	1	1	2	2	2	—	—	—	3	4	4	—	—	—	—	5,6	5,6
Ghana	6	1	1	1	1	1	2	2	2	3	4	4	4	—	5	5	6	6
Hungary	5	1	1	2	2	2	—	—	—	3	4	4	—	—	—	—	5	6
India	5	1	1	1	1	1	1	—	1	2	3	3	3	2	—	—	4,5	5
Israel	6	1	1	1	1	1	1	2	2	2	3	3	—	4	—	—	5	6
Italy	3	1	1	2	2	2	3	—	—	2	2	2	2	2	3	3	3	3
Italy	7	1	1	2	2	2	3	—	—	4	5	5	5	—	6	—	6,7	7

274

Japan	6	1	1,2	2	2	2	—	—	3	4	4	4	—	5	4	5,6	6
Korea	5	1	1,2	2	2	2	3	3	3	4	4	4	—	5	4	5	5
Lebanon	8	1	1	2	2	—	3	3	4	5	5	6	7	—	6	8	8
Mexico	3	1	1	1	1	1	1	—	2	2	2	2	2	2	2	3	3
Netherlands	5	1	2	2	2	—	—	—	3	4	4	4	—	—	5	3	3
New Zealand	4	1	2	2	2	2	—	—	—	3	3	3	—	—	4	5	5
Peru	3	1	1	1	1	—	—	—	—	2	2	2	2	—	4	4	4
Philippines	3	1	1	1	1	2	1	1	2	2	2	2	2	2	2	3	3
Poland	6	1	1	2	2	—	—	—	4	3	3	—	5	6	6	3	3
Puerto Rico	5	1	—	2	2	3	—	—	3	—	—	3	3	—	6	6	6
Senegal	3	1	—	1	1	—	—	—	3	2	2	3	—	2	—	4	4,5
South Africa	5	1	1	2	2	2	1	1	2	4	4	4	2	5	5	3	3
South Africa	3	1	1	1	1	1	2	2	3	2	2	2	3	3	3	5	5
Soviet Union	6	1	1	2	2	—	1	1	3	4	4	4	4	—	3	3	3
Spain	7	1	1	2	2	3	—	—	4	5	5	5	5	6	4	5	6
Sweden	7	1	1	2	2	—	3	3	4	4	5	4	5	5	3	6	7
Taiwan	5	1	—	2	2	—	—	—	3	4	4	3	—	3	5	6	7
Thailand	5	1	1	1	1	1	—	—	2	3	3	3	3	3	—	4	5
Turkey	4	1	1	2	2	2	—	—	—	3	3	3	3	—	—	4	5
United States	4	1	1	2	2	2	2	—	—	3	3	3	—	4	—	4	4
Venezuela	4	1	1	2	2	2	—	—	3	3	3	3	3	3,4	4	4	4
West Germany	7	1	1	2	2	—	—	4	3	4	4	—	4	—	5	6	7

*The table includes only those foods that could be grouped on the basis of the information given. Foods belonging to the same group are marked by the same number. Foods belonging to the same group are marked by the same number; thus the numbers do not indicate order of groups. If a food component appears in several groups for some reason, it is given all the respective numbers.

†Costa Rica, Guatemala, Honduras, Nicaragua, Panama, El Salvador.

Appendix 7
Dietary Guidelines for All Healthy Americans
Over 2 Years Old*#

1. Eat a variety of foods.

2. Maintain healthy weight.

3. Choose a diet low in fat, saturated fat, and cholesterol.

4. Choose a diet with plenty of vegetables, fruits, and grain products.

5. Use sugars in moderation.

6. Use salt and sodium in moderation.

7. If you drink alcoholic beverages, do so in moderation. (Children, adolescents, and pregnant women should abstain).

---

*From USDA. Nutrition and Your Health: Dietary Guidelines for Americans. HG-232, 1990
#Not intended for infants whose food and nutrient needs are different from those of older children and adults. Guidelines for infants are:
  - Mother's milk is the best food for nearly all infants.
  - To help prevent tooth decay in newly growing teeth, infants should not use as pacifiers nursing bottles containing any beverage other than water.
  - Babies are generally not given solid foods until they are 4 to 6 months old when foods are gradually introduced.
  - Salt and sugar are not needed and should not be added to an infant's food as inducements to eat.

Additional recommendations to reduce the risk
for specific health problems:

Dental cavities	Ensure access to fluoride. Moderate between-meal consumption of foods containing sugars, especially for children.
Osteoporosis	Increase consumption of foods high in calcium (particularly low fat dairy products), especially by adolescents and young women.
Iron deficiency anemia	Consume good sources of iron (like lean red meats, fish, and iron-enriched cereals), especially by children, adolescents, and women of child-bearing age.

Appendix 8
Classification of Carbohydrates

Carbohydrate	Occurrence	Characteristics
Monosaccharides (simple sugars)		
Hexoses		
Glucose	Honey, fruits, corn syrup, sweet grapes, and sweet corn; hydrolysis of starch and of cane sugar	Physiologically the most important sugar; the "sugar" carried by the blood and the principal one used by tissues
Fructose	Honey, ripe fruits, and some vegetables; hydrolysis of sucrose inulin	Can be changed to glucose in the liver and intestine; an intermediate metabolite in glycogen breakdown
Galactose	Not found free in nature; digestive end product of lactose hydrolysis	Can be changed to glucose in the liver; synthesized in body to make lactose; constituent of glycolipids
Mannose	Legumes; hydrolysis of plant mannosans and gums	Constituent of polysaccharide of albumins, globulins, and mucoids
Pentoses		
Arabinose	Derived from gum arabic and plum and cherry gums; not found free in nature	Has no known physiologic function in man; used in metabolism studies of bacteria
Ribose	Derived from nucleic acid of meats and seafoods	Structural element of nucleic acids, ATP, and coenzymes (NAD and FAD)
Ribulose	Formed in metabolic processes	Intermediate in direct oxidative pathway of glucose breakdown
Xylose	Wood gums, corncobs, and peanut shells; not found free in nature	Very poorly digested and has no known physiologic function; used medicinally as a diabetic food
Oligosaccharides (2-10 sugar units)		
Disaccharides		
Sucrose	Cane and beet sugar, maple syrup, molasses, and sorghum	Hydrolyzed to glucose and fructose; a nonreducing sugar
Maltose	Malted products and germinating cereals; an intermediate product of starch digestion	Hydrolyzed to two molecules of glucose; a reducing sugar; does not occur free in tissue
Lactose	Milk and milk products; formed in body from glucose nature	Hydrolyzed to glucose and galactose; may occur in urine during pregnancy; a reducing sugar
Trisaccharides		
Raffinose	Cottonseed meal, molasses, and sugar beets and stems	Only partially digestible but can be hydrolyzed by enzymes of intestinal bacteria to glucose, fructose, and galactose
Melizitose	Honey, poplars, and conifers	Composed of one fructose unit and two glucose units

(continued)

Appendix 8 *(continued)*

Carbohydrate	Occurrence	Characteristics
Polysaccharides (more than 10 sugar units)		
Digestible		
Glycogen	Meat products and seafoods	Polysaccharide of the animal body, often called animal starch; storage form of carbohydrate in body, mainly in liver and muscles
Starch	Cereal grains, unripe fruits, vegetables, legumes, and tubers	Most important food source of carbohydrate; storage form of carbohydrate in plants; composed chiefly of amylose and amylopectin; hydrolyzable to glucose
Dextrin	Toasted bread; intermediate product of starch digestion	Formed in course of hydrolytic breakdown of starch
Partially digestible		
Inulin	Tubers and roots of dahlias, artichokes, dandelions, onions, and garlic	Hydrolyzable to fructose; used in physiologic investigation for determination of glomerular filtration rate
Mannosan	Legumes and plant gums	Hydrolyzable to mannose but digestion incomplete; further splitting by bacteria may occur in large bowel
Indigestible*		
Cellulose	Skins of fruits, outer coverings of seeds, and stalks and leaves of vegetables	Not subject to attack of digestive enzyme in man, thus an important source of "bulk" in diet; may be partially split to glucose by bacterial action in large bowel
Hemicellulose and pectin	Woody fibers and leaves	Less polymerized than cellulose; may be digested to some extent by microbial enzymes, yielding xylose

*Another nomenclature for indigestible polysaccharides is <u>dietary fiber</u>. The two groups are:
  A. Insoluble dietary fibers (cellulose, lignin and cutin) which are the most abundant organic compounds in the world. They help prevent constipation, colon cancer, and diverticulosis, but not hypercholesterolemia.
  B. Soluble dietary fibers (hemicellulose, pectins, gums, and algal polysaccharides) which are useful in decreasing serum cholesterol and in regulating blood glucose levels.

Appendix 9
Classification of Proteins

Protein	Occurrence	Characteristics
Simple proteins		
Albumins	Blood (serum albumin); milk (lactalbumin); egg white (ovalbumin); lentils (legumelin); kidney beans (phaseolin); wheat (leucosin)	Globular protein; soluble in water and dilute salt solutions; precipitated by saturation with ammonium sulfate solution; coagulated by heat; found in plant and animal tissues
Globulins	Blood (serum globulin); muscle (myosin); potato (tuberin); Brazil nuts (excelsin); hemp (edestin); lentils (legumin)	Globular protein; sparingly soluble in water; soluble in dilute neutral solutions; precipitated by dilute ammonium sulfate and coagulated by heat; distributed in both plant and animal tissues
Glutelins	Wheat (glutenin); rice (oryzenin)	Insoluble in water and dilute salt solutions; soluble in dilute acids; found in grains and cereals
Prolamines	Wheat and rye (gliadin); corn (zein); rye (secaline); barley (hordein)	Insoluble in water and absolute alcohol; soluble in 70% alcohol; high in amide nitrogen and proline; occur in grain seeds
Protamines	Sturgeon (sturine); mackerel (scombrine); salmon (salmine); herring (clupeine)	Soluble in water; not coagulated by heat; strongly basic; high in arginine; associated with DNA and occur in sperm cells
Histones	Thymus gland, pancreas; nucleoproteins (nucleohistone)	Soluble in water, salt solutions, and dilute acids; insoluble in ammonium hydroxide; yields large amounts of lysine and arginine; combined with nucleic acids within cells
Scleroproteins	Connective tissues and hard tissues	Fibrous protein; insoluble in all solvents and resistant to digestion
Collagen	Connective tissues, bones, cartilage, and gelatin	Resistant to digestive enzymes but altered to digestible gelatin by boiling water, acid, or alkali; high in hydroxyproline
Elastin	Ligaments, tendons, and arteries	Similar to collagen but cannot be converted to gelatin
Keratin	Hair, nails, hooves, horn, and feathers	Partially resistant to digestive enzymes; contains large amounts of sulfur, as cystine
Conjugated proteins		
Nucleoproteins	Cytoplasm of cells (ribonucleoprotein); nucleus of chromosomes (deoxyribonucleoprotein); viruses and bacteriophages	Contains nucleic acids, nitrogen, and phosphorus; present in chromosomes and in all living forms as a combination of protein with either RNA or DNA

(continued)

Appendix 9 *(continued)*

Protein	Occurrence	Characteristics
Mucoprotein or Glycoprotein	Saliva (mucin); egg white (ovomucoid) Bone (osseomucoid); tendons (tendomucoid); cartilage (chondromucoid)	Proteins combined with amino sugars, sugar acids, and sulfates Containing more than 4% hexosamine, mucoproteins; if less than 4%, glycoproteins
Phospho-proteins	Milk (casein); egg yolk (ovovitellin)	Phosphoric acid joined in ester linkage to protein
Chromo-proteins	Hemoglobin; myoglobin; flavoproteins; respiratory pigments; cytochromes	Protein compounds with nonprotein pigments such as heme; colored proteins
Lipopro-teins	Serum lipoprotein; brain, nerve tissues, milk, and eggs	Water-soluble proteins conjugated with lipids; found dispersed widely in all cells and all living forms
Metallo-proteins	Ferritin; carbonic anhydrase; ceruloplasmin	Proteins combined with metallic atoms that are not parts of a nonprotein prosthetic group

Derived proteins

Proteans	Edestan (from elastin) and myosan (from myosin)	Results from short action of acids or enzymes; insoluble in water
Proteoses	Intermediate products of protein digestion	Soluble in water; uncoagulated by heat, and precipitated by saturated ammonium sulfate; result from partial digestion of protein by pepsin or trypsin
Peptones	Intermediate products of protein digestion	Same properties as proteoses except that they cannot be salted out; of smaller molecular weight than proteoses
Peptides	Intermediate products of protein digestion	Two or more amino acids joined by a peptide linkage; hydrolyzed to individual amino acids*

*Classification of amino acids according to essentiality:

Nonessential Amino Acids	Essential Amino Acids	Estimated Requirements for adults (mg/kg/day)
Alanine	Histidine	8-12
Asparagine	Isoleucine	10
Cysteine	Leucine	14
Cystine	Lysine	12
Glutamic acid	Methionine	13 (plus cystine)
Glycine	Phenylalanine	14 (plus tyrosine)
Hydroxylysine	Threonine	7
Hydroxyproline	Tryptophan	3.5
Proline	Valine	10
Serine		
Tyrosine		

Appendix 10
Classification of Lipids

Lipid	Occurrence	Characteristics
Simple lipids		
Triglycerides, neutral fats	Adipose tissue, butterfat, lard, suet, fish oils, olive oil, corn oil, etc.	Esters of three molecules of fatty acids and one molecule of glycerol; the fatty acids may all be be different
Waxes	Beeswax, head oil of sperm whale, cerumen, carnauba oil, and lanolin	Composed of esters of fatty acids with alcohol other than glycerol; of industrial and medicinal importance
Compound lipids		
Phospholipids (phosphatides)	Chiefly in animal tissues	Substituted fats consisting of phosphatidic acid; composed of glycerol, fatty acid, and phosphoric acid bound in ester linkage to a nitrogenous base
Lecithin	Brain, egg yolk, and organ meats	Phosphatidyl choline or serine; phosphatide linked to choline; a lipotropic agent; important in fat metabolism and transport; used as emulsifying agent in food industry
Cephalin	Occurs predominantly in nervous tissue	Phosphatidyl ethanolamine; phosphatide linked to serine or ethanolamine; plays a role in blood clotting
Plasmalogen	Brain, heart, and muscle	Phosphatidal ethanolamine or choline; phosphatide containing an aliphatic aldehyde
Lipositol	Brain, heart, kidneys, and plant tissues together with phytic acid	Phosphatidyl inositol; phosphatide linked to inositol; rapid synthesis and degradation in brain; evidence for role in cell transport processes
Sphingomyelin	Nervous tissue, brain, and red blood cells	Sphingosine-containing phosphatide; yields fatty acid, choline, sphingosine, phosphoric acid, and no glycerol; source of phosphoric acid in body tissue
Glycolipids		
Cerebroside	Myelin sheaths of nerves, brain, and other tissues	Yields on hydrolysis fatty acids, sphingosine, galactose (or glucose), but not fatty acid; includes kerasin and phrenosin
Ganglioside	Brain, nerve tissue, and other selected tissues, notably spleen	Contains a ceramide linked to hexose (glucose or galactose), neuraminic acid, sphingosine, and fatty acids
Sulfolipid	White matter of brain, liver, and testicle; also plant chloroplast	Sulfur-containing glycolipid; sulfate present in ester linkage to galactose

(continued)

Lipid	Occurrence	Characteristics
Proteolipids	Brain and nerve tissues	Complexes of protein and lipids having solubility properties of lipids

Terpenoids and steroids

Lipid	Occurrence	Characteristics
Terpenes	Essential oils, resin acids, rubber, plant pigments such as carotenes and lycopenes, vitamin A, and camphor	Large group of compounds made up of repeating isoprene units; vitamin A of nutritional interest; fat-soluble vitamins E and K also related chemically to terpenes

Sterols

Lipid	Occurrence	Characteristics
Cholesterol, ergosterol, & 7-dehydro-cholesterol	Cholesterol found in egg yolk, dairy products, and animal tissues; ergosterol found in plant tissues, yeast, and fungi; 7-dehydrocholesterol found in animal tissues and underneath skin	Cholesterol, a constituent of bile acids and precursor of vitamin D; ergosterol and 7-dehydrocholesterol, converted to vitamin D_2 and D_3, respectively, on irradiation

Sex hormones

Lipid	Occurrence	Characteristics
Androgens, estrogens	Ovaries and testes	
Adrenal corti-cal steroids	Adrenal cortex, blood	

Derived lipids

Lipid	Occurrence	Characteristics
Fatty acids*	Occur in plant and animal foods; also exist in complex forms with other substances	Obtained from hydrolysis of fats; usually contain an even number of carbon atoms and are straight chain derivatives

*Classification of fatty acids is based on the length of the carbon chain (short, medium, or long); number of double bonds (unsaturated, mono- or polyunsaturated); or essentiality in the diet (essential or nonessential). A current designation is based on the position of the endmost double bond counting from the methyl (CH_3) carbon, called the omega end. The most important omega fatty acids are:

Omega-6 fatty acids	linoleic and arachidonic acids
Omega-3 fatty acids	linolenic, eicosapentaenoic, and docosahexaenoic acids

Sample nomenclature for fatty acids according to its chemical characteristics are:

Butyric acid	4:0 (carbon length:no. of double bond)
Palmitic acid	16:0
Oleic acid	18:1 (9) indicating position of double bond
Linoleic acid	18:2 (9,12)
Linolenic acid	18:3 (9,12,15)
Arachidonic acid	20:4 (5,8,11,14)
Eicosapentaenoic acid	20:5 (5,8,11,14,17)
Docosahexaenoic acid	22:6 (4,7,10,13,16,19)

Appendix 11
Summary of Digestive Enzymes

Source & Enzyme	Substrate	Products
Mouth		
Salivary α-amylase	Cooked starch	Dextrins, maltose, and maltriose
Stomach		
Gastric lipase	Emulsified fat	Fatty acids and glycerol
Pepsin	Proteins and polypeptides	Polypeptides and amino acids
Rennin	Casein of milk	Calcium caseinate
Pancreas		
Carboxypeptidase A	Proteins and polypeptides	Aromatic or branch chain amino acids
Carboxypeptidase B	Proteins and polypeptides	Basic side chain amino acids
Chymotrypsin	Proteins and polypeptides	Polypeptides, proteoses and peptones
Deoxyribonuclease	DNA	Mononucleotides
Elastase	Elastin and other protein	Neutral aliphatic amino acids
Cholesterol esterase	Cholesteryl esters	Cholesterol; fatty acids
Pancreatic α-amylase	Cooked starch	Same as salivary α-amylase
Pancreatic lipase	Fat and triglycerides	Glycerides, fatty acids, and glycerol
Phospholipase A	Lecithin	Lysolecithin
Ribonuclease	RNA	Mononucleotides
Trypsin	Proteins and polypeptides	Polypeptides, peptones, proteoses
Small intestines		
Aminopeptidase	Polypeptides	N-terminal amino acids
Dipeptidase	Dipeptides	Two amino acids
Enterokinase	Trypsinogen	Trypsin
Intestinal lipase	Monoglycerides	Glycerol and fatty acids
Isomaltase	Dextrins	Glucose
Lactase	Lactose	Glucose, galactose
Maltase	Maltose	Glucose
Nucleosidase	Nucleosides	Purines, pyrimidines, and pentose
Sucrase	Sucrose	Glucose, fructose

Appendix 12
Utilization of Carbohydrates

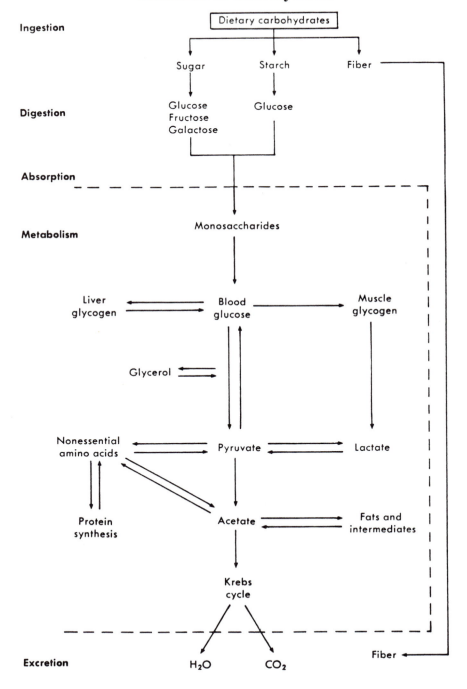

Ingestion · Digestion · Absorption · Metabolism · Excretion

Dietary carbohydrates → Sugar, Starch, Fiber

Sugar → Glucose, Fructose, Galactose

Starch → Glucose

Monosaccharides → Blood glucose

Liver glycogen ⇄ Blood glucose ⇄ Muscle glycogen

Glycerol ⇄

Nonessential amino acids ⇄ Pyruvate ⇄ Lactate

Protein synthesis

Acetate ⇄ Fats and intermediates

Krebs cycle → H_2O, CO_2

Fiber

Appendix 13
Utilization of Proteins

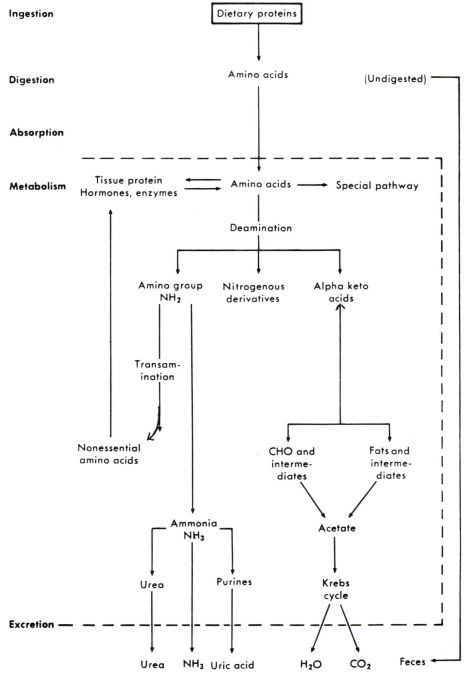

Ingestion

Dietary proteins

Digestion

Amino acids   (Undigested)

Absorption

Metabolism

Tissue protein
Hormones, enzymes   Amino acids ⟶ Special pathway

Deamination

Amino group NH_2 Nitrogenous derivatives   Alpha keto acids

Transamination

Nonessential amino acids

CHO and intermediates   Fats and intermediates

Ammonia NH_3 Acetate

Urea   Purines   Krebs cycle

Excretion

Urea NH_3 Uric acid H_2O CO_2 Feces

Appendix 14
Utilization of Fats

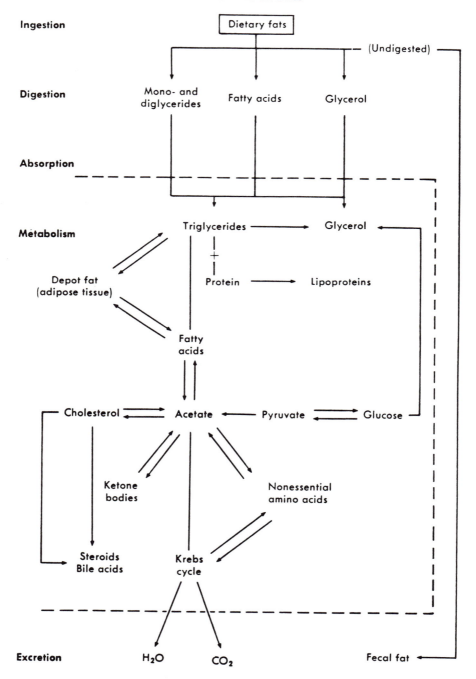

Appendix 15
Interrelationship of Carbohydrate, Protein, and Fat

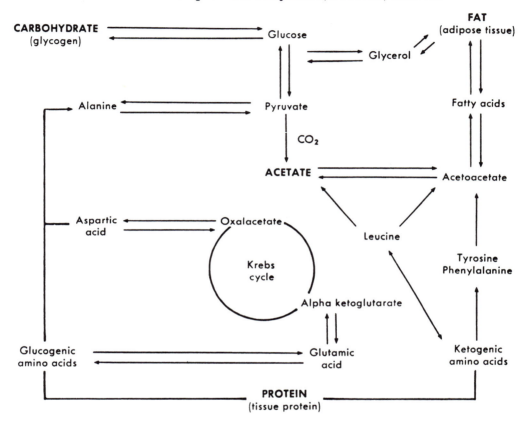

Appendix 16
Summary of Vitamins

Vitamin	Major Functions	Signs of Deficiency	Food sources
Fat-soluble vitamins			
Vitamin A	Maintenance of skin and mucous membranes; component in visual process; immune stimulation	Poor growth; nightblindness xerophthalmia; keratomalacia; Bitot's spots; follicular hyperkeratosis; reduced resistance to infection	Liver; dark green and deep yellow fruits and vegetables
Vitamin D	Mineralization of bones and teeth; intestinal absorption and regulation of calcium and phosphate	Rickets; costochondral beading; bowed legs; epiphyseal enlargement; muscle weakness; osteomalacia	Sunlight exposure; fortified milk and milk products; cod liver oil
Vitamin E	Antioxidant; prevents peroxidation of polyunsaturated lipids; free radical scavenger	Hemolytic anemia of newborn; increased fragility of red blood cells; ceroid pigment deposits	Oils high in polyunsaturated fatty acids; wheat germ; seeds
Vitamin K	Synthesis of prothrombin and clotting factors II, VII, IX, and X	Bleeding tendency (especially in newborns); ecchymosis; epistaxis	Green leafy vegetables; liver; vegetable oils
Water-soluble vitamins			
Vitamin C	Reducing agent; collagen synthesis; helps in wound healing and resistance to infection; iron absorption	Scurvy; easy bruising; joint tenderness; muscle ache; slow wound healing; petechiae; bleeding gums	Citrus fruits; tomatoes; papaya; raw cabbage; green pepper
Vitamin B_1 (Thiamin)	Coenzyme in carbohydrate fat and protein metabolism; promotes normal functioning of the nervous system	Beriberi; peripheral edema; polyneuritis; high-output cardiac failure; anorexia; paresthesias; tender muscles	Lean pork; wheat germ; whole and enriched cereals; legumes
Vitamin B_2 (Riboflavin)	Part of flavin coenzymes required in cellular oxidation; essential for growth	Cheilosis; glossitis; photophobia; angular stomatitis; seborrhea; magenta tongue; corneal vascularization	Milk and dairy products; liver; dark green vegetables; organ meats
Vitamin B_6 (Pyridoxine)	Cofactor for many enzymes in metabolism of protein and amino acids; functions in hemoglobin synthesis	Anemia; irritability; convulsions; depression; skin lesions; seborrheic dermatitis; glossitis	Liver; pork; poultry; whole grain; fortified cereals; bananas; legumes
Vitamin B_{12} (Cobalamin)	Maintenance of nerve tissue and normal blood formation; nucleic acid synthesis; recycling of tetrahydrofolate	Megaloblastic anemia; glossitis; spinal cord degeneration; peripheral neuropathy	Liver; meat; fish; poultry; eggs; (not present in plant foods)

288

Appendix 16 *(continued)*

Vitamin	Major Functions	Signs of Deficiency	Food sources
Niacin	Part of coenzymes for oxidation/reduction reactions, release of energy and biosynthesis of fatty acids	Pellagra; pigmented dermatitis; inflammation of mucous membranes; diarrhea; weakness; depression	Lean meats; fish; poultry; whole grains; peanuts; organ meats
Folate	Cofactor for synthesis of purine and pyrimidine; transfer of single carbon; red blood cell maturation	Megaloblastic anemia; gastrointestinal disturbances; glossitis; stomatitis; diarrhea	Dark green leafy vegetables; whole grains; legumes; nuts; organ meats
Pantothenic Acid	Component of coenzyme A; functions in release of energy from carbohydrate, protein, and fat	Fatigue; malaise; insomnia; abdominal cramps; burning paresthesias; impaired coordination; depression	Liver; egg; meat; fish; poultry; whole grains; fresh vegetables
Biotin	Coenzyme for carboxylation reactions; plays a role in carbohydrate and fat metabolism	Dermatitis; neuritis; anorexia; nausea; vomiting; glossitis; insomnia; thin hair; depression	Liver; milk; egg; kidney; mushrooms; bananas; strawberries

Usual Daily Dose Ranges for Oral Vitamin Administration:

	Prophylactic	Low Dose	High Dose
Biotin, mg	-	10	-
Folic acid, mg	2.5-10	5-10	10-20
Niacin, mg	10	10-100	100-500
Pantothenate, mg	100	100-200	200-600
Vitamin A, IU	5,000	5,000-30,000	100,000-200,000
Vitamin D, IU	500-1000	5,000	10,000-15,000
Vitamin E, mg	3-15	10-100	400-600
Vitamin K_1, mg	5-10	5-10	10-20
Vitamin B_1, mg	3-10	10-100	100-600
Vitamin B_2, mg	1-5	5-10	10-100
Vitamin B_6, mg	20	20-50	50-300
Vitamin B_{12}, μg*	5-50 monthly	100-250 weekly	Up to 500 weekly
Vitamin C, mg	100	100-200	Up to 3000

*Intramuscular
Data from Marks, John.: <u>The Vitamins. Their Role in Medical Practice</u>. Boston: MTP Press Limited, 1985.

Appendix 17
Summary of Minerals

Mineral	Major Functions	Signs of Deficiency	Food Sources
Calcium	Structure of bones and teeth; nerve transmission; blood clotting; muscle contraction	Stunted growth; rickets; osteomalacia; osteoporosis; muscle cramping; tetany; possibly hypertension	Milk; cheese; sardines with bones; mustard greens; kale
Chloride	Constituent of gastric juice; major anion of extracellular fluid; enzyme activator; acid-base balance	Mental apathy; muscle cramps; usually accompanied with sodium depletion	Table salt; seafoods; meats
Chromium	Insulin cofactor; glucose and energy metabolism; stimulates fat and cholesterol synthesis	Insulin resistance; glucose intolerance; impaired growth; elevated serum lipids	Liver; cheese; meat; whole-grain cereals
Cobalt	Constituent of vitamin B_{12}	Only as vitamin B_{12} deficiency; pernicious anemia	Organ and muscle meats; milk
Copper	Absorption and use of iron; enzyme cofactor; electron transport; myelin sheath of nerves; maybe part of RNA	Anemia; disturbance of bone formation; impairment of cardiovascular system; neutropenia; kinky hair	Liver; shellfish; nuts; whole grain cereals; legumes; organ meats
Fluoride	Structure of teeth enamel; reduces dental caries	Dental caries; possibly growth depression;	Drinking water; tea; seafood
Iodine	Constituent of thyroid hormones	Goiter; depressed thyroid function; cretinism	Iodized salt; seafoods; marine fish
Iron	Constituent of hemoglobin and the cytochrome enzymes involved in oxygen and electron transport	Microcytic and hypochromic anemia; growth retardation; decreased serum iron; easy fatigability	Liver; lean meats; legumes; egg yolk; fortified cereals and breads
Magnesium	Activates enzymes; nerve impulse transmission and muscle contraction; constituent of bones and teeth	Neuromuscular irritability; weakness; spasms; apathy; growth failure; behavioral disturbances	Whole grains; nuts, legumes; green leafy vegetables; seafoods
Manganese	Constituent of enzymes in mucopolysaccharide metabolism and fat synthesis	Scaly dermatitis; retarded hair/nail growth; weight loss	Nuts; legumes; unrefined cereals dried fruits
Molybdenum	Enzyme cofactor in sulfur and purine metabolism; oxidation/reduction process	Dietary deficiency not observed in humans	Milk, organ meats; legumes; whole-grain cereals

Appendix 17 *(continued)*

Mineral	Major Functions	Signs of Deficiency	Food Sources
Phosphorus	Structure of bones and teeth; component of phospholipids, and nucleic acids; acid-base balance; energy metabolism	Demineralization of bone; weakness; poor growth. paresthesia of hands and feet; seizures	Milk; cheese; egg; meats; whole-grain cereals; legumes
Potassium	Major cation of intracellular fluid; regulates acid-base & water balance, osmotic pressure, nerve transmission	Muscle weakness; nausea; cardiac arrhythmias; heart failure; glycogen depletion; respiratory failure	Many fruits; nuts; meats; milk; vegetables; potatoes; cereals
Selenium	Antioxidant; constituent of glutathione oxidase; associated with vitamin E and fat	Cardiac myopathy; increased fragility of red blood cells; muscle tenderness	Meat; seafoods; grains; milk; vegetables
Sodium	Major cation of extracellular fluid; regulates body fluid volume, pH, and osmolarity; influences nerve irritability and muscle contraction	Abdominal cramps; nausea; vomiting; apathy; muscle contraction; palpitation; confusion	Table salt (NaCl); processed foods; abundant in most foods except for fruits
Sulfur	Constituent of coenzyme A, certain amino acids, hair, cartilage, thiamin, biotin	No dietary deficiency if protein intake is adequate	All foods rich in protein - meat, milk, legumes
Zinc	Constituent of many enzymes; cell replication; connective tissue synthesis; immune system function	Dermatitis; impaired wound healing; taste changes; depressed immunocompetence; sexual immaturity	Seafood; eggyolk; liver; meat; oysters; cereal germ

Daily oral therapeutic dosages for mineral deficiency:

Calcium	1-1.5 gm bid
Chromium	200 µg (chromium chloride)
Copper	2-3 mg (copper sulfate)
Iodine	50 µg (potassium iodide)
Fluoride	1-2 mg (sodium fluoride)
Iron	325 mg tid (ferrous sulfate)
Magnesium	250-500 mg bid to qid (magnesium oxide)
Molybdenum	300 µg
Phosphorus	1-1.5 mmol/kg
Selenium	100-200 µg
Zinc	60 mg elemental zinc (zinc sulfate 220 mg)

Data from Weinsier, R. et al.: Handbook of Clinical Nutrition. 2nd ed., St. Louis, MO, 1989.

(continued)

Appendix 18
Median Weights and Heights for
Children from Birth to 18 Years

Age	Males				Females			
	Weight		Height		Weight		Height	
	kg	lb	cm	in	kg	lb	cm	in
Months								
1	4.29	9.4	54.6	21.5	3.98	8.8	53.5	21.1
3	5.98	13.2	61.1	24.1	5.40	11.9	59.5	23.4
6	7.85	17.3	67.8	26.7	7.21	15.9	65.9	25.9
9	9.18	20.2	72.3	28.5	8.56	18.8	70.4	27.7
12	10.15	22.3	76.1	30.0	9.53	21.0	74.3	29.3
18	11.47	25.2	82.4	32.4	10.82	23.8	80.9	31.9
Years								
2	12.34	27.1	86.8	34.2	11.80	26.0	86.8	34.2
3	14.62	32.2	94.9	37.4	14.10	31.0	94.1	37.0
4	16.69	36.7	102.9	40.5	15.96	35.1	101.6	40.0
5	18.67	41.1	109.9	43.3	17.66	38.9	108.4	42.7
6	20.69	45.5	116.1	45.7	19.52	42.9	114.6	45.1
7	22.85	50.3	121.7	47.9	21.84	48.0	120.6	47.5
8	25.30	55.7	127.0	50.0	24.84	54.6	126.4	49.8
9	28.13	61.9	132.2	52.0	28.46	62.6	132.2	52.0
10	31.44	69.2	137.5	54.1	32.55	71.6	138.3	54.4
11	35.30	77.7	143.3	56.4	36.95	81.3	144.8	57.0
12	39.78	87.5	149.7	58.9	41.53	91.4	151.5	59.6
13	44.95	98.9	156.5	61.6	46.10	101.4	157.1	61.9
14	50.77	111.7	163.1	64.2	50.28	110.6	160 4	63.1
15	56.71	124.8	169.0	66.5	53.68	118.1	161.8	63.7
16	62.10	136.6	173.5	68.3	55.89	123.0	162.4	63.9
17	66.31	145.9	176.2	69.4	56.69	124.7	163.1	64.2
18	68.88	151.5	176.8	69.6	56.62	124.6	163.7	64.4

Data from the National Health Survey: NCHS Growth Curves for Children. Birth-18
Years, United States. In Vital and Health Statistics, Series 11, no. 124, DHEW
Publication No. (PHS) 78-1650.

Appendix 19
Average Weights for Men and Women
Aged 18-74 Years

| | Height | | Weight in Pounds by Age Group in Years | | | | | |
	Ft	In	18-24	25-34	35-44	45-54	55-64	65-74
Men	5	2	130	141	143	147	143	143
	5	3	135	145	148	152	147	147
	5	4	140	150	153	156	153	151
	5	5	145	156	158	160	158	156
	5	6	150	160	163	164	163	160
	5	7	154	165	169	169	168	164
	5	8	159	170	174	173	173	169
	5	9	164	174	179	177	178	173
	5	10	168	179	184	182	183	177
	5	11	173	184	190	187	189	182
	6	0	178	189	194	191	193	186
	6	1	183	194	200	196	197	190
	6	2	188	199	205	200	203	194
Women	4	9	114	118	125	129	132	130
	4	10	117	121	129	133	136	134
	4	11	120	125	133	136	140	137
	5	0	123	128	137	140	143	140
	5	1	126	132	141	143	147	144
	5	2	129	136	144	147	150	147
	5	3	132	139	148	150	153	151
	5	4	135	142	152	154	157	154
	5	5	138	146	156	158	160	158
	5	6	141	150	159	161	164	161
	5	7	144	153	163	165	167	165
	5	8	147	157	167	168	171	169

Data from the National Center for Health Statistics: Weight by Height and Age
for Adults 18-74 Years, United States, 1971-1974. In Vital and Health Statistics, Series II, no. 208, DHEW Publication No. (PHS) 79-1656.

Appendix 20-A
Acceptable Weights for Men and Women#

Height*		Weight in pounds**	
Ft	In	19 to 34 yrs	35 yrs & over
5	0	97-128	108-138
5	1	101-132	111-143
5	2	104-137	115-148
5	3	107-141	119-152
5	4	111-146	122-157
5	5	114-150	126-162
5	6	118-155	130-167
5	7	121-160	134-172
5	8	125-164	138-178
5	9	129-169	142-183
5	10	132-174	146-188
5	11	136-179	151-194
6	0	140-184	155-190
6	1	144-189	159-205
6	2	148-195	164-210
6	3	152-200	168-216
6	4	156-205	173-222
6	5	160-211	177-228

*Height without shoes   **Weight without clothes
#USDA. Nutrition and Your Health: Dietary Guidelines
for Americans. HG-232, 1990.

Criteria for a healthy weight:

1. Weight is within the acceptable range for the height
   and age group

2. Waist-to-hip ratio (WHR) is less than 0.8 for women
   and less than 0.95 for men, where

   WHR =   Waist measurement
            Hip measurement

3. No weight-related medical problems or family history
   of such problems

Appendix 20-B
1983 Metropolitan Height-Weight Tables

Men

Height Ft in		Small Frame	Medium Frame	Large Frame
5	2	128-134	131-141	138-150
5	3	130-136	133-143	140-153
5	4	132-138	135-145	141-156
5	5	134-140	137-148	144-160
5	6	136-142	139-151	146-164
5	7	138-145	142-154	149-168
5	8	140-148	145-157	152-172
5	9	142-151	148-160	155-176
5	10	144-154	151-163	158-180
5	11	146-157	154-166	161-184
6	0	149-160	157-170	164-188
6	1	152-164	160-174	168-192
6	2	155-168	164-178	172-197
6	3	158-172	167-182	176-202
6	4	162-176	171-187	181-207

Women

Height Ft in		Small Frame	Medium Frame	Large Frame
4	10	102-111	109-121	118-131
4	11	103-113	111-123	120-134
5	0	104-115	113-126	122-137
5	1	106-118	115-129	125-140
5	2	108-121	118-132	128-143
5	3	111-124	121-135	131-147
5	4	114-127	124-138	134-151
5	5	117-130	127-141	137-155
5	6	120-133	130-144	140-159
5	7	123-136	133-147	143-163
5	8	126-139	136-150	146-167
5	9	129-142	139-153	149-170
5	10	132-145	142-156	152-173
5	11	135-148	145-159	155-176
6	0	138-151	148-162	158-179

Weights at ages 25-59 based on lowest mortality. Weight in pounds in indoor clothing (5 lb for men and 3 lb for women); shoes with 1 inch heels. Data from 1979 Build Study, Society of Actuaries and Association of Life Insurance Medical Directors of America. Courtesy of the Metropolitan Life Insurance Company, 1983.

Appendix 21
Estimation of Frame Size and Stature

A. Body Frame According to Wrist Size

Wrap the fingers of one hand around the opposite wrist. If the thumb and middle finger

        Overlap by 1 cm = small frame

        Touch = medium frame

        Cannot touch by 1 cm = large frame

B. Body Frame According to Height:Wrist Circumference ("r")

	Large	Medium	Small
Males, "r" values	< 9.6	9.6-10.4	> 10.4
Females, "r" values	< 9.9	9.9-10.9	> 10.9

Where "r" = Height (cm) divided by wrist circumference (cm)

C. Body Frame According to Elbow Breadth

	Males			Females		
Age	Large	Medium	Small	Large	Medium	Small
18-24	>7.7	6.6-7.7	<6.6	>6.5	5.6-6.5	<5.6
25-34	>7.9	6.7-7.9	<6.7	>6.8	5.7-6.8	<5.7
35-44	>8.0	6.7-8.0	<6.7	>7.1	5.7-7.1	<5.7
45-54	>8.1	6.7-8.1	<6.7	>7.2	5.7-7.2	<5.7
54-55	>8.1	6.7-8.1	<6.7	>7.2	5.8-7.2	<5.8
65-74	>8.1	6.7-8.1	<6.7	>7.2	5.8-7.2	<5.8

To measure elbow breadth, extend arm forward and bend forearm upward at 90 degrees with fingers pointing up and inside of wrist toward the body. Measure the breadth with a sliding caliper (in cm) across the elbow joint on the two prominent bones on either side.

D. Stature from Knee Height Measurement

Men   Height (cm) = $(2.03 \times \text{knee height}_{cm}) - (0.04 \times \text{age}_{yr} + 64.19)$

Women Height (cm) = $(1.83 \times \text{knee height}_{cm}) - (0.24 \times \text{age}_{yr} + 84.88)$

Use a broad-blade caliper to get knee height measurement. The subject lies on the back with the knee bent to a 90 degree angle. Press the sliding blade of the caliper against the thigh about 2 inches behind the kneecap and hold the caliper shaft in line with the shaft of the tibia. Two readings should agree within $\pm$ 0.5 cm.

Sources: Grant, J.P.: Handbook of Total Parenteral Nutrition, W.B. Saunders Company, 1980, p.15; Frisancho, A.R.: New standards of weight and body composition by frame and height for assessment of nutritional status of adults and the elderly," Am J Clin Nutr, 40:808, 1984; Chumlea, W.C. et al.: Estimating stature from knee height for persons 60 to 90 years of age, J Am Geriatr Soc, 33:116, 1985.

Appendix 22
Reference Values for Triceps Skinfold Thickness*

Age	Males (mm Percentile)						Females (mm Percentile)				
	10th	25th	50th	75th	90th		10th	25th	50th	75th	90th
18-74	6.0	8.0	11.0	15.0	20.0		13.0	17.0	22.0	28.0	34.0
18-24	5.0	7.5	9.5	14.0	20.0		11.0	14.0	18.0	24.0	30.0
25-34	5.5	8.0	12.0	16.0	21.5		12.0	16.0	21.0	26.5	33.5
35-44	6.0	8.5	12.0	15.5	20.0		14.0	18.0	23.0	29.5	35.5
45-54	6.0	8.0	11.0	15.0	20.0		15.0	20.0	25.0	30.0	36.0
55-64	6.0	8.0	11.0	14.0	18.0		14.0	19.0	25.0	30.5	35.0
65-74	5.5	8.0	11.0	15.0	19.0		14.0	18.0	23.0	28.0	33.0

*Developed from data collected during the NHANES I, 1971 to 1974.
From Bishop, C.W., P.E. Bowen and S.J. Ritchey. Norms for nutritional assessment of American adults by upper arm anthropometry. Am. J. Clin. Nutr. 34:2530, 1981. (adapted with permission)

Triceps skinfold: With the arm relaxed and the elbow flexed at 90° angle, grasp the skin and subcutaneous tissue at the midpoint of the upper arm between the acromion and the olecranon processes of the scapula and the ulna. Measure with a caliper while the fold is still held with the hand to release skin tension. Take three measurements to the nearest 0.5 mm and average the results.

Appendix 23
Reference Values for Midarm Muscle Circumference*

Age	Males (cm Percentile)						Females (cm Percentile)				
	10th	25th	50th	75th	90th		10th	25th	50th	75th	90th
18-74	24.8	26.3	27.9	29.5	31.4		19.0	20.2	21.8	23.6	25.8
18-24	24.4	25.8	27.2	28.9	30.8		18.5	19.4	20.6	22.1	23.6
25-34	25.3	26.5	28.0	30.0	31.7		18.9	20.0	21.4	22.9	24.9
35-44	25.6	27.1	28.7	30.3	32.1		19.2	20.6	22.0	24.0	26.1
45-54	24.9	26.5	28.1	29.8	31.5		19.5	20.7	22.2	24.3	26.6
55-64	24.4	26.2	27.9	29.6	31.0		19.5	20.8	22.6	24.4	26.3
65-74	23.7	25.3	26.9	28.5	29.9		19.5	20.8	22.5	24.4	26.5

*Developed from data collected during the NHANES I, 1971 to 1974.
From Bishop, C.W., P.E. Bowen and S.J. Ritchey. Norms for nutritional assessment of American adults by upper arm anthropometry. Am. J. Clin. Nutr. 34:2530, 1981. (adapted with permission)

Mid-upper arm: Allow the arm to hang relaxed at the side. Using a tape measure, get the arm circumference (in cm) at the midpoint of the upper arm. The tape should be maintained in a horizontal position touching the skin and following the contours of the limb, but not compressing underlying tissue. Calculate the mid-arm muscle circumference (MAMC) with the formula: MAMC,cm = mid-arm circumference,cm - TSF,mm x 0.314

Appendix 24
Estimation of Energy and Protein
Requirements of Adults

Energy Requirement:

Method I.
1. Determine basal or resting energy expenditure (BEE or REE) from the Harris Benedict formula
    Male: BEE = 66.47 + (13.75 x Wt) + (5 x Ht) - (6.76 x Yr)
    Female: BEE = 655.10 + (9.56 x Wt) + (1.85 x Ht) - (4.68 x Yr)
        Where: Wt is actual weight in kilogram
               Ht is height in centimeters (height in inches x 2.54)
               Yr is age in years

2. Adjustment for activity = BEE x activity factor below
    Bed rest   1.0-1.1   Moderate   1.6-1.7
    Very light   1.2-1.3   Heavy   1.9-2.1
    Light   1.4-1.5   Strenuous or 2.2-2.4
                               exceptional
    (Use lower factor for females; higher factor for males)

3. Provision for illness = BEE x stress or injury factor below
    No illness/nonstress   1.0
    Convalescence, mild malnutrition,   1.1
        Post-operative (no complication)
    Mild illness, noncatabolic
        Confined to bed   1.2
        Ambulatory/out of bed   1.3
    Infections & stress, catabolic
        Mild   1.2-1.3
        Moderate   1.4-1.5
        Severe, hypercatabolic   1.6-1.8
        Sepsis   2.0-2.2
    Burns, <20% body surface   1.2-1.4
           20-40% body surface   1.5-1.7
           >40% body surface   1.8-2.0
    Fracture, long bone   1.2-1.3
    Respiratory/renal failure   1.4-1.5
    COPD   1.4-1.8
    Cancer with chemotherapy or   1.5-1.6
        radiation, cardiac cachexia
    Surgery, minor/elective   1.1-1.2
    Surgery, major   1.2-1.3
    Trauma, skeletal/blunt   1.3-1.4
    Trauma, multiple/head injury   1.5-1.6

4. Kilocalories for total energy expenditure (TEE)
    Weight maintenance TEE = BEE x activity factor and stress/injury factor
    Weight gain: Add 500 kcal/day to gain at the rate of 1 lb per week
    Weight loss: Subtract 500 kcal/day to lose at the rate of 1 lb per week

(continued)

Appendix 24 *(continued)*

Method II. Quick Method. Calorie allowances per kg (or lb) body weight
for different activity levels and stress conditions:

Activity level:	kcal/kg BW	kcal/lb BW
Bed patient	25	11
Very light activity	30	14
Light activity	35	16
Moderate activity	40	18
Active/heavy work	45	20
Streneous/exceptional	50	23

Stress condition:		
Overweight/weight reduction	20	9
Nonstress, bed rest	25	11
Mild stress, bed rest	30	14
ambulatory	35	16
Moderate stress, bed rest	35	16
ambulatory	40	18
Severe stress, polytrauma, hypermetabolic, sepsis	45	20
Surgery, elective/minor	32	14.5
Surgery, major, bed rest	35	16
ambulatory	38	17.5
Burn, major, bed rest	45-50	20-23
ambulatory	55-60	25-27
Cancer	35-45	16-20
Predialysis	40-50	18-23
Hemodialysis	35	16
Peritoneal dialysis	30	14

Protein requirement:

1. Normal requirement: 0.8-1.0 gm/kg body weight

2. Requirement during illness or stress (gm/kg body weight)

Mild stress	1.1-1.2	Acute renal failure,	0.3-0.5
Moderate stress	1.3-1.4	Chronic renal failure	0.55-0.6
Severe stress	1.5-1.7	Hemodialysis	1.0-1.2
Polytrauma, infection	1.8-2.4	Peritoneal dialysis	1.2-1.5
Severe sepsis, major burn head injury	2.5-3.0	Post renal transplant	1.5-2.0
		COPD	1.2-1.5
Surgery, minor/elective	1.2-1.3	Hepatitis, cirrhosis	1.5-2.0
Surgery, major	1.4-1.5	Depleted protein stores,	1.6-1.7
Cancer, malabsorption syndromes, tuberculosis	1.2-1.5	decubiti, long-bone fractures, draining	
Acute respiratory failure	1.3-1.4	wounds	

Appendix 25
Interpretations and Equations for
Assessing Nutritional Status

Albumin
      Interpretation: >3.5 gm/dl, acceptable
                      2.8-3.4 gm/dl, mild depletion
                      2.1-2.7 gm/dl, moderate depletion
                      <2.1 gm/dl, severe depletion

Prealbumin
      Interpretation: >15 mg/dl, acceptable
                      10-15 mg/dl, mild depletion
                      5-10 mg/dl, moderate depletion
                      <5 mg/dl, severe depletion

Serum transferrin
      Interpretation: >200 mg/dl, acceptable
                      150-200 mg/dl, mild depletion
                      100-149 mg/dl, moderate depletion
                      <100 mg/dl, severe depletion

Transferrin, calculated from total iron-binding capacity (TIBC)
      Transferrin, mg/dl $= \dfrac{\text{TIBC } (\mu g/dl)}{1.45}$

      Interpretation: >170 mg/dl, acceptable
                      <170 mg/dl, deficient

      (Transferrin values determined from TIBC and are lower than
      those obtained by radioimmunodiffusion, but may be elevated
      in patients with severe iron deficiency anemia).

Total iron-binding capacity (TIBC)
      Interpretation: 250-350 µg/dl, normal
                       >400 µg/dl, indicative of iron deficiency

Total lymphocyte count (TLC), (cells/mm^3)
      TLC $= \dfrac{\text{\% lymphocytes } \times \text{ white blood cells (WBC)}/mm^3}{100}$

      Interpretation: >2000/mm^3, acceptable
                      1200-2000/mm^3, mild depletion
                      800-1199/mm^3, moderate depletion
                      <800/mm^3, severe depletion

(continued)

Appendix 25 *(continued)*

Creatinine:height index (CHI)

$$\text{CHI} = \frac{\text{24-hr urinary creatinine (mg)}}{\text{expected 24-hr urinary creatinine (mg)}} \times 100\%$$

Interpretation: >90%, acceptable
80-90%, mild depletion
60-79%, moderate depletion
<60%, severe depletion

Nitrogen balance $= \dfrac{\text{Protein intake,gm}}{6.25} - (\text{Urinary urea nitrogen} + 4*)$

*Value represents an estimate of the unmeasured
nitrogen lost in sweat, hair, skin, and stool

Protein loss, gm $=$ (Urinary urea nitrogen + 4) x 6.25

Prognostic Nutritional Index (PNI)

PNI $=$ 158 - 16.6 (Alb) - 0.78 (TSF) - 0.2 (TFN) - 5.8 (DH)

Where: Alb = serum albumin (gm/dl); TSF = triceps skinfold (mm)
TFN = transferrin level (mg/dl); DH = delayed hypersensitivity skin test

Interpretation: <30, low risk of mortality and morbidity
30-50, intermediate risk
>50, high risk

Triceps skinfold thickness (TSF), mm
Interpretation: >50th percentile, acceptable
40-50th percentile, mild fat depletion
25-39th percentile, moderate fat depletion
<25th percentile, severe fat depletion

Mid-arm circumference (MAC),cm
Interpretation: >50th percentile, acceptable
40-50th percentile, mild fat depletion
25-39th percentile, moderate fat depletion
<25th percentile, severe fat depletion

Mid-arm muscle circumference (MAMC),cm
MAMC,cm = MAC,cm - (TSF,mm x 0.314)

Interpretation: >85%, acceptable
76-85%, mild depletion
65-75%, moderate depletion
<65%, severe depletion

Fat-free mass (FFM), prediction from 24-hr urinary creatinine excretion
FFM (kg) = 29.08 creatinine (gm/dl) + 7.38

Appendix 25 *(continued)*

Weight:height ratio or Body Mass Index (BMI)

$$BMI = \frac{Weight\ (kg)}{Height^2\ (meters)}$$

    19-34 years old: 19-25, acceptable
                       >25, unacceptable
    35 years & over: 21-27, acceptable
                       >27, unacceptable

Relative body weight (RBW), as % of desirable weight

$$RBW = \frac{Actual\ weight}{Desirable\ body\ weight} \times 100$$

    Interpretation: <70, severe underweight
                    70-79, moderate underweight
                    80-89%, mild underweight
                    90-110%, acceptable
                    111-120%, overweight
                    >120% obese

Weight change, as % of usual weight

$$\%\ weight\ change = \frac{Present\ weight}{Usual\ weight} \times 100$$

    Interpretation: >120%, significant weight gain
                    110-120%, moderate weight gain
                    90-109%, acceptable
                    85-89%, mild weight loss
                    75-84%, moderate weight loss
                    <75%, severe weight loss

        10% unplanned or recent weight loss is a
        risk factor for malnutrition
        20% unplanned or recent weight loss is a
        high risk for surgical patients

Weight change, as % of usual weight over time

$$\%\ weight\ loss = \frac{Usual\ weight - present\ weight}{Usual\ weight} \times 100$$

	Significant loss	Severe loss
Interpretation: 1 week	1-2 %	>2 %
1 month	5 %	>5 %
3 month	7.5 %	>7.5 %
6 month	10 %	>10 %

Stature, from knee height:

    Men (cm)   = (knee height,cm x 2.02) - (age,yr x 0.04) + 64.19
    Women (cm) = (knee height,cm x 1.83) - (age,yr x 0.24) + 84.88

Appendix 26
Physical Assessment of Nutritional Status

Body Area	Normal Appearance	Signs associated with Malnutrition
Hair	Shiny; firm; not easily plucked	Lack of natural shine; hair dull and dry; thin and sparse; hair fine, silky and straight; color changes; can be easily plucked
Face	Skin color uniform; smooth, pink, and healthy appearance; not swollen	Skin color loss (depigmentation); skin dark over cheeks and under eyes; lumpiness or flakiness of skin of nose and mouth; swollen face; enlarged parotid glands; scaling of skin around nostrils (nasolabial seborrhea)
Eyes	Bright, clear, shiny; no sores at corners of eyelids; membranes pink and moist. No prominent blood vessels, sclera or mound of tissue	Eye membranes are pale (pale conjunctivae); redness of membranes; Bitot's spots; redness and fissuring of eyelid corners; dryness of eye membranes (conjunctival xerosis); cornea has dull appearance (corneal xerosis); cornea is soft (keratomalacia); scar on cornea; ring of fine blood vessels around cornea (circumcorneal injection)
Lips	Smooth, not chapped or swollen	Redness and swelling of mouth or lips (cheilosis), especially at corners of mouth (angular fissures and scars)
Tongue	Deep red in appearance; not swollen or smooth	Swelling; scarlet and raw tongue; magenta (purplish color) tongue; swollen sores; hyperemic and hypertrophic papillae; and atrophic papillae
Teeth	No cavities; no pain; bright	May be missing or erupting abnormally; gray or black spots (fluorosis); cavities (caries)
Gums	Healthy; red; do not bleed; not swollen	"Spongy" and bleed easily; recession of gums
Glands	Face not swollen	Thyroid enlargement (front of neck); parotid enlargement (cheeks become swollen

Appendix 26 *(continued)*

Nails	Firm, pink	Nails are spoon-shape (koilonychia); brittle, ridged nails
Skin	No signs of rashes, swellings, dark or light spots	Dryness of skin (xerosis); sandpaper feel of skin (follicular hyperkeratosis); flakiness of skin; skin swollen and dark; red swollen pigmentation of exposed areas (pellagrous dermatosis); excessive lightness or darkness of skin (dyspigmentation); Black and blue marks due to skin bleeding (petechiae); lack of fat under skin
Muscular & skeletal system	Good muscle tone; some fat under skin; can walk or run without pain	Muscles have "wasted" appearance; baby's skull bones are thin and soft (craniotabes); round swelling of front and side of head (frontal and parietal); swelling of ends of bones (epiphyseal enlargement); small bumps on both sides of chest wall (on ribs) -- beading of ribs; baby's soft spot on head does not harden at proper time (persistently open anterior fontanelle); knock-knees or bow-legs; bleeding into muscle (musculoskeletal hemorrhages); cannot get up or walk properly
Cardiovascular system	Normal heart rate and rhythm; no murmurs; normal blood pressure for age	Rapid heart rate (above 100 tachycardia); enlarged heart; abnormal rhythm; elevated blood pressure
Gastrointestinal system	No palpable organs or masses (in children liver edge may be palpable	Liver enlargement; enlargement of spleen (usually indicates other associated diseases)
Nervous	Psychological stability; normal reflexes	Mental irritability and confusion; burning and tingling of hands and feet (paresthesia); loss of position and vibratory sense; weakness and tenderness of muscles (may result in inability to walk); decrease and loss of ankle and knee reflexes.

From Christakis, G.: Nutritional Assessment in Health Programs. Am. J. Public Health. 63 (Suppl.1):19, 1973, with permission.

Appendix 27
Biochemical Assessment of Nutritional Status

Nutrient (unit)	Age (years)	Deficient	Marginal	Acceptable
*Hemoglobin (gm/100 ml)	6-23 mos.	Up to 9.0	9.0- 9.9	10.0+
	2-5	Up to 10.0	10.0-10.9	11.0+
	6-12	Up to 10.0	10.0-11.4	11.5+
	13-16 M	Up to 12.0	12.0-12.9	13.0+
	13-16 F	Up to 10.0	10.0-11.4	11.5+
	16+ M	Up to 12.0	12.0-13.9	14.0+
	16+ F	Up to 10.0	10.0-11.9	12.0+
	Pregnant (6+ mos.)	Up to 9.5	9.5-10.9	11.0+
*Hematocrit (% Packed cell volume)	Up to 2	Up to 28	28-30	31+
	2-5	Up to 30	30-33	34+
	6-12	Up to 30	30-35	36+
	13-16 M	Up to 37	37-39	40+
	13-16 F	Up to 31	31-35	36+
	16+ M	Up to 37	37-43	44+
	16+ F	Up to 31	31-37	33+
	Pregnant	Up to 30	31-32	33+
*Serum Albumin (gm/100 ml)	Up to 1	-	Up to 2.5	2.5+
	1-5	-	Up to 3.0	3.0+
	6-16	-	Up to 3.5	3.5+
	16+	Up to 2.8	2.8-3.4	3.5+
	Pregnant	Up to 3.0	3.0-3.4	3.5+
*Serum Protein (gm/100 ml)	Up to 1	-	Up to 5.0	5.0+
	1-5	-	Up to 5.5	5.5+
	6-16	-	Up to 6.0	6.0+
	16+	Up to 6.0	6.0-6.4	6.5+
	Pregnant	Up to 5.5	5.5-5.9	6.0+
*Serum Ascorbic Acid (mg/100 ml)	All ages	Up to 0.1	0.1-0.19	0.2+
*Plasma Vitamin A (µg/100 ml	All ages	Up to 10	10-19	20+
*Plasma Carotene (µg/100 ml)	All ages	Up to 20	20-39	40+
	Pregnant	-	40-79	80+
*Serum Iron (µg/100 ml)	Up to 2	Up to 30	-	30+
	2-5	Up to 40	-	40+
	6-12	Up to 50	-	50+
	12+ M	Up to 60	-	60+
	12+ F	Up to 40	-	40+
*Transferrin Saturation (%)	Up to 2	Up to 15.0	-	15.0+
	2-12	Up to 20.0	-	20.0+
	12+ M	Up to 20.0	-	20.0+
	12+ F	Up to 15.0	-	15.0+
‡Serum Folacin (ng/ml)	All ages	Up to 2.0	2.1-5.9	6.0+

Appendix 27 *(continued)*

Nutrient (unit)	Age (years)	Criteria of Status		
		Deficient	Marginal	Acceptable
‡Serum Vitamin B_{12} (pg/ml)	All ages	Up to 100	–	100+
*Thiamin in Urine	1-3	Up to 120	120-175	175+
	4-5	Up to 85	85-120	120+
	6-9	Up to 70	70-180	180+
	10-15	Up to 55	55-150	150+
	16+	Up to 27	27-65	65+
	Pregnant	Up to 21	21-49	50+
*Riboflavin in Urine	1-3	Up to 150	150-499	500+
(µg/gm creatinine)	4-5	Up to 100	100-299	300+
	6-9	Up to 85	85-269	270+
	10-16	Up to 70	70-199	200+
	16+	Up to 27	27-79	80+
	Pregnant	Up to 30	30-89	90+
‡RBC Transketolase TPP-effect (ratio)	All ages	25+	15-25	Up to 15
‡RBC Glutathione Reductase-FAD-effect (ratio)	All ages	1.2+	–	Up to 1.2
‡Tryptophan Load (mg Xanthurenic acid excreted)	Adults (Dose:100 mg per kg BW)	25+(6 hr) 75+(24 hr)	– –	Up to 25 Up to 75
‡Urinary Pyridoxine	1-3	Up to 90	–	90+
(µg/gm creatinine)	4-6	Up to 80	–	80+
	7-9	Up to 60	–	60+
	10-12	Up to 40	–	40+
	13-15	Up to 30	–	30+
	16+	Up to 20	–	20+
*Urinary N'methyl	All ages	Up to 0.2	0.2-5.59	0.6+
nicotinamide (mg/gm creatinine)	Pregnant	Up to 0.8	0.8-2.49	2.5+
‡Urinary Pantothenic Acid (µg)	All ages	Up to 200	–	200+
Plasma Vitamin E (mg/100 ml)	All ages	Up to 0.2	0.2-0.6	0.6+
‡Transaminase Index (ratio)				
EGOT[a]	Adult	2.0 +	–	Up to 2.0
EGPT[b]	Adult	1.25+	–	Up to 1.25

From Christakis, G.:Nutritional Assessment in Health Programs. Am J. Public Health. 63 (Suppl 1):34, 1973, with permission.

*Adapted from the Ten State Nutrition Survey; ‡Criteria may vary with different methodology; [a] Erythrocyte glutamic oxalacetic transaminase; [b] Erythrocyte glutamic pyruvic transaminase.

Appendix 28
Plasma Lipid Concentrations and Association with Coronary Artery Disease

(In mg/dL)

Age (yr)	CAD risk Percentile	Total Cholesterol Normal 50	Mod 75	High 90	HDL Cholesterol High 5	Normal 50	Low 95	Triglycerides * 50	* 95
Men									
5 - 19		155	170	185	35	55	75	58	111
20 - 24		165	185	205	30	45	65	78	165
25 - 29		180	200	225	30	45	65	88	204
30 - 34		190	215	240	30	45	60	102	253
35 - 39		200	225	250	30	45	60	109	316
40 - 44		205	230	250	25	45	65	123	318
45 - 69		215	235	260	30	50	70	117	261
70 +		205	230	250	30	50	75	115	239
Women									
5 - 19		160	175	190	35	55	70	68	120
20 - 24		170	190	215	35	55	80	80	161
25 - 34		175	195	220	35	55	80	75	168
35 - 39		185	205	230	35	55	80	83	205
40 - 44		195	215	235	35	60	90	86	191
45 - 49		205	225	250	35	60	85	94	223
50 - 54		220	240	265	35	60	90	103	223
55 +		230	250	275	35	60	95	111	271

Reproduced by permission from Weinsier, Roland., Heimburger, Douglas C., and Butterworth, Charles.: Handbook of Clinical Nutrition, ed. 2, St. Louis, 1989, The C.V. Mosby Co.
*Adapted from the Lipid Research Clinics' Population Studies Data
#An independent relationship between triglyceries and coronary artery disease has not been established.

Ratio of Total Cholesterol to HDL Cholesterol:
Goal for men   ≤5.0
Goal for women   ≤4.5

LDL cholesterol = total cholesterol - (triglycerides + HDL)
5

Appendix 29
Expected 24-Hour Urinary Creatinine Excretion*

Men[a]			Women[b]		
Height		Creatinine	Height		Creatinine
ft	in	mg	ft	in	mg
5	2	1290	4	10	782
5	3	1320	4	11	802
5	4	1360	5	0	826
5	5	1390	5	1	848
5	6	1430	5	2	872
5	7	1470	5	3	894
5	8	1510	5	4	923
5	9	1550	5	5	950
5	10	1600	5	6	983
5	11	1640	5	7	1010
6	0	1690	5	8	1040
6	1	1740	5	9	1080
6	2	1780	5	10	1110
6	3	1830	5	11	1140
6	4	1890	6	0	1170

From Bistrian, B.R.: Nutritional assessment and therapy of protein-calorie malnutrition in the hospital. J Am Diet Assoc, 71:395, 1977. Adapted with permission.

*For adults less than or equal to age 54. Decrease value by 10% per decade for older persons.

[a]Creatinine coefficient (men)   = 23 mg/kg ideal body weight/24 hours
[b]Creatinine coefficient (women) = 18 mg/kg ideal body weight/24 hours

$$\text{Creatinine-height index} = \frac{\text{24-hour urinary creatinine excretion}}{\text{expected urinary creatinine excretion (for same height)}}$$

Interpretation:
>90%   = Adequate muscle mass
80-90% = Mild depletion
60-79% = Moderate depletion
<60%   = Severe depletion

Appendix 30
Reference Values for Normal Blood Constituents

Physical measurements
  Specific gravity   1.025-1.030
  Reaction   pH 7.35-7.45
  Bleeding time   1-5 minutes
  Coagulation time, venous blood   4-12 minutes
  Prothrombin time, plasma   14-18 seconds
  Erythrocyte sedimentation rate
    Men   1-13 mm/hr
    Women   1-20 mm/hr
                           (Slightly higher in children
                          and during pregnancy)
  Osmolality, serum   275-295 mOsmol/kg
  Viscosity, serum   1.4-1.8 times water
Hematology
  Cells, differential count
    Basophils $0\%-1\%/mm^3$
    Eosinophils $1\%-4\%/mm^3$
    Lymphocytes $25\%-35\%/mm^3$ (higher in children)
    Monocytes $3\%-7\%/mm^3$
    Neutrophils $50\%-65\%/mm^3$ (lower in children)
  Erythrocytes (RBCs) $4.2-5.9 \; mil/mm^3$
  Leukocytes (WBCs) $4300-10,800/mm^3$
  Thrombocytes (platelets) $150,000-350,000/mm^3$
  Reticulocytes   0.5%-2.5% red cells
  Hematocrit (vol% red cells)
    Men   40%-54%
    Women   37%-47%
    Newborn   49-54%
    Children (varies with age)   35%-49%
  Hemoglobin
    Men   13.5-17.5 g/dL
    Women   12-16 g/dL
    Newborn   16.5-19.5 g/dL
    Children (varies with age)   10-18 g/dL
  Hemoglobin, glycosylated   4.0-7.0%
  Mean corpuscular volume (MCV) $82-98 \; um^3/cell$
  Mean corpuscular hemoglobin (MCH) 27-32 pg/RBC
  Mean corpuscular hemoglobin
    concentration (MCHC)   32-36%
  Volume, whole blood   70-100 ml/kg
  Total protein, serum   6-8.4 g/dL
  Albumin, serum   3.5-5.0 g/dL
  Globulin, serum   1.3-2.7 g/dL
                            2.3-3.5 g/dL
    Alpha$_1$ 0.2-0.4 g/dL
                            2-5% of total
    Alpha$_2$ 0.5-0.9 g/dL
                            7-14% of total

Appendix 30 *(continued)*

Beta	0.6-1.1 g/dL
	9-15% of total
Gamma	0.7-1.7 g/dL
	11-21% of total
Albumin/globulin ratio	1.8-2.5
Ceruloplasmin, plasma	27-37 mg/dL
Ferritin, serum	
Men	20-200 ng/mL
Women	20-150 ng/mL
Iron deficiency	<10 ng/mL
Borderline	13-20 ng/mL
Iron excess	>400 ng/L
Fibrinogen, plasma	200-400 mg/dL
Prealbumin, serum	16.5-40.2 mg/dL
Protein C, plasma	80-144%
Transferrin, serum	220-400 mg/dL

Nitrogen constituents

Amino acid nitrogen, blood	4-8 mg/dL
Ammonia, blood	40-70 ug/dL
Ammonia, plasma	15-49 ug/dL
Creatine, serum	0.2-0.8 mg/dL
Creatinine, serum	0.6-1.5 mg/dL
Nonprotein nitrogen, blood	20-40 mg/dL
Urea nitrogen, blood	10-20 mg/dL
Urea, blood	21-43 mg/dL
Uric acid, blood	2.5-5 mg/dL

Amino acids, plasma

Alanine	2.3-5.1 mg/dL
Alpha-aminobutyric acid	0.2-0.4 mg/dL
Arginine	0.4-1.3 mg/dL
Asparagine	0.2-0.8 mg/dL
Aspartic acid	0.01-0.07 mg/dL
Citrulline	0.2-0.6 mg/dL
Cysteine and cystine	1.1-1.3 mg/dL
Glutamic acid	0.2-1.2 mg/dL
Glutamine	4-7 mg/dL
Glycine	1.7-3.3 mg/dL
Histidine	0.3-1.2 mg/dL
Isoleucine	0.4-1.1 mg/dL
Leucine	0.7-1.7 mg/dL
Lysine	1.5-2.2 mg/dL
Methionine	0.2-0.3 mg/dL
Ornithine	0.3-0.8 mg/dL
Phenylalanine	0.7-2.0 mg/dL
Phosphoethanolamine	0-0.6 mg/dL
Phosphoserin	0-0.1 mg/dL
Proline	1.1-3.6 mg/dL
Serine	0.6-1.4 mg/dL
Taurine	0.4-1.3 mg/dL
Threonine	0.9-2.4 mg/dL
Tryptophan	1.0-1.2 mg/dL

(continued)

Appendix 30 *(continued)*

Tyrosine	0.4-0.7 mg/dL
Valine	1.5-3.1 mg/dL

Carbohydrates

Glucose,blood	
Fasting, adult	70-110 mg/dL
>60 yr	80-115 mg/dL
2 hr postprandial	<120 mg/dL
Fructose	6-8 mg/dL
Glycogen	5-6 mg/dL
Hexoses	70-105 mg/dL
Hexuronates (as glucuronic acid)	0.4-1.4 mg/dL
Pentose (total	2-4 mg/dL

Lipids

Cephalin	0-30 mg/dL
Cholesterol, serum	
Total	150-240 mg/dL
Esters	100-180 mg/dL
Free	50-60 mg/dL
LDL cholesterol	60-180 mg/dL
HDL cholesterol	30-80 mg/dL
Fats, neutral	150-300 mg/dL
Fatty acids, serum	
Total	190-420 mg/dL
Free	8-30 mg/dL
Glycerol, free	0.29-1.72 mg/dL
Lecithin	100-200 mg/dL
Lipids, serum (total)	450-850 mg/dL
Phospholipids, serum (total)	230-300 mg/dL
Plasmalogen	7-8 mg/dL
Sphingomyelin	10-50 mg/dL
Triglycerides	40-150 mg/dL

Minerals

Base, serum (total)	145-155 mEq/L
Aluminum, plasma	13-17 ug/dL
Arsenic, blood	0.2-6.2 ug/dL
Bromide, plasma	300 ug/dL
Cadmium	0.1-0.7 ug/dL
Calcium, serum	9.0-11.0 mg/dL
	(Varies with protein concentration)
Calcium, ionized, serum	4.25-5.25 mg/dL
Chloride, serum	340-376 mg/dL
Chromium, plasma	0.15 ug/dL
Cobalt, plasma	0.7-6 ug/dL
Copper	100-200 ug/dL
Fluoride	20-100 ug/dL
Iodine, serum	3.5-8.0 ug/dL
Iron, serum	
Men	50-160 ug/dL
Women	40-150 ug/dL
Iron binding capacity, serum	
Total	250-410 ug/dL

Appendix 30 *(continued)*

Saturation	20-55%
Lead, blood	50 ug/dL or less
Lithium, serum	0.8-1.2 mEq/L
Magnesium, serum	1.8-3.0 mg/dL
Manganese, plasma	1-2 ug/dL
Mercury, whole blood	<5.0 ug/dL
Molybdenum, plasma	1.3 ug/dL
Nickel, plasma	2-4 ug/dL
Phosphorus, inorganic, serum	3.0-4.5 mg/dL
Potassium, serum	14-20 mg/dL
Selenium	7-30 ug/dL
Silicon, plasma	500 ug/dL
Sodium, serum	310-340 mg/dL
Sulfates, inorganic, serum	2.5-5.0 mg/dL
Vanadium, plasma	0.5-2.3 ug/dL
Zinc, plasma	100 ug/dL

Vitamins

Ascorbic acid, serum	0.4-1.5 mg/dL
white blood cells	25-40 mg/dL
Carotenoids	60-180 ug/dL
Folate, serum	1.8-9.0 ng/mL
erythrocytes	150-450 ng/mL
Retinoids, serum	
Retinal	<10 ug/L
Retinol	360-1,200 ug/L
Riboflavin	20 ug/dL
Thiamin, serum	0-3 ug/dL
Vitamin A, serum	20-80 ug/dL
Vitamin B_6, plasma	3.6-18 ng/mL
Vitamin B12, serum	180-900 pg/mL
Vitamin D, 1,25-dihydroxy	26-65 pg/mL
25-hydroxy	8-55 ng/mL
Vitamin E, serum	5.0-50 ug/mL
Vitamin K, prothrombin time	10-15 seconds

Organic acids

Acetoacetic acid	0.8-2.8 mg/dL
Alpha-ketoglutaric acid	0.2-1.0 mg/dL
Citric acid	1.4-3.0 mg/dL
Lactic acid	8-17 mg/dL
Malic acid	0.1-0.9 mg/dL
Pyruvic acid	0.4-2 mg/dL
Succinic acid	0.1-0.6 mg/dL
Ketone bodies	0.3-2 mg/dL

Enzymes

Aldolase	1.3-8.2 U/L
Amylase, serum	25-125 mU/dL
Creatine kinase (CK), serum	
Men	38-174 U/L
Women	96-140 U/L
Lactate dehydrogenase (LD)	45-90 mU/mL (30^0)
	100-190 mU/mL (37^0)

(continued)

Appendix 30 *(continued)*

Lipase, serum	450-850 mg/dL
Phosphatase, serum	
Acid	0.11-0.60 mU/mL (37^0)
Alkaline	20-90 mU/mL (30^0)
	(Values higher in children)
Transaminase, serum	
SGOT or AST	7-40 units/mL (37^0)
SGPT or ALT	5-35 units/mL (37^0)

Hormones

Adrenocorticotropic hormone (ACTH)	25-100 pg/mL
Aldosterone, supine	3-10 ng/dL
Calcitonin	
Men	0-14 pg/mL
Women	0-28 pg/mL
Corticosterone, plasma or serum	0.13-2.3 ug/dL
Cortisol, plasma or serum	
8 A.M.	5-23 ug/dL
4 P.M.	3-15 ug/dL
Estradiol, plasma or serum	
Men	8-36 pg/mL
Women, follicular	10-90 pg/mL
midcycle	100-500 pg/mL
luteal	50-240 pg/mL
postmenopausal	10-30 pg/mL
Estrogens, serum	
Men	40-115 pg/mL
Women, cycle 1-10 d	61-394 pg/mL
11-20 d	122-437 pg/mL
21-30 d	156-350 pg/mL
Estrone, serum	
Men	30-170 pg/mL
Women, follicular	20-150 pg/mL
Follicle-stimulating hormone (FSH)	
Men	3-18 mU/mL
Women, premenopausal	4-30 mU/mL
midcycle peak	10-90 mU/mL
pregnancy	low to detectable
postmenopausal	40-250 mU/mL
Growth hormone, serum or plasma	
Children	Over 10 ng/mL
Men	<2 ng/mL
Women	<10 ng/mL
Insulin, plasma (fasting)	5-25 mU/mL
Luteinizing hormone (LH)	
Men	6-23 mU/mL
Women, follicular	5-30 mU/mL
midcycle	75-150 mU/mL
postmenopausal	30-200 mU/mL
Parathyroid hormone	<25 pg/mL
Progesterone, serum	
Men	0.12-0.3 ng/mL

Appendix 30 *(continued)*

Women, follicular	0.02-0.9 ng/mL
luteal	6.0-30.0 ng/mL
Prolactin	2-15 ng/mL
Prolactin, serum	
Men	1-20 ng/mL
Women	1-25 ng/mL
Somatomedin C	
Men	0.34-1.9 U/mL
Women	0.45-2.2 U/mL
Testosterone, plasma	
Men	275-875 ng/dL
Women	23-75 ng/dL
Pregnant	38-190 ng/dL
Thyroxine (T_4), serum	5-12 ug/dL
>60 yr Men	5.0-10.0 ug/dL
Women	5.5-10.5 ug/dL
Thyroxine binding globulin (TBG)	15-34 ug/mL
Transcortin, serum	
Men	1.5-2.0 mg/dL
Women, follicular	1.7-2.0 mg/dL
luteal	1.6-2.1 mg/dL
postmenopausal	1.7-2.5 mg/dL
Triiodothyronine (T_3), total	120-195 ng/dL
>60 yr Men	105-175 ng/dL
Women	108-205 ng/dL
Triiodothyronine (T_3), uptake	25-38%
<u>Blood gases</u>	
CO_2-combining power	50-65 vol%
	21-28 mEq/L
CO_2 content	
Serum	50-70 vol% (21-30 mEq/L)
Whole blood	40-60 vol% (18-27 mEq/L)
CO_2 tension	18-40 mm Hg
O_2 capacity, whole blood	16-27 vol%
	(varies with hemoglobin)
O_2 content	
Arterial blood	15-23 vol%
Venous blood	10-16 vol%
O_2 saturation	
Arterial blood	94%-96%
Venous blood	60%-85%

Compiled from Leavelle, Dennis E.: Interpretative Data for Diagnostic Laboratory Tests. Reference Laboratory of the Mayo Clinic, Rochester, MN, 1986; Linder, Maria C.: Nutritional Biochemistry and Metabolism with Clinical Applications. New York: Elsevier Science Publishing Company, 1985, pp. 152-153; Normal Laboratory Values, N Engl J Med 314:39-49, 1986; Weinsier, Roland L., Heimburger, Douglas C. and Butterworth, Charles C.: Handbook of Clinical Nutrition. 2nd ed. St. Louis, The C.V. Mosby Company, 1989, pp. 371-373; Wyngaarden, James B. and Lloyd H. Smith.: Cecil Textbook of Medicine. 18 ed. Philadelphia, W.B. Saunders Company, 1988, pp. 2395-2401.

Appendix 31
Normal Reference Values for Urine

Physical measurements

Specific gravity	1.008-1.030
Reaction	pH 5.5-8.0 (varies with diet)
Volume	800-1500 ml/24 hours
Total solids	55-70 gm/L
Osmolality	300-800 mOsm/kg
Overhydration	<100 mOsm/kg
Dehydration	>800 mOsm/kg
Creatinine clearance	70-135 ml/min/1.73 m^2 at age 20
	(decreased by 6 ml/min/decade)
Glomerular filtration rate	90-130 ml/min/1.73 m^2 at age 20
	(decreased by 4 ml/min/decade)

Organic constituents

Acetone (ketone) bodies	3-15 mg/24 hours
Albumin	<80 mg/d at rest
	<150 mg/d ambulatory
Ammonia nitrogen	140-1500 mg/24 hours
Bile	None
Bilirubin, total	None
Biotin	24-81 ug/24 hours
Catecholamines, free	<280 ug/24 hours
Coproporphyrin	34-234 ug/24 hours
Cortisol	10-100 ug/24 hours
Creatine	Under 100 mg/day or less
	than 6% of creatinine
Creatinine	
Men	14-26 mg/kg/d
Women	11-20 mg/kg/d
Cystine or cysteine	None
Dopamine	65-400 ug/24 hours
Epinephrine	0-15 ug/24 hours
Glucose	<250 mg/24 hours
Hemoglobin	None
Hippuric acid	0.1-1.0 gm/24 hours
Homogentisic acid	None
Homovanillic acid (HVA)	<15 mg/24 hours
5-Hydroxyindoleacetic acid	2-8 mg/24 hours
(5-HIAA)	(women lower than men)
Hydroxyproline, total	15-45 mg/24 hours
Indican	4-20 mg/24 hours
17-Ketosteroids	
Men	9-22 mg/24 hours
Women	6-15 mg/24 hours
Metanephrine	<1.3 mg/24 hours
Nitrogen, total	10-17 gm/24 hours
Norepinephrine	0-100 ug/24 hours
Oxalate	20-60 mg/24 hours

Appendix 31 *(continued)*

Porphobilinogen	0-2.0 mg/24 hours
Porphyrins	
Coproporphyrin	50-250 ug/24 hours
Uroporphyrin	10-30 mcg/24 hours
Pregnanetriol	<2.0 mg/24 hours
Protein, total	50-80 mg/24 hours (at rest)
Purine bases	6-14 mg/24 hours
Riboflavin (fasting)	80-269 ug/g creatinine
Sugar	None (in some persons, 2-3 mg per 24 hr after a heavy meal)
Sulfate, organic	60-200 mg/24 hours
Testosterone	
Men	50-135 ug/hours
Women	2-12 ug/hours
Urea	20-35 gm/24 hours
Uric acid	<750 mg/24 hours (diet dependent)
Urobilinogen	<4 mg/24 hours
Uroporphyrin	0-30 ug/day
Vanillylmandelic acid (VMA)	<9 mg/24 hours

Inorganic constituents

Aluminum	0-32 ug/24 hours
Arsenic	5-50 ug/24 hours
Cadmium	<3.0 ug/24 hours
Calcium	
Low Ca diet	<150 mg/24 hours
Usual diet	<300 mg/24 hours
Chloride (as NaCl)	10-15 gm/24 hours (Varies with intake)
Chromium	<8.0 ug/24 hours
Copper	15-60 ug/24 hours
Iron	100-300 ug/24 hours
Lead	<80 ug/24 hours
Magnesium	75-150 mg/24 hours
Mercury	<20 ug/24 hours
Phosphorus, inorganic	0.4-1.3 gm/24 hours (varies with intake)
Potassium	0.8-3.9 gm/24 hr (Varies with intake)
Selenium	<35 ug/24 hours
Sodium	3-6 gm/24 hours (Varies with intake)
Sulfur, total	1.5-3.0 gm/24 hours
Zinc	300-600 ug/24 hours

Compiled from Leavelle, Dennis E.: Interpretative Data for Diagnostic
Laboratory Tests. Reference Laboratory of the Mayo Clinic, Rochester,
MN, 1986; Normal Laboratory Values, N Engl J Med 314:39-49, 1986;
Wyngaarden, James B and Lloyd H. Smith. Cecil Textbook of Medicine. 18 ed.
Philadelphia, W.B. Saunders Company, 1988, pp. 2395-2401.

Appendix 32
Dietary Fiber in Selected Foods

Food	Serving Size	Fiber (gm)	Food	Serving Size	Fiber (gm)
Breakfast Cereals			Pineapple	1/2 c	1.1
All-Bran	1/3 c	8.5	Plum, damson	5	0.9
Bran Buds	1/3 c	7.9	Prune	3	3.0
Bran Chex	2/3 c	4.6	Raisins	1/4 c	3.1
Cheerios-type	1-1/4 c	1.1	Raspberries	1/2 c	3.1
Corn Bran	2/3 c	5.4	Strawberries	1 c	3.0
Cornflakes	1-1/4 c	0.3	Watermelon	1 c	0.4
Cracklin' Bran	1/3 c	4.3	**Vegetables (cooked)**		
Frosted Mini Wheats	4 pcs	2.1	Asparagus	1/2 c	1.0
Graham Crackos	3/4 c	1.7	Beans, string	1/2 c	1.6
Grape Nuts	1/4 c	1.4	Broccoli	1/2 c	2.2
Honey Bran	7/8 c	3.1	Brussels sprouts	1/2 c	2.3
Nutri-Grain	3/4 c	1.8	Cabbage	1/2 c	1.4
Oatmeal	3/4 c	1.6	Carrots	1/2 c	2.3
100% Bran	1/2 c	8.4	Cauliflower	1/2 c	1.1
Raisin Bran-type	3/4 c	4.0	Corn, canned	1/2 c	2.9
Rice Krispies	1 c	0.1	Kale leaves	1/2 c	1.4
Shredded Wheat	2/3 c	2.6	Parsnip	1/2 c	2.7
Special K	1-1/3 c	0.2	Peas	1/2 c	3.6
Sugar Smacks	3/4 c	0.4	Potato, w/o skin	1 med	1.4
Tasteeos	1-1/4 c	1.0	Potato, w/ skin	1 med	2.5
Total	1 c	2.0	Spinach	1/2 c	2.1
Wheat Chex	2/3 c	2.1	Squash, summer	1/2 c	1.4
Wheat germ	1/4 c	3.4	Turnip	1/2 c	1.6
Wheaties	1 c	2.0	Zucchini	1/2 c	1.8
Fruits			**Vegetables (raw)**		
Apple, w/o skin	1 med	2.7	Bean sprout	1/2 c	1.5
Apple, w/ skin	1 med	3.5	Celery, diced	1/2 c	1.1
Apricot, fresh	3 med	1.8	Cucumber	1/2 c	0.4
Apricot, dried	5 halves	1.4	Lettuce, sliced	1 c	0.9
Banana	1 med	2.4	Mushrooms, sliced	1/2 c	0.9
Blueberries	1/2 c	2.0	Onions, sliced	1/2 c	0.8
Cantaloupe	1/4 melon	1.0	Pepper, green	1/2 c	0.5
Cherries, sweet	10	1.2	Tomato	1 med	1.5
Dates	3	1.9	Spinach	1 c	1.2
Grapefruit	1/2	1.6	**Legumes (cooked)**		
Grapes	20	0.6	Baked beans	1/2 c	8.8
Orange	1	2.6	Dried peas,	1/2 c	4.7
Peach, w/ skin	1	1.9	Kidney beans,	1/2 c	7.3
Peach, w/o skin	1	1.2	Lentils	1/2 c	3.7
Pear, w/ skin	1/2 lg	3.1	Lima beans	1/2 c	4.5
Pear, w/o skin	1/2 lg	2.5	Navy beans	1/2 c	6.0

Source: Lanza, Elaine and Ritva B. Butrum: A critical review of food fiber analysis and data, J Am Diet Asso 86:732, 1986. (Adapted with permission)

Appendix 33
Alcohol and Caloric Content of Alcoholic Beverages

Beverage - Serving	Weight gm	Alcohol gm	CHO gm	Calories
Ale, mild - 8 fl oz	230	8.9	8.0	98
Ale, mild - 12 fl oz	345	13.4	12.0	147
Anisette - 1 cordial glass	20	7.0	7.0	74
Beer - 8 fl oz	240	8.7	9.0	99
Beer - 12 fl oz	360	13.1	13.2	148
Benedictine - 1 cordial glass	20	6.6	6.6	69
Brandy - 1 brandy glass	30	10.5	-	73
Champagne, dry - 1 champagne gl	135	13.0	3.0	105
Champagne, sweet - champagne gl	135	13.0	17.0	160
Cider, fermented - 6 fl oz	180	9.4	1.8	71
Creme de menthe - 1 cordial gl	20	7.0	6.0	67
Curacao - 1 cordial glass	20	6.0	6.0	54
Daiquiri - 1 cocktail	100	15.1	5.2	122
Eggnog - 4 fl oz punch cup	123	15.0	18.0	335
Gin, 80% proof - 1 jigger	42	14.0	tr	97
Gin rickey - 4 fl oz	120	21.0	1.3	150
Highball - 8 fl oz	240	24.0	-	166
Madeira wine - 1 wine glass	100	15.0	1.0	105
Manhattan - 1 cocktail	100	19.2	7.9	164
Martini - 1 cocktail	100	18.5	0.3	140
Mint julep - 10 fl oz	300	29.2	2.7	212
Muscatel wine - 1 wine glass	100	15.0	14.0	158
Old-fashioned - 4 fl oz	100	24.0	3.5	179
Planter's punch - 4 fl oz	100	21.5	7.9	175
Port wine - 1 sherry glass	30	4.0	5.0	50
Rum, 80% proof - 1 jigger	42	14.0	tr	97
Rum sour - 4 fl oz	100	21.5	-	165
Sauterne, calif - 1 wine glass	100	10.5	4.0	84
Sherry, dry - 1 wine glass	60	9.0	4.8	84
Tom collins - 10 fl oz	300	21.5	9.0	180
Vermouth, dry - 1 wine glass	100	15.0	1.0	105
Vermouth, sweet, 1 wine glass	100	18.0	12.0	167
Vodka, 80% proof - 1 jigger	42	14.0	tr	97
90% proof - 1 jigger	42	15.9	tr	110
Whiskey, 80% proof - 1 jigger	42	14.0	tr	97
100% proof - 1 jigger	42	17.9	tr	124

Source: Pennington, Jean A. and Helen Nichols Church. 14 ed. Bowe's and Church's Food Values of Portions Commonly Used, p.196. Philadelphia, J.B. Lippincott Company, 1985 (adapted with permission).
*One gram (cc) alcohol = 7 calories. Alcohol is metabolized by the body as fat. It has negligible or a slightly lowering effect on blood sugar. In dietary calculations, alcohol is considered as fat.

Appendix 34
Cholesterol and Fatty Acid Content
of Selected Foods
(per 100 gm edible portion)

Food Item	CHOL (mg)	SFA (g)	MFA (g)	PFA (g)
Cereal Grains				
Barley, bran	0	1.0	0.6	2.7
Corn, germ	0	3.9	7.6	18.0
Oats, germ	0	5.6	11.1	12.4
Rice, bran	0	3.6	7.3	6.6
Wheat bran	0	0.7	0.7	2.4
Wheat germ	0	1.9	1.6	6.6
Wheat, hard	0	0.4	0.3	1.2
Dairy and Eggs				
Cheese, cheddar	105	21.1	9.0	0.9
Cheese, Roquefort	90	19.3	8.5	1.3
Cream, half and half	37	7.2	3.3	0.4
Cream, heavy whipping	137	23.0	10.7	1.4
Creamer, imitation	0	1.5	4.3	3.8
Egg, whole	548	3.4	4.5	1.4
Eggyolk	1,602	9.9	13.2	4.3
Eggwhite	0	0.0	0.0	0.0
Ice cream, medium-rich	59	10.0	4.6	0.6
Ice milk	8	1.6	0.8	0.1
Milk, whole	14	2.1	1.0	0.1
Milk, 2%	8	1.2	0.6	0.1
Milk, 1%	4	0.7	0.3	-
Sherbet	7	1.2	0.6	0.1
Yogurt, low-fat	6	1.0	0.4	0.3
Fats and Oils				
Butter	219	50.5	23.4	3.0
Coconut oil	0	86.5	5.8	1.8
Cod liver oil	570	17.6	51.2	25.8
Corn oil	0	12.7	24.2	58.7
Cottonseed oil	0	25.9	17.8	51.9
Herring oil	766	19.2	60.3	16.1
Lard, rendered	95	39.6	45.1	11.8
Margarine, corn, 80% fat	0	12.6	29.6	33.8
Mayonnaise, commercial	57	11.8	22.7	41.3
MCT oil	0	94.5	0.0	0.0
Menhaden oil	521	33.6	32.5	29.5
Olive oil	0	13.5	73.7	8.4
Palm oil	0	49.3	37.0	36.6
Palm kernel	0	81.4	11.4	1.6
Peanut oil	0	16.9	46.2	32.0
Rapeseed oil (Canola)	0	6.8	55.5	33.3
Rice bran oil	0	19.7	39.3	35.0
Safflower oil	0	9.1	12.1	74.5

SFA=saturated fatty acid; MFA=monounsaturated fatty acid; PFA=polyunsaturated fatty acid

Salmon oil	485	23.8	39.7	29.9
Sesame oil	0	14.2	39.7	41.7
Shortening, vegetable	0	24.7	44.5	26.1
Soybean, partly hydrogenated	0	14.9	43.0	37.6
Sunflower oil	0	10.3	19.5	65.7
Walnut oil	0	9.1	22.8	63.3
Wheat germ oil	0	18.8	15.1	61.7
Fish and Seafoods				
Clam, hardshell	31	0.6	tr	tr
Crab, blue	78	0.2	0.2	0.5
Haddock	63	0.1	0.1	0.2
Halibut, Pacific	32	0.3	0.8	0.7
Lobster, northern	95	0.2	0.2	0.2
Mackerel, Atlantic	80	3.6	5.4	3.7
Mussel, blue	38	0.4	0.5	0.6
Oyster, eastern	47	0.6	0.2	0.7
Perch, white	80	0.6	0.9	0.7
Pike, northern	39	0.1	0.2	0.2
Pike, walleye	86	0.2	0.3	0.4
Salmon, chum	74	1.5	2.9	1.5
Scallop, Atlantic	37	0.1	0.1	0.3
Shrimp, unspecified	147	0.2	0.1	0.4
Swordfish	39	0.6	0.8	0.2
Trout, rainbow	57	0.6	1.0	1.2
Tuna, bluefin	38	1.7	2.2	2.0
Fruits/Vegetables				
Avocado	**0**	**2.4**	**9.6**	**2.0**
Coconut, fresh	**0**	**29.7**	**1.4**	**0.4**
Peas, blackeye, chick, cked	**0**	**0.2**	**0.5**	**1.1**
Peas, split or lentils	**0**	**0.2**	**0.2**	**0.5**
Soybeans, dry, cooked	**0**	**0.9**	**1.3**	**3.3**
Meats (cooked)				
Bacon, regular, cooked	85	17.4	23.7	5.8
Beef, approx. 6% fat	66	2.8	2.8	0.4
Beef, approx. 30% fat	94	13.3	15.7	1.3
Bologna, beef	56	11.7	13.3	1.1
Chicken, Cornish hen, turkey, light meat, no skin	89	1.2	1.1	0.9
Duck, goose, no skin	92	4.4	4.0	1.5
Frankfurter, all beef	48	12.0	14.4	1.2
Frankfurter, beef, pork	50	10.7	13.7	2.7
Lamb, approx. 8% fat	84	2.7	3.4	0.6
Lamb, approx. 36% fat	98	16.8	14.7	2.1
Pork, approx. 24% fat	82	9.1	11.5	2.8
Salami, dry	77	11.9	16.0	3.7
Veal, approx. 6% fat	99	2.3	2.9	0.5
Veal, approx. 25% fat	101	9.2	0.2	1.3

From USDA Provisional Table on the Content of Cholesterol, Fatty Acids, and Other Fat Components in Selected foods. Nutrient Data Research Branch, Human Nutrition Information Service, HNIS/PT-103, May 1986.

Appendix 35
Average Caffeine Content of Selected Foods (mg)

Coffee beverage, per 5 fl oz

Drip, automatic	137
Drip, nonautomatic	124
Instant	60
Instant decaffeinated	3
Percolated, automatic	117
Percolated, nonautomatic	108

Coffee flavored (from instant mixes), per 6 fl oz

Cafe amaretto	60
Cafe francais	52
Cafe vienna	57
Irish mocha mint	27
Orange cappuccino	74
Sunrise	37
Suisse mocha	40

Coffee instant dry powder

Decaffeinated, 1 tsp	3
Regular/freeze-dried, 1 tsp	60

Tea beverage, per 5 fl oz

Black, 1 min brew	28
Black, 3 min brew	42
Black, 5 min brew	46
Decaffeinated	1
Green, 1 min brew	14
Green, 3 min brew	27
Green, 5 min brew	31
Instant	33
Mint flavor, 5 min brew	50
Orange & spice, 5 min brew	45
Oolong, 1 min brew	13
Oolong, 3 min brew	30
Oolong, 5 min brew	40

Tea instant dry powder

Lemon flavored, 1 tsp	38
Regular, 1 tsp	32

Soft drinks, per 12 fl oz

Aspen	36
Big Red	38
Big Red, diet	38
Canada Dry	30
Coca Cola	45
Dr. Pepper	40
Kick	31
Mellow Yello	53
Mountain Dew	54
Mr. Pibb	41
Pepsi Cola	38
Pepsi Light	36
Royal Crown Cola	36
Royal Crown with a Twist	21
Shasta Cola	44
Tab	45

Foods containing chocolate

Baking choc, 1 oz	35
Choc brownie, 1-1/4 oz	8
Choc cake, 1/16 of 9" cake	14
Chocolate candy	
Choc, german sweet, 1 oz	8
Choc kisses, 6 pieces	5
Crunch Bar (Nestle), 1 oz	7
Golden Almond, 1 oz	5
Kit Kat, 1.5 oz	5
Krackel Bar, 1.2 oz	5
Milk chocolate	6
Mr. Goodbar, 1.65 oz	6
Semi-sweet, Bakers 1 oz	12
Special dark, 1 oz	23
Sweet dark choc, 1 oz	20
Choc flavored chips, 1/4 c	12
Choc ice cream, 2/3 c	5
Choc milk, 8 fl oz	5
Choc pudding, 1/2 c	6
Choc syrup, 2 T	4
Cocoa beverage, 6 fl oz	5
Cocoa, dry powder, 1 T	11
Cocoa, dry, Hershey, 1 oz	70
Cocoa mix, Hershey, 1 pkt	5
Cocoa mix, Nestle, 1 oz	4
Cocoa mix w/marshmallows, Nestle, 1 oz	4

Source: Pennington, Jean A. and Helen Nichols Church.: 14th ed. Bowe's and Church's Food Values of Portions Commonly Used, p. 223-224. Philadelphia: J.B. Lippincott Company, 1985. (Adapted with permission).

Appendix 36
Protein Food Mixtures in the World

Product	Country	Composition
Bal-Ahar	India	Mixed wheat flour, peanut flour, chickpea, vitamins, calcium
Bal-Amul	India	Ground cereal, soybean flour, legumes, dry skim milk
Cerealina	Brazil	Soya bean flour, dry skim milk, maize, and vitamins
Colombinara	Colombia	Flour mixture of soya bean and rice, with vitamins and minerals
CSM	United States	Precooked maize, defatted soybean flour, dry skim milk, calcium, vitamins
Duryea	Colombia	Mixed soya bean flour and maize, skim milk powder
Faffa	Ethiopia	Soya bean flour, skim milk powder, legume, and teff
Fortifex	Brazil	Maize, defatted soybean flour, riboflavin, thiamin, vitamin A, calcium carbonate
Incaparina	Guatemala	Cottonseed flour, ground corn, Torula yeast, calcium, vitamin A
Milpro	India	Beverage mixture of animal milk, ground nut isolate, and vegetable oil
Miltone	India	Buffalo milk, ground nut isolate, vitamins, minerals, hydrolyzed starch syrup
MPF	India	Peanut flour, chickpea flour, vitamin A, thiamin, riboflavin, calcium carbonate
Poluk	Thailand	Beverage mixture of soya milk, skim milk and butterfat
Pronutro	South Africa	Mixture of maize, peanut, soybean, dry skim milk, wheat germ, vitamins, minerals
Protamin	India	Mixture of ground nut and chickpea, with vitamins and minerals
Protone	South Africa	Maize, skim milk powder, yeast, vitamins, and minerals
Puma	Guyana	Beverage containing vegetable protein, sugar, and vitamins
Sekmana	Turkey	Mixture of soya flour, dry skim milk, chick pea, and wheat flour
Superamine	Algeria	Wheat, chickpea, lentils, dry skim milk, sugar, and vitamin D
Super Maeu	Mozambique	Finely ground maize, soya bean flour, and dry skim milk
Supro	Kenya	Mixture of maize and barley flour, yeast, and dry skim milk
Vitabean	Singapore	Beverage containing soya milk, vitamins, and minerals
Vitasoy	Hongkong	Beverage containing vegetable protein, sugar, and vitamins
Yoo Hoo	Iran	Beverage containing skim milk, whey, vitamins and minerals

Appendix 37
Composition of Milk and Selected Formulas
for Infant Feeding

	Kcal per oz	Pro gm	CHO gm	Fat gm	Fe mg	Ca mg	P mg	Na mg	K mg	Cl mg	Renal Solute Load**
Human milk	22	11	68	38	1.5	333	133	161	507	390	97
Cow's milk	20	33	48	37	1	1200	946	506	1365	994	310
Advance	16	20	55	27	12	510	390	230	900	520	128
Enfamil*	20	15	70	37	12	458	312	182	718	417	98
Enfamil Premature*	20	20	74	34	12	1104	552	260	687	562	125
Enfamil Premature*	24	24	88	41	12	1323	667	312	823	677	150
Isomil	20	18	68	37	12	700	500	320	950	430	122
Isomil SF	20	20	68	36	12	700	500	320	770	590	131
Lofenalac	20	22	86	26	12.5	625	469	312	677	469	132
MBF	20	27	60	32	-	937	625	171	360	-	176
MSUD Diet Powder‡	20	14	90	28	12	687	375	260	688	520	100
Nursoy	20	22	66	37	13	630	420	198	693	370	136
Nutramigen	20	19	90	26	12.5	625	417	312	729	573	124
Phenyl-free‡	25	42	140	14	25	1042	1042	833	2812	1917	330
Portagen	20	23	77	31	12.5	625	469	365	833	573	145
Premee SMA	20	20	86	44	NA	750	400	322	741	NA	175
Pregestimil	20	19	69	38	12.5	625	488	260	729	573	122
Product 3200A‡	20	22	86	26	12.5	625	469	312	677	469	132
Product 3200K‡	20	20	67	35	12.5	625	495	240	812	552	127
Product 3232A‡	20	19	90	28	12.5	625	417	286	729	573	123
Product 80056‡	20	0	83	26	12.5	625	344	188	708	417	NA
Prosobee	20	20	67	35	12.5	625	495	240	812	552	127
RCF	-	20	0	36	1.5	700	500	320	770	590	131
Similac 13*	13	12	46	23	7.8	410	310	190	620	400	83
Similac 20*	20	15	72	36	12	510	390	230	800	500	105
Similac 24*	24	22	85	43	15	730	560	350	1100	740	152
Similac 27	27	25	96	48	2	810	620	380	1200	820	170
Similac 24 LBW	24	22	85	45	3	730	560	360	1220	900	161
Similac PM 60/40	20	16	69	38	1.5	400	200	160	580	400	96
Similac 20 SP	20	18	72	37	2.5	1200	600	310	940	640	128
Similac 24 SP	24	22	86	44	3.0	1440	720	380	1120	710	154
SMA	20	15	72	36	12.5	440	320	150	562	372	92
SMA 24	24	18	86	43	14.4	510	336	179	663	451	110
SMA 27	27	20	97	49	16.2	564	378	202	753	508	122
Soyalac	20	21	68	37	12.8	640	186	299	780	461	134

**Renal solute load = (Protein,gm x 4) + Na,mEq + K,mEq + Cl,mEq; *Formula with iron;
‡These formulas are for specific metabolic disorders; certain nutrients may be low or absent
from the formula. Information on exact composition is available from the manufacturer.
Manufacturers: Loma Linda (Soyalac); Mead Johnson Nutritionals (Enfamil, Lofenalac, MSUD,
Nutramigen, Phenyl-free, Portagen, Pregestimil, Product 3200AB, Product 3200K, Product 3232A,
Product 80056, Prosobee); Ross Laboratories (Advance, Isomil, RCF, Similac); Wyeth-Ayerst
(Nursoy, SMA)

Appendix 38
Composition of Oral and Intravenous Electrolyte Solutions

A. Oral Solutions
(Electrolyte content in mEq/L)

	Glucose gm	Na	K	Cl	Cit-rate	Bicar-bonate	mOsm/kg water
Gastrolyte	20	90	20	80	30	-	NA
Hydralyte	12	84	10	59	-	10	NA
Infalyte	20	50	20	40	-	30	NA
Lytren	20	50	25	45	30	-	220
Pedialyte	25	45	20	35	30	-	250
Pedialyte RS	25	75	20	65	30	-	305
Pediatric Maintenance	50	25	-	20	(560 mg/L sodium lactate)		
Rehydralyte	25	75	20	65	30	-	305
Resol*	20	50	20	50	34	-	265
WHO solution	18	90	20	80	-	30	333

*Also contains magnesium (4 mEq/L) and phosphate (4 mEq/L)

B. Intravenous Solutions
(Electrolyte content in mEq/L)

	Na	K	Ca	Mg	Cl	Lactate	Acetate	Gluconate	mOsm/kg water
Isolyte S	140	5	-	3	98	-	29	23	295
Normosol-R	140	5	-	3	98	-	27	23	295
Plasma-Lyte R	140	10	5	3	103	8	47	-	312
Ringer's	147	4	4	-	156	-	-	-	310
Ringer's, lactated	130	4	3	-	109	28	-	-	272
Concentrates:‡									
Hyperlyte	25	40.5	5	8	33.5	-	40.6	5	6015
Hyperlyte CR	25	20	5	5	30	-	30	-	5500
Lypholyte II	35	20	4.5	5	35	-	29.5	-	6200
Multilyte-20	25	20	5	5	30	-	25	-	4205
TPN Electrolytes	35	20	4.5	5	35	-	29.5	-	6200
TPN Electrolytes II	15	18	4.5	5	35	-	7.5	-	3400

‡Electrolyte concentrates are for compounding of IV admixtures and are not used for direct infusion. Osmolarity is based on the concentrate; electrolyte concentrations are when diluted in one liter.

Manufacturers: Abbott Laboratories (Normosol, Pediatric Maintenance, Ringer's, TPN electrolytes); Baxter (Plasma-Lyte R, Ringer's); Jayco (Hydralyte); Kendall McGaw (Hyperlyte, Hyperlyte CR, Isolyte-S, Ringer's,); LyphoMed (Lypholyte, Multilyte-20); Mead Johnson (Lytren); Pennwalt (Infalyte); Ross (Pedialyte, Pedialyte RS, Rehydralyte); USV Labs (Gastrolyte); Wyeth-Ayerst (Resol)

Appendix 39
Proprietary Formulas for Enteral Nutrition

| Product name | kcal per ml | Composition Per Liter | | | | | mOsm per kg | Vol (ml) to meet RDA |
		Pro gm	CHO gm	Fat gm	Na mg	K mg		
Monomeric (elemental) Products								
Amin-Aid	2.0	19	366	46	345	234	700	NA
Criticare HN	1.06	38	222	3	634	1323	650	1892
Hepatic Aid II	1.2	44	168	36	338	234	560	NA
Peptamen	1.0	40	127	39	500	1250	260	2000
Pepti 2000	1.0	40	189	10	680	1150	490	1600
Reabilan	1.0	31	131	39	690	1248	350	2250
Reabilan HN	1.3	58	157	52	990	1638	490	1875
Tolerex	1.0	21	226	>2	468	1172	550	1800
Travasorb Hepatic	1.1	29	215	15	235	882	600	2100
Travasorb HN	1.0	45	175	14	920	1170	560	2000
Travasorb Renal	1.35	23	271	18	tr	tr	590	2100
Travasorb STD	1.0	30	190	14	920	1170	560	2000
Vital HN	1.0	41	183	11	462	1320	500	1500
Vivonex HN	1.0	44	210	1	529	1170	810	3000
Vivonex Standard	1.0	21	231	1	460	1170	550	1800
Vivonex. T.E.N.	1.0	38	106	3	460	780	630	2000
Polymeric Products								
Milk-based, lactose-containing:								
C.I.B.	1.1	60	136	36	966	2808	694	1373
Compleat regular	1.07	43	128	43	1300	1400	405	1500
Meritene liquid	1.0	58	110	32	880	2600	500	1250
Meritene powder	1.06	69	119	34	1100	2800	690	1040
Sustacal Powder	1.01	64	187	>2	960	1920	700	800
Sustagen	1.7	111	312	17	1030	3328	1100	960
Fiber-containing, lactose-free:								
Compleat modified	1.07	43	141	37	670	1400	300	1500
Enrich	1.06	40	162	37	835	1543	480	1391
Glucerna	1.0	42	94	56	928	1561	375	1420
Jevity	1.06	44	152	37	930	1564	310	1320
Newtrition Isofiber	1.25	50	160	40	920	1560	310	1250
Profiber	1.0	40	132	40	736	1248	300	1500
Sustacal w/ Fiber	1.06	46	148	35	651	1300	480	1420
Ultracal	1.04	43	121	45	917	1585	310	1180
Vitaneed	1.0	35	125	40	500	1250	310	2000

Appendix 39 *(continued)*

| Product name | kcal per ml | Composition Per Liter | | | | | mOsm per kg | Vol (ml) to meet RDA |
		Pro gm	CHO gm	Fat gm	Na mg	K mg		
Lactose-free, low calorie (<1 kcal/ml):								
Citrotein	0.7	41	122	2	710	710	480	NA
Entrition Half Str.	0.5	18	68	18	350	600	120	NA
Introlite	0.53	22	71	18	920	1560	200	1320
Newtrition Half Str.	0.53	22	70	18	345	585	150	2000
Pre-Attain	0.5	20	60	20	340	575	150	750
Lactose-free, normocaloric (1-1.2 kcal/ml):								
Attain	1.0	35	125	40	500	250	300	2000
Attain L.S.	1.0	40	120	40	200	1150	240	1600
Compleat modified	1.07	43	141	37	670	1400	300	1500
Ensure	1.06	37	145	37	835	1543	470	1920
Ensure HN	1.06	44	140	35	917	1543	470	1335
Entralife	1.06	35	137	35	834	1543	450	NA
Entrition	1.0	35	136	35	710	1200	300	2000
Entrition HN	1.0	44	114	41	920	1580	300	1300
Entrition RDA	1.0	36	135	35	800	1333	300	1500
Isocal	1.06	34	135	44	530	1320	270	1900
Isocal HN	1.06	44	124	45	930	1610	270	1250
Isolife	1.02	42	138	34	800	1500	300	1300
Isosource	1.25	43	175	42	720	1680	300	1500
Newtrition Isotonic	1.06	40	144	36	690	1170	300	1250
Nutren 1.0	1.0	40	127	38	500	1250	300	1500
Osmolite	1.06	37	145	38	625	1000	300	1890
Osmolite HN	1.06	44	141	37	917	1543	300	1320
Precision HN	1.05	44	216	1	980	910	525	2850
Precision Isotonic	1.0	29	144	30	780	960	300	1560
Precision LR	1.1	26	248	2	700	888	530	1710
Reabilan	1.0	31	131	39	690	1248	350	2250
Resource	1.06	37	145	37	688	1160	430	1893
Lactose-free, normocaloric, high protein:								
Isosource HN	1.28	53	171	43	720	1680	300	1500
Isotein HN	1.2	68	156	34	620	1070	300	1770
Newtrition HN	1.24	60	160	40	690	1170	310	1250
Replete	1.0	62	113	33	500	1560	350	1500
Sustacal Liquid	1.01	61	140	23	930	2100	650	1080
Lactose-free, hypercaloric, high protein:								
Comply	1.5	60	180	60	1020	1725	410	1060
Ensure Plus	1.5	54	197	53	1126	2294	600	1600
Ensure Plus HN	1.5	62	200	50	1168	1793	650	950
Isocal HCN	2.0	75	200	102	800	1700	560	1000
Magnacal	2.0	70	250	80	1000	1250	590	1000
Newtrition One & Half	1.5	63	200	50	1035	1755	550	1000

(continued)

Appendix 39 *(continued)*

| Product name | kcal per ml | Composition Per Liter | | | | | mOsm per kg | Vol (ml) to meet RDA |
		Pro gm	CHO gm	Fat gm	Na mg	K mg		
Nutren 1.5	1.5	60	170	68	750	1875	510	1000
Nutren 2.0 Liquid	2.0	80	196	106	1000	2500	710	750
Resource Plus	1.5	55	200	53	899	1740	600	1420
Sustacal HC	1.5	61	190	58	850	1480	650	1200
TwoCal HN	2.0	84	217	91	1042	2293	690	960
Lactose-free, low fat:								
Citrotein	0.7	41	122	2	710	710	480	--
Criticare HN	1.06	38	222	3	634	1323	650	1892
Precision HN	1.05	44	216	1	980	910	525	2850
Precision LR	1.1	26	248	2	700	888	530	1710
Ross SLD	0.7	38	137	>1	835	835	545	1200
Sustacal Powder	1.01	64	187	>2	960	1920	700	800
Tolerex	1.0	21	226	>2	468	1172	550	1800
Vivonex HN	1.0	44	210	1	529	1170	810	3000
Vivonex Standard	1.0	21	231	1	460	1170	550	1800
Vivonex. T.E.N.	1.0	38	106	3	460	780	630	2000

Specialized Formulas

Product name	kcal per ml							
Diabetes Mellitus:								
Glucerna	1.0	42	94	56	928	1561	375	1420
Respiratory failure:								
Pulmocare	1.5	62	104	91	1310	1902	490	950
Liver disease, with BCAA:								
Hepatic Aid II	1.2	44	168	36	338	234	560	NA
Travasorb Hepatic	1.1	29	215	15	235	882	600	2100
Renal disease:								
Replena	2.0	30	253	95	776	1105	615	950
Renal failure, with EAA:								
Amin-Aid	2.0	19	366	46	345	234	700	NA
Travasorb Renal	1.35	23	271	18	tr	tr	590	2100
Malabsorption, with high MCT:								
Portagen	1.0	35	114	48	468	1248	320	NA
Travasorb MCT	1.5	49	123	33	350	1000	312	NA
Cardiac, low sodium:								
Lonalac	1.01	54	75	56	40	1958	360	NA
Stress or trauma:								
Impact	1.0	56	132	28	1080	1280	375	1500
Stresstein	1.2	70	170	28	650	1100	910	2000
Traum-Aid HBC	1.0	67	198	15	618	1380	760	3000
Traumacal	1.5	82	142	68	1180	1390	490	2000
Vivonex T.E.N.	1.0	38	206	3	460	780	630	2000

Appendix 39 *(continued)*

Modular Supplements

| Product Name | Per 100 gm Powder or 100 ml Liquid | | | | | |
	Pro	CHO	Fat	Na	K	kcal
Modular protein:						
Casec	88	0	2	150	10	370
Gevral	60	27	2	192	50	367
Nutrisource Protein	76	8	7	270	570	402
Promix RDP	75	5	4	230	825	360
Promod	75	9	9	180	900	424
Propac	75	6	8	225	500	395
Modular carbohydrate:						
L.C.,liquid CHO	0	62	0	62	7	250
Moducal	0	95	0	55	7	380
Nutrisource carbohydrate	0	80	0	2	1	320
P.C.,pure CHO	0	96	0	15	7	400
Polycose Liquid	0	50	0	70	6	200
Polycose Powder	0	94	0	110	10	380
Sumacal	0	95	0	100	0	380
Modular fat:						
High MCT suppl.	0	0	48			612
Lipomul Oral	0	0	100			600
MCT Oil	0	0	92			830
Microlipid	0	0	50			450
Nutrisource LCT	0	0	24			216
Nutrisource MCT	0	0	24			201

Manufacturers: Clintec Nutrition Company (C.I.B.,Entrition, Entrition HN, Entrition RDA, Half Strength Entrition, Nutren 1.0, Nutren 1.5, Nutren 2.0, Peptamen, Replete, Travasorb MCT, Travasorb Hepatic, Travasorb Renal, Travasorb STD); Kendall McGaw Laboratories (Amin-Aid, Hepatic Aid, Traum-Aid); Lederle Laboratories (Gevral); Mead Johnson (Casec, Criticare HN, Isocal, Isocal HN, Lonalac, MCT Oil, Moducal, Portagen, Sustacal, Sustacal with Fiber, Sustagen, Traumacal, Ultracal); Navaco Laboratories (Entralife, Isolife, L.C. Liquid Carbohydrate, P.C. Pure Carbohydrate, High MCT Supplement, Promix RDP); Norwich Eaton Pharmaceuticals (Tolerex, Vivonex HN, Vivonex Standard, Vivonex T.E.N.); O'Brien KMI (Isofiber, Newtrition Isotonic, Newtrition HN, Newtrition One & Half); Ross Laboratories (Enrich, Ensure, Ensure HN, Ensure Plus, Ensure Plus HN, Glucerna, Jevity, Osmolite, Osmolite HN, Polycose, Promod, Pulmocare, Replena, Ross SLD, TwoCal HN, Vital HN); Sandoz Nutrition (Citrotein, Compleat Regular, Compleat Modified, Impact, Isosource, Isosource HN, Isotein HN, Meritene, Nutrisource Carbohydrate, Nutrisource LCT, Nutrisource MCT, Nutrisource Protein, Precision HN, Precision Isotonic, Precision LR, Resource, Stresstein); Sherwood Medical (Attain, Attain L.S., Comply, Magnacal, Microlipid, Pepti-2000, Pre-Attain, Profiber, Propac, Sumacal, Vitaneed); Upjohn Company (Lipomul Oral).

Appendix 40
Selected Amino Acid Solutions for Parenteral Nutrition

General Amino Acid Solutions	Pro-cal-amine 3%	Ami-no-syn 5%	Troph-Am-ine 6.0%	Pre-Am-ine 8.5%	Tra-va-sol 8.5%	Ami-nos-yn II 10%	Nov-am-ine 15%
Amino acid concentration	3.0%	5.0%	6.0%	8.5%	8.5	10%	15%
Total nitrogen (g/100 ml)	0.46	0.79	0.93	1.43	1.43	1.53	2.37
Essential amino acids (mg/100 ml)							
Histidine	85	150	290	240	372	300	894
Isoleucine	210	360	490	590	406	660	749
Leucine	270	470	840	770	526	1000	1040
Lysine	220	360	490	620	492	1050	1180
Methionine	160	200	200	450	492	172	749
Phenylalanine	170	220	290	480	526	298	1040
Threonine	120	260	250	340	356	400	749
Tryptophan	46	80	120	130	152	200	250
Valine	200	400	470	560	390	500	960
Nonessential amino acids (mg/100 ml)							
Alanine	210	640	320	600	1760	993	2170
Arginine	290	490	730	810	880	1018	1470
Proline	340	430	410	950	356	722	894
Serine	180	210	230	500		530	592
Tyrosine		44	140		34	270	39
Glycine	420	640	220	1190	1760	500	1040
Glutamic acid			300			738	749
Aspartic acid			190			700	434
Cysteine	<20		<20	<20			
Electrolytes (mEq/L)							
Sodium	35			10	70	45.3	
Potassium	24	5.4			60		
Magnesium	5				10		
Chloride	41		<3	<3	70		
Acetate	47	86	56	73	141	71.8	151
Phosphate (mM/1)	3.5			10	30		
Osmolarity (mOsm/L)	735	500	525	810	1160	873	1388

Appendix 40 *(continued)*

Disease-Specific Amino Acid Solutions	Renal Failure				Stress			Liver
	Amin-ess	Amin-osyn RF	Neph-rAm-ine	Ren-Amin	Bran-nch Amin	Fre-Amine HBC	Amin-osyn HBC	Hep-atAm-ine
Amino acid concentration	5.2%	5.2%	5.4%	6.5%	4.0%	6.9%	7.0%	8.0%
Nitrogen (g/100 ml)	0.66	0.79	0.65	1.0	0.44	0.97	1.12	1.2
Essential amino acids (mg/100 ml)								
Histidine	412	429	250	420	–	160	154	240
Isoleucine	525	462	560	500	1380	760	789	900
Leucine	825	726	880	600	1380	1370	1576	1100
Lysine	600	535	640	450	–	410	265	610
Methionine	825	726	880	500	–	250	206	100
Phenylalanine	825	726	880	490	–	320	228	100
Threonine	375	330	400	380	–	200	272	450
Tryptophan	188	165	200	160	–	90	88	66
Valine	600	528	640	820	1240	880	789	840
Nonessential amino acids (mg/100 ml)								
Alanine	–	–	–	560	–	400	660	770
Arginine	–	600	–	630	–	580	507	600
Cysteine	–	–	<20	–	–	<20	–	<20
Glycine	–	–	–	300	–	330	660	900
Proline	–	–	–	350	–	630	448	800
Serine	–	–	–	300	–	330	221	500
Tyrosine	–	–	–	40	–	–	33	–
Electrolytes (mEq/L)								
Acetate	50	105	44	60	–	57	72	62
Chloride	–	–	<3	31	–	<3	≤40	<3
Phosphate (mM/L)	–	–	–	–	–	–	–	10
Potassium	–	5.4	–	–	–	–	–	–
Sodium	–	–	5	–	–	10	7	10
Osmolarity (mOsm/L)	416	475	435	600	316	620	665	785

Manufacturers: Abbott (Aminosyn, Aminosyn II Aminosyn RF, Aminosyn HBC); Clintec Nutrition (Aminess, BranchAmin, RenAmin, Travasol); KabiVitrum (Novamine); Kendal McGaw (FreAmine, FreAmine HBC, HepatAmine, NephrAmine, Procalamine, TrophAmine).

(continued)

Appendix 41
Intravenous Fat Emulsions

	Intra-lipid 10%	Lipo-syn II 10%	Lipo-syn III 10%	Nutri-lipid 10%	Soya-cal 10%
Fat Source (%)					
Soybean oil	10	5	10	10	10
Safflower oil		5			
Fatty acid content (%)					
Linoleic	50	65.8	54.5	49-60	49-60
Oleic	26	17.7	22.4	21-26	21-26
Palmitic	10	8.8	10.5	9-13	9-13
Linolenic	9	4.2	8.3	6-9	6-9
Stearic	3.5	3.4	4.2	3-5	3-5
Egg yolk phospho-lipid (%)	1.2	1.2	1.2	1.2	1.2
Glycerin (%)	2.25	2.5	2.5	2.21	2.21
Calories/ml	1.1	1.1	1.1	1.1	1.1
Osmolarity (mOsm/L)	260	276	292	280	280

Manufacturers: Alpha Therapeutic (Soyacal); Abbott Laboratories (Liposyn);
Clintec Nutritional (Intralipid); Kendall McGaw (Nutrilipid).

Appendix 42
Suggested Intravenous Vitamin Formulation*

	Adults & Older Children[a]	Infants and Children under 11 years[b]
Vitamin A, IU	3300	2300
Vitamin D, IU	200	400
Vitamin E, IU	10	7
Vitamin K, mg	-	0.2
Vitamin C, mg	100	80
Vitamin B_1, mg	3	1.2
Vitamin B_2, mg	3.6	1.4
Vitamin B_6, mg	4	1
Vitamin B_{12}, ug	5	1
Folic acid, ug	400	140
Niacin, mg	40	17
Biotin, ug	60	20
Pantothenic acid, mg	15	5

*American Medical Association, Nutrition Advisory Group.
[a]M.V.I.-12, M.V.I. Plus, M.V.C. 9 + 3, Berocca PN; [b]M.V.I. Pediatric

Appendix 43
Caloric Values and Osmolarities of
Intravenous Dextrose Solutions

Percent Dextrose	Calories Per Liter	Calculated Osmolarity
2.5	85	126
5	170	250
7.7	260	390
10	340	505
11.5	390	580
20	680	1010
25	850	1330
30	1020	1515
38	1290	1920
38.5	1310	1945
40	1360	2020
50	1700	2525
60	2040	3030
70	2380	3530

Reprinted with permission from McEvoy, G.K.: AHFS (American Hospital Formulary Service) drug information 90. American Society of Hospital Pharmacists, Inc., Bethesda, MD, 1990:1442.

Appendix 44
Nutritional Intervention in Inborn Errors of Metabolism

Disorder or Enzyme Deficiency	Nutritional Intervention
Disorders in Amino Acid Metabolism	
Alkaptonuria	Phenylalanine and tyrosine restriction; ascorbic acid supplementation
Arginase deficiency	Protein-free diet; supplementation with amino acids, except arginine
Argininemia	Protein restriction; essential amino acids and ornithine supplementation
Arginosuccinic aciduria	Protein restriction; arginine and sodium benzoate supplements
Beta-methylcrotonylglycinuria	Leucine restriction
Branched chain a-ketoaciduria	BCAA (branched chain amino acid) restriction and thiamin supplementation
Branched chain transaminase deficiency	Protein restriction
Carbamylphosphate synthetase deficiency	Protein restriction; arginine and sodium benzoate supplementation
Chediak-Higashi syndrome	Ascorbic acid supplementation
Citrullinemia	Protein restriction; essential amino acids, arginine, and benzoic acid supplementation
Cystathionine synthetase deficiency	Methionine restriction; pyridoxine, folic acid, and cysteine supplementation
Cystathioninuria	Pyridoxine supplementation
Glutaric acidemia I	Protein restriction
Glutaric acidemia II	Protein and fat restriction; riboflavin and carnitine supplementation
Glutathionine synthetase deficiency	Vitamin E
Histidinemia	Histidine restriction
Homocystinuria	Methionine restriction with supplemental cystine, betaine, and pyridoxine
Hydroxy-methyl glutaryl CoA deficiency	Protein restriction
Hyperornithinemia	Protein and arginine restriction; lysine and pyridoxine supplementation
Hyperphenylalaninemia	Phenylalanine restriction
Hyperprolinemia	Proline restriction
Hypervalinemia	Valine restriction
Isovaleric acidemia	Protein and/or leucine restriction; glycine supplementation
B-ketothiolase deficiency	Moderate protein and isoleucine restriction
Leucine-induced hypoglycemia	Moderate protein (leucine) restriction; small, frequent feedings
Lysine intolerance	Protein restriction
Maple syrup urine disease	Leucine, valine, and isoleucine restriction; thiamin supplementation
Methylcrotonyl CoA carboxylase def.	Leucine restriction
Methylmalonic acidemias	Protein restriction; vitamin B_{12} supplementation
Multiple carboxylase deficiency	Protein restriction; biotin supplementation
Ornithine transcarbamylase deficiency	Protein restriction; arginine, essential amino

(continued)

335

Appendix 44 *(continued)*

Disorder or Enzyme Deficiency	Nutritional Intervention
	acids, and benzoic acid supplementation
Phenylketonuria	Phenylalanine restriction; tyrosine supplementation
Propionic acidemia	Isoleucine, methionine, threonine, and valine restriction; biotin supplementation
Propionyl CoA carboxylase deficiency	Protein restriction; biotin supplementation
Pyroglutaric acidemia	Protein restriction; alkali
Tyrosinemia	Phenylalanine and tyrosine restriction; high calorie diet; vitamin D supplementation with rickets
Disorders in Carbohydrate Metabolism	
Fructose-1,6-diphosphatase deficiency	Fructose restriction; frequent glucose feeding; folate supplementation
Fructose-1-phosphate aldolase def.	Exclusion of fructose, sucrose, and sorbitol
Galactosemia	Exclusion of galactose and lactose
Glucose-6-phosphatase deficiency	High carbohydrate; frequent feeding
Glucose 6-phosphate dehydrogenase def.	Avoidance of fava beans
Glycerate dehydrogenase deficiency	High phosphate diet; pyridoxine supplementation
Glycogen storage disease	
Type I (glucose-6-phosphatase def)	Frequent feeding; high carbohydrate intake
Type III (amylo-1,6-glucosidase def)	Frequent glucose feeding; high protein intake
Type V (muscle phosphorylase def)	Intravenous glucose; high carbohydrate intake
Type VI (liver phosphorylase def)	Frequent glucose feedings
Type VIII (phosphorylase kinase def)	Avoidance of fasting; high protein intake
Pyruvate carboxylase deficiency	Frequent feeding; biotin and thiamin supplements
Pyruvate dehydrogenase deficiency	Ketogenic diet; thiamin supplementation
Disorders in Lipid Metabolism	
Abetalipoproteinemia	Low fat diet with medium chain triglycerides (MCT); vitamin A, E, and K supplementation
Acyl-CoA dehydrogenase deficiency	Fat restriction; riboflavin and carnitine suppl.
Apolipoprotein C-II deficiency	Moderate fat restriction
Familial cholesterol ester deficiency	Restricted fat diet
Familial hyperlipoproteinemias	Restriction of saturated fatty acids and cholesterol; nicotinic acid
Type I (hyperchylomicronemia)	Low fat, high protein diet; use of medium chain triglycerides (MCT); no alcohol; weight control
Type II (hypercholesterolemia)	Saturated fat and cholesterol restriction; use of unsaturated fats (MUFA & PUFA); nicotinic acid
Type III (broad beta disease)	Cholesterol restriction; no concentrated sweets; PUFA preferred; weight control/maintenance
Type IV (hyperprebetalipoproteinemia)	Weight control; moderate cholesterol and saturated fat restriction; controlled carbohydrate
Type V (mixed hyperlipidemia)	Calorie, carbohydrate, saturated fat, and cholesterol restriction; nicotinic acid; no alcohol
Glucocerebrosidase deficiency	Iron and vitamin supplementation
Hypobetalipoproteinemia	Long chain triglycerides; vitamins A, E, and K
Lipoprotein lipase deficiency	Low fat diet
Refsum's disease	Phytanic acid restriction
β-sitosterolemia	Plant sterol restriction
Tangier disease	Fat restriction

Appendix 44 *(continued)*

Disorder or Enzyme Deficiency	Nutritional Intervention
Disorders in Nucleic Acid Metabolism	
Adenine phosphoribosyltransferase def.	Dietary purine restriction; high fluid intake
Gout	Weight reduction; low purine; high fluids; alcohol restriction; alkalinized urine
Myoadenylate deaminase deficiency	High ribose diet
Orotic aciduria	Large doses of uridine
Xanthinuria (xanthine oxidase def)	Purine restriction; high fluid intake; alkali
Disorders in Transport	
Abetalipoproteinemia	Long chain triglyceride restriction; MCT and vitamins A, D, E, and K supplementation
Acrodermatitis enteropathica	Zinc supplementation
Cystinosis	Methionine restriction; cysteamine, vitamin C, vitamin D, and phosphate supplementation
Cystinuria	High fluid; bicarbonate to alkalinize urine
Dibasic aminoaciduria	Protein restriction; arginine supplementation
Fanconi syndrome	Vitamin D and phosphate supplementation; control of acidosis
Folic acid transport defect	Parenteral folate supplementation
Glucose-galactose malabsorption	Glucose and galactose restriction; fructose substituted for glucose
Glutamate-aspartate transport defect	Glutamine supplementation
Hartnup disease	Nicotinamide supplementation; high protein intake
Hypobetalipoproteinemia	Long chain triglyceride (LCT) restriction; use of MCT; vitamins A, D, E, and K supplementation
Hypomagnesemia, idiopathic	Magnesium supplementation
Hypophostatemic rickets	Phosphorus and vitamin D supplementation
Lactose intolerance (primary alactasia)	Lactose restriction
Menkes kinky hair syndrome	Parenteral copper administration
Methionine malabsorption	Methionine restriction; cysteine supplementation
Pseudohypoaldosteronism, type I	Sodium supplementation
Pseudohypoaldosteronism, type II	Chloride restriction
Renal tubular acidosis, type I	Potassium and bicarbonate supplementation
Renal tubular acidosis, type II	Potassium restriction
Sucrose-isomaltose intolerance	Sucrose restriction
Transcobalamin II deficiency	Vitamin B_{12} parenterally
Vitamin D-dependent rickets, type I	Vitamin D (1,25 DHCC)
Other Disorders	
Congenital erythropoietic porphyria	B-carotene supplementation
Ehlers-Danlos syndrome	Ascorbic acid supplementation
Ferrochelatase deficiency	Caloric restriction; β-carotene supplementation
Hereditary coproporphyria	High carbohydrate diet
Hydroxykynureninuria	Nicotinic acid supplementation
Hypophosphatasia	Phosphate supplementation
Methemoglobinemia	Diet free of nitrate and nitrite
Porphyria (acute, intermittent)	High carbohydrate with glucose supplementation
Porphyria cutanea tarda	Low alcohol; pyridoxine and vitamin E suppl.
Pyridoxine-dependent seizures	Pyridoxine parenterally
Wilson's disease	Copper restriction

Appendix 45
Common Prefixes, Suffixes, and Symbols

Prefixes

a, an	without; as avitaminosis
ab	away from; as abnormal
ad	near, toward; as adrenal
ana	upward; as anabolism
anti	against; as antibiotic
auto	self ; as autodigestion
bio	life; as biology
calor	heat; as calorimeter
cata	downward; as catabolism
chole	bile, gall; as cholagogue
chroma	color; as chromatosis
co	together; as coenzyme
di	two, double; as diplopia
dis	ill, negative; as disease
dys	difficult; as dyspepsia
ec	outside; as ectopic
encephal	brain; as encephalogram
endo	inside; as endogenous
exo	outside; as exogenous
hemo	blood; as hemopoiesis
hyper	excessive; as hyperacid
hypo	little; as hypofunction
im	not; as immature
in	not; as incurable
inter	between; as interstitial
intra	within; as intravascular
meta	change; as metaplasia
necro	dead; as necrosis
para	beside; as paravertebral
peri	around; as pericardium
post	after; as postmortem
pre	before; as prenatal
syn	union; as synthesis

Suffixes

algia	pain; as neuralgia
ase	enzyme; as amylase
cide	kill; as bactericide
clysis	drenching; as venoclysis
cule	small; as molecule
cyte	cell; as erythrocyte
ectomy	cut off; as appendectomy
emesis	vomiting; as hematemesis
emia	blood; as anemia
esthesia	sensation; as anesthesia
ism	condition; as alcoholism

itis	inflammation; as appendicitis
lysis	destruction; as hemolysis
malacia	softening; as osteomalacia
oma	tumor, swelling; as adenoma
opsy	to view; as biopsy
osis	condition; as tuberculosis
pathy	disease of; as neuropathy
penia	poverty; as leucopenia
phagia	to eat; as polyphagia
phil	to love; as basophil
phobia	fear of; as photophobia
pnea	breath; as hyperpnea
poiesis	to produce; as hemopoiesis
ptysis	to spit; as hemoptysis
rrhea	to discharge; as diarrhea
tomy	to cut; as vagotomy
trophy	growth; as hypertrophy
uria	urine; as glucosuria

Symbols

(+)	significant; uncommon
+	plus; positive; present
++	trace or notable reaction
+++	moderate amount or reaction
++++	large amount or reaction
(-)	insignificant
--	minus; negative; absent
±	more or less; with or without;
=	equal to
≠	not equal; unequal
≡	identical
≢	not identical
↑ or Λ	elevated; above; enlarged
↓ or V	decreased; below; depressed
↗	increasing
↘	decreasing
⇒	implies; implication
>	greater than; leads to
<	less than; caused by
≯	not greater than
≮	not less than
≥	greater than or equal
≤	less than or equal
~	about; approximately
≈	approximately equal
::	proportionate to
Δ	change
∴	therefore

Appendix 46
Common Abbreviations in Medical Records

a	ante; before	bid	bis in die; twice daily
aa	each; of each	bilat	bilateral
AAA	aromatic amino acid	BKA	below knee amputation
Abd	abdominal; abdomen	BM	bowel movement; bone marrow
ABG	arterial blood gases	BMI	body mass index
ac	ante cibum; before meals	BMR	basal metabolic rate
ACF	acute care facility	BMT	bone marrow transplantation
ACTH	adrenocorticotropic hormone	bp	boiling point
ADH	antidiuretic hormone	BP	blood pressure
ADI	average or acceptable daily intake	BPH	benign prostatic hypertrophy
ADL	activities of daily living	BR	bed rest
ad lib	ad libitum; as desired	BRP	bathroom privileges
Adm	admission	BS	blood sugar
ADMR	average daily metabolic rate	BSA	body surface area
ADR	adverse drugs reaction	BSL	blood sugar level
AF	atrial fibrillation	BSP	bromosulphalein
A/G	albumin-globulin ratio	BTL	bilateral tubal ligation
AHD	arteriosclerotic heart disease	BUN	blood urea nitrogen
AID	acute infectious disease	BV	blood volume
AIDS	acquired immune deficiency syndrome	BW	body weight
		Bx	biopsy
AKA	above knee amputation	c	cum; with
alb	albumin	C	centigrade
alk	alkaline	C_{cr}	creatinine clearance
ALS	amyotrophic lateral sclerosis	Ca	calcium; cancer; carcinoma
AMA	arm muscle area	CA	chronological age
amp	ampule	CAD	coronary artery disease
amt	amount	CAH	chronic active hepatitis
AODM	adult onset diabetes mellitus	Cal	large calorie
AP	anterior-posterior; angina pectoris	CALD	chronic active liver disease
		cap	capsule
APC	arterial premature contraction	CAPD	continuous ambulatory peritoneal dialysis
approx	approximately		
Aq	aqua; water	CAT	computerized axial tomography
ARC	aids related complex	cath	catheterize
ARDS	adult respiratory distress syndrome	CBC	complete blood count
		CBD	common bile duct
ARF	acute renal failure; acute rheumatic fever	cc	cubic centimeter
		CC	chief complaint
A.R.T.	accredited record technician	CCF	cephalin-cholesterol flocculation
ASHD	arteriosclerotic heart disease	CCK	cholecystokinin
as tol	as tolerated	CCU	coronary care unit
A & W	alive and well	cd	cane die; daily
B	born; basophils	CHD	coronary heart disease
Ba	barium	CHF	congestive heart failure
BCAA	branched-chain amino acids	CHI	creatinine height index
BCG	bacillus Calmette-Guerin	CHO	carbohydrate
BEE	basal energy expenditure	Chol	cholesterol

(continued)

Appendix 46 *(continued)*

chr	chronic	DL	danger list
ck	check	DM	diabetes mellitus
CK	creatine kinase	DN	do not resuscitate
Cl	chloride	D_2O	deuterium or heavy water
cm	centimeter	DOA	dead on arrival
CNS	central nervous system	DOE	dyspnea on exertion
c/o	complains of	DOS	day of surgery
CO_2	carbon dioxide	DPM	discontinue previous medication
COLD	chronic obstructive lung disease	DPT	diphtheria, pertussis, tetanus
comp	compound	dr	dram; drachm; 3.8 gm
conc	concentration	DR	delivery room
con	continued	DRG	diagnostis related groups
COPD	chronic obstructive pulmonary disease	D/S	dextrose and saline
		DSD	dry sterile dressing
C.O.T.A.	certified occupational therapy assistant	DT	delirium tremens
		d/t	due to
Cpd	compound	D.T.R.	dietetic technician registered
CPK	creatine phosphokinase	DU	duodenal ulcer
CPN	central parenteral nutrition	DVT	deep vein thrombosis
CPR	cardiopulmonary resuscitation	DW	distilled water
Creat	creatinine	Dx	diagnosis
CRF	chronic renal failure	e	et; and
CRI	chronic renal insufficiency	ea	each
crit	hematocrit	EAA	essential amino acid
C & S	culture and sensitivity	E, EOS	eosinophils
C/S	cesarean section	ECG, EKG	electrocardiogram
CSF	cerebrospinal fluid	ED	emergency department
CT	computerized tomography	EDC	expected date of confinement
C.T.R.S.	certified therapeutic recreation specialist	EEG	electroencephalogram
		EFA	essential fatty acid
CV	cardiovascular	Elix	elixir
CVA	cerebral vascular accident	ENT	ear, nose, and throat
CVP	central venous pressure	ER	emergency room
CVS	cardiovascular system	ESR	erythrocyte sedimentation rate
Cw	crutch walking	ESRD	end-stage renal disease
d	daily	ETOH	ethyl alcohol
db	diabetic	exp	expired
DBW	desirable body weight	Expl Lap	exploratory laparotomy
D & C	dilatation and curettage	ext	external
D/C	discontinue; discharge	extr	extract
DF	dietary fiber	F	father; female; Fahrenheit
DI	diabetes insipidus	FA	fatty acid
Diag, Dx	diagnosis	FBS	fasting blood sugar
diff	differential	fdg	feeding
dil	dilute	Fe	iron
disc	discontinue	FFA	free fatty acid
Disch	discharge	FH	family history; fetal heart
DJD	degenerative joint disease	Fib	fibrillation
DKA	diabetic ketoacidosis	fld	fluid
dl	deciliter	fl oz	fluid ounce
		FMH	family medical history

FSH	follicle stimulating hormone	hx	hospitalization; history
ft	foot or feet	I	iodine
FTT	failure to thrive	IBD	inflammatory bowel disease
F/U	follow-up	ibid	same as before
FUO	fever of unknown origin	IBW	ideal body weight
Fx	fracture	Ict	icterus index
GA	gastric analysis	ICU	intensive care unit
gal	gallon	I & D	incision and drainage
GB	gallbladder	IDDM	insulin-dependent diabetes
GBD	gallbladder disease		mellitus
GE	gastroenteritis; gastroenterology	IDL	intermediate-density lipoprotein
GBS	gallbladder series	IF	intrinsic factor
GC	gonococcal count	IHD	ischemic heart disease
GE	gastroenteritis	IM	intramuscular
GFR	glomerular filtration rate	Imp	impression
GI	gastrointestinal	IMV	intermittent mechanical ventilation
GIT	gastrointestinal tract	incl	include
gm	gram; 15.43 grains	int	internal
GN	glomerulonephritis	I & O	intake and output
gr	grain	IPPB	intermittent positive pressure
GTF	glucose tolerance factor		breathing
gtt(s)	gutta; drop(s)	irrig	irrigation
GTT	glucose tolerance test	IU	international unit
GU	genitourinary	IV	intravenous
Gyn	gynecology	IVH	intravenous hyperalimentation
h	hour	IVP	intravenous pyelogram
H & H	hemoglobin and hematocrit	J	joule
H & P	history and physical	K	potassium
HA	headache; hyperalimentation	kcal	kilocalories
Hb, Hgb	hemoglobin	kg	kilogram
HBP	high blood pressure	kJ	kilojoule
Hct	hematocrit	KUB	kidney, ureter, and bladder
HCVD	hypertensive cardiovascular	L	liter
	disease	LAP	laparotomy
HDL	high-density lipoprotein(s)	lat	lateral
HEN	home enteral nutrition	lb	pound
HH	hiatal hernia	LBBB	left bundle branch block
HIV	human immunodeficiency virus	LBP	low back pain
H & N	head and neck	LBW	low birth weight
HO	house officer	LCT	long chain triglyceride
H/O	history of	LDH	lactate dehydrogenase
HOB	head of bed	LDL	low-density lipoprotein
HNV	has not voided	LES	lower esophageal sphincter
H & P	history and physical	LFT	liver function test
HPI	history of present illness	LH	luteinizing hormone
HPN	home parenteral nutrition	liq	liquid
HPT	hyperparathyroidism	LLE	left lower extremity
HR	heart rate	LLL	left lower lobe
hs	hora somni; at bedtime	LLQ	left lower quadrant
Ht	height	LMP	last menstrual period
HTN	hypertension	LOC	loss of consciousness

(continued)

LOS	length of stay		NDF	no diagnostic findings
LP	lumbar puncture		NE	niacin equivalent
L.P.N.	licensed practical nurse		NEFA	nonesterified fatty acid
LR	labor room		neg	negative
LTT	lactose tolerance test		ng	nanogram
LUE	left upper extremity		N/G, NG	nasogastric
LUL	left upper lobe		NIDDM	noninsulin dependent diabetes
LUQ	left upper quadrant			mellitus
lym	lymphocyte		nil	nothing
lytes	electrolytes		NKA	no known allergy
m	minim; meter; male		NP	neuropsychiatry
M	mother; monocyte; male		N.P.	nurse practitioner
MAC	midarm circumference		NPH	neutral protamine Hagedorn
MAMC	midarm muscle circumference		NPN	nonprotein nitrogen
MAO	monoamine oxidase		NPO	nil per os; nothing by mouth
M & N	one et nocte; day and night		NS, NSS	normal saline solution
MCFA	medium chain fatty acid		NSR	normal sinus rhythm
mcg	microgram		N & T	nose and throat
MCH	mean corpuscular hemoglobin		NTG	nitroglycerin
MCHC	mean corpuscular hemoglobin		NTS	ontropical sprue
	concentration		N & V	nausea and vomiting
MCT	medium chain triglyceride		NWB	no weight bearing
MCV	mean corpuscular volume		O_2	oxygen
MDR	minimum daily requirement		OB	obstetrics; occult blood
mEq	milliequivalent		OBS	organic brain syndrome
Mg	magnesium		od	daily
mg	milligram		O.D.	oculus dexter; right eye
MI	mitral insufficiency; myocardial		OGTT	oral glucose tolerance test
	infarction		oint	ointment
ml	milliliter		OM	omne mone; every day
mM	millimole		ON	omne nocte; every night
Mn	manganese		OOB	out of bed
MO	mineral oil; month		OOR	out of room
M.O.	medical officer		O & P	ova and parasites
MOM	milk of magnesia		OPD	outpatient department
mOsm	milliosmole		ophth	ophthalmology
M & R	measure and record		OR	operating room
M.R.A.	medical record administrator		ORIF	open reduction internal
MRI	magnetic resonance imaging			fixation
MS	mitral stenosis; multiple		Orth(o)	orthopedics
	sclerosis		O.S.	oculus sinister; left eye
M.T.	medical technologist		OT	occupational therapy
MVA	motor vehicle accident		OTC	over the counter
MVI	multiple vitamin infusion		O.T.R.	occupational therapist registered
MVR	mitral valve replacement		O.U.	both eyes; each eye
n	nocte; night; normal		oz	ounce
N	nitrogen		p	post; after
Na	sodium		P	pulse; phosphorus
NAD	no apparent distress		PA	posterior-anterior (x-ray
N.B.	newborn			ilm);pernicious anemia
NC	noncontributory		P.A.	physician assistant

PAC	premature atrial contraction
PAF	paroxysmal atrial fibrillation
PAME	preanesthesia medical exam
Pap smear	Papanicolaou smear
PAT	pregnancy at term; paroxysmal atrial tachycardia
path	pathology
PBI	protein-bound iodine
pc	post cibum; after meals
PCM	protein calorie malnutrition
PCV	packed cell volume
PE	physical examination
Ped	pediatrics
PEG	percutaneous endoscopic gastrostomy
PEM	protein-energy malnutrition
PER	protein efficiency ratio
PERRLA	pupils are equal, round, regular, react to light & accomodation
pg	picogram
pH	hydrogen ion concentration
PH	past history
PI	present illness
PID	pelvic inflammatory disease
PKU	phenylketonuria
PM	post mortem
PMD	private medical doctor
PMH	past medical history
PMI	post myocardial infarction
PMP	previous menstrual period
PMS	premenstrual syndrome
PND	paroxysmal nocturnal dyspnea
PNI	prognostic nutritional index
po	per os; by mouth; orally
POMR	problem-oriented medical record
pos	positive
Post	posterior
pp	postprandial; postpartum
PPBS	post prandial blood sugar
PPD	purified protein derivative
PPN	peripheral parenteral nutrition
pr	per rectum
prn	prore nata; whenever necessary
Pro	protein
prog	prognosis
PS	pulmonary stenosis
PSE	portal systemic encepalopathy
PSP	phenolsulfonphthalein
P/S ratio	polyunsaturated:saturated fatty acid ratio
pt	patient

PT	physical therapy; prothrombin time
PTA	prior to admission
PTB	pulmonary tuberculosis
PTH	parathyroid hormone
PTT	partial thromboplastin time
PU	peptic ulcer
PUD	peptic ulcer disease
PUFA	polyunsaturated fatty acid
PVA	peripheral venous alimentation
PVC	premature ventricular contractions
PVD	peripheral vascular disease
PWB	partial weight bearing
PZI	protamine zinc insulin
q	quaque; every
qd	quaque die; every day
qh	quaque hora; every hour
qid	quater in die; four times a day
ql	quantum libit; as much as desired
qn	quaque nocte; every night
qns	quantity not sufficient
qod	every other day
qoh	every other hour
qon	every other night
qs	quantum sufficiat; quantity sufficient
qt	quart
R	right; rectal
RA	rheumatoid arthritis
RAI	radio active isotope
RBBB	right bundle branch block
RBC, rbc	red blood cell
RBP	retinol binding protein
R.D.	registered dietitian
RDA	recommended dietary allowance
RE	retinol equivalent
REE	resting energy expenditure
RF	renal failure; rheumatic fever
RHD	rheumatic heart disease
RLE	right lower extremity
RLL	right lower lobe
RLQ	right lower quadrant
R.N.	registered nurse
R/O	rule out
ROM	range of motion
ROS	review of systems
R.P.T.	registered physical therapist
RQ	respiratory quotient
RR	recovery room; respiratory rate
RT	radiation therapy
R.T.	respiratory therapist
RTA	renal tubular acidosis
RTC	return to clinic

(continued)

RUE	right upper extremity		THA	total hip arthroplasty
RUL	right upper lobe		TIA	transient ischemic attacks
RUQ	right upper quadrant		TIBC	total iron-binding capacity
Rx	treatment; take		tid	three times a day
s	without		tinct	tincture
SAH	subarachnoid hemorrhage		TKA	total knee arthroplasty
SBE	subacute bacterial endocarditis		TLC	total lung capacity; total
SBO	small bowel obstruction			lymphocyte count
sc	subcutaneous		TNA	total nutrient admixture
SCI	spinal cord injury		T.O.	telephone order
SDA	specific dynamic action		TP	total protein
sed rat	sedimentation rate		TPN	total parenteral nutrition
SGOT	serum glutamic oxaloacetic		TPR	temperature, pulse, respiration
	transaminase		Trach	tracheostomy
SGPT	serum glutamic pyruvic		TSF	triceps skinfold
	transaminase		TSH	thyroid stimulating hormone
SH	social history		TTT	thymol turbidity test
sibs	brothers and sisters		TUR	transurethral resection
SIDS	sudden infant death syndrome		TURP	transurethal prostatectomy
sig	sign; write or label		TWE	tap water enema
SL	sublingual		Tx	treat
SLE	systemic lupus erythematosis		U/A	urinary analysis
SOAP	subjective, objective, assess-		UGI	upper gastrointestinal
	ment, plan		UIBC	unsaturated iron-binding capacity
SOB	shortness of breath		URI	upper respiratory infection
Sol	solution		Urol	urology
S.O.S.	if it is necessary		USP	United States Pharmacopoeia
S/P	status postop		UTI	urinary tract infection
spec	specimen		UUN	urinary urea nitrogen
sp gr	specific gravity		VC	vital capacity
ss	one half		VD	venereal disease
S & S	signs and symptoms		VF	ventricular fibrillation
SSE	soapsuds enema		VH	vaginal hysterectomy
SSS	subscapular skinfold		vit	vitamin
Staph	staphylococcus		VLDL	very low-density lipoprotein
stat	immediately		VMA	vanillylmandelic acid
STD	sexually transmitted disease		VO	verbal order
Strep	streptococcus		VNS	visiting nurse service
supp	suppository		VP	venous pressure
S.W.	social worker		VPC	ventricular premature contraction
Sx	symptoms		VS	vital signs
Sy	syphilis		VT	ventricular tachycardia
T3	triiodothyronine		WB	weight-bearing
T4	thyroxine		WBC	white blood count; white blood cell
T & A	tonsils and adenoids		wdwn	well developed, well nourished
tab	tablet		WF	white female
TB, TBC	tuberculosis		WM	white male
TBW	total body weight		WNL	within normal limits
TCR	turn, cough, and rebreathe		wt, wgt	weight
TF	tube feeding		WU	work-up
TG	triglyceride		YO	year old
U.R.	utilization review		Zn	zinc

Appendix 47
Agencies and Organizations with Nutrition-Related Activities

Administration on Aging, 330 Independence Avenue SW, Washington, DC 20201

Al-Anon Family Group Headquarters, 1372 Broadway, New York, NY 10018

Alcoholics Anonymous Inc., 468 Park Avenue South, New York, NY 10016

Alcoholics Anonymous World Services, P.O. Box 459, Grand Central Station, New York, NY 10163

Allergy Foundation of America, 801 Second Avenue, New York, NY 10017

American Academy of Allergy and Immunology, 611 East Wells Street, Milwaukee, WI 53202

American Academy for Cerebral Palsy and Developmental Medicine, P.O. Box 11086, Richmond, VA 23230

American Academy of Pediatrics, 141 Northwest Point Boulevard, Elk Grove Village, Evanston, IL 60009

American Anorexia/Bulimia Association Inc., 133 Cedar Lane, Teaneck, NJ 07666

American Association for World Health, U.S. Committee for the World Health Organization, 2001 S Street NW, Suite 530, Washington, DC 20009

American Board of Nutrition, 9650 Rockville Pike, Bethesda, MD 20814

American Cancer Society, 777 Third Avenue, New York, NY 10017

American Celiac Society, 45 Gifford Avenue, Jersey City, NJ 07304

American College of Nutrition, 345 Central Park Avenue, # 207 Scarsdale, NY 10583

American Council on Science and Health, 1995 Broadway, New York, NY 10023

American Dental Association, 211 East Chicago Avenue, Chicago IL 60611

American Diabetes Association, National Service Center, 1660 Duke Street, Alexandria, VA 22313

American Dietetic Association, 216 West Jackson, Chicago, IL 60604

American Digestive Disease Society, 7720 Wisconsin Avenue, Bethesda, MD 20814

American Epilepsy Society, 179 Allyn Street, Suite 304, Hartford, CT 06103

American Geriatrics Society, 770 Lexington Avenue, Suite 400, New York, NY 10021

American Heart Association, 7320 Greenville Avenue, Dallas, TX 75231

American Home Economics Association, 2010 Massachusetts Avenue NW, Washington, DC 20036

American Hospital Association, 840 North Lake Shore Drive, Chicago, IL 60611

American Institute for Cancer Research, 803 West Broad Street, Falls Church, VA 22046

American Institute of Baking, 400 Ontario Street, Chicago, IL 60611

American Institute of Nutrition, 9650 Rockville Pike, Bethesda, MD 20814

American Lung Association, 1740 Broadway, New York, NY 10019

American Medical Association, Nutrition Information Service, 535 North Dearborn Street, Chicago, IL 60610

American National Red Cross, Food and Nutrition Consultant, National Headquarters, Washington, DC 20006

American Parkinson Disease Association, 116 John Street, Suite 417, New York, NY 10038

American Pediatric Society, 450 Clarkson Avenue, Brooklyn, NY 11207

American Public Health Association, 1015 15th Street NW, Washington, DC 20005

American School Food Service, 5600 S. Quebec Street, Suite 300 B, Englewood, CO 80111

American Society for Clinical Nutrition, 9650 Rockville Pike, Bethesda, MD 20814

American Society for Hospital Food Service Administrators, 840 North Lakeshore Drive, Chicago, IL 60611

American Society for Parenteral and Enteral Nutrition, 8605 Cameron Street, Suite 500, Silver Spring, MD 20910

Anorexia Nervosa and Related Eating Disorders, P.O. Box 5102, Eugene, OR 97405

Arthritis Foundation, 1314 Spring Street NW, Atlanta, GA 30309

Association of Official Analytical Chemists, 1111 North 19th Street, Arlington, VA 22209

(continued)

Asthma and Allergy Foundation of America, 1717 Massachusetts Avenue, Washington DC 20036
Center for Science in the Public Interest, 1501 16th Street NW, Washington, DC 20036
Cereal Institute, 135 South LaSalle Street, Chicago, IL 60603
Child Nutrition Forum, 1319 F Street NW, Suite 500, Washington, DC 20004
Community Nutrition Institute, 2001 S Street NW, Washington, DC 20009
Cystic Fibrosis Foundation, 6931 Arlington Road, #200, Bethesda, MD 20814
Dietary Managers Association, 400 East 22nd Street, Lombard, IL 60148
Epilepsy Foundation of America, 4351 Garden City Drive, Landover, MD 20785
European Federation of the Associations of Dietitians, Tak Van Poortvlietstraat 3,
    NL-5344, GZ Oss, Netherlands
Food and Agricultural Organization, 345 Park Avenue South, New York, NY 10016
Food and Drug Administration, Parklane Building, 5600 Fishers Lane, Rockville, MD 20857
Food and Drug Law Institute, 1200 New Hampshire Avenue NW, Washington, DC 20036
Food and Nutrition Board, National Research Council, 2101 Constitution Avenue,
    Washington, DC 20418
Food Research and Action Center, 2011 I Street NW, Washington, DC 20006
Ford Foundation, 320 East 43rd Street, New York, NY 10017
Gluten Intolerance Group, P.O. Box 23053, Seattle, WA 98102-0353
Hospital, Institution and Educational Food Service Society, 4410 West Roosevelt Road,
    Hillside, IL 60162
Institute of Food Technologists, 221 North La Salle Street, Chicago, IL 60601
Institute of Nutrition of Central America and Panama (INCAP), Apartado Postal 1188,
    Guatemala, Guatemala.
International College of Applied Nutrition, P.O. Box 386, La Habra, CA 90631
Joint Commission on Accreditation of Healthcare Organizations, 875 North Michigan Avenue,
    Chicago, IL 60611
Kellogg Foundation, 400 North Avenue, Battle Creek, MI 49016
La Leche League International, Inc., 9616 Minneapolis Avenue, Franklin Park, IL 60131
Leukemia Society of America, Inc., 733 Third Avenue, New York, NY 10017
Lupus Foundation of America, 1717 Massachussetts Avenue SW, Suite 203, Washington, DC 20036
March of Dimes Birth Defects Foundation, 1275 Mamaroneck Avenue, White Plains, NY 10605
Meals for Millions/Freedom from Hunger Foundation, 1800 Olympic Boulevard, P.O. Drawer 680,
    Santa Monica, CA 90406
Muscular Dystrophy Association Inc., 810 Seventh Avenue, New York, NY 10019
National Academy of Sciences/National Research Council (NAS/NRC), 2101 Constitution
    Avenue NW, Washington, DC 20418
National Association for Down's Syndrome, P.O. Box 4542, Oak Brook, IL 60522
National Association of Anorexia Nervosa and Associated Disorders, Inc., Box 271, Highland
    Park, IL 60035
National Cancer Foundation, 1 Park Avenue, New York, NY 10016
National Cancer Institute, Cancer Information Service, Building 31, Bethesda, MD 20892
National Celiac-Sprue Society, 5 Jeffrey Road, Wayland, MA 01778
National Center for Health Statistics (NCHS), U.S. Department of Health and Human Services,
    Public Health Service, 3700 East West Highway, Hyattsville, MD 20782
National Child Nutrition Project, 1501 Cherry Street, Philadelphia, PA 19102
National Clearinghouse for Alcohol Information, Box 2345, Rockville, MD 20850
National Council on the Aging, 600 Maryland Avenue SW, W. Wing 100, Washington, DC 20024
National Council on Alcoholism, 12 W. 21st Street, New York, NY 10010
National Council for International Health, 1701 K Street NW, Suite 600, Washington, DC 20006

National Dairy Board, P.O. Box 1022, Fairview, NJ 07022-9962
National Dairy Council, 6300 N. River Road, Rosemont, IL 60018
National Diabetes Information Clearing House, Westwood Building, Room 603, Bethesda, MD 20205
National Down's Syndrome Society, 141 Fifth Avenue, New York, NY 10010
National Easter Seal Society, 2023 West Ogden Avenue, Chicago, IL 60612
National Foundation --- March of Dimes, 1275 Mamaroneck Avenue, White Plains, NY 10605
National Foundation for Cancer Research, 7315 Wisconsin Avenue, Bethesda, MD 20014
National Foundation for Ileitis and Colitis Inc., 444 Park Avenue S, New York, NY 10016
National Foundation for Long Term Health Care, 1200 15th Street, NW Washington, DC 20005
National High Blood Pressure Education Program, 120/80 National Institutes of Health,
    Bethesda, MD 20892
National Institutes of Diabetes, Digestive and Kidney Diseases, National Institutes of
    Health, 900 Rockville Pike, Bethesda, MD 20892
National Institute of Hypertension Studies, 12007 Linwood Avenue, Detroit, MI 48206
National Kidney Foundation, 2 Park Avenue, New York, NY 10016
National Livestock and Meat Board, 444 N. Michigan Avenue, Chicago, IL 60611
National Multiple Sclerosis Society, 205 East 42nd Street, New York, NY 10017
National Nutrition Consortium Inc, 1635 P Street NW, Suite 1, Washington, DC 20036
Nutrition Education Association, P.O. Box 20301, 3647 Glen Haven, Houston TX 77225
Nutrition Foundation, Inc., 1126 Sixteenth Street NW, Suite 111, Washington, DC 20036
Nutrition Institute of America, 200 W 86th Street, Suite 17A, New York, NY 10024
Nutrition for Optimal Health Association, P.O. Box 380, Winnetka, IL 60093
Nutrition Today Society, 428 East Preston Street, Baltimore, MD 21202
Overeaters Anonymous, 2190 190th Street, Torrance, CA 90504
Pan American Health Organization, 525 23rd Street NW, Washington, DC 20037
Parkinson's Disease Foundation Inc, 640 West 168th Street, New York, NY 10032
Prader-Willi Syndrome Association, 6490 Excelsion Boulevard, E-102, St. Louis Park, MN 55426
Price-Pottenger Nutrition Foundation, P.O. Box 2614, La Mesa, CA 92041
Sister Kenny Institute, 800 E. 28th Street at Chicago Avenue, Minneapolis, MN 55407
Society for Nutrition Education, 1700 Broadway, Suite 300, Oakland, CA 94612
Society for the Protection of the Unborn Through Nutrition, 17 North Wabash, Suite 603,
    Chicago, IL 60602
Superintendent of Documents, U.S. Government Printing Office, Washington, DC 20402
United Cerebral Palsy Association Inc, 66 East 34th Street, New York, NY 10016
United Ostomy Association, 36 Executive Park, Suite 120, Irvine, CA 92714
United Parkinson Foundation, 360 W Superior Street, Chicago, IL 60610
United Scleroderma Foundation Inc, P.O. Box 350, Watsonville, CA 95077
USDA Cooperative Extension Service, Washington, DC 20250
USDA Food and Consumer Services, 6505 Belcrest Road, Hyattsville, MD 20782
USDA Food and Nutrition Service (FNS), Child Nutrition Division, 3101 Park Center Drive,
    Alexandria, VA 22302
USDA Food Safety and Inspection Service (FSIS), 14th and Independence Avenue, SW,
    Washington, DC 20250
USDA Human Nutrition Information Service (HNIS), 6505 Belcrest Road, Hyattsville, MD 20782
USDA Nutrition Program, Consumer and Food Economics Division, Agricultural Research
    Service, Hyattsville, MD 20782
USDA National School Lunch Program, Food and Nutrition Service, Washington, DC 20250
USDA School Breakfast Program, Food and Nutrition Service, 3101 Park Center Drive
    Alexandria, VA 22302

(continued)

Appendix 47 *(continued)*

USDA Special Food Supplemental Program for Women, Infants, and Children (WIC), Food and Nutrition Service, 3101 Park Center Drive, Room 1017, Alexandria, VA 22302

USDA Supplemental Food Programs Division, Food and Nutrition Service, 3101 Park Center Drive, Room 1017, Alexandria, VA 22302

U.S. Government Printing Office, The Superintendent of Documents, Washington, DC 20402

Vitamin Information Bureau Inc, 664 North Michigan Avenue, Chicago, IL 60611

World Health Organization (WHO), CH-1211 Geneva 27, Switzerland

Worldwatch Institute, 1776 Massachusetts Avenue NW, Washington, D.C. 20036

TRADE ORGANIZATIONS:

Abbott Laboratories, 14th Street, Sheridan Road, North Chicago, IL 60064

ABC Corporation, 1330 Avenue of the Americas, New York, NY 10019

Alpha Therapeutic Corporation, 5555 Valley Boulevard, Los Angeles, CA 90032

American Egg Board, 1460 Renaissance Street, Park Ridge, IL 60068

American McGaw, Division of Travenol, 1425 Lake Cook Road, Deerfield, IL 60015

American Meat Institute, P.O. Box 3556, Washington, DC 20007

American Institute of Baking, 400 East Ontario Street, Chicago, IL 60611

Anglo-Dietetics Ltd, P.O. Box 333, Wilton, CT 06897

Baxter Healthcare Corporation, 1 Baxter Parkway, Deerfield, IL 60015

Best Foods, Division of CPC International, Englewood Cliffs, NJ 07623

Biosearch Medical Products Inc, 35 Industrial Parkway, P.O. Box 1700, Somerville, NJ 08876

Borden Company, 350 Madison Avenue, New York, NY 10017

California Raisin Advisory Board, P.O. Box 5335, Fresno, CA 93755

Campbell Soup Company, Food Service Products Division, 385 Memorial Avenue, Camden, NJ 08103

Carnation Company, Health Care Services Division, 1425 Lake Cook Road, Los Angeles, CA 90036

Cheesebrough-Pond's Inc, 33 Benedict Place, Greenwich, CT 06830

Clintec Nutrition Company, P.O. Box 760, 1425 Lake Cook Road, Deerfield, IL 60015

Delmark Food Service Company, (Division of Sandoz) 5320 West 23rd, Minneapolis, MN 55416

Del Monte Corporation, Consumer and Education Services, Box 3757, San Franscisco, CA 94119

Doyle Pharmaceutical Company, (Division of Sandoz) 5320 West 23rd, Minneapolis, MN 55416

Del Monte Teaching Aids, P.O. Box 9075, Clinton, IA 52736

Dietary Specialties Inc, P.O. Box 227, Rochester, NY 14601

Eli Lilly and Company, Medical Department, 307 East McCarty, Indianapolis, IN 46225

Ener-G Foods Inc, 6901 Fox Avenue South, Seattle, WA 98124

Evaporated Milk Association, 288 North La Salle Avenue, Chicago, IL 60601

Featherweight, Chicago Dietetic Supply Inc, P.O. Box 529, La Grange, IL 60525

Fleischmann's Margarines, Standard Brands Inc, 625 Madison Avenue, New York, NY 10022

Florida Citrus Commission, Box 148, Lakeland, FL 33802

Food Sciences Corporation, 821 East Gate Drive, Mt. Laurel, NJ 08054

General Foods Corporation, Consumer Center, 250 North Street, White Plains, NY 10602

General Mills Inc, 9200 Wayxata Boulevard, Minneapolis, MN 55426

Gerber Products Company, 445 State Street, Fremont, MI 49412

Hauck Inc, P.O. Box, 1065, Roswell, GA 30775

Henkel Corporation, Dietary Specialties, 4620 West 77th, Minneapolis, MN 55436

H. J. Heinz, Consumer Relations, P.O. Box 57, Pittsburgh, PA 15230

Hunt-Wesson Foods, Educational Services, 1645 West Valencia Drive, Fullerton, CA 92634
John Hancock Life Insurance Company, 200 Berkley Street, Boston, MA 02117
KabiVitrum Inc, 1311 Harbor Bay Parkway, Alameda, CA 94501
Keene (Vicam) Pharmaceuticals, 333 South Mocking Bird, P.O. Box 7, Keene, TX 76058
Kellogg Company, Dept. of Home Economics Services, Battle Creek, MI 49016
Kendall McGaw Laboratories Inc, P.O. Box 25080, 2525 McGaw Avenue, Irvine, CA 92714
Lactaid, P.O. Box 111, Pleasantville, NJ 08232
Lederle Laboratories, 1 Cyanamid Plaza, Wayne, NJ 07470
Loma Linda Food Co, 11503 Pierce Street, Riverside, CA 92505
McDonald's Action Packs, Box 14317, Dayton, OH 45414
Mead Johnson Nutritionals, 2400 West Lloyd Expressway, Evansville, IN 47721-0001
Med-Diet Laboratories Inc, P.O. Box 27251, Golden Valley, MN 55427
Metropolitan Life Insurance Company, Health and Welfare Division, 1 Madison Avenue,
    New York, NY 10010
Nasco, Nutrition Teaching Aids, 901 Janesville Avenue, Fort Atkinson, WI 53538
National Commission on Egg Nutrition, 205 Touvy Avenue, Park Ridge, IL 60668
Navaco Laboratories, 512 Ash Avenue, Mc Allen, TX 78501
Norwich Eaton Pharmaceuticals, P.O. Box 191, 17 Eaton Avenue, Norwich, NY 13815-0191
Numed Corporation, 1400 Fairfield Road South, Minnetonka, MN 55343
O'Brien/KMI, Dept 9567, 320 Charles Steet, Cambridge, MA 02141
Peanut Association, 342 Madison Avenue, New York, NY 10017
Pillsbury Company, Minneapolis, MN 55402
Potato Board, 1385 South Colorado Boulevard, Denver, CO 80222
Poultry and Egg National Board, 250 West 57th Street, New York, NY 10010
Procter and Gamble Educational Services, P.O. Box 14009, Cincinnati, OH 45214
Roche Laboratories, Division of Hoffman-LaRoche Inc, 340 Kingsland Street, Nutley, NJ 07110
Ross Laboratories, 625 Cleveland Avenue, Columbus, OH 43216
Sandoz Nutrition Corporation, 5320 West 23rd Street, P.O. Box 370, Minneapolis, MN 55440
Saron Pharmacal Corp, 1640 Central Avenue, St. Petersburg, FL 33712
Sherwood Medical Company, 1831 Olive Street, St. Louis, MO 63103
Sunkist Growers, P.O. Box 2706, Los Angeles, CA 90054
Travenol Laboratories, 1425 Lake Cook Road, Deerfield, IL 60015
UpJohn Company, 7000 Portage Road, Kalamazoo, MI 49001
USV Laboratories, 1 Scarsdale Road, Tuckahoe, NY 10707
Wheat Flour Institute, 309 West Jackson Boulevard, Chicago, IL 60606
Wyeth-Ayerst Laboratories, P.O. Box 8299, Philadelphia, PA 19101

Appendix 48
Sources of Nutrition Information

BOOKS

Anderson, Judith V., and Marian R. Van Nicorp. 1989. *Basic Nutrition Facts: A Nutrition Reference.* Lansing, MI: Michigan Department of Public Health and Michigan State University Bulletin Office.

Armstrong, F. B. 1989. *Biochemistry.* 3rd Edition. New York: Oxford University Press.

Backus, Karen. 1990. *Medical and Health Information Directory.* Vol. 1, *Organizations, Agencies and Institutions.* Detroit, MI: Gale Research, Inc.

Beare-Rogers, Joyce. 1988. *Dietary Fat Requirements in Health and Development.* Champaign, IL: American Chemists' Society.

Bender, A. E., and L. J. Brookes. 1987. *Body Weight Control: The Physiology, Clinical Treatment and Prevention of Obesity.* New York: Churchill Livingstone.

Bloch, Abby S. 1990. *Nutrition Management of the Cancer Patient.* Rockville, MD: Aspen Publishers, Inc.

Bodinski, Lois H. 1987. *The Nurse's Guide to Diet Therapy.* New York: John Wiley & Sons.

Boyle, Marie A., and E. N. Whitney. 1989. *Personal Nutrition.* St. Paul, MN: West Publishing Co.

Brinkley, Roger W. 1988. *Modern Carbohydrate Chemistry.* New York: Marcel Dekker.

Brostoff, Jonathan, and Stephen J. Challacombe. 1987. *Food Allergy and Intolerance.* Philadelphia: Bailliere Tindall.

Brown, Judith E. 1990. *The Science of Human Nutrition.* San Diego, CA: HBJ Publishers.

Burtis, Grace, Judi Davis, and Sandra Martin. 1988. *Applied Nutrition and Diet Therapy.* Philadelphia: W. B. Saunders Co.

Burton, Benjamin T., and Willis R. Foster. 1988. *Human Nutrition* (formerly *The Heinz Handbook of Nutrition*). Philadelphia: McGraw-Hill Book Co.

Cataldo, Corinne Balog, Jacque Nyenheris, and Eleanor Noss Whitney. 1989. *Nutrition and Diet Therapy: Principles and Practice.* 2nd Edition. St. Paul, MN: West Publishing Co.

Chan, James C., and John R. Gill. 1990. *Kidney and Electrolyte Disorders.* New York: Churchill Livingstone.

Clark, Kristine, Richard Parr, and William Castelli. 1988. *Evaluation and Management of Eating Disorders: Anorexia, Bulimia, and Obesity.* Champaign, IL: Life Enhancement Publications.

Clark, Nancy. 1990. *Sports Nutrition Guidebook.* Champaign, IL: Leisure Press Co.

Dickerson, John W. T., and Lee A. Harry. 1988. *Nutrition in the Clinical Management of Disease.* 2nd Edition. Baltimore: Edward Arnold.

Debruyne, Linda K., and Sharon Rady Rolfes. 1989. *Life Cycle Nutrition: Concept Through Adolescence.* St. Paul, MN: West Publishing Co.

Diabetes Treatment Centers of America. 1989. *Current Trends in Diabetes Management.* Nashville, TN: Diabetes Treatment Centers of America.

Dreher, Mark L. 1987. *Handbook of Dietary Fiber: An Applied Approach.* New York: Marcel Dekker.

Eastham, R. D. 1985. *Biochemical Values in Clinical Medicine.* 7th Edition. Bristol: John Wright & Sons Ltd.

Escot-Stump, Sylvia. 1988. *Nutrition and Diagnosis-Related Care.* Philadelphia, PA: Lea & Febiger.

Feldman, Elaine B. 1988. *Essentials of Clinical Nutrition.* Philadelphia: F. A. Davies Co.

Frankie, Riva T. 1987. *Obesity and Weight Control: The Health Professional's Guide to Understanding and Treatment.* Rockville, MD: Aspen Publishers, Inc.

Frisancho, A. R. 1990. *Anthropometric Standards for the Assessment of Growth and Nutritional Status.* MI: The University of Michigan Press.

Gallagher-Allred, Charlotte R. 1989. *Nutritional Care of the Terminally Ill.* Rockville, MD: Aspen Publishers, Inc.

Garrison, Robert, and Elizabeth Somer. 1985. *The Nutritional Desk Reference.* New Canaan, CT: Keats Publishing.

Gibson, R. S. 1990. *Principles of Nutritional Assessment.* New York: Oxford University Press.

Gines, Deon J. 1990. *Nutrition Management in Rehabilitation.* Rockville, MD: Aspen Publishers, Inc.

Grand, Richard J., James L. Sutphen, and William H. Dietz, Jr. 1987. *Pediatric Nutrition: Theory and Practice.* Boston, MA: Butterworth Publishers.

Guthrie, Helen A., with Robin S. Bagby. 1989. In-

Appendix 48 *(continued)*

troductory Nutrition. 7th Edition. St. Louis, MO: Times Mirror/Mosby College Publishing Co.

Halpern, Seymour L. 1987. *Quick Reference to Clinical Nutrition: A Guide for Physicians.* 2nd Edition. Philadelphia: J. B. Lippincott.

Hamilton, Betty, and Barbara Guidos. 1984. *Medical Acronyms, Symbols, and Abbreviations.* New York: Neal-Schuman Publishers, Inc.

Hamilton, Eva May, and Frank S. Sizer. 1988. *Nutrition: Concepts and Controversies.* 4th Edition. St. Paul, MN: West Publishing Co.

Hamilton, Eva May, and Sareen-Stepnick Gropper. 1987. *The Biochemistry of Human Nutrition—A Desk Reference.* St. Paul, MN: West Publishing Co.

Huyck, N. L., and M. M. Rowe. 1990. *Managing Clinical Nutrition Services.* Rockville, MD: Aspen Publishers, Inc.

Herrman-Zcudins, Mindy, and Riva Tougher-Decker. 1989. *Nutrition Support in Home Health.* Rockville, MD: Aspen Publishers, Inc.

Hodges, Patricia A. M., and Connie E. Vickery. 1988. *Effective Counseling Strategies for Dietary Management.* Rockville, MD: Aspen Publishers, Inc.

Hui, Y. H. 1988. *Handbook of Enteral and Parenteral Feedings.* New York: John Wiley & Sons.

Hunt, Sara M., and James L. Groff. 1990. *Advanced Nutrition and Human Metabolism.* St. Paul, MN: West Publishing Co.

International Life Sciences Institute. 1990. *Present Knowledge in Nutrition.* 6th Edition. Washington, DC: ILSI.

Iowa Dietetic Association. 1990. *Simplified Diet Manual: Study Guide to the Sixth Edition.* Ames, Iowa: State University Press.

Jeejeebhoy, Kursheed. 1988. *Current Therapy in Nutrition.* Philadelphia: B. C. Decker, Inc.

Kaufman, Mildred. 1990. *Nutrition in Public Health: A Handbook for Developing Programs and ·Services.* Rockville, MD: Aspen Publishers, Inc.

Kemm, J. R. 1985. *Vitamin Deficiency in the Elderly: Prevalence, Clinical Significance and Effects on Brain Function.* Boston, MA: Blackwell Scientific Publications.

Kinney, John M., K. N. Jeejeebhoy, Graham L. Hill, and Oliver E. Owen. 1988. *Nutrition and Metabolism in Patient Care.* Philadelphia, PA: W. B. Saunders Co.

Kreut, L. R., A. Palmer, and D. Narins. 1987. *Nutrition in Perspective.* 2nd Edition. Englewood Cliffs, NJ: Prentice-Hall, Inc.

Krall, Leo P., and Richard S. Beaser. 1989. *Joslin Diabetes Manual.* Philadelphia: Lea & Febiger.

Lang, Carol E. 1987. *Nutritional Support in Critical Care.* Rockville, MD: Aspen Publishers, Inc.

Langford, Herbert, and Barbara Levine. 1990. *Contemporary Issues in Clinical Nutrition.* Vol. 12, *Nutrition Factors in Hypertension.* New York: Alan R. Liss, Inc.

Lawrence, Ruth A. 1989. *Breastfeeding: A Guide for the Medical Profession.* St. Louis, MO: The C. V. Mosby Co.

Leavelle, Dennis E. 1986. *Interpretative Data for Diagnostic Laboratory Tests.* Rochester, MN: Mayo Medical Laboratories.

Livingston, G. E. 1989. *Nutritional Status Assessment of the Individual.* Trumbull, CT: Food and Nutrition Press, Inc.

Logan, Carolyn M., and Katherine M. Rice. 1987. *Logan's Medical and Scientific Abbreviations.* Philadelphia: J. B. Lippincott Co.

Mayo Foundation. 1988. *Mayo Clinic Diet Manual.* Philadelphia, PA: B. C. Decker, Inc.

Mead, James F., Roslyn B. Alfin-Slater, David R. Howton, and George Popjak. 1986. *Lipids, Chemistry, Biochemistry and Nutrition.* New York: Plenum Press.

Messerli, Franz H. 1987. *Current Clinical Practice.* Philadelphia, PA: W. B. Saunders Co.

Moore, Mary Courtney. 1988. *Pocket Guide to Nutrition and Diet Therapy.* St. Louis, MO: The C. V. Mosby Company.

Morley, J. E., Z. Glick, and L. Z. Rubenstein. 1990. *Geriatric Nutrition: A Comprehensive Review.* New York: Raven Press.

Mòsby's Medical, Nursing, and Allied Health Dictionary. 1990. 3rd Edition. St. Louis, MO: The C. V. Mosby Co.

National Research Council. 1990. *Diet and Health,* Washington, DC: National Academy Press.

National Research Council. 1989. *Recommended Dietary Allowances.* 10th Edition. Washington, DC: National Academy Press.

Natow, Annette B., and Jo-Ann Heslin. 1986. *Nutritional Care of the Older Adult.* New York: Macmillan Publishing Co.

New Hampshire Dietetic Association. 1986. *Diet*

(continued)

Appendix 48 *(continued)*

Manual for Long-Term Care Facilities. Concord, NH: Dietetic Association.

Nieman, D. C., D. E. Butterworth, and C. N. Nieman. 1990. *Nutrition.* Dubuque, IA: WCB Publishers.

Obert, Jessie Craig. 1986. *Community Nutrition.* New York: John Wiley & Sons.

Osborne, D. R., and P. Voogt. 1978. *The Analysis of Nutrients in Foods.* New York: Academic Press.

Owen, A., and R. Frankie. 1986. *Nutrition in the Community.* St. Louis, MO: Times Mirror/Mosby Publication Co.

Paige, David M. 1988. *Clinical Nutrition.* 2nd Edition. St. Louis, MO: The C. V. Mosby Co.

Pemberton, Cecilia M., Karen E. Moxness, Mary J. German, Jennifer K. Nelson, and Clifford F. Gastineau. 1988. *Mayo Clinical Diet Manual. A Handbook for Practitioners.* Philadelphia, PA: B. C. Decker, Inc.

Pennington, Jean A., and Helen Nichols Church. 1989. *Bowes and Church's Food Values of Portions Commonly Used.* 15th Edition. Philadelphia: J. B. Lippincott Co.

Philips, G. D., and C. L. Odgers. 1986. *Parenteral and Enteral Nutrition: A Practical Guide.* 3rd Edition. New York: Churchill Livingstone.

Pipes, Peggy L. 1988. *Nutrition in Infancy and Childhood.* 4th Edition. St. Louis, MO: The C. V. Mosby Co.

Powers, Margaret A. 1987. *Handbook of Diabetes Nutritional Management.* Rockville, MD: Aspen Publishers, Inc.

Rakel, Robert E. 1990. *Conn's Current Therapy.* Philadelphia, PA: W. B. Saunders Co.

Rambeau, J. L., and M. D. Caldwell. 1984 and 1986. Clinical Nutrition. Vol. I, *Enteral and Tube Feeding.* Vol. II, *Parenteral Nutrition.* Philadelphia, PA: W. B. Saunders Co.

Ravel, Richard. 1989. *Clinical Laboratory Medicine.* 5th Edition. Chicago, IL: Yearbook Medical Publishers, Inc.

Renner-McCaffrey, Jo. 1988. *Quality Assurance in Hospital Nutrition Services.* Rockville, MD: Aspen Publishers, Inc.

Roe, Daphne A. 1989. *Handbook on Drug and Nutrient Interactions: A Problem-Oriented Reference Guide.* The American Dietetic Association.

Rolfes, S. R., and L. K. DeBruyne. Edited by E. N.

Whitney. 1990. *Life Span Nutrition: Conception Through Life.* St. Paul, MN: West Publishing Co.

Schlichtig, Robert, and Stephen M. Ayres. 1988. *Nutritional Support of the Critically Ill.* Chicago, IL: Yearbook Medical Practices, Inc.

Schreiner, J. E. 1990. *Nutrition Handbook for Aids.* 2nd Edition. Aurora, CO: Carrot Top Nutrition Resources.

Schroeder, S. A., M. A. Krupp, L. M. Tierney, and S. J. McPhee. 1990. *Current Medical Diagnosis and Treatment 1990.* Norwalk, CT: Appleton and Lange.

Shils, Maurice E., and Vernon R. Young. 1988. *Modern Nutrition in Health and Disease.* 7th Edition. Philadelphia, PA: Lea & Febiger.

Silberman, Howard. 1989. *Parenteral and Enteral Nutrition.* 2nd Edition. Norwalk, CT: Appleton & Lange.

Simko, Margaret D., Catherine Cowell, and Maureen S. Hreha. 1989. *Practical Nutrition: A Quick Reference for the Health Care Practitioner.* Rockville, MD: Aspen Publishers, Inc.

Skipper, Annalynn. 1989. *Dietitian's Handbook of Enteral and Parenteral Nutrition.* Rockville, MD: Aspen Publishers, Inc.

Smith, Kenneth T. 1988. *Trace Minerals in Foods.* New York: Marcel Dekker.

Snetselaar, Linda G. 1988. *Nutrition Counselling Skills: Assessment, Treatment and Evaluation.* 2nd Edition. Rockville, MD: Aspen Publishers, Inc.

Snow, Teepa L. 1987. *Handbook of Geriatric Practice Essentials.* Rockville, MD: Aspen Publishers, Inc.

Snyder, David L. 1988. *Dietary Restriction and Aging.* New York: Alan R. Liss.

Somogyi, J. C. 1988. *Malnutrition—A Problem of Industrial Societies.* Basel, Switzerland: Karger Co.

Spittel, John A., Jr. 1985. *Clinical Medicine.* New York: Harper & Row, Publishers.

Spratto, George R. 1990. *Nurse's Drug Reference: NDR '90.* Albany, NY: Delmar Publishers.

Stare, Frederick J., Robert E. Olson, and Elizabeth M. Whelan. 1989. *Balanced Nutrition: Beyond the Cholesterol Scare.* Boston, MA: Bob Adams.

Surgeon General's Report on Nutrition and Health.

Appendix 48 *(continued)*

1988. DDHS Publication no. (PHS) 88-50211. Washington, DC: DDHS.

Tepperman, J., and H. Tepperman. 1987. *Metabolism and Endocrine Physiology.* 5th Edition. Chicago, IL: Yearbook Medical Publishers.

The American Dietetic Association. 1988. *Manual of Clinical Dietetics.* Chicago, IL: American Dietetic Association.

Tver, David F., and P. Russell. 1989. *The Nutrition and Health Encyclopedia.* 2nd Edition. New York: Van Nostrand Reinhold.

USDA Food Composition Tables. No. 8-17. Washington, DC: Superintendent of Documents, Government Printing Office.

USPDI. 1989. *Drug Information for the Health Care Professional.* 9th Edition. Rockville, MD: United States Pharmacopeia Convention, Inc.

Vahouney, George V., and David Kritchewsky. 1986. *Dietary Fiber: Basic and Clinical Aspects.* New York: Plenum Press.

Walser, MacKenzie, Anthony L. Imbembo, Simeon Margolis, and Gloria A. Elfert. 1984. *Nutrition Management. The Johns Hopkins Handbook.* Philadelphia, PA: W. B. Saunders Co.

Wardlaw, Gordon M., and Paul M. Insel. 1990. *Perspectives in Nutrition.* St. Louis, MO: Times Mirror/C. V. Mosby Co.

Watson, Ronald R. 1985. *Handbook of Nutrition in the Aged.* Boca Raton, FL: CRC Press.

Weinser, Ronald R., Douglas C. Heimburger, and Charles E. Butterworth, Jr. 1989. *Handbook of Clinical Nutrition.* 2nd Edition. St. Louis, MO: C. V. Mosby Co.

Werbach, Melvyn R. 1987. *Nutritional Influences on Illness—A Sourcebook of Clinical Research.* Tarzana, CA: Third Line Press.

Whitney, E. N., E. M. Hamilton, and S. R. Rolfes. 1990. *Understanding Nutrition.* 5th Edition. St. Paul, MN: West Publishing Co.

Williams, Sue Rodwell. 1989. *Essentials of Nutrition and Diet Therapy.* 5th Edition. St. Louis, MO: Times Mirror/C. V. Mosby Co.

Winick, Myron. 1989. *Nutrition, Pregnancy and Early Infancy.* Baltimore, MD: Williams & Wilkins.

Worthington-Roberts, Bonnie S. (Sue Rodwell Williams, Editor). 1989. *Nutrition in Pregnancy and Lactation.* 4th Edition. St. Louis, MO: Times Mirror/Mosby Co.

Zeman, Francis J., and Denise M. Ney. 1988. *Applications of Clinical Nutrition.* Englewood Cliffs, NJ: Prentice-Hall.

JOURNALS AND REVIEWS

Aging
American Family Physician
American Health
American Heart Journal
American Journal of Clinical Nutrition
American Journal of Digestive Diseases
American Journal of Epidemiology
American Journal of Gastroenterology
American Journal of Medicine
American Journal of Nursing
American Journal of Public Health
Annals of Internal Medicine
Annals of Nutrition and Metabolism
Annual Reviews of Medicine
Annual Reviews of Nutrition
Archives of Internal Medicine
British Journal of Nutrition
British Medical Journal
Cancer
Canadian Medical Association Journal
Cereal Chemistry
Circulation
Clinical Nutrition
Consultant
Current Concepts in Nutrition
Diabetes
Diabetes Care
Diabetes Educator
Diabetes Forecast
Ecology of Food and Nutrition
Epidemiology
Food and Drug Administration Consumer
Federation Proceedings
Food Technology
Gastroenterology
Geriatrics
Hospital Practice
Human Nutrition: Applied Nutrition
Human Nutrition: Clinical Nutrition
International Journal of Vitamin Research
Journal of Applied Physiology
Journal of Clinical Endocrinology and Metabolism

(continued)

353

Journal of Clinical Investigation
Journal of Food Composition and Analysis
Journal of Food Protection
Journal of Food Science
Journal of Food Technology
Journal of General Internal Medicine
Journal of Gerontology
Journal of Home Economics
Journal of Nutrition
Journal of Nutrition Education
Journal of Nutrition for the Elderly
Journal of Nutrition Research
Journal of Parenteral and Enteral Nutrition
Journal of Pediatrics
Journal of Renal Nutrition
Journal of Surgical Research
Journal of the American Dietetic Association
Journal of the American Geriatric Society
Journal of the American College of Nutrition
Journal of the American Medical Association
Journal of the Canadian Dietetic Association
Journal of the National Cancer Institute
Lancet
Mayo Clinic Proceedings
Medical Clinics of North America
Metabolism
Modern Health Care
New England Journal of Medicine
Nutrition Abstracts and Reviews
Nutrition and Metabolism
Nutrition Forum
Nutrition Reviews
Nutrition Today
Pediatric Clinics of North America
Pediatrics
Postgraduate Medicine
Proceedings for the Society for Experimental Biology and Medicine
Proceedings of the Nutrition Society
Public Health Reports
Science
Scientific American
Seminars in Oncology
Surgery
Topics in Clinical Nutrition
Vitamins and Hormones
WHO Chronicle
World Review of Nutrition and Dietetics

MISCELLANEOUS: NEWSLETTERS, LEAFLETS, AND BOOKLETS

ACHS News and Views
AICR Newsletter
Clinical Management
CNI Weekly Report
Consulting Nutritionists
Contemporary News
Contemporary Nutrition
Currents in Food, Nutrition, and Health
Dairy Council Digests
Diet and Nutrition Newsletter
Dietetic Currents
Drug-Nutrient Interactions
FDA Consumer
Food Action
Food and Nutrition News
Food Insight
Harvard Medical School Health Letter
Health and Nutrition Newsletter (Santa Clara Medical Society and San Jose Peninsula CDA)
Healthline
Hospital Food and Nutrition Focus
National Dairy Council
NCAF Newsletter
Nutrition and the MD
Nutrition Clinics
Nutrition Counselor
Nutrition Forum
Nutrition News
Nutrition Perspectives (UC Cooperative Extension)
Nutrition Research Newsletter
Nutrition Week
Obesity and Health
Rapport
RD
Science News
Seminars in Nutrition
Tufts University Diet and Nutrition Letter
U.C. Berkeley Wellness Letter
Various publications of major drug/food corporations and universities.

SELECTED SOURCES FOR SOFTWARE AND AUDIOVISUAL AIDS*

AccuPEN-PC (Assessment, Meal Planning, E/P Feedings)